OCCUPATIONAL
SCIENCE FOR
OCCUPATIONAL
THERAPY

OCCUPATIONAL SCIENCE FOR OCCUPATIONAL THERAPY

EDITED BY

Doris Pierce, PhD, OTR/L, FAOTA

ENDOWED CHAIR IN OCCUPATIONAL THERAPY
EASTERN KENTUCKY UNIVERSITY
RICHMOND, KENTUCKY

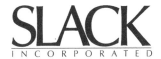

www.Healio.com/books

ISBN: 978-1-55642-933-0

Copyright © 2014 by SLACK Incorporated

Chapter opener illustrations by Stan Pierce.

SLACK Incorporated uses a review process to evaluate submitted material. Prior to publication, educators or clinicians provide important feedback on the content that we publish. We welcome feedback on this work.

Published by: SLACK Incorporated
               6900 Grove Road
               Thorofare, NJ 08086 USA
               Telephone: 856-848-1000
               Fax: 856-848-6091
               www.Healio.com/books

Contact SLACK Incorporated for more information about other books in this field or about the availability of our books from distributors outside the United States.

Library of Congress Cataloging-in-Publication Data

Occupational science for occupational therapy / edited by Doris Pierce.
     p. ; cm.
  Includes bibliographical references and index.
  ISBN 978-1-55642-933-0 (hardback : alk. paper)
  I. Pierce, Doris E., editor of compilation.
  [DNLM: 1. Occupational Therapy. WB 555]
  RM735.3
  615.8'515--dc23
                    2013030731

For permission to reprint material in another publication, contact SLACK Incorporated. Authorization to photocopy items for internal, personal, or academic use is granted by SLACK Incorporated provided that the appropriate fee is paid directly to Copyright Clearance Center. Prior to photocopying items, please contact the Copyright Clearance Center at 222 Rosewood Drive, Danvers, MA 01923 USA; phone: 978-750-8400; Web site: www.copyright.com; email: info@copyright.com

Printed in the United States of America.

Last digit is print number: 10 9 8 7 6 5 4 3 2 1

DEDICATION

This book is dedicated to our students,
whose caring and innovative work will unfold into the future
the potential of occupation to enrich lives.

CONTENTS

ACKNOWLEDGMENTS

I would like to acknowledge, first and foremost, the chapter authors of *Occupational Science for Occupational Therapy,* who contributed their stellar research work to this book's intent to articulate how occupational science supports occupational therapy. Most of them labor in a world where book chapters count for little, yet they valued and supported this effort. Without them, this book would not exist.

I would also like to acknowledge the great researchers and leaders of occupational therapy who have so inspired my own vision of occupational science, without whom the science would not have come to be: Drs. Elizabeth Yerxa, Ruth Zemke, Florence Clark, and Diane Parham. Each has given differently and tirelessly to provide occupational therapy with a science that clarifies and evolves the field's potent concepts, strengthens practice effectiveness, and leverages the profession to a new height of maturation. These are the shoulders upon which this work stands.

I owe a debt of gratitude to the Society for the Study of Occupation: USA (SSO:USA), which has provided me with the intellectual home within which to enjoy discussing, debating, celebrating, and being surprised by the continual unfolding of occupational science. My colleagues at the SSO:USA provide me with a sense of disciplinary community, without which I would not have undertaken this project.

The enthusiasm of my colleagues at Eastern Kentucky University, as they do their curriculum and teaching work within our baccalaureate program in occupational science, has provided me with an ongoing and inspiring testimony to the potential of the science for our field. It is an honor and a privilege to hold an endowed chair within such a large, creative, and dedicated occupational therapy department. Many thanks go to the Kentucky Legislature for this investment in occupational therapy, which, among other projects, has provided me with the time to prepare this book. I would also like to acknowledge my graduate assistants, who, over several years, have patiently supported my efforts to produce a book that is both useful and well referenced: Lisabeth Mobley, Kris Howard, Nicole Sheffield, Eric Hamm, and Emily Fintel.

I extend my gratitude to my family for their part in completing this book: my husband, Gregory Roberts, who is my rock; my daughter, Celeste Roberts, who gives me the occupational therapy student's perspective; my sister, Cindy Pierce-Roberts, who keeps me creative and inspired; and my father, Stan Pierce, this book's artist.

In addition, I would like to express my appreciation to SLACK Incorporated, for its willingness to invest in an occupational science book that targets such a radical outcome as bringing the potential of occupational science to bear within occupational therapy. I would especially like to thank my editor, Brien Cummings, for his patience and persistence in bringing this book to light. May your gamble be rewarded!

Lastly, I acknowledge the devotion of my two American white shepherds, Mercury and Mink, who have kept me company through all my writing and reminded me that, once in a while, one does need to go outside.

ABOUT THE EDITOR

Doris Pierce, Ph.D., OTR/L, FAOTA is Eastern Kentucky University's Endowed Chair in Occupational Therapy. She began her career with a BS in Occupational Therapy from Ohio State University, followed by an MA in Occupational Therapy and a PhD in Occupational Science from the University of Southern California. She has been a pediatric therapist for 30 years, trained at Ayres Clinic, and operated a private practice in the greater Los Angeles area for more than 10 years, serving infants and children in home, school, aquatic, and therapeutic riding settings.

Dr. Pierce is a leading occupational scientist. Above all, she is centrally concerned with examining and strategically developing the theoretical potential of occupational science to support the knowledge base needs of occupational therapy. On a broad level, her work has explored research methods; international differences and similarities in the valued occupations of elder women; and key constructs of occupation such as co-occupation, occupation-based practice, and the relations between the productive, pleasurable, and restorative dimensions of occupation. Her initial occupational science research was responsive to her clinical interests in early childhood play, play objects in the natural settings of children, and mothering of children who are typically developing as well as developmentally challenged. Her current research focuses on the occupations of youth at risk and the development of occupational therapy transition services to secondary students with disabilities. She has directed several research and training projects in this area and is currently completing a mixed methods study for the Ohio Department of Education on the intervention processes and outcomes in occupational therapy transition services for secondary students with high-incidence disabilities.

Dr. Pierce has worked steadily throughout her career to support the maturation of the discipline of occupational science. She chaired the charter group and served in a series of positions to build the first research society in occupational science and therapy, the Society for the Study of Occupation: USA. Dr. Pierce delivered the 10th Ruth Zemke Lecture in Occupational Science in 2011 as she was at work on *Occupational Science for Occupational Therapy*, as can be seen in the congruence of the perspectives presented in these two works.

In 2000, Dr. Pierce accepted the Endowed Chair in Occupational Therapy at Eastern Kentucky University, a full-time research position created through a matching funds initiative of the Kentucky Legislature. Since then, she has dedicated her work to an occupational science and occupational therapy response to the needs of youth at risk. Dr. Pierce is proud of her cultural heritage, rooted in farming families of both eastern Kentucky and central Ohio. She also lives her passion for occupation as a dedicated wife, the proud mother of a daughter nearing completion of her occupational therapy degree, an amazed grandmother, an enthusiastic event planner, a heartfelt singer, and a writer reaching beyond her profession.

Contributing Authors

Karen Atler, PhD, OTR (Chapter 16)
Assistant Professor
Occupational Therapy Department
Colorado State University
Fort Collins, Colorado

Carolyn M. Baum, PhD, OTR/L, FAOTA (Chapter 9)
Professor of Occupational Therapy,
    Neurology, and Social Work
Washington University School of Medicine
St. Louis, Missouri

Michele Berro, MA, OTR/L (Chapter 26)
Clinical Manager
Rancho Los Amigos National Rehabilitation Center
Downey, California

Catana Brown, PhD, OTR/L, FAOTA (Chapter 22)
College of Health Sciences—Occupational Therapy
Midwestern University
Glendale, Arizona

Wannipa Bunrayong, PhD (Chapter 11)
Associate Professor
Chiang Mai University
Chiang Mai, Thailand

Florence A. Clark, PhD, OTR/L, FAOTA (Chapter 25)
Associate Dean and Professor
Division of Occupational Science and
    Occupational Therapy
Ostrow School of Dentistry of USC
Los Angeles, California

Donna Colaianni, PhD, OTR/L, CHT (Chapter 27)
Assistant Professor
Division of Occupational Therapy
West Virginia University
Morgantown, West Virginia

Lisa Tabor Connor, PhD (Chapter 9)
Assistant Professor
Program in Occupational Therapy
Departments of Radiology and Neurology
Washington University School of Medicine
St. Louis, Missouri

Susan Corr, DipCOT, MPhil, PhD (Chapter 20)
Visiting Professor of Occupational Therapy
University of Northampton
Head of Research and Development
Leicestershire Partnership NHS Trust
Leicester, England

Lisa Deshaies, OTR/L, CHT (Chapter 26)
Clinical Specialist
Rancho Los Amigos National Rehabilitation Center
Downey, California

Joanne Phillips Estes, MS, OTR/L (Chapter 24)
Department of Occupational Therapy
Xavier University
Cincinnati, Ohio

Elaine Fehringer, MA, OTR/L (Chapter 28)
Eastern Kentucky University
Richmond, Kentucky

Erin R. Foster, OTD, MSCI (Chapter 9)
Assistant Professor in Occupational Therapy,
    Neurology, and Psychiatry
Washington University School of Medicine
St. Louis, Missouri

Betty Risteen Hasselkus, PhD, OTR, FAOTA (Chapter 3)
Emeritus Professor
University of Wisconsin—Madison
Madison, Wisconsin

Mary W. Hildebrand, OTD, OTR/L (Chapter 9)
Assistant Professor
Department of Occupational Therapy
East Carolina University
Greenville, North Carolina

Claudia List Hilton, PhD, OTR/L, FAOTA (Chapter 13)
Assistant Professor
Department of Occupational Therapy
School of Health Professions
University of Texas Medical Branch
Galveston, Texas

Clare Hocking, PhD, NZROT (Chapter 11)
Professor
Auckland University of Technology
Auckland, New Zealand

Jeanne Jackson, PhD, OTR, FAOTA (Chapter 25)
Vice Dean of Clinical Therapies
Professor and Chair
Department of Occupational Science and
    Occupational Therapy
University College Cork
Cork, Ireland

Hans Jonsson, OT(reg), PhD (Chapter 18)
Associate Professor
Division of Occupational Therapy
Karolinska Institutet
Stockholm, Sweden

Gillian King, PhD (Chapter 8)
Senior Scientist
Bloorview Research Institute and University of Toronto
Toronto, Ontario, Canada

Sheama Krishnagiri, PhD, OTR/L, FAOTA (Chapter 4)
San Jose State University
San Jose, California

Mary Law, PhD, FCAOT, FCAHS (Chapter 8)
Professor
School of Rehabilitation Science and
    CanChild Centre for Childhood Disability Research
McMaster University
Hamilton, Canada

Amy Marshall, PhD, OTR/L (Chapter 28)
Department of Occupational Therapy
Eastern Kentucky University
Richmond, Kentucky

Phyllis J. Meltzer, PhD, MSG, MS (Chapter 17)
Founder
Life Course Publishing
Redondo Beach, California

Matthew Molineux, BOccThy, MSc, PhD (Chapter 10)
Professor and Head of Occupational Therapy
School of Rehabilitation Sciences
Griffith University
Gold Coast, Australia

Alexandra Palombi, BSc OT (hons), MSC OT (Chapter 20)
Istituto Chirurgico Ortopedico Traumatologico, GIOMI
Latina, Italy

Pollie Price, PhD, OTR/L (Chapter 23)
Associate Professor
Division of Occupational Therapy
University of Utah
Salt Lake City, Utah

Ingrid Provident, EdD, OTR/L (Chapter 27)
Assistant Professor
Master of Occupational Therapy Program
Program Coordinator
Post-Professional Doctorate (OTD) Program
Chatham University
Pittsburgh, Pennsylvania

Elizabeth A. Pyatak, PhD, OTR/L (Chapter 25)
Assistant Professor
Division of Occupational Science and
    Occupational Therapy
University of Southern California
Los Angeles, California

Phuanjai Rattakorn, PhD (Chapter 11)
Assistant Professor
Chiang Mai University
Chiang Mai, Thailand

Melisa Rempfer, PhD (Chapter 22)
Department of Psychology
University of Missouri—Kansas City
Kansas City, Missouri

Wendy Rickard, PhD (Chapter 10)
University of Exeter Medical School
Exeter, United Kingdom

Charlotte Brasic Royeen, PhD, OTR/L, FAOTA (Chapter 6)
Professor of Occupational Science and
    Occupational Therapy
Edward and Margaret Doisy College of Health Science
Saint Louis University
St. Louis, Missouri

Debbie Laliberte Rudman, PhD, OT Reg (ON) (Chapter 12)
Associate Professor
School of Occupational Therapy and
    Graduate Program in Health and
    Rehabilitation Sciences (Occupational Science Field)
University of Western Ontario
London, Ontario, Canada

Anne Shordike, PhD, OTR/L (Chapter 11)
Professor
Occupational Therapy Department
Eastern Kentucky University
Richmond, Kentucky

Diane L. Smith, PhD, OTR/L, FAOTA (Chapter 13)
Chair and Assistant Professor
Department of Occupational Therapy
University of Missouri
Columbia, Missouri

Jenny Strong, BOccThy, MOccThy, PhD (Chapter 10)
Professor of Occupational Therapy
School of Health and Rehabilitation Sciences
The University of Queensland
Brisbane, Queensland, Australia

Karen Summers, MS, OTR/L (Chapter 28)
Occupational Therapist
Model Laboratory School
Eastern Kentucky University
Richmond, Kentucky

Soisuda Vittayakorn, BS (Chapter 11)
Associate Professor
Chiang Mai University
Chiang Mai, Thailand

*Gail Whiteford, BAppSc (Occ Therapy),
MHSc (Occ Therapy), PhD (Chapter 14)*
Pro Vice Chancellor (Social Inclusion)
Macquarie University
New South Wales, Australia

Alison Wicks, PhD, MHSc(OT), BAppSc(OT) (Chapter 19)
Associate Professor in Occupational Therapy
University of Canberra
Bruce, Australian Capital Territory
Director
Australasian Occupational Science Centre
Visiting Fellow
Australian Health Services Research Institute
University of Wollongong
New South Wales, Australia

Timothy J. Wolf, OTD, MSCI, OTR/L (Chapter 9)
Assistant Professor
Program in Occupational Therapy
Department of Neurology
Washington University School of Medicine
St. Louis, Missouri

Wendy H. Wood, PhD, OTR, FAOTA (Chapter 5)
Professor and Head
Department of Occupational Therapy
Colorado State University
Fort Collins, Colorado

*Valerie A. Wright St-Clair, PhD, MPH, DipProfEthics,
DipBusStudies, DipOccTherapy (Chapter 11)*
Associate Professor
Department of Occupational Science and Therapy
School of Rehabilitation and Occupation Studies
Faculty of Health and Environmental Sciences
Auckland University of Technology
Auckland, New Zealand

*Elizabeth J. Yerxa, EdD, LhD (Hon.), ScD (Hon.),
DMed (Hon.), OTR, FAOTA (Foreword)*
Distinguished Professor Emerita
Division of Occupational Science and
    Occupational Therapy
University of Southern California
Los Angeles, California

FOREWORD

You who will read this book are about to be launched on an exciting adventure of exploration, discovering new ideas ("detective work") and how they can be used to improve the lives of human beings. You will find inspiration here and gain respect for those who ventured into the unknown, uncharted process of becoming researchers, finding thrills, satisfactions, "a-ha!" moments, and inevitable frustrations. That is how occupational science is done.

One of the profound gratifications of being a teacher is discovering that your students and younger colleagues have gone far beyond you in their thinking and creative vision. In this respect, we teach to make ourselves obsolete. This work goes far beyond what I imagined when the development of occupational science began, on two sides of the planet, in the late 1980s.

These studies validate the fruitfulness, complexity, and inexhaustibility of the idea of occupation for the development of theory, research, education, and practice. Some of these works demonstrate how research emanating from this idea can enlighten other disciplines besides our own and contribute to the universe of knowledge represented by universities.

This research in occupational science encompasses many dimensions of the occupational human, from the biological to the psychological, social, cultural, political, and spiritual. Occupation is viewed as a universal phenomenon that influences and is influenced by the environment or context in which it is done. Occupational science seeks to answer the question "What is it that we need to know about occupation so that we can contribute new understanding and improve the lives of our fellow human beings?" No wonder one author compared occupation to a precious gem, one with seemingly unlimited facets.

As these researchers have viewed the world through the lenses of occupation, they have discovered unforeseen treasures. For example, they have identified new populations and venues for professional intervention, expanding practice; developed new theoretical models to enhance our understanding of occupation and to guide practice; formulated new concepts such as "lifestyle redesign," "occupational justice," "paradox of freedom," etc., to explain what they have discovered and make it understandable to the wider world; constructed new instruments to measure important specifics of occupation; revealed hidden needs for occupational therapy in previously served populations; formulated new roles for occupational therapists (e.g., as advocates for change in public policy or as architects of environments that nourish human capability); and, finally, they have employed innovative research methods that pay respect to the ethical foundations of occupational therapy. Rather than separating science from practice, these studies demonstrate the evolutionary process of discovering new ideas (science) and translating these into practice.

As you read this book, you might feel overwhelmed by the prospect of doing research. But please recognize that the most important part of any study is the idea that launches it and the openness of the researcher to see with fresh, unbiased eyes no matter what appears, whether it is a clinical event, a personal incident, an idea from the literature, or one's own research.

It is not widely understood that the people who contribute the breakthroughs and revolutionary ideas to a discipline often are not the elders, such as I, but the newcomers such as you. Why? Because at this stage of your career you are truly open and without allegiance to any person, group, theory, or "politically correct" paradigm. And you have been deeply immersed in literature during the years of your higher education while free of the pressures to conform to our field's conventional wisdom.

A case in point is Einstein. He formulated the special theory of relativity when he was only 26 years old and newly immersed in the content of physics. Relativity theory is considered his most creative work because it generated a scientific revolution such as the world has never seen. Yet in his later years, according to Dyson (1995), a contemporary professor of physics, Einstein exhibited extraordinary hostility to the idea of black holes, now considered one of the most exciting and important consequences of his theory.

Dyson (1995) concluded from the case of Einstein and others that science is an art form practiced by free spirits. It flourishes when the scientist freely uses the tools at hand, unrestrained by preconceived notions of what science ought to be. That sounds like a student who selected occupational therapy as a career or the character of an occupational therapist engaged in reflective practice.

As many of these authors described the actual doing of research, they mentioned feelings of frustration and times of deep discouragement along with their need to persist, no matter how difficult the terrain. Thus, when you begin to think about what you will study, energize yourself by choosing something you care about deeply. Some of my research was generated by my anger at seeing people in a clinical setting being reduced to nonhuman parts and being made to conform to a culture that ignored their interests and motivations. I was viewing practice through the lenses of an occupational scientist.

If you choose an issue that you care about, you will more likely be able to withstand the frustration and overcome the barriers that inevitably arise when doing research. Sometimes outrage is a powerful motivator fueled by the thought "something needs to be done about this." I call that beginning point a clinical irritation, but it can also arise from something I've read in the literature, experienced in daily life, or discussed with a colleague. Controversy can also be a powerful motivator for research (see Chapter 25).

Arnold Beisser (1989), totally paralyzed just as he was about to enter his residency as a medical student, described his experience:

> I felt cut off from the elemental functions and activities that grounded me. I was quite literally separated from the earth, for while I spent my time in an iron lung, in bed, or in a wheelchair, my feet never really touched the ground …
>
> But, more important, I believe, was being separated from many of the elemental routines that occupy people. … I felt no longer connected with the familiar roles I had known in family, work, sports. My place in the culture was gone. (p. 166)

You, as young, open, free spirits infected with the need to know much, much more about occupation, will create new ideas that will enable people like Arnold Beisser to achieve competence, experience a decent quality of life, reclaim their resources, and rediscover their place in the culture.

I congratulate Doris Pierce and her selected cadre of researchers for demonstrating the richness, complexity, diversity, and some of the potential of occupational science. This book is a promising beginning to a journey of exploration that will contribute new and unlimited knowledge to our exciting, demanding, and unfinished profession and to science as a whole. May your fresh vision, grounded in occupation, create and test new ideas that will make the world a better place because we will know much, much more about the occupational human living in the real world.

References

Beisser, A. (1989). *Flying without wings: Personal reflections on being disabled.* New York, NY: Doubleday.

Dyson, F. (1995). Introduction: The scientist as rebel. In J. Cornwall (Ed.), *Nature's imagination: The frontiers of scientific vision* (pp. 1–11). Oxford, United Kingdom: Oxford University Press.

—*Elizabeth J. Yerxa, EdD, LhD (Hon.), ScD (Hon.),*
DMed (Hon.), OTR, FAOTA
Distinguished Professor Emerita
Division of Occupational Science and
Occupational Therapy
University of Southern California
Los Angeles, California

INTRODUCTION

Welcome

Welcome to *Occupational Science for Occupational Therapy*! This book marks a new phase in the evolution of both our science and our profession. The primary intent of the book is to articulate how different types of occupational science research support occupational therapy. For too long, the science and the profession have been considered separate efforts. They are not. They are highly related. They birth and require each other.

Occupational Science for Occupational Therapy is uniquely research based. Every invited chapter in this book reports either a single study or a multistudy research program. The work of researchers in the 23 invited chapters of this volume demonstrates the very best of what occupational science offers to occupational therapy. The book also moves firmly away from presenting theories and models that are unsupported by research within our field. In this book, we insist on regarding occupational therapy as actively involved in producing a science highly responsive to its knowledge needs, instead of as a profession that consumes and applies research that is produced within other disciplines and for other purposes.

The most valued audience of *Occupational Science for Occupational Therapy* is occupational therapy students. They are our future. It is critical that students are provided with a solid scientific foundation for understanding occupation within their practice. Occupation-based practice will define, sustain, and inspire future practitioners, despite any changes that may occur in our culture and its many systems.

Beyond my hopes for the practice lives of our students, I also know that some students will pursue their curiosity about occupation and practice into lives of research. For this reason, *Occupational Science for Occupational Therapy* illustrates the wide variety of research methods in occupational science. In each contributed chapter, researchers also share the occupational experience of research: the passions, frustrations, adaptations, decisions, and satisfactions that are so much a part of being a researcher. Usually, the research process is reduced to a cut-and-dried report, as if it had not been an ongoing and emotional puzzle to the researcher. For the sake of our future researchers, *Occupational Science for Occupational Therapy* uncovers the occupation of research as it is experienced by researchers.

Organization of the Book

Occupational Science for Occupational Therapy is organized in a very structured way. Chapter 1 provides an orientation to key concepts in occupational science, to prepare the reader for the rest of the book. Then, four types of occupational science are introduced, one section at a time. Each section begins with an overview chapter that describes a particular type of occupational science and then offers several exemplar chapters from leading occupational science researchers. Each section addresses a distinctly different type of occupational science: descriptive, relational, predictive, and prescriptive. To respond to occupational therapy's strong interest in interventions, the book section on prescriptive occupational science includes a greater number of contributed chapters than the other book sections. Throughout the book, the contributed chapters offer the unique insights of a star-studded cast of occupational scientists, as well as exercises for trying out their ideas. *Occupational Science for Occupational Therapy* concludes with an editor's summary chapter that reviews the strengths of the science, the forces that partition occupational science from occupational therapy, and the commitment made to the profession to generate knowledge of occupation that would support practice.

Occupational science is developing rapidly in the degree to which it is able to honor its founding promise to produce knowledge of occupation to support practice. Whether you are a seasoned researcher, an experienced practitioner, or an entry-level student, *Occupational Science for Occupational Therapy* offers you a fresh, inspiring, data-based, and organized understanding of how the new discipline of occupational science is contributing to the unique knowledge base of the profession of occupational therapy.

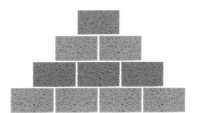

Occupational Science
A Powerful Disciplinary Knowledge Base for Occupational Therapy

Doris Pierce, PhD, OTR/L, FAOTA

WHAT IS OCCUPATIONAL SCIENCE?

A Discipline

A key issue from the beginning of occupational science has been whether it would be a discipline or an interdisciplinary focus of study (Pierce, 2012; Pierce et al., 2010). At its debut, occupational science was presented as an emergent discipline (Clark et al., 1991). Disciplines have distinguishing features: a core problem, a specific intent, a body of work, research societies, journals, and academic departments awarding disciplinary degrees (Good, 2000; Heilbron, 2003; Powell, O'Malley, Muller-Wille, Calvert, & Dupre, 2007). Well-known sociologist of professions and disciplines, Andrew Abbott (1988, 2001, 2004) adds one further characteristic: fully mature disciplines are self-sufficient in producing the number of PhDs required to fully staff the academic departments of the discipline.

As occupational science has grown, it has increasingly demonstrated these disciplinary hallmarks. The core problem is occupation. The intent is to support occupational therapy through research into occupation. Occupational therapy has responded by increasing its emphasis on occupation-based practice. The numbers of occupational science articles and books have increased significantly since the discipline was launched. There are many national or regional occupational science research societies as well as a virtual international society. Many academic occupational therapy departments have added occupational science to their department name. There are five occupational science doctoral programs and an even greater number of occupational science baccalaureate programs. But, fully staffing academic departments with faculty who have occupational science degrees? Although these numbers have slowly crept upward, it will be many years before this last marker of a mature discipline will be reached.

A Response to the Knowledge Base Needs of Occupational Therapy

From the beginning, the intent of occupational science has been to produce knowledge of occupation that will inform and strengthen occupational therapy practice

Pierce, D. (Ed.).
Occupational Science for Occupational Therapy (pp. 1-10).
© 2014 SLACK Incorporated.

(Clark et al., 1991; Yerxa et al., 1989). That is, in order for practice to be effective in applying occupation to improve lives, we need to understand how it is experienced and perceived by our clients, how it is shaped by other factors, how it develops, and how it is best used to make change. Some professions are well supported by academic disciplines from which they can import the knowledge they need in order to understand their primary approach to intervention. Anatomy and kinesiology inform physical therapy's focus on restoring bodily movement. Chemistry informs pharmacy's design and dispensing of prescribed medications. Physics informs engineering. For occupational therapy, however, there is not an existing discipline that studies occupation and can provide it with the science it requires. Human doing is a broad, holistic concept that no science has previously studied in depth. For this reason, occupational science has been created out of occupational therapy to produce the knowledge needed by practice. *Occupational Science for Occupational Therapy* offers a thorough overview of progress thus far in the production of four types of knowledge necessary to strengthen practice.

WHO IS AN OCCUPATIONAL SCIENTIST?

I have often heard people ask, "Who is an occupational scientist?" It is an interesting question. An occupational scientist is a person who engages in research on occupation and self-identifies as an occupational scientist. The clearest case, of course, is that of a person with a research degree in occupational science. Such a degree requires years of work that demonstrates not only the commitment of an entire research career to the study of occupation, but also the surrender of whatever advantages might have been secured by pursuing a research degree in a more established discipline. So, it is pretty safe to say that a person with a terminal degree in occupational science is an occupational scientist. Most, but not all, people with terminal degrees in occupational science are also occupational therapists. This, too, is logical, given the intent of occupational science to develop the knowledge base of occupational therapy. Most people with occupational science doctorates are occupational therapists who have decided that the best way they can contribute to occupational therapy is through research on occupation. They carefully choose research questions that will best contribute to the development of occupational science. They constantly consider the unfolding of occupational science by reading newly published work, collaborating with other occupational scientists, and discussing new research at occupational science meetings. They are not only prepared in the discipline, but also remain actively engaged in its evolution.

Some researchers who self-identify as occupational scientists have research degrees in other fields. Again, they are often, but not always, occupational therapists. Their occupational science research most often examines the relation of occupation to the primary extradisciplinary concepts of the field in which they have been prepared. This type of occupational science is explored in Chapters 7 through 14 of *Occupational Science for Occupational Therapy*, in the section on Level 2, relational research. Of course, occupational scientists trained in other disciplines also do research that is not focused on occupation, which does not contribute key knowledge to our understanding of occupation. Occupational scientists with degrees in other fields vary greatly in the degree to which they are engaged with occupational science, because they are of course most involved with the discipline in which they received their research degrees. Their selected research topics must meet two objectives: they must be strategic questions for occupational science, as well as a good fit to current work in their original discipline. This interface keeps occupational science responsive to the theories and interests of other disciplines. It can also confuse the emerging identity of the new science and dilute its focus on occupation.

Sometimes someone will recognize the usefulness of research from another discipline and declare that researcher to be an occupational scientist (Wright-St Clair, 2012). This happened with Csikszentmihalyi's (1975, 1988) wonderful work on optimal experience, or flow. I do not think, however, that Csikszentmihalyi would identify himself as an occupational scientist. Certainly, he has not attempted to choose strategic occupational science research questions, joined in occupational science discourse through publications in occupational science venues, or given presentations at occupational science meetings. I am pretty sure he considers himself a psychologist. In fact, he is recognized as a primary thinker in the subdiscipline of positive psychology. This is also where his students' work is located. Although researchers may have multiple disciplinary identities, those identities are personal, self-conceived, and expressed in patterns of publishing and disciplinary interactions. One cannot be declared by others to be a part of a discipline with which one is only marginally aware or involved.

I also think that novice researchers, such as occupational therapy students completing master's theses that address occupation, are occupational scientists. Everyone must start somewhere! Some students will develop from their thesis experience into career researchers in occupational science. I did a master's thesis on the development of early childhood play (Pierce, 1991). I was very fortunate to have as my thesis advisor Dr. Elizabeth Yerxa, who provided the Foreword for this book. In my dissertation research, I further developed this topic, guided by Dr. Diane Parham (Pierce, 2000; Pierce, Myers, & Munier, 2009). I did not realize when I chose my master's thesis topic that I was setting my feet on a long road of research projects. For students reading this now, perhaps you are also at this place in your career?

Even therapists who are not formally running research projects are, in some ways, occupational scientists. They are constantly testing predictions in regard to occupation in their daily practice. Often, they are trying prescriptions of occupation as they seek solutions to client problems. These are not formal research processes that produce publishable results that are shared to help develop knowledge. Still, they include queries very much focused on occupation, trials of occupation, and reflections on discoveries about occupation. I believe there is an occupational scientist in the heart of every occupational therapist. Many use that fascination with occupation as a powerful guide to artful practice.

WHAT ABOUT INTERDISCIPLINARITY?

Some have suggested that occupational science is not a unique discipline, but an interdisciplinary endeavor (Clark, 2006; Laliberte Rudman et al., 2008); interdisciplinarity is "an adjective describing the interaction among two or more different disciplines" (Smelser, 2004, p. 53). The key point here is that it is an interaction. That is, to engage in an interdisciplinary collaboration, exchange, or research project, one must have a discipline to bring to the table. Unfortunately, occupational therapy's history as a profession that imports knowledge from other disciplines muddies its understandings of the meaning of interdisciplinarity. The use of interdisciplinary knowledge is prevalent in professional schools, where this diversity of knowledge is balanced by a focus on very specific professional outcomes (Garber, 2001; Smelser, 2004). In that context, interdisciplinary perspectives and collaborations are generally viewed as positive, open-minded, and indicating potential to disseminate work beyond one's own discipline. In mature disciplines, however, interdisciplinarity has also been viewed as a threat to the focused productivity of a scholar, as risky in terms of career progression, and as the mark of a declining discipline (Keith, 2000; Smelser, 2004; Turner, 2004).

Interdisciplinary studies programs are areas of research that combine the perspectives of multiple disciplines to examine a specific topic (Garber, 2001). Interdisciplinary studies programs have evolved over time, initially focusing on regional studies (e.g., European studies), then adding historical period studies (e.g., Renaissance studies), and then programs addressing particular populations (e.g., African American studies). Within academia, interdisciplinary programs struggle. Usually, they do not have their own faculty members, depend on cross-listed courses that draw on the resources of other academic units, and produce few graduates. No examples of occupational science interdisciplinary studies programs are known to this author.

The idea that occupational science might evolve into an interdisciplinary studies focus, rather than a discipline of its own, is a concept that was woven into the science by its Australasian founders, who completed their occupational science doctoral research in the academic departments of other disciplines. For example, Ann Wilcock completed her doctorate in community medicine, which led to a focus within occupational science on the relations of occupation to community health and social justice at population levels. Dr. Wilcock was also instrumental in starting *The Journal of Occupational Science: Australia*, which has a strong orientation to publishing research on occupation by an interdisciplinary array of researchers. Now called *The Journal of Occupational Science*, the editorial intent has remained the same. The *Journal* does not publish research on occupational therapy, excluding all Level 4, prescriptive research addressing applications of occupation. Over nearly 20 years as the discipline's only journal, the editorial stance of the *Journal* has exerted strong pressures against occupational science's intent to develop knowledge that will actively support the profession of occupational therapy. It does, however, provide an excellent publication outlet for occupational scientists studying the relation of occupation to the primary concepts of other disciplines, especially for those researchers whose disciplinary preparation has not been in occupational science. Many occupational science researchers focus their research at the intersection of occupational science with other disciplines. Their research addresses the relations of occupation to the primary concepts of other fields, such as identity, disability, justice, or culture. Chapters 7 through 14 of this book provide an overview and exemplars of this relational, interdisciplinary level of occupational science research.

WHAT IS OCCUPATION?

Already in the young discipline of occupational science, many definitions of occupation have been proposed (Clark et al., 1991). This fascination with defining key concepts, and the development of thinking that results from that effort, is typical of healthy disciplines. As the editor of *Occupational Science for Occupational Therapy*, I am, of course, most comfortable with the definition that I have offered. Actually, my definition of occupation is unique in proposing that we require two definitions: a definition of occupation at the level of richly contexted individual experience and a definition of activity at the level of cultural ideas (Pierce, 2001).

An occupation is a specific individual's personally constructed, nonrepeatable experience. That is, an occupation is a subjective event in perceived temporal, spatial, and sociocultural conditions that are unique to that one-time occurrence. An occupation has a shape, a pace, a beginning and an ending, a shared or solitary aspect, a cultural meaning to the person, and an infinite number of other perceived contextual qualities.

An activity is an idea held in the minds of people and in their shared cultural language. An activity is a culturally defined and general class of human actions. The common sense meanings of activities, such as play or cooking, enable us to communicate about generalized categories of occupational experiences in a broad, accessible way. An activity is not experienced by a specific person, it is not observable as an occurrence, and it is not located in a fully existent temporal, spatial, and sociocultural context. (p. 139)

To emerge from its early growth without narrowing its focus to only one of these two levels, either contexted individual experiences of occupation or generalized cultural ideas of activities, occupational science must reconcile and become sophisticated in moving between these two very different aspects of its work as a discipline. Dickie, Cutchin, and Humphry (2006) and others (Hocking, 2012; Kinsella, 2012; Magalhaes, 2012) have expressed concerns that occupational science is too individualistic in its focus, rejecting occupational science research that focuses on the unique subjective experience that individuals have in their own lives. Their mistake is in assuming a forced choice between the two, instead of moving to the more sophisticated understanding that both views are valuable within occupational science (Pierce, 2001; Rudman, 2012).

Understanding the meanings, experiences, and contextual dimensions of occupation as individuals perceive them is critical knowledge for occupational therapists, who work primarily within the life circumstances of single individuals and their families. Further, this epistemological stance, that individuals are the authors and most accurate interpreters of their own occupations, is radical in its fit to occupational therapy's valuing of the voices and choices of its clients (Yerxa, 1991b, 1992). This focus on the experience of individuals in their everyday lives may be one of the distinct offerings of occupational science, distinguishing it from such sciences as anthropology and sociology, whose research is focused largely at the levels of cultures and institutions. Discounting research strongly based in the individual perspectives of those studied is a mistake, although the critique of individualism is important. Occupational science does need to understand the broad cultural shaping of activity ideas then impact occupational experience. Thus far, however, research beyond individual experiences of occupation has been largely limited to the importation of extradisciplinary theories with which to examine occupation.

THE HISTORY OF OCCUPATIONAL SCIENCE

Emergence of Occupational Science From Occupational Therapy

Occupational science was birthed from, and in response to the needs of, occupational therapy (Clark & Larson, 1993; Clark et al., 1991; Clark, Wood, & Larson, 1998; Larson, Wood, & Clark, 2003; Lunt, 1997; Primeau, Clark, & Pierce, 1989; Yerxa et al., 1989; Zemke & Clark, 1996). It was formed in congruence with the beliefs and values of the earliest founders of the profession (Clark & Larson, 1993; Clark et al., 1998; Larson et al., 2003; Yerxa, 1992). It emerged from calls for such a science by occupational therapy leaders. Mary Reilly's (1962, 1974) occupational behavior theory guided the emerging focus of the science. Her students Gary Kielhofner and Janice Burke (1977) described occupational therapy's historical knowledge base crisis as a paradigm shift away from biomechanical approaches and toward a more holistic, occupation-focused paradigm. Gail Fidler (1981) also recognized this shift. In her Slagle Lectureship, Elnora Gilfoyle (1984) described a similar transformation of the profession in response to a changing culture, calling for a "science of occupation" (p. 578). Elizabeth Yerxa (1966, 1981, 1991a, 1991b, 1992, 1993, 1995, 1998a, 1998b, 2000a, 2000b, 2009) repeatedly expressed her concern that occupational therapy required a unique and ethical knowledge base focused on occupation, in order to become an autonomous, authentic, and self-directed profession.

First Origin of Occupational Science

Officially, the first origin of occupational science was in the Occupational Therapy Department of the University of Southern California (USC) and began with the opening of the PhD in Occupational Science Program in 1989 (Kantartzis & Molineux, 2012; Pierce, 2012). But, years of work within that department laid the way to that milestone event.

Dr. Elizabeth Yerxa assumed the chair of the department in 1976. Building on the long-term focus of the department on occupation in practice, her dream was to launch a science of occupation that provided occupational therapy with the unique knowledge base of an autonomous profession. An initial PhD proposal was developed by the department in the 1970s, but the University declined approval. Academia was changing; to garner support for a new PhD, highly productive researchers were needed. Building the research capacity of the department became a key strategy of Dr. Yerxa's leadership. She also advocated to the profession that qualitative research approaches offered an ethical match to occupational therapy's valuing of the lives and voices of patients.

During the 1980s, Dr. Yerxa required all of her faculty members, who were by then highly engaged in quite different research areas, to meet intensively to conceptualize the new science and design the first PhD program to train its scientists. She transformed her faculty from a group of independent researchers into a powerful team questing after a new discipline (Yerxa, 2000a). My first academic job was as the project specialist supporting this work group. A series of leading researchers provided the team with consultations on content, methods, funding, publishing, interdisciplinary collaborations, and the process of shaping a unique discipline. As the design of the PhD program took shape, a grant proposal to the Bureau of Maternal and Child Health (MCH) to support the new program with additional faculty members and student stipends was also prepared. The PhD was approved by the University, and the grant from MCH was awarded. Dr. Yerxa retired amid celebration of the new discipline she had worked so hard to bring into being.

Dr. Florence Clark accepted the department chair position prior to the start of the PhD Program in Occupational Science in the fall of 1989. All seven students in the first class of the new program were occupational therapists, and I was one of them. It was an exciting time. Professors and students explored together a world of research and methods that we hoped held answers to our project of creating a science of occupation. Supported by MCH, the annual Occupational Science Symposium was launched. Coordinating the yearly Symposium was another of my part-time jobs in those early years. The first keynote was by Mihalyi Csikszentmihalyi, who had been a consultant during the program development phase. At that time, the faculty found his research into optimal experience and his use of experiential sampling methods rich with examples and broad guidance in regard to how to undertake a science of occupation.

Once the PhD Program in Occupational Science began, the profession clamored to know more. Dr. Yerxa guided the first publication in 1989 of an occupational science special issue in *Occupational Therapy in Health Care*. In 1991 (Clark et al.), the debut article on occupational science in the *American Journal of Occupational Therapy* appeared, articulating the potential of a basic science of occupation to support the knowledge base of occupational therapy. Of course, there was then some push back from competing universities, producing a highly unusual exchange in the *American Journal of Occupational Therapy* that criticized and defended the usefulness of a descriptive science to a profession whose focus was intervention (Carlson & Dunlea, 1995; Clark et al., 1993; Mosey, 1992). Despite these challenges, occupational science was on its way at USC, with a new group of PhD students and another Occupational Science Symposium added each year.

Second Origin of Occupational Science

As occupational science continued to unfold in southern California, interest in the new science was also growing in Australia. In 1993, under the leadership of Ann Wilcock, the *Journal of Occupational Science: Australia* began publication, developing articles by drawing together interdisciplinary perspectives on occupation. The following year, USC's PhD Program in Occupational Science had its first graduate: Dr. Sheama Krishnagiri (Chapter 4). A series of PhD graduates began to emerge from USC, anxious to see whether or not occupational therapy departments would welcome them with academic appointments (Chapters 5, 17, 23, 25). In 1996, the first occupational science book, *Occupational Science: The Evolving Discipline*, was published, edited by Zemke and Clark and including Symposium keynotes, PhD seminar papers, and early studies. In 1996, I was thrilled to graduate after 7 years of full-time study and accepted an appointment at Creighton University. Also in 1996, Dr. Wilcock completed her PhD in Community Medicine in Australia. She quickly converted her dissertation into the second book to be published in occupational science, *An Occupational Perspective of Health* (1998). Soon, Dr. Wilcock began mentoring a new set of occupational scientists with a uniquely interdisciplinary and community health conceptualization of occupation (Whiteford, Townsend, & Hocking, 2000; Chapters 11, 14, 19).

This difference in the envisioned intent of the science at its two primary historical origins continues today. American occupational science is more focused on strategic disciplinary research that will support the autonomy and effectiveness of occupational therapy. The Australian perspective emphasizes occupation at the population level, the relation of occupation to justice, the need for policy change in regard to large-scale patterns of occupation, and interdisciplinary research. Such significant differences in the expressed purpose of the discipline produce creative tensions in the maturation of the science, requiring occupational science to reach a transcending and integrative standpoint in regard to the unfolding of the discipline and its relation to the profession.

A Growing Body of Theory and Research

The transcending hallmark of a mature discipline is its produced body of theory and research (Abbott, 1988, 2001, 2004; Pierce, 2012). The growth of occupational science since its beginning is easily seen in dramatic increases in the publication of books and articles in occupational science.

As just described, the first two books in occupational science came from their two origins: *Occupational Science: The Evolving Discipline*, edited by Ruth Zemke and Florence Clark (1996) and *An Occupational Perspective of Health* written by Ann Wilcock (1998). In the 2000s, books began to be published more frequently. Three introductory-level books for occupational therapy students were released in 2003 and 2004: *Occupation by Design: Building Therapeutic Power* by myself (2003), *The Meaning of Everyday Occupation* by Betty Hasselkus (2002), and *Introduction to Occupation: The Art and Science of Living* by Charles Christiansen and Elizabeth Townsend (2004). The year 2004 also saw two new types of books in occupational science. *Mothering Occupations: Challenge, Agency, and Participation*, edited by Susan Esdaile and Jane Olsen (2004), was the first collection of research on a particular type of occupation. *Occupation for Occupational Therapists*, by Matthew Molineux (2004), was the first book written specifically for therapists. In 2004, Gail Whiteford and Valerie Wright-St Clair published a highly theoretical collection, titled *Occupation and Practice in Context*. Ann Wilcock's second edition of *An Occupational Perspective of Health* was released in 2006. In 2008, Moses Ikiugu published a fascinating essay on the ecological impacts of human occupation, titled *Occupational Science in the Service of Gaia*. Katherine Matuska and Charles Christiansen published *Life Balance: Multidisciplinary Theories and Research* in 2009, introducing an interdisciplinary collection as a new mode of publication in occupational science, focusing on occupation and time use. In 2011, the second edition of *The Meaning of Everyday Occupation*, by Betty Hasselkus, was published. Most recently, additional theoretical collections have been published by Cutchin and Dickie (2012), *Transactional Perspectives on Occupation*, and by Whiteford and Hocking (2012), *Occupational Science: Society, Inclusion, Participation*. This rapid increase in the number of books being published in occupational science is a clear indicator of the discipline's growth. Now *Occupational Science for Occupational Therapy* joins this list. This book provides a synthesis of the diversity of occupational science in regard to how that research supports practice. Many of the leading scholars who have published or contributed to books in occupational science thus far are included here.

The growth of occupational science research has also been well documented in three studies. Molke, Laliberte Rudman, and Polatajko (2004) compared occupational science publications in 1990 and 2000. During that time, publications quadrupled in number, were more widely published, used a greater variety of methods, included more international authors, and added the new concept of occupational justice. Glover (2009) completed a statistical examination of occupational science articles over 11 years, 1996 through 2006, finding similar results: an increased numbers of articles, an increased proportion of quantitative articles as well as qualitative-only studies, and an increase in articles not focused on people with disabilities. Glover also found an association between publishing in the *Journal of Occupational Science* and interdisciplinary authorship.

Lastly, I and a group of my colleagues (Pierce et al., 2010) analyzed the contents of presentations in the first 5 years of research presented at the Society for the Study of Occupation: USA, which spanned the years 2002 to 2006. In the 108 data-based presentations, the most studied groups were adult women without disabilities, followed by 46% of studies addressing occupations of people with either disabilities or disadvantages. Research focused on one of four themes, in descending order of frequency: personal experiences of occupation, the context of occupation, changes in occupation, and descriptions of specific craft or daily living activities. Approximately 12% of work presented focused on individual interpretations of personal experiences, 67% looked at occupation within groups of people with shared characteristics, and 21% examined co-occupations in dyad, group, or community interactive sequences.

In the early years of the young science, occupational scientists of various backgrounds often declared what occupational science is, or ought to be. The time for making such statements about the future of the discipline without the support of data on research trends has passed (Laliberte Rudman et al., 2008). This book marks that change by being firmly centered on research work within the science.

The Disciplinary Culture of Occupational Science

Beyond the development of a knowledge base, an additional important hallmark of the maturation of occupational science is its manifestation of a disciplinary culture (Abbott, 1988, 2001). Like the pipes, cables, and foundations that underlie a city's streets, the organizations, academic structures, and one dedicated journal that have been created by occupational science over the past 25 years provide the necessary foundation upon which the discipline is built (Macaulay, 1976; Pierce, 2012).

The first academic degree in occupational science was the PhD in Occupational Science at USC. Many of the graduates of this first program have taken appointments across the United States and globally, supporting the further development of occupational science within academia. Additional doctoral programs focused on occupation have begun, all within occupational therapy departments: PhDs in Occupational Science at the University of North Carolina, Chapel Hill, and the University of Western Ontario; a ScD in Occupational Science at Towson University; and a PhD in Occupation and Rehabilitation Science at the University of Colorado. Several departments, including my own at Eastern Kentucky University, offer baccalaureate programs in occupational science that provide excellent preparation for graduate programs in occupational therapy. A further, and perhaps most symbolic, change in academia is the renaming of occupational therapy departments to include the term *occupational science*. Clearly, the culture of this young discipline is spreading rapidly through occupational therapy academia.

A key manifestation of the culture of a discipline is its journals. The *Journal of Occupational Science* has been in publication for nearly 20 years. In 1993, it began as the *Journal of Occupational Science: Australia*. In keeping with the leadership of Ann Wilcock, its editorial intent is interdisciplinary, and it does not publish research related to interventions. Articles are "welcomed, from anthropologists, ethnologists, human geographers, occupational scientists and therapists, psychologists, sociologists, and social biologists; any discipline, in fact, which has a humanistic view and could contribute to the study of occupation" (*Journal of Occupational Science*, front matter). There have also been occupational science special issues in other journals, including the *American Journal of Occupational Therapy*, *Scandinavian Journal of Occupational Therapy*, and *Work*.

Disciplinary culture is also expressed in ongoing organizations that provide researchers with opportunities to hear and share disciplinary work. The first of these was USC's annual Occupational Science Symposium, which began in 1989 and featured speakers selected in response to a theme. In this way, the perspectives of great scholars were brought to the attention of occupational scientists, including Andrew Abbott, Mary Catherine Bateson, Jerome Bruner, Mihalyi Csikszentmihalyi, Jane Goodall, Steven Hawking, and many others. In 1995, the annual Japanese Occupational Science Seminar began, and in 1997, the Australasian Symposium began.

The Society for the Study of Occupation: USA was planned in 1999 at the USC Symposium, was chartered there in 2000, and held its first annual meeting in 2002. This ushered in a new organizational mode for occupational science: a research society, presenting a fully peer-reviewed program of research and theory. Regional occupational science organizations now exist all over the world: the Canadian Society for Occupational Science, Occupational Science Europe, the Japanese Society for the Study of Occupation, and others. The International Society for Occupational Science provides a virtual, global occupational science organization (Wicks, 2012). Together, these social structures carry forward the disciplinary culture of occupational science through their support of the discourse, dissemination, and scholarly success of occupational scientists.

OCCUPATIONAL SCIENCE FOR OCCUPATIONAL THERAPY: AN OVERVIEW

As occupational science has developed, different theorists have advocated for different visions of the focus of the young science, depending on their own theoretical perspectives. At this point in the maturation of the discipline, it

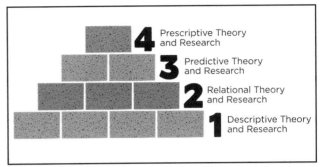

Figure 1-1. The four interdependent levels of theory and science.

is time to turn from imagining the future of occupational science to examining how it is being expressed in research. It is also no longer necessary to argue why one vision of occupational science may be better than another. Clearly, occupational science has multiple intents.

Occupational Science Under Construction: Four Types of Knowledge

In this book, occupational science is presented across four levels of research on occupation: descriptive, relational, predictive, and prescriptive (Dickoff, James, & Weidenbach, 1968; Pierce, 2012). I would like to acknowledge Elizabeth Yerxa for first bringing this elegant nursing theory to my attention in 1985. Like occupational therapy, nursing has had to reconcile the need for different types of theory. Nursing still uses this transcending notion that sciences have different, and even multiple, key purposes (Meleis, 2005). Unlike many meta-theories with which I have over the years become intrigued, explored in research, and then set aside along my own path, this one has retained for me its original utility and elegance. Understanding occupational science across differing but related levels allows a more diversified and nuanced conceptualization of the science than does any single-level approach (Figure 1-1).

In the 10th Ruth Zemke Lecture in Occupational Science, *Promise* (2011, 2012), I was inspired by the work of children's author and illustrator David Macaulay (1973, 1976, 1983), to present the idea of a multileveled science through the metaphor of construction. That is, I see occupational science as having levels that depend on each other's adequacy for their own stability. Level 1, descriptive research, provides the science with a solid base; Level 2 research is built on Level 1 concepts; and so on. This is a novel perspective for occupational therapy, which has always focused on the fourth and most complex theoretical level, the therapeutic applications of occupation, rarely considering how unclear descriptive, relational, and predictive knowledge of occupation might be undermining the success of research and interventions at the applied level.

Different sciences sometimes focus more on one level than another. Biology is highly descriptive, economics is interested in prediction, and nursing cares most about prescriptive research to guide interventions. Yet, in order to be considered useful in people's lives, sciences need all four levels of theory to some degree, even if that science must be borrowed.

Level 1: Description of Key Concepts and Dynamics of Occupation

Level 1, or descriptive, occupational science theory and research, is described in *Occupational Science for Occupational Therapy* in Chapters 2 through 6. Descriptive research names and explains the basic concepts of a science. In this way, descriptive research can be considered a foundation upon which the rest of the science rests. If the descriptive work is not deeply developed, levels of research that study how those factors relate to other concepts, unfold in larger patterns, or can be applied will be weakened. Descriptive occupational science provides occupational therapists with an understanding of how their clients see, experience, and organize their occupations.

Level 2: Relations Between Occupation and Key Concepts of Other Disciplines

Level 2, or relational, research is strong in occupational science. You will see, in Chapters 7 through 14, how research relating occupation to the primary concepts of other disciplines has seen explosive growth. Level 2 research has especially drawn on the theoretical perspectives of more mature disciplines to study occupation in relation to disability, identity, and culture. Yet, like a wide structure resting on a narrow foundation, the rapid growth of Level 2 research in comparison to other levels challenges occupational science's clarity of focus and intent.

Level 3: Predicting Large Patterns of Occupation

Level 3, or predictive, occupational science is, as yet, relatively undeveloped (Chapters 15 through 20). Predictive research in occupational science attempts to describe occupation in broad patterns, across time and development, over large spaces, and in differing sociocultural conditions. There may be several explanations for why Level 3 research is limited thus far in occupational science. Level 3, predictive, research may require a greater development of Level 1, descriptive, research before it can produce research on larger patterns of occupation. Also, the large sample studies that would best fit predictive research questions require quantitative methods, which are less common in occupational science (Glover, 2009). The predictive occupational science

research that we have at present is probably most helpful to occupational therapists by illustrating what may be expected or measured in the unfolding of developmental patterns of occupation, whether in regard to play, retirement, or other types of occupations.

Level 4: Prescriptive Research on the Applications of Occupation

Level 4, or prescriptive, occupational science is intervention research (Chapters 21 through 28). Prescriptive occupational science is the most complex level and is highly sensitive to the adequacy of development of its supporting levels. This level has also developed rapidly, however, supported by its excellent match to the interests of occupational therapy. Prescriptive occupational science research helps therapists understand the thinking and effectiveness behind occupation-based practice, as well as providing occupation-based assessments.

BEING THE NEWEST OCCUPATIONAL THERAPISTS OFF THE LOT

For occupational therapy students using *Occupational Science for Occupational Therapy* as a learning tool, I extend to you a heartfelt wish that what you find here will support and encourage you as you enter, or continue, the work of your profession. Know how fortunate you are that you are being prepared at a time when you have occupational science to undergird your thinking and practice! You will be the best therapist your faculties can prepare. As I always tell entry-level students, you are like beautiful new sports cars. You are the newest, most up-to-date occupational therapists off the lot. But be humble: most therapists you meet were prepared differently than you were, and they certainly have much to teach you. Someday, you will be the experienced, classic therapist trained 20 years before, looking at a new student and realizing how differently prepared he or she is from you. Always take time to reflect, as you read this book and in all the years of your practice. Reflection and continued learning are the roads to greatness for a therapist. As you work your way through *Occupational Science for Occupational Therapy*, also consider the passions, commitments, and adventures of the scientists included here. For some of you, the path of research will also be in your future.

REFERENCES

Abbott, A. (1988). *Discipline and profession*. Chicago, IL: University of Chicago Press.

Abbott, A. (2001). *Chaos of disciplines.* Chicago, IL: University of Chicago Press.

Abbott, A. (2004, January). *Becoming discipline: From occupational therapy to occupational science.* Paper presented at the Occupational Science Symposium XVI: Creating an Academic Discipline that Supports Practice, Los Angeles, CA.

Carlson, M., & Dunlea, A. (1995). The issue is: Further thoughts on the pitfalls of partition: A response to Mosey. *American Journal of Occupational Therapy, 49,* 73-81. doi:10.5014/ajot.49.1.73

Christensen, C., & Townsend, E. (Eds.). (2004). *Introduction to occupation: The art and science of living.* Upper Saddle River, NJ: Prentice Hall.

Clark, F. (2006). One person's thought on the future of occupational science. *Journal of Occupational Science, 13*(3), 167-179. doi:10.1080/14427591.2006.9726513

Clark, F., & Larson, E. (1993). Developing an academic discipline: The science of occupation. In H. Hopkins & H. Smith (Eds.), *Willard and Spackman's occupational therapy* (8th ed., pp. 44-57). Philadelphia, PA: J. B. Lippincott.

Clark, F., Parham, D., Carlson, M. E., Frank, G., Jackson, J., Pierce, D., . . . Zemke, R. (1991). Occupational science: Academic innovation in the service of occupational therapy's future. *American Journal of Occupational Therapy, 45,* 300-310. doi:10.5014/ajot.45.4.300

Clark, F., Wood, W., & Larson, E. (1998). Occupational sceince: Occupational therapy's legacy for the 21st century. In M. Neistadt & E. Crepeau (Eds.), *Willard and Spackman's occupational therapy* (9th ed., pp. 13-21). Philadelphia, PA: J. B. Lippincott.

Clark, F., Zemke, R., Frank, G., Parham, D., Neville-Jan, A., Hendricks, C., . . . Abreu, B. (1993). Dangers inherent in the partition of occupational therapy and occupational science. *American Journal of Occupational Therapy, 47*(2), 184-186. doi:10.5014/ajot.47.2.184

Csikszentmihalyi, M. (1975). *Beyond boredom and anxiety: Experiencing flow in work and play.* San Francisco, CA: Jossey-Bass.

Csikszentmihalyi, M., & Csikszentmihalyi, I. (1988). *Optimal experience: Psychological studies of flow in consciousness.* New York, NY: Cambridge University Press.

Cutchin, M., & Dickie, V. (2012). *Transactional perspectives on occupation.* New York, NY: Springer.

Dickie, V., Cutchin, M., & Humphry, R. (2006). Occupation as a transactional experience: A critique of individualism in occupational science. *Journal of Occupational Science, 13,* 83-93. doi:10.1080/14427591.2006.9686573

Dickoff, J., James, P., & Weidenbach, E. (1968). Theory in practice discipline: Part I. Practice oriented theory. *Nursing Research, 17*(5), 387-480.

Esdaile, S., & Olsen, J. (2004). *Mothering occupations: Challenge, agency, and participation.* Philadelphia, PA: F.A. Davis.

Fidler, G. (1981). From crafts to competence. *American Journal of Occupational Therapy, 35,* 567-573. doi:10.5014/ajot.35.9.567

Garber, M. (2001). Coveting your neighbor's discipline. *Chronicle of Higher Education, 47,* 18-19.

Gilfoyle, E. (1984). Eleanor Clarke Slagle Lectureship, 1984: Transformation of a profession. *American Journal of Occupational Therapy, 38,* 575-584.

Glover, J. (2009). The literature of occupational science: A systematic, quantitative examination of peer-reviewed publications from 1996 to 2006. *Journal of Occupational Science, 16*(2), 92-103. doi:10.1080/14427591.2009.9686648

Good, G. (2000). The assembly of geophysics: Scientific disciplines as frameworks of consensus. *Studies in History and Philosophy of Modern Physics, 31,* 259-292. doi:10.1016/S1355-2198(00)00018-6

Hasselkus, B. R. (2002). *The meaning of everyday occupation.* Thorofare, NJ: SLACK Incorporated.

Hasselkus, B. R. (2011). *The meaning of everyday occupation* (2nd ed.). Thorofare, NJ: SLACK Incorporated.

Heilbron, J. (2003). A regime of disciplines: Toward a historical sociology of disciplinary knowledge. In C. Camic & H. Joas (Eds.), *The dialogical turn: New roles of sociology in the postdisciplinary age.* New York, NY: Rowman and Littlefield.

Hocking, C. (2012). Occupations through the looking glass: Reflecting on occupational scientists' ontological assumptions. In G. Whiteford & C. Hocking (Eds.), *Occupational science: Society, inclusion, participation* (pp. 54-66). Oxford, United Kingdom: Wiley-Blackwell.

Ikiugu, M. (2008). *Occupational science in the service of Gaia.* Baltimore, MD: Publish America.

Kantartzis, S., & Molineux, M. (2012). Understanding the discursive development of occupation: Historico-political perspectives. In G. Whiteford & C. Hocking (Eds.), *Occupational science: Society, inclusion, participation* (pp. 38-53). Oxford, United Kingdom: Wiley-Blackwell.

Keith, B. (2000). Taking stock of the discipline: Some reflections on the state of American sociology. *The American Sociologist, 31,* 5-14. doi:10.1007/s12108-000-1001-4

Kielhofner, G., & Burke, J. (1977). Occupational therapy after 60 years: An account of changing identity and knowledge. *American Journal of Occupational Therapy, 31,* 675-688.

Kinsella, E. (2012). Knowledge paradigms in occupational science: Pluralistic perspectives. In G. Whiteford & C. Hocking (Eds.), *Occupational science: Society, inclusion, participation* (pp. 69-85). Oxford, United Kingdom: Wiley-Blackwell.

Laliberte Rudman, D., Dennhardt, S., Fok, D., Huot, S., Molke, D., Park, A., & Zur, B. (2008). A vision for occupational science: Reflecting on our disciplinary culture. *Journal of Occupational Science, 15*(3), 136-146. doi:10.1080/14427591.2008.9686623

Larson, E., Wood, W., & Clark, F. (2003). Occupational science: Building the science and practice of occupation through an academic discipline. In H. Hopkins & H. Smith (Eds.), *Willard and Spackman's occupational therapy* (8th ed., pp. 15-26). Philadelphia, PA: J. B. Lippincott.

Lunt, A. (1997). Occupational science and occupational therapy: Negotiating the boundary between a discipline and a profession. *Journal of Occupational Science: Australia, 4,* 56-61.

Macaulay, D. (1973). *Cathedral: The story of its construction.* Boston, MA: Houghton Mifflin.

Macaulay, D. (1976). *Underground.* Boston, MA: Houghton Mifflin.

Macaulay, D. (1983). *Mill.* Boston, MA: Houghton Mifflin.

Magalhaes, L. (2012). What would Paulo Freire think of occupational science? In G. Whiteford & C. Hocking (Eds.), *Occupational science: Society, inclusion, participation* (pp. 8-22). Oxford, United Kingdom: Wiley-Blackwell.

Matuska, K., & Christiansen, C. (2009). *Life balance: Multidisciplinary theories and research.* Thorofare, NJ: SLACK Incorporated.

Meleis, A. I. (2005). Foreword. In B. J. Daly, D. Speedy, V. Jackson, & C. Lambert (Eds.), *Professional nursing: Concepts, issues, and challenges.* New York, NY: Springer Publishing.

Molineux, M. (Ed.). (2004). *Occupation for occupational therapists.* Oxford, United Kingdom: Blackwell.

Molke, D. K., Laliberte Rudman, D., & Polatajko, H. J. (2004). The promise of occupational science: A developmental assessment of an emerging academic discipline. *Canadian Journal of Occupational Therapy, 71*(5), 269-280.

Mosey, A. C. (1992). The issue is: Partition of occupational science and occupational therapy. *American Journal of Occupational Therapy, 46,* 851-853. doi:10.5014/ajot.46.9.851

Pierce, D. (1991). Early object rule acquisition. *American Journal of Occupational Therapy, 45,* 438-450.

Pierce, D. (2000). Maternal management of the home as an infant/toddler developmental space. *American Journal of Occupational Therapy, 54,* 290-299. doi:10.5014/ajot.54.3.290

Pierce, D. (2001). Untangling occupation and activity. *American Journal of Occupational Therapy, 55,* 138-146. doi:10.5014/ajot.55.2.138

Pierce, D. (2003). *Occupation by design: Building therapeutic power.* Philadelphia, PA: F. A. Davis.

Pierce, D. (2011, October). *Promise: The 10th Ruth Zemke lecture in occupational science.* Keynote for SSO:USA Meeting, Park City, UT.

Pierce, D. (2012). Promise. *Journal of Occupational Science, 19*(4), 298-311. doi:10.1080/14427591.2012.667778

Pierce, D., Atler, K., Baltisberger, J., Fehringer, E., Hunter, E., Malkawi, S., & Parr, T. (2010). Occupational science: A data-based American perspective. *Journal of Occupational Science, 17*(4), 204-215. doi:10.1080/14427591.2010.9686697

Pierce, D., Myers, C., & Munier, V. (2009). Informing early intervention through an occupational science description of infant-toddler interactions with home space. *American Journal of Occupational Therapy, 63,* 273-287. doi:10.5014/ajot.63.3.273

Powell, A., O'Malley, M., Muller-Wille, S., Calvert, J., & Dupre, J. (2007). Disciplinary baptisms: A comparison of the naming stories of genetics, molecular biology, genomics and systems biology. *History and Philosophy of the Life Sciences, 29,* 5-32.

Primeau, L., Clark, F., & Pierce, D. (1989). Occupational therapy alone has looked upon occupation: Future applications of occupational science to pediatric occupational therapy. *Occupational Therapy in Health Care, 6,* 19-32.

Reilly, M. (1962). 1961 Eleanor Clarke Slagle Lecture: Occupational therapy can be one of the great ideas of 20th-century medicine. *American Journal of Occupational Therapy, 16,* 1-9.

Reilly, M. (1974). *Play as exploratory learning.* Beverly Hills, CA: Sage Publications.

Rudman, D. (2012). Governing through occupation: Shaping expectations and possibilities. In G. Whiteford & C. Hocking (Eds.), *Occupational science: Society, inclusion, participation* (pp. 100-116). Oxford, United Kingdom: Wiley-Blackwell.

Smelser, N. (2004). Interdisciplinarity in theory and practice. In C. Camic & H. Joas (Eds.), *The dialogical turn: New roles of sociology in postdisciplinary age* (pp. 43-64). New York, NY: Rowman and Littlefield Publishers.

Turner, S. (2004). The maturity of social theory. In C. Camic & H. Joas (Eds.), *The dialogical turn: New roles of sociology in the postdisciplinary age* (pp. 141-170). New York, NY: Rowman and Littlefield Publishers.

Whiteford, G., & Hocking, C. (Eds.). (2012). *Occupational science: Society, inclusion, participation.* Oxford, United Kingdom: Wiley-Blackwell.

Whiteford, G., Townsend, E., & Hocking C. (2000). Reflections on a renaissance of occupation. *Canadian Journal of Occupational Therapy, 67,* 61-69.

Whiteford, G., & Wright-St Clair, V. (Eds.) (2004). *Occupation and practice in context.* Sydney, NSW: Elsevier Churchill Livingstone.

Wicks, A. (2012). The International Society for Occupational Science: A critique of its role in facilitating the development of occupational science through international networks and intercultural dialogue. In G. Whiteford & C. Hocking (Eds.), *Occupational science: Society, inclusion, participation* (pp. 163-183). Oxford, United Kingdom: Wiley-Blackwell.

Wilcock, A. A. (1998). *An occupational perspective of health.* Thorofare, NJ: SLACK Incorporated.

Wilcock, A. A. (2006). *An occupational perspective of health* (2nd ed.). Thorofare, NJ: SLACK Incorporated.

Wright-St Clair, V. (2012). The case for multiple research methodologies. In G. Whiteford & C. Hocking (Eds.), *Occupational science: Society, inclusion, participation* (pp. 137-151). Oxford, United Kingdom: Wiley-Blackwell.

Yerxa, E. (1966). Eleanor Clarke Slagle Lecture: Authentic occupational therapy. *American Journal of Occupational Therapy, 21,* 1-9.

Yerxa, E. (1981). A "developmental assessment" of occupational therapy research in 1981. *American Journal of Occupational Therapy, 35,* 820-821. doi:10.5014/ajot.35.12.820

Yerxa, E. (1991a). Occupational therapy: An endangered species or an academic discipline in the 21st century? *American Journal of Occupational Therapy, 45,* 680-685. doi:10.5014/ajot.45.8.680

Yerxa, E. (1991b). Seeking a relevant, ethical, and realistic way of knowing for occupational therapy. *American Journal of Occupational Therapy, 45,* 199-204. doi:10.5014/ajot.45.3.199

Yerxa, E. (1992). Some implications of occupational therapy's history for its epistemology, values, and relation to medicine. *American Journal of Occupational Therapy, 46,* 79-83. doi:10.5014/ajot.46.1.79

Yerxa, E. (1993). Occupational science: A new source of power for participants in occupational therapy. *Journal of Occupational Science, 1,* 3-10. doi:10.1080/14427591.1993.9686373

Yerxa, E. (1995). Nationally speaking: Who is the keeper of occupational therapy's practice and knowledge? *American Journal of Occupational Therapy, 49,* 295-299. doi:10.5014/ajot.49.4.295

Yerxa, E. (1998a). Health and the human spirit for occupation. *American Journal of Occupational Therapy, 52,* 412-418. doi:10.5014/ajot.52.6.412

Yerxa, E. (1998b). Occupation: The keystone of a curriculum for a self-defined profession. *American Journal of Occupational Therapy, 52,* 365-372. doi:10.5014/ajot.52.5.365

Yerxa, E. (2000a). Confessions of an occupational therapist who became a detective. *British Journal of Occupational Therapy, 63,* 192-200.

Yerxa, E. (2000b). Occupational science: A renaissance of service to humankind through knowledge. *Occupational Therapy International, 7,* 87-98.

Yerxa, E. (2009). Infinite distance between the I and the it. *American Journal of Occupational Therapy, 63*(4), 490-497. doi:10.5014/ajot.63.4.490

Yerxa, E., Clark, F., Frank, G., Jackson, J., Parham, D., Pierce, D., . . . Zemke, R. (1989). An introduction to occupational science, a foundation for occupational therapy in the 21st century. *Occupational Therapy in Health Care, 6,* 1-18.

Zemke, R., & Clark, F. (1996). *Occupational science: The evolving discipline.* Philadelphia, PA: F. A. Davis.

I

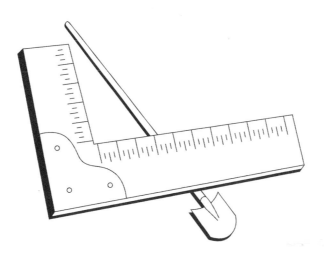

Level 1 Research

How Does Occupational Science Provide Descriptive Knowledge to Strengthen Occupational Therapy?

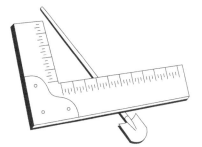

Occupational Science Research Describing Occupation

Doris Pierce, PhD, OTR/L, FAOTA

DESCRIPTIVE RESEARCH: THE INITIAL VISION OF OCCUPATIONAL SCIENCE

When occupational science began, the focus was on developing an understanding of occupation (Clark et al., 1991). That is, we initially targeted Level 1 factor-identifying, descriptive research on occupation (Dickoff, James, & Weidenbach, 1968). The science was conceptualized as basic and descriptive. The profession was expressing a widening realization that descriptive research on the core concept and primary modality of occupational therapy was extremely limited (Fidler, 1981; Rogers, 1984). Yerxa (1987, 1995) argued repeatedly that a true profession requires a unique body of knowledge that is not duplicated by any other profession. Thus, the founders of occupational science began with the notion that occupational therapy required an in-depth theoretical description of occupation itself. As Yerxa (1987) expressed it, an academic discipline that described occupation would help clients because, "we are often in the position of dealing with incapacity, trying

to reduce it although we don't know nearly enough about *capacity*" (p. 416). Later, in occupational science's debut article in the *American Journal of Occupational Therapy*, the same focus on descriptive knowledge of occupation was expressed. "Occupational science is to occupational therapy what anatomy and physiology are to medicine" (Clark et al., 2001, p. 307). Because the science was viewed as largely descriptive, it began with qualitative methods.

PRECURSORS TO OCCUPATIONAL SCIENCE RESEARCH AT LEVEL 1

A Historical Interest in Craft Occupations

Prior to the launch of occupational science in 1989, little research describing occupation had been done within occupational therapy. A search through occupational therapy's archive, the Wilma West Library, produced very little research descriptive of occupation. In its earliest

Pierce, D. (Ed.).
Occupational Science for Occupational Therapy (pp. 13-21).
© 2014 SLACK Incorporated.

days, however, occupational therapy had a strong interest in crafts as occupations. Herbert Hall (1923) published an article shortly after occupational therapy began, discussing a debate between himself and Dr. Dunton (both influential founders) of the relative merits of wooden toy making as an occupational therapy intervention. Also of interest was a four-article series that described Mexican trades and crafts in fair detail (Knox, 1931, 1932a, 1932b, 1932c). At the time of these publications, occupational therapy was borrowing knowledge from master craftsmen to create interventions that used pottery, basketry, weaving, leatherwork, woodwork, and copper. Occupational therapy's interest in crafts at that time was in the production of goods that would provide income for inpatients and support their skilled livelihood following discharge. Early efforts to describe craft occupations were intended to increase therapists' understanding of the process used for different types of craft work. In some places, master craftsman were included in occupational therapy educational programs so that students would be skilled in the crafts they used as therapy. Even when I was in school in the 1970s, we still took a class in the industrial technology department, where we learned woodworking and other crafts. This focus on craft production in practice is greatly reduced in occupational therapy today.

Centering on Activities of Daily Living

Since its inception, occupational therapy has also focused on enabling everyday activities for people with disabilities. To illustrate this long-standing focus, here is a sampling of how this was addressed in early editions of *Willard and Spackman's Occupational Therapy*, a classic occupational therapy text for many generations of therapists.

In the 1954 edition, Edgerton described "activities aimed at training or retraining the patient to be able to care for his personal needs in self-toileting, dressing and grooming and self-reliance at the dining table, the telephone and in travel by public conveyance" (p. 54). Wagner (1954) listed self-help activities such as feeding, dressing, writing, and typing. In the fourth edition, Spackman (1971) described eight functions of occupational therapy, one of which was "to teach self-help activities, those of daily living such as eating, dressing, writing, the use of adaptive equipment and prostheses" (p. 2). Zimmerman (1971) described activities of daily living programs for patients in rehabilitation settings, advocating that, for adult women, occupational therapists begin to extend their concerns beyond self-help devices, splints, and prostheses and strength training to address homemaking and home evaluations.

These historical excerpts demonstrate the centrality of everyday self-care activities to occupational therapy's professional identity. Because little research in occupational therapy has been descriptive of occupation in people without disability, however, there has not been much of a knowledge base to support therapists' practice in this area. Until recently, a therapist's understanding of these critical daily activities has generally been left to the therapist's common sense, life experience, and intuition.

Occupational Therapy's Developmental Perspective on Occupation

The fertile soil from which occupational science grew was Mary Reilly's (1962, 1974) theory of occupational behavior. Reilly carried on the tradition of Adolf Meyer (1922), who provided the earliest categorical description of occupations as "work and play and rest and sleep" (p. 7). Reilly's work was centered in the longstanding interests of occupational therapy in play as an intervention (Bundy, 1990; Clark, 1979a, 1979b). Occupational behavior described an original perspective on the developmental progression of occupation, from play exploration to competence and adult achievement. Reilly's theory drew largely from psychological theories of play progression and human motivation, but also brought together perspectives from evolutionary biology, anthropology, sociology, primatology, and systems theory. Mary Reilly's many graduate students went on to expand occupational behavior into play-based therapeutic approaches (Florey, 1971, 1981; Robinson, 1977) and systems models (Kielhofner & Burke, 1980) that began to explore occupation as it was experienced by people not impacted by disability.

In Mary Reilly's work, the logic of a developmental approach to understanding occupation was especially drawn from the play theories of Piaget and Gesell. This "ages and stages" approach was, and continues to be, broadly accepted in Western science. Certainly, in occupational therapy, it is a pillar of therapeutic thinking to move a client from one developmental phase to the next. For this reason, some occupational scientists in the early years focused on play in their research, reasoning that a good beginning place would be to study occupation in its younger or more creative forms (Blanche, 2007; Knox, 1997, 2008; Pierce, 1996).

SEARCHING FOR EXTRADISCIPLINARY DESCRIPTIVE WORK ON OCCUPATION

The emergence of occupational science in the United States was also influenced by extradisciplinary descriptive research related to occupation. In the mid-1980s, under the direction of Dr. Elizabeth Yerxa, the work group developing the PhD Program in Occupational Science at the University of Southern California embarked on a search for theory and research that promised insights into the nature of occupation. Emanating from disciplines beyond occupational therapy, the research that they found primarily examined occupation in relation to phenomenon of interest to the originating discipline; description of occupation was not the focus (Clark et al., 1991). Still, it was exciting to explore the universe of possibilities for understanding the central concept of the profession. The dawning realization that such an important aspect of human life was so little studied was even more exciting! Such a significant knowledge gap was a testimony to the need for occupational science. Further, the profession's best descriptions of typical occupation at that time used either a focus on specific subparts of occupation, such as sensory processes, or used systems models to combine concepts from multiple fields into a theoretical collage. The idea of doing original research that would really dig into and describe occupation using methods specifically fit to that effort was a new frontier.

Flow Theory: Describing Optimal Experience

The faculty group that developed the PhD in Occupational Science used a very deliberately selected series of consultations to cultivate their understanding of their project. They were quite aware of the methodological and epistemological challenges ahead of them. They required a science that would be responsive to occupational therapists' need for descriptions of everyday occupations and that those descriptions would be accurate enough to support effective therapeutic applications.

Among the many extradisciplinary theories examined, flow theory held great potential for occupational science, in terms of both its substance and its methods. Flow theory was produced by Csikszentmihalyi (1975; Csikszentmihalyi & Csikszentmihalyi, 1988) from a series of studies of groups of people experiencing the same type of occupation, including writing, playing the piano, ocean cruising, mountain climbing, television watching, everyday work, sports, and burglary. The central concept of the theory is that there is a state of optimal experience between boredom and anxiety that is created by a just-right match of perceived challenge and perceived skill. That state of flow includes a loss of sense of time and self, an immersed engagement in the occupation at hand, a deep enjoyment, and a close link to creativity.

During Dr. Csikszentmihalyi's consult, the group developing the PhD asked him a key question: "How can one measure subjective experience in an objective way?" His reply was "very carefully." Flow theory was created and refined using a method called *experience sampling method* (ESM). Stated very simply, ESM used randomized cuing of research participants to immediately complete a brief questionnaire regarding their experience at that moment. Dr. Csikszentmihalyi served as the first keynote speaker for the Occupational Science Symposium, which was funded by the Bureau of Maternal and Child Heath to support the development of the new science (Csikszentmihalyi, 1993). His ESM methods were used in several occupational science dissertations (e.g., a study of boredom in adolescents by Farnworth [1998]). Other interesting studies of flow were also later completed (Jonsson & Persson, 2006; Persson, Eklund, & Isaacson, 1999). Inevitably, the consideration of how flow might be used to improve the effectiveness of intervention was much discussed (Wright, 2004). Due to the initial focus of occupational science on descriptive work, however, no Level 4 research using flow theory or ESM methods was produced.

Chimpanzee Occupations

The work of Dr. Jane Goodall had a strong impact on the development of occupational science. In 1986, Goodall published her major research report, *The Chimpanzees of Gombe: Patterns of Behavior*. Based on 30 years of naturalistic observation of a community of wild-living chimpanzees, this massive tome detailed the occupational patterns of the nonhuman primates most closely related to humans. It described their thinking, family patterns, communications, ranging, feeding, hunting, aggression, friendly behavior, grooming, dominance, sexual behavior, territoriality, object manipulation, and social awareness as it was expressed over the 30 years of study. Further, it demonstrated the potential of an ethological approach to the study of occupation.

This comprehensive portrayal of primate life inspired the faculty work group that was attempting to sketch out the tentative boundaries of the new science. As the organizer of the Occupational Science Symposium, I recruited Dr. Goodall as the second keynote speaker in that series. Later, she accepted a joint appointment in occupational therapy and anthropology at the University of Southern California. In the anthropology department, The Jane Goodall Archive was created to house her Gombe video data and make it available to other researchers. I worked there as a graduate assistant for 2 years. Because Dr. Goodall wanted occupational therapists to become involved in enrichment of living conditions for captive chimpanzees, The Jane Goodall Fellowship was created to support an occupational science PhD student. That Fellowship was accepted by Wendy Wood, whose subsequent work with chimpanzees is reported in Chapter 5.

THE DEVELOPMENT OF OCCUPATIONAL SCIENCE DESCRIPTIVE RESEARCH

As occupational science began, it immediately had to confront existing categorizations of occupation. Occupational therapy was accustomed to directly and rather uncritically adopting cultural notions regarding types of occupation, such as work, play, and self-care. Primeau (1996) was one of the first occupational scientists to begin analyzing these categories, arguing that dichotomizing occupation into separate types was a false logic. In my own work (Pierce, 2001, 2003), I have carried forward this theoretical question, arguing that occupations do not fall into separate categories, but are each an experiential blend of productivity, pleasure, and restoration.

Mundane and Creative Occupations

A study of research reported at the Society for the Study of Occupation: USA documented the interest of occupational scientists in common everyday activities as well as creative occupations (Pierce et al., 2010). Occupational scientists have published several studies related to crafts (Dickie, 1996, 2003; Frank, 1996; Riley, 2008), but few in relation to self-care of people without disability or a need for caregiving (Hannam, 1997; Moore, 1996; Royeen, 2010). This finding echoes the documented historical interest of occupational therapy in crafts, as well as in daily living activities. In Chapter 6, Charlotte Royeen's work offers an elegant and methodologically innovative study of morning routines.

Elder Occupations

In keeping with the increasing demographic of elders in industrialized nations around the globe, occupational science has focused a significant portion of its descriptive research on the occupations of elders. Of these studies, I have found most informing Ludwig's (1998) study of routine in older women, which turns on its head the cultural idea that elders organize their lives through rigid routines. She found, instead, that routines are unpackaged with age, becoming more flexible and fluid.

Female Occupations

Occupational science has strongly invested in descriptive research on female occupations (Pierce et al., 2010; Primeau, 2000). Hocking (2012) has argued that this is due to a gender bias, and perhaps that is true. We should dig deeper, however, to understand why occupational science has overemphasized female occupations and perspectives to this degree. First, researchers in occupational science are predominantly female. Second, researchers in occupational science often take a feminist standpoint, bringing out the unique voices of those who are not well represented within patriarchal systems. Third, female researchers may also be more interested in the occupations particularly important in their own lives. Fourth, occupational science has inherited from occupational therapy a long-held interest in daily living and craft occupations, as well as a special interest

in women's occupations of caregiving. Fifth, it is easier to recruit women than men into studies. It is likely that a combination of these factors has created this gender gap in occupational science research.

One of the earliest books in occupational science was Esdaile and Olsen's (2004) edited collection on mothering. The book followed a special issue of the *American Journal of Occupational Therapy* on maternal work that was edited by an occupational scientist (Larson, 2000a). Betty Hasselkus' work (Chapter 3) adds descriptive research on caregiving that is well fit to the needs of occupational therapy to understand those they serve as well as those with whom they collaborate to provide care. Additional occupational science research on caregiving includes two studies of caregiving by grandmothers (Ludwig, Hattjar, Russell, & Winston, 2007; Marken, Pierce, & Baltisberger, 2010), studies of caregiving for children and adults with disability (Heward, Molineux, & Gough, 2006; Scoggin, 1999), a study of mothering at two different life stages (Francis-Connolly, 2000), and my own study of how mothers manage the home play spaces of infants and toddlers (Pierce, 2000).

Co-Occupations

Co-occupation is a concept that has emerged from occupational science. It is central to our understanding of occupation, expanding it to a more complex and dynamic level. Beyond the theoretical importance of co-occupation itself, the discovery and research development of original concepts also demonstrates the maturation of a science. The production of new ideas through ongoing and related research moves occupational science away from its dependence on borrowing fully developed theories from older sciences, investing instead in the much more difficult work of research that tests and evolves innovative theory in order to make a fresh contribution to the universe of knowledge.

Co-occupation refers to the uniquely interactive occupations of more than one individual, where the expressions of those occupations are closely shaping each other (Pierce, 2009). Good examples would be the occupations of a nursing mother and child, a pair of tennis players, or a teacher and student. Co-occupations occur in a responsive and continual shaping and matching of occupations. It is easy to see how this insight into occupation is centered in the confluence of occupational science's research investment in descriptive work on mothering and caregiving (Evans & Rodger, 2008; Pierce & Frank, 1992). It is also rooted in a strong interest in the temporal dimension of occupation, capturing the sequenced, active quality of co-occupations. Sufficient research on co-occupation had been completed by 2009 to warrant a special issue of the *Journal of Occupational Science* (Mahoney & Roberts, 2009; Persch, Pizur-Barnekow, Cashen, & Pickens, 2009; Pickens & Pizur-Barnekow, 2009; Pierce, 2009; Pizur-Barnekow & Knutson, 2009; Price & Stephenson, 2009).

Occupational Context

Occupational science has always held a strong interest in the contextual dimensions of occupation (Pierce, 2001; Pierce et al., 2010). As the discipline matures, it is important to balance occupational science's strong emphasis on the social dimension of occupational context with descriptive research into the spatial and temporal dimensions of occupation (Farnworth, 2004; Kantartzis & Molineux, 2012; Pierce, 2000, 2001, 2003). Occupational science has been strongly influenced by its sister discipline of anthropology to focus on sociocultural aspects of occupation. This has produced some outstanding descriptive research that gives occupational science significant depth with regard to social and cultural aspects of occupational context (Rudman, 2012; Segal & Hinojosa, 2006) (see Chapter 7). For anthropology, this focus is a necessity, since its primary disciplinary concept is culture. For occupational science, however, this strong focus on the sociocultural dimension is not as logical. Like our overemphasis of female occupations, overemphasizing the social dimension of occupations leaves a gap in our understanding.

Notably, a few occupational science researchers have focused their work on the spatial dimensions of occupation (Hocking, 1997, 2000; Howell & Pierce, 2000; Hunter, 2008; Huot & Rudman, 2010; Peralta-Catipon, 2009; Pierce, 1991; Rowles, 1991, 2008). A slightly larger number of studies have examined the temporal dimension of occupation (Erlandsson & Eklund, 2006; Farnworth, 1998, 2000; Humphry & Wakeford, 2006; Larson, 2000a, 2000b, 2003, 2004; Larson & von Eye, 2010; Ludwig, 1998; Pentland, Harvey, & Walker, 1998; Primeau, 1998; Segal, 2004; Singleton & Harvey, 1995; Stanley, 1995; Walker, 2001; Yerxa & Locker, 1990). More rare is research that examines the spatial and temporal context simultaneously (Alsaker et al., 2006; Kroksmark et al., 2006; Lynch, 2009; Pierce, Myers, & Munier, 2009; Zemke, 2004).

LEVEL 1 QUESTIONS FOR OCCUPATIONAL SCIENCE

In truth, although occupational science started out to make its primary contribution to occupational therapy by describing occupation itself, descriptive occupational science research is not extensive (Pierce et al., 2010). This base level, the understanding of occupation itself, is the foundation of the science. Any effort to explore the relations of occupation to other concepts (Level 2), its wider patterns across time or population groups (Level 3), or its applications in practice (Level 4) depend entirely on the depth of development of a corpus of Level 1, descriptive occupational science. With that in mind, what descriptions of occupation are most pressing to describe and why (Yerxa, 2005)?

What About Male Occupations?

For the sake of equity, it is evident that the occupations of males require attention. As discussed here, occupational science has been, for many reasons, particularly interested in the occupations of women. Only a few studies of the occupations of males without disability have been reported (Beagan & Saunders, 2005; Wada & Beagan, 2006). Research into the male experience and perspective would be highly informing to occupational science. The degree of contrast provided by such research can be expected to produce new insights into occupation.

Description of the Occupations of Which Population Would Best Serve Practice?

Description of critical occupations in populations important to occupational therapy at this time would be a strategic support to practice. For example, studies of successful in-home living by fragile elders would be beneficial to therapists providing home-based care to elders.

Will We Describe Less Positive Occupations?

It is important that we produce more studies of occupations that are disrupted, deviant, violent, aggressive, or self-damaging. So far, occupational science has been drawn toward more useful and enjoyable occupations. This is an unacknowledged bias that probably derives from occupational therapy's special interest in occupations that are therapeutic. Beyond bringing greater balance to the science, research on less positive occupations would be especially useful to those who are working with people experiencing such negative-impact occupations.

Can We Develop Descriptive Research on the Occupations of Sleep and Restoration?

Lastly, occupational science would be well guided to launch significant studies of sleep and restoration (Green, 2008; Pierce, 2003). A few studies of quiet, restorative occupations have been completed, but few have attempted to study sleep (Gibbs & Klinger, 2011; Howell & Pierce, 2000; Nurit & Michal, 2003). An outstanding example of what occupational science research into sleep might yield is provided by an extradisciplinary scholar. Rosenblatt (2006) studied couple bed-sharing across age, illness/wellness, and a variety of relationships. Often dismissed as a state of unconsciousness, sleep is an occupation of unrivaled prevalence, cross-cultural engagement, and dominance in daily individual patterns (Kryger, Roth, & Dement, 2005; Pierce & Summers, 2011). It makes up one third of all human lives! Sleep is also the occupation with the strongest tie to health. It is the occupation without which we would the soonest die, yet we live in a sleep-sick society. Sleep has fascinating neurological, developmental, psychological, and cultural patterns. Sleep has its own medical specialty and a specific set of medical diagnoses, something that is rare for any type of occupational dysfunction. Many of occupational therapy's clients have sleep disturbances, often untreated, that contribute to their life challenges. Sleep has incredible theoretical potential for occupational science and theoretical potential for occupational therapy.

SECTION CHAPTERS ILLUSTRATING LEVEL 1, DESCRIPTIVE OCCUPATIONAL SCIENCE RESEARCH

This section of *Occupational Science for Occupational Therapy* showcases some of the most outstanding Level 1 descriptive research in this young science. In some of this work, such as Betty Hasselkus' research on caregiving (Chapter 3) or Charlotte Royeen's descriptions of morning routines (Chapter 6), the usefulness to occupational therapists of a stronger understanding of these particular occupations is obvious. Sheama Krishnagiri's research on mating and dating in people of different ages and abilities/disabilities pushes into areas of descriptive occupational science that remain largely unexplored: shared, intimate, and coupled occupations (Chapter 4). Wendy Wood's work describing contextual influences on the occupations of nonhuman primates and people with Alzheimer's takes occupational science out of the box of intra-individual experience to help us understand occupation in its spatial, temporal, and sociocultural dimensions (Chapter 5). Of course, this selection of descriptive occupational science research is only a sample of Level 1 occupational science. There is certainly much excellent work focused on the description of occupations that has not been included in this book. Provided here, however, is an especially strong, well-designed, and promising set of examples of descriptive occupational science research, each of which required many years of career commitment from their authors.

REFERENCES

Alsaker, S., Jakobsen, K., Magnus, E., Bendixen, H. J., Kroksmark, U., & Nordell, K. (2006). Everyday occupations of occupational therapy and physiotherapy students in Scandinavia. *Journal of Occupational Science, 13*, 17-26. doi:10.1080/14427591.2006.9686567

Beagan, B., & Saunders, S. (2005). Occupations of masculinity: Producing gender through what men do and don't do. *Journal of Occupational Science, 12*(3), 161-169. doi:10.1080/14427591.2005.9686559

Blanche, E. I. (2007). The expression of creativity through occupation. *Journal of Occupational Science, 14*, 21-29. doi:10.1080/14427591.2007.9686580

Bundy, A. (1990). Free play of preschoolers: Synthesis and annotations of the literature describing developmental theory. In A. Bundy, N. Predergst, J. Steffan, & D. Thorn (Eds.), *Reviews of selected literature on occupation and health* (pp. 5-68). Rockville, MD: American Occupational Therapy Foundation.

Clark, F., Azen, S. P., Carlson, M., Mandel, D., LaBree, L., Hay, J., . . . Lipson, L. (2001). Embedding health-promoting changes into the daily lives of independent-living older adults: Long-term follow-up of occupational therapy intervention. *Journal of Gerontology: Psychological Sciences and Social Sciences, 56B*, 60-63. doi: 10.1093/geronb/56.1.P60

Clark, F. A., Parham, D., Carlson, M. E., Frank, G., Jackson, J., Pierce, D., . . . Zemke, R. (1991). Occupational science: Academic innovation in the service of occupational therapy's future. *American Journal of Occupational Therapy, 45*, 300-310. doi:10.5014/ajot.45.4.300

Clark, P. N. (1979a). Human development through occupation: Theoretical frameworks in contemporary occupational therapy practice, part 1. *American Journal of Occupational Therapy, 33*, 505-514.

Clark, P. N. (1979b). Human development through occupation: A philosophy and conceptual model for practice, part 2. *American Journal of Occupational Therapy, 33*, 577-585.

Csikszentmihalyi, M. (1975). *Beyond boredom and anxiety: Experiencing flow in work and play.* San Francisco, CA: Jossey-Bass.

Csikszentmihalyi, M. (1993). Activity and happiness: Towards a science of occupation. *Journal of Occupational Science, 1*, 38-42. doi:10.1080/14427591.1993.9686377

Csikszentmihalyi, M., & Csikszentmihalyi, I. (1988). *Optimal experience: Psychological studies of flow in consciousness.* New York, NY: Cambridge University Press.

Dickie, V. (1996). Craft production in Detroit: Spatial, temporal, and social relations of work in the home. *Journal of Occupational Science, 3*(2), 65-71. doi:10.1080/14427591.1996.9686409

Dickie, V. (2003). Establishing worker identity: A study of people in craft work. *American Journal of Occupational Therapy, 57*, 250-261. doi:10.5014/ajot.57.3.250

Dickoff, J., James, P., & Weidenbach, E. (1968). Theory in practice discipline: Part I. Practice oriented theory. *Nursing Research, 17*(5), 387-480.

Edgerton, W. (1954). Activities in occupational therapy. In H. Willard & C. Spackman (Eds.), *Principles of occupational therapy* (pp. 43-60). Philadelphia, PA: J. B. Lippincott.

Erlandsson, L., & Eklund, M. (2006). Levels of complexity in patterns of daily occupations: Relationship to women's well-being. *Journal of Occupational Science, 13*, 27-36. doi:10.1080/14427591.2006.9686568

Esdaile, S., & Olsen, J. (2004). *Mothering occupations: Challenge, agency, and participation.* Philadelphia, PA: F. A. Davis.

Evans, J., & Rodger, S. (2008). Mealtimes and bedtimes: Windows to family routines and rituals. *Journal of Occupational Science, 15*(2), 98-104. doi:10.1080/14427591.2008.9686615

Farnworth, L. (1998). Doing, being, and boredom. *Journal of Occupational Science, 5*, 140-146. doi:10.1080/14427591.1998.9686442

Farnworth, L. (2000). Time use and leisure occupations of young offenders. *American Journal of Occupational Therapy, 54*, 315-325. doi:10.5014/ajot.54.3.315

Farnworth, L. (2004). Time use and disability. In M. Molineux (Ed.), *Occupation for occupational therapists* (pp. 46-65). Oxford, United Kingdom: Blackwell Publishing.

Fidler, G. (1981). From crafts to competence. *American Journal of Occupational Therapy, 35*, 567-573. doi:10.5014/ajot.35.9.567

Florey, L. (1971). An approach to play and play development. *American Journal of Occupational Therapy, 25,* 275-280.

Florey, L. (1981). Studies of play: Implications for growth, development, and for clinical practice. *American Journal of Occupational Therapy, 35,* 519-524. doi:10.5014/ajot.35.8.519

Francis-Connolly, E. (2000). Toward an understanding of mothering: A comparison of two motherhood stages. *American Journal of Occupational Therapy, 54,* 281-289. doi:10.5014/ajot.54.3.281

Frank, G. (1996). Crafts production and resistance to domination in the late 20th century. *Journal of Occupational Science, 3*(2), 56-64. doi: 10.1080/14427591.1996.9686408

Gibbs, L., & Klinger, L. (2011). Rest is a meaningful occupation for women with hip and knee osteoarthritis. *OTJR: Occupation, Participation, and Health, 31,* 143-150. doi:10.3928/15394492-20101122-01

Goodall, J. (1986). *The chimpanzees of Gombe: Patterns of behavior.* Cambridge, MA: Belknap Press of Harvard University Press.

Green, A. (2008). Sleep, occupation and the passage of time. *British Journal of Occupational Therapy, 71*(8), 339-347.

Hall, H. J. (1923). In defense of toys. *Archives of Occupational Therapy, 2,* 43-46.

Hannam, D. (1997). More than a cup of tea: Meaning construction in an everyday occupation. *Journal of Occupational Science, 4*(20), 69-74. doi:10.1080/14427591.1997.9686423

Heward, K., Molineux, M., & Gough, B. (2006). A grounded theory analysis of the occupational impact of caring for a partner who has multiple sclerosis. *Journal of Occupational Science, 13*(3), 188-197. doi:10.1080/14427591.2006.9726515

Hocking, C. (1997). Person-object interaction model: Understanding the use of everyday objects. *Journal of Occupational Science, 4,* 27-35. doi:10.1080/14427591.1997.9686418

Hocking, C. (2000). Having and using objects in the Western world. *Journal of Occupational Science, 7*(3), 148-157. doi:10.1080/144275 91.2000.9686478

Hocking, C. (2012). Occupations through the looking glass: Reflecting on occupational scientists' ontological assumptions. In G. Whiteford & C. Hocking (Eds.), *Occupational science: Society, inclusion, participation* (pp. 54-66). Oxford, United Kingdom: Wiley-Blackwell.

Howell, D., & Pierce, D. (2000). Exploring the forgotten restorative dimension of occupation: Quilting and quilt use. *Journal of Occupational Science, 7*(2), 68-72. doi:10.1080/14427591.2000.9686467

Humphry, R., & Wakeford, L. (2006). An occupation-centered discussion of development and implications for practice. *American Journal of Occupational Therapy, 60,* 258-267. doi:10.5014/ajot.60.3.258

Hunter, E. G. (2008). Legacy: The occupational transmission of self through actions and artifacts. *Journal of Occupational Science, 15,* 48-54. doi:10.1080/14427591.2008.9686607

Huot, S., & Rudman, D. L. (2010). The performances and places of identity: Conceptualizing intersections of occupation, identity, and place in the process of migration. *Journal of Occupational Science, 17*(2), 68-77. doi:10.1080/14427591.2010.9686677

Jonsson, H., & Persson, D. (2006). Towards an experiential model of occupational balance: An alternative perspective on flow theory analysis. *Journal of Occupational Science, 13,* 62-73. doi:10.1080/14 427591.2006.9686571

Kantartzis, S., & Molineux, M. (2012). Understanding the discursive development of occupation: Historico-political perspectives. In G. Whiteford & C. Hocking (Eds.), *Occupational science: Society, inclusion, participation* (pp. 38-53). Oxford, United Kingdom: Wiley Blackwell.

Kielhofner, G., & Burke, J. P. (1980). A model of human occupation, part 1. Conceptual framework and content. *American Journal of Occupational Therapy, 34,* 572-581. doi:10.5014/ajot.34.9.572

Knox, M. (1931). Mexican trades and crafts. *Occupational Therapy and Rehabilitation, 10,* 319-327.

Knox, M. (1932a). Mexican trades and crafts. *Occupational Therapy and Rehabilitation, 11,* 213-225.

Knox, M. (1932b). Mexican trades and crafts II. *Occupational Therapy and Rehabilitation, 11,* 45-64.

Knox, M. (1932c). Mexican trades and crafts III: Carving: Weaving. *Occupational Therapy and Rehabilitation, 11,* 135-146.

Knox, S. (1997). Knox Preschool Play Scale. In D. Parham & L. Fazio (Eds.), *Play in occupational therapy for children* (pp. 35-51). St. Louis, MO: Mosby Year Book.

Knox, S. (2008). Development and current use of the revised Knox Preschool Play Scale. In D. Parham & L. Fazio (Eds.), *Play in occupational therapy for children* (2nd ed., pp. 55-70). London, England: Elsevier.

Kroksmark, U., Nordell, K., Bendixen, H. J., Magnus, E., Jakobsen, K., & Alsaker, S. (2006). Time geographic method: Application to studying patterns of occupation in different contexts. *Journal of Occupational Science, 13,* 11-16. doi:10.1080/14427591.2006.9686566

Kryger, M., Roth, T., & Dement, W. (Eds.). (2005). *Principles and practice of sleep medicine* (4th ed.). Philadelphia, PA: Elsevier Saunders.

Larson, E. A. (2000a). Mothering: Letting go of the past ideal and valuing the real. *American Journal of Occupational Therapy, 54*(3), 249-251. doi:10.5014/ajot.54.3.249

Larson, E. A. (2000b). The orchestration of occupation: The dance of mothers. *American Journal of Occupational Therapy, 54,* 269-280. doi:10.5014/ajot.54.3.269

Larson, E. A. (2003). Shaping the temporal patterns of our lives: The social coordination of occupation. *Journal of Occupational Science, 10,* 80-89. doi:10.1080/14427591.2003.9686514

Larson, E. A. (2004). The time of our lives: The experience of temporality in occupation. *Canadian Journal of Occupational Therapy, 71,* 24-35.

Larson, E., & von Eye, A. (2010). Beyond flow: Temporality and participation in everyday activities. *American Journal of Occupational Therapy, 64,* 152-163. doi:10.5014/ajot.64.1.152

Ludwig, F. M. (1998). The unpackaging of routine in older women. *American Journal of Occupational Therapy, 52*(3), 168-175. doi:10.5014/ajot.52.3.168

Ludwig, F. M., Hattjar, B., Russell, R. L., & Winston, K. (2007). How caregiving for grandchildren affects grandmothers' meaningful occupations. *Journal of Occupational Science, 14,* 40-51. doi:10.1080 /14427591.2007.9686582

Lynch, H. (2009). Patterns of activity of Irish children aged five to eight years: City living in Ireland today. *Journal of Occupational Science, 16,* 44-49. doi:10.1080/14427591.2009.9686641

Mahoney, W., & Roberts, E. (2009). Co-occupation in a day program for adults with developmental disabilities. *Journal of Occupational Science, 16,* 170-179. doi:10.1080/14427591.2009.9686659

Marken, D., Pierce, D., & Baltisberger, J. (2010). Grandmothers' use of routines to manage custodial care of young children. *Occupational and Physical Therapy in Geriatrics, 28,* 360-375. doi:10.3109/027031 81.2010.535119

Meyer, A. (1922). The philosophy of occupation therapy. *Archives of Occupational Therapy, 1,* 1-10.

Moore, A. (1996). Feasting as occupation: The emergence of ritual from everyday activities. *Journal of Occupational Science, 3,* 5-15. doi:10.1 080/14427591.1996.9686403

Nurit, W., & Michal, A. (2003). Rest: A qualitative exploration of the phenomenon. *Occupational Therapy International, 10,* 227-238. doi:10.1002/oti.187

Pentland, W., Harvey, A. S., & Walker, J. (1998). The relationships between time use and health and well-being in men with spinal cord injury. *Journal of Occupational Science, 5,* 14-25. doi:10.1080/14427591.1998.9686431

Peralta-Catipon, T. (2009). Statue square in a liminal sphere: Transforming space and place in migrant adaptation. *Journal of Occupational Science, 16,* 32-37. doi:10.1080/14427591.2009.9686639

Persch, A., Pizur-Barnekow, K., Cashen, S., & Pickens, N. (2009). Heart rate variability of activity and occupation during solitary and social engagement. *Journal of Occupational Science, 16,* 163-169. doi:10.1080/14427591.2009.9686658

Persson, D., Eklund, M., & Isaacson, A. (1999). The experience of everyday occupations and its relation to sense of coherence: A methodological study. *Journal of Occupational Science, 6,* 13-26. doi:10.1080/14427591.1999.9686447

Pickens, N., & Pizur-Barnekow, K. (2009). Co-occupation: Extending the dialogue. *Journal of Occupational Science, 16,* 151-156. doi:10.1080/14427591.2009.9686656

Pierce, D. (1991). Early object rule acquisition. *American Journal of Occupational Therapy, 45,* 438-450. doi:10.5014/ajot.45.5.438

Pierce, D. (1996). *Infant space, infant time: Development of infant interactions with the physical environment, from 1 to 18 months.* Dissertation Abstracts International.

Pierce, D. (2000). Maternal management of the home as an infant/toddler developmental space. *American Journal of Occupational Therapy, 54,* 290-299. doi:10.5014/ajot.63.3.273

Pierce, D. (2001). Occupation by design: Dimensions, creativity, and therapeutic power. *American Journal of Occupational Therapy, 55,* 249-259. doi:10.5014/ajot.55.3.249

Pierce, D. (2003). *Occupation by design: Building therapeutic power.* Philadelphia, PA: F. A. Davis.

Pierce, D. (2009). Co-occupation: The challenges of defining concepts original to occupational science. *Journal of Occupational Science, 16,* 273-287. doi:10.1080/14427591.2009.9686663

Pierce, D., Atler, K., Baltisberger, J., Fehringer, E., Hunter, E., Malkawi, S., & Parr, T. (2010). Occupational science: A data-based American perspective. *Journal of Occupational Science, 17*(4), 204-215. doi:10.1080/14427591.2010.9686697

Pierce, D., & Frank, G. (1992). A mother's work: Two levels of feminist analysis. *American Journal of Occupational Therapy, 46,* 972-980. doi:10.5014/ajot.63.3.273

Pierce, D., Myers, C., & Munier, V. (2009). Informing early intervention through an occupational science description of infant-toddler interactions with home space. *American Journal of Occupational Therapy, 63,* 273-287. doi:10.5014/ajot.63.3.273

Pierce, D., & Summers, K. (2011). Rest and sleep. In T. Brown & V. Stoeffel (Eds.), *Occupational therapy in mental health: A vision for participation* (pp. 736-754). Philadelphia, PA: F. A. Davis.

Pizur-Barnekow, K., & Knutson, J. (2009). A comparison of personality dimensions and behavior changes that occur during solitary and co-occupation. *Journal of Occupational Science, 16,* 157-162. doi:10.1080/14427591.2009.9686657

Price, P., & Stephenson, S. (2009). Learning to promote occupational development through co-occupation. *Journal of Occupational Science, 16,* 180-186. doi:10.1080/14427591.2009.9686660

Primeau, L. (1996). Work and leisure: Transcending the dichotomy. *American Journal of Occupational Therapy, 50,* 569-577. doi:10.5014/ajot.50.7.569

Primeau, L. (1998). Orchestration and play within families. *American Journal of Occupational Therapy, 52*(3), 188-193. doi:10.5014/ajot.52.3.188

Primeau, L. (2000). Household work: When gender ideologies and practices interact. *Journal of Occupational Science, 7,* 118-127. doi:10.1080/14427591.2000.9686474

Reilly, M. (1962). Occupational therapy can be one of the great ideas of 20th-century medicine. *American Journal of Occupational Therapy, 16,* 1-9.

Reilly, M. (1974). *Play as exploratory learning.* Beverly Hills, CA: Sage Publications.

Riley, J. (2008). Weaving an enhanced sense of self and collective sense of self through creative textile-making. *Journal of Occupational Science, 15*(2), 63-73. doi:10.1080/14427591.2008.9686611

Robinson, A. (1977). Play: The arena for acquisition of rules of competent behavior. *American Journal of Occupational Therapy, 31,* 248-253.

Rogers, J. C. (1984). Why study human occupation? *American Journal of Occupational Therapy, 38*(1), 47-49. doi: 10.5014/ajot.38.1.47

Rosenblatt, P. (2006). *Two in a bed: The social system of couple bed sharing.* Albany, NY: State University of New York Press.

Rowles, G. (1991). Beyond performance: Being in place as a component of occupational therapy. *American Journal of Occupational Therapy, 45,* 265-271. doi:10.5014/ajot.45.3.265

Rowles, G. (2008). Place in occupational science: A life course perspective on the role of environmental context in the quest for meaning. *Journal of Occupational Science, 15*(3), 127-135. doi:10.1080/14427591.2008.9686622

Royeen, C. B. (2010). Towards an emerging understanding of morning routines: A preliminary study using developing methods in arts based inquiry. *Irish Journal of Occupational Therapy, 38*(1), 30-42.

Rudman, D. (2012). Governing through occupation: Shaping expectations and possibilities. In G. Whiteford & C. Hocking (Eds.), *Occupational science: Society, inclusion, participation* (pp. 100-116). Oxford, United Kingdom: Wiley-Blackwell.

Scoggin, A. E. (1999). Caregiving as an occupation: Developmental intervention for a group of hospitalized Peruvian children. *Journal of Occupational Science, 6,* 34-41. doi:10.1080/14427591.1999.9686449

Segal, R. (2004). Family routines and rituals: A context for occupational therapy interventions. *American Journal of Occupational Therapy, 58,* 499-508. doi:10.5014/ajot.58.5.499

Segal, R., & Hinojosa, J. (2006). The activity setting of homework: An analysis of three cases and implications for occupational therapy. *American Journal of Occupational Therapy, 60,* 50-59. doi:10.5014/ajot.60.1.50

Singleton, J. F., & Harvey, A. (1995). Stage of lifecycle and time spent in activities. *Journal of Occupational Science, 2,* 3-12. doi:10.1080/14427591.1995.9686391

Spackman, C. (1971). Occupational therapy—its relation to allied medical services. In H. Willard & C. Spackman (Eds.), *Willard and Spackman's occupational therapy* (4th ed., pp. 1-12). Philadelphia, PA: J. B. Lippincott.

Stanley, M. (1995). An investigation into the relationship between engagements in valued occupations and life satisfaction for elderly south Australians. *Journal of Occupational Science, 2*(3), 100-114. doi:10.1080/14427591.1995.9686400

Wada, M., & Beagan, B. (2006). Values concerning employment-related and family-related occupations: Perspectives of young Canadian male medical students. *Journal of Occupational Science, 13*(2), 117-125. doi:10.1080/14427591.2006.9726504

Wagner, E. (1954). Occupational therapy for amputees. In H. Willard & C. Spackman (Eds.), *Principles of occupational therapy* (pp. 285-300). Philadelphia, PA: J. B. Lippincott.

Walker, C. (2001). Occupational adaptation in action: Shift workers and their strategies. *Journal of Occupational Science, 8,* 17-24. doi:10.1080/14427591.2001.9686481

Wright, J. (2004). Occupation and flow. In M. Molineux (Ed.), *Occupation for occupational therapists* (pp. 66-77). Oxford, United Kingdom: Blackwell Publishing.

Yerxa, E. (1987). Nationally speaking: Research: the key to the development of occupational therapy as an academic discipline. *American Journal of Occupational Therapy, 41,* 415-419. doi:10.5014/ajot.41.7.415

Yerxa, E. (1995). Nationally speaking: Who is the keeper of occupational therapy's practice and knowledge? *American Journal of Occupational Therapy, 49,* 295-299. doi:10.5014/ajot.49.4.295

Yerxa, E. (2005). Learning to love the questions. *American Journal of Occupational Therapy, 59,* 108-112. doi:10.5014/ajot.59.1.108

Yerxa, E., & Locker, S. (1990). Quality of time use by adults with spinal cord injuries. *American Journal of Occupational Therapy, 44*(4), 318-326. doi:10.5014/ajot.44.4.318

Zemke, R. (2004). Time, space, and the kaleidoscope of occupation. *American Journal of Occupational Therapy, 58*(6), 608-620. doi:10.5014/ajot.58.6.608

Zimmerman, M. (1971). Occupational therapy in the A.D.L program. In H. Willard & C. Spackman (Eds.), *Willard and Spackman's occupational therapy* (4th ed., pp. 217-256). Philadelphia, PA: J. B. Lippincott.

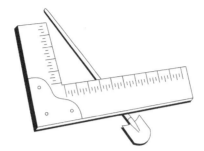

3

The Occupation of Caregiving

Betty Risteen Hasselkus, PhD, OTR, FAOTA

For 7 years of my career in occupational therapy, I was the occupational therapist in a hospital-based home-care program for older people. We were part of the Veterans Administration system of health care, and, as such, we were able to follow our clients for literally years—getting to know the clients and their family caregivers intimately over time.

After 7 years, I left the program to go back to graduate school for a doctoral degree. But the influence of the home-care experience remained strong on my emerging scholarship and research. My graduate work ultimately culminated in a doctoral dissertation study with the title, "Family Caregivers for the Elderly at Home: An Ethnography of Meaning and Informal Learning."

My dissertation research on family caregivers for the elderly in the community proved to be a jumping-off place for an extended research program that has focused on the caregiving experiences of family members and professionals. The four studies described and discussed in this chapter focus on aspects of the caregiving experience—by family members, occupational therapists, physicians, and day-care staff members. New understandings that arose from the these studies include concepts of family caregivers as practitioners, the meaning of occupation in dementia

caregiving, negotiations between professional and family caregivers, and key dimensions of meaning in the doing of occupational therapy.

At the same time, while pursuing and deepening my research focus on professional and family caregiving, I gradually honed my skills in, and became committed to, the paradigm of interpretive research (see Frank & Polkinghorne, 2010). Of the studies reported here, two are ethnographic and two are phenomenological. Interpretive research (also referred to as *qualitative research*) is based on a view of the world as subjective and context dependent; the goals are to gain understandings of perspectives and phenomena, bringing us closer to our world. The researcher is part of the research process—not as an outside observer but as an integral and contributing part of the study—its goals, methods, results, and interpretations. The "data" are textual, not numerical.

In ethnography, the researcher seeks to gain understanding of people's perspectives in situations or life contexts within a cultural framework. So, for example, in my dissertation research, I used ethnographic interview techniques to gain understanding of the cultural meanings that the participant-caregivers used to organize their behaviors

Pierce, D. (Ed.).
Occupational Science for Occupational Therapy (pp. 23-36).
© 2014 SLACK Incorporated.

and interpret their experiences. Alternatively, phenomenological research aims to understand the nature of the lived experiences of a social phenomenon (Van Manen, 1990). In the second study reported here, Virginia Dickie and I (1994) asked occupational therapists to describe satisfying and dissatisfying experiences of practice. The data in phenomenology are detailed descriptions of the experiences as they were lived, getting us as close as possible to understanding the essence of that experience. The purpose of the new understandings and insights gained from ethnographic and phenomenological research is, in the broadest terms, to bring us closer to our lifeworld (Van Manen, 1990) and to help us "understand the complexities of being human" (Frank & Polkinghorne, 2010, p. 52). Specifically, the research program on caregiving described here is intended to enhance our understandings of the nature and experience of human caregiving as represented by both formal and informal systems of care.

A RESEARCH PROGRAM ON CAREGIVING

Study 1: Family Caregivers for the Elderly at Home: An Ethnography of Meaning and Informal Learning

In 1979, Shanas startled the Western world of geriatric health care with the statistic that 80% of all caregiving for the elderly in the United States was provided by family members in the community. The previously held misconception that most older people were being cared for in skilled nursing facilities was exposed as a falsehood. Gerontologists began to pay attention to the family caregiver in elder care, initially focusing on concepts such as kinship patterns and caregiving routines and tasks (Clark & Rakowski, 1983; Kivitt, 1985), and then broadening to address the subjective experiences of caregiving (i.e., concepts such as burden, future outlook, and protective caregiving) (Bowers, 1987; Rakowski & Clark, 1985; Zarit, Todd, & Zarit, 1986).

At the same time, emerging research findings in geriatrics revealed tensions between family caregivers and professional health workers in a variety of settings (Kaye, 1985; Litwak, 1985; Simmons, Ivry, & Seltzer, 1985). Litwak described coordination between formal and informal care systems for older people as a balancing act, implying a back-and-forth process of negotiation of responsibilities and decision making throughout care. Hofer (1985) called for better integration of the formal and informal care systems and for increased recognition by professionals of the family's authority. Bowers (1987) study of family perspectives on nursing home care revealed family beliefs that good care was dependent on family participation and that professional staff did not have the skills or background necessary to provide quality care.

The purpose of this study was to gain understanding of the cultural meanings and informal learning embedded in the context of family caregiving for the elderly in the community (Hasselkus, 1988, 1989; Hasselkus & Ray, 1988). The significance of the study was based on the assumption that a greater understanding of the cultural meaning systems and informal learning processes of family caregivers in the community would enhance formal health providers' abilities to work together with caregivers, thus better supporting the family as a caring unit.

Method

A series of four 1-hour ethnographic interviews (Spradley, 1979) was conducted with each of the 15 family caregivers in their homes. All caregivers were adults (14 female, one male) related by blood or marriage to their care-receivers and not receiving monetary reimbursement for their caregiving services. Of the 15 caregivers, nine were spouses, four were daughters, one was a daughter-in-law, and one was a sister. All care-receivers (age range 63 to 99 years) required personal and/or instrumental care on a daily basis.

Conducting a series of interviews with each caregiver provided a type of prolonged engagement, persistent observation, and opportunities to check with participants for validation across the interviews (Guba, 1981). All interviews were tape recorded and transcribed verbatim. The first two or three of the four interviews in each series were used to gather descriptions of the domains of the caregiving, using descriptive questions ("Can you begin by telling me what your day is like?") and structural questions ("Tell me more about what you do in the morning to 'get him up'"). A card-sorting task (with each domain on a separate card) was used in the final interviews to clarify, validate, and augment the meaning of emerging domains. For example, during one caregiver's last interview, I handed her a small stack of cards, each one with a domain printed on it that had been revealed in the previous interviews, and asked her to sort the cards by how difficult or easy each was. As she was sorting through the cards, making small piles, she suddenly pounced on one card, exclaiming, "This is the most difficult of all!" The card said, "Thinking of things for him to do." The caregiver's spontaneous exclamation during the card-sorting provided strong validation of the domain and much deeper understanding for me, the researcher, about its meaning to the caregiver.

On the basis of my sense that it had a good fit with the data, Donald Schön's (1983) model of reflection in action was used to organize the data for analysis. The family caregiver was conceptualized as a reflective practitioner, and the transcribed interview data were coded into domains of problem situations (e.g., eating, finances, dressing, going out, getting things done, night problems). A computer database management program, Notebook II (1985), was used to organize the coded problem situations into text fields using Schön's model—Naming, Framing, Action, and Judgment. With the interview texts thus organized, it was possible to further analyze the data for themes of meaning in the caregiving.

Results

Five themes of meaning in the cultural context of family caregiving for the elderly were derived from the interview narratives. The themes of meaning blended together to form a framework of reflective practice for the family caregiver (Schön, 1983). A sense of tension often existed between the caregivers and the health professionals, stemming from disparities between each other's reflective practices.

Themes of Meaning

The Sense of Self reflected data about the caregiver's personal needs, beliefs about her or his own capabilities, and, for some, a conscious sense of having special knowledge: "I just figure we'll work it out between us... nobody knows her better than I do." The Sense of Managing (including not managing) was pervasive in the interviews, with the routines and tasks of the caregiving often judged by standards of orderliness and cleanliness: "I wash everything up good, and I'm sure I kill germs, and then I'm satisfied." The Sense of Future often focused on a possible worsening of the care-receiver's condition, but, for some, a sense of doom was focused strongly on the caregiver's own lasting power: "I worry about what's going to happen... and I pray every night that the Lord will let me take care of her." The Sense of Fear and Risk was strongly represented in the caregiver's fear of change or anything that might cause a change: "Now he's got a sore on the other foot, so now I'm worried about that one." The Sense of Change in Role and Responsibility was reflected in caregivers' statements about changes in long-time relationships between family members: "It's like I'm not married, I'm not divorced, I'm not widowed, I'm kind of in limbo."

Caregiver-Health Professional Tension

These caregivers' contextualized views of their caregiving experiences, as synthesized into the five themes of meaning, were often the basis for tension between the caregivers and the health professionals in the narratives. Caregivers recounted stories of telling a health practitioner "what works," showing the professional "how," and critiquing and modifying the instructions and recommendations of a professional ("They told me to let him do some of those things himself [washing up, dressing], but he's so slow and he gets up so late it'd be forever. He'd never get his breakfast"). They came up with their own reasons and even diagnoses for the situation and symptoms ("My grandfather died of Alzheimer's, and I don't think that's what this is"). More rarely, a caregiver would concede to the authority of the professional worker ("We do what the professionals tell us to"). Some described a certain amount of mutuality between caregiver and professional ("The nurse and I are watchin' her feet.... She got an open area on there that we been bathin' with Betadine").

Discussion

Within the framework of reflective practice proposed by Schön (1983), the caregiver names that to which she or he will attend (the problem situation), frames the context (meaning) in which it will be attended to, takes action based on that framing, and makes a judgment about that action. The care-receivers, other family members, and health professionals, too, have their own frameworks of reflective practice.

Litwak (1985) presented a theory of agency-family cooperation as a balancing act of shared tasks. Schön's (1983) concept of reflective practice moves beyond the focus on the visible tasks of caregiving to the more invisible meanings of the situation (i.e., the way the situations are framed and actions are judged). In reflective practice, the emphasis is on problem setting, "the process by which we define the decisions to be made, the ends to be achieved, the means which may be chosen" (Schön, 1983, pp. 39-40). The narrative data of this study revealed the presence of family caregiver meanings that were often discordant with the professional health providers' understandings of the situation. The results support Bowers' (1987) findings of the need for professional practitioners and family caregivers to share perspectives and understandings of the invisible work of caregiving. The use of descriptive questions at the start of assessments and interviews (e.g., "Would you start by telling me what your day is like?") would convey to a family member the importance of her or his perspective (Hasselkus, 1990).

Schön suggests that, within the tradition of health professions, the professional makes a claim to ownership of special knowledge "rooted in techniques and theories derived from scientific research" (1983, p. 288). Waitzkin and Stoeckle (1976) propose that too often this ownership of special knowledge is purposefully guarded as a means of maintaining control over the professional-client relationship. The results of this study suggest that family caregivers, too, have a personal sense of ownership of the knowledge of caregiving. A meaningful and workable reflective contract between lay and professional practitioners is proposed as an approach that facilitates a partnership between family and professional in the caregiving process. For occupational therapists, the themes of meaning derived from these interview data are strongly relevant to practice in the community; the therapist and family caregiver would want to work reflectively to achieve a harmonious approach to support the caregiver's sense of self and sense of managing, as well as to ease the sense of fear, risk, future decline, and changes in roles and responsibilities. The findings point to the need for better understanding of the meanings of both informal and formal caregiving and of the relationship between family practitioners and health professionals in the health care process.

Study 2: Doing Occupational Therapy: Dimensions of Satisfaction and Dissatisfaction

The purpose of this study was to gain understanding of the nature of satisfying and dissatisfying practice in occupational therapy. While Study 1 focused on understanding the meanings of informal family caregiving for older people, Study 2 followed with an aim to better understand the formal caregiving experience as represented by occupational therapists. The prominent theme of tension between family caregivers and professionals found in Study 1 led to the interest in understanding the formal/informal dynamics more fully.

Virginia Dickie and I planned and carried out this study together with funding from the American Occupational Therapy Foundation (Hasselkus & Dickie, 1994). Using a phenomenological research approach, we asked 148 occupational therapists to describe especially satisfying and dissatisfying experiences of practice (Flanagan, 1954). In effect, we were asking therapists to construct a narrative or story that represented the lived experience of a practice situation (Bruner, 1986). Diekelmann (1991) described narratives in nursing as emancipatory and empowering and useful for revealing what she called the invisible part of our practices. In the same year, Mattingly (1991) asserted that narrative thinking (storying, emplotment) is fundamental to the clinical reasoning of occupational therapists. Understandings about the nature of doing occupational therapy can bring therapists closer to their world of therapy, can assist therapists to minimize dissatisfying and maximize satisfying therapeutic experiences, and can help in career decisions and career counseling for individuals considering occupational therapy as a professional career.

Method

In the phenomenological research view, knowledge is not essentially theoretical but instead resides in practice and in our encounters with the world through involved activity (Allen, Benner, & Diekelmann, 1986). For this study, we purchased (from the American Occupational Therapy Association) a random sample of 200 registered occupational therapists living in the United States. Of the 148 respondents (74% response rate), 139 were women and nine were men, and ages ranged from 24 to 70 years, with a median age of 36. The proportion of advanced degrees (40 master's degrees and two doctoral degrees) in the sample was significantly greater than that of the 1990 American Occupational Therapy Association survey data

($df = 2$, critical value $= 6.00$, $X^2 = 13.70$, $p = .05$); no statistically significant difference was present for age or gender.

After a small response rate of 32 from our initial mailed survey (24 completed, eight blank), and in consultation with the survey research lab on the University of Wisconsin-Madison campus, we decided to seek responses from the remainder of the sample by telephone (123 completed), and one more mailed response was received. All written and recorded telephone responses were transcribed and entered into a computer database for storage and analysis.

For the analysis of the data, we used a process that included initial parallel reading of a subset of 24 responses, feedback from two expert consultants on our tentative ideas for units of meaning, and ultimate consensus on an emerging code list of categories. Subsequently, in our organization of all 148 responses for coding, satisfying and dissatisfying narratives were unlinked, and each was treated as a separate entity. Using the text-oriented data management software program Tally (Bowyer, 1991), we coded the data from all respondents, each of us doing half (74) of the responses.

We met again for what Van Manen (1990) called *phenomenological reflection*. We compared, clustered, and synthesized our coded data and emerging themes into unifying concepts, and ultimately derived three overarching dimensions of meaning from the data: change, community, and craft. Dimensionality includes the "parts, attributes, interconnections, context, processes, and implications" of a phenomenon (Schatzman, 1991, p. 309). The process of analysis moved from an initial identification of many coded categories and individual distinctions to grouping categories into these three broad dimensions followed by an iterative in-depth return to the richness within each dimension. Finally, we each incorporated the cases the other had coded into our analysis for comparison and final interpretations.

Results

Storytelling is the ordering of a succession of events into a narrative whole with a beginning, a middle, and an end (Kermode, 1967; Ricoeur, 1984). The therapists' narratives often began with a description of the medical and social contexts of a clinical situation as first encountered, then moved through actions that were taken, and concluded with a discussion of the results. According to Kermode (1967), it is the end of a story that gives the story significance and its sense of harmony or disharmony—concepts analogous to satisfaction and dissatisfaction.

Stories of Change

The dimension of change is strongly linked to the ends of the therapists' stories, and it figures prominently as a sense of satisfying or dissatisfying closure in the narratives. Being able to help a patient regain previous capabilities in daily activities—especially when significant barriers had to be overcome ("the patient was *totally* nonfunctional"; "we really worked hard")—was a source of great satisfaction. A lost battle meant a story that ended without the expected change, without the return to prior functional life. Sometimes, a patient's improvement reached a plateau much earlier than the therapist expected, and the therapist expressed dismay that the change was less than she or he had hoped for. A perceived inability to make any difference was a compelling theme of dissatisfaction in narratives of change. Regarding one patient who had a degenerative neurological disease, the therapist said she "worked and worked and worked with her and got her to where she could do these things [feed herself, dress herself, etc.] and then the family thought they were being a benefit to her by helping her out and that just made her slide backwards... that was real sad."

Dissatisfaction from bringing about a negative change, or the therapist's perception of actually causing harm to a patient, was less commonly described, but when it occurred, the narrative was filled with anguish. As one respondent said about her work in a cardiac rehab program, "After 5 minutes of working with one patient, he coded and did not survive. I always wondered if the activity I had him do could have contributed to his death. I had reported heart arrhythmias to nursing during treatment, and they advised me that this was not unusual for this patient and to continue treatment. Since this experience, I have always preferred not to work in cardiac rehab or in an ICU." Sometimes, the sense of dissatisfaction with the ending led to more dramatic personal consequences, such as quitting a job, taking a 3-month break from work, or actually leaving the profession.

Stories of Community

The dimension of community encompassed the interpersonal or relational aspects of occupational therapy practice. In contrast to the strong emphasis on the story endings within change, in community, the focus was more on the story as a whole and the harmony or disharmony among all of the people who took part in the narrative.

In stories of satisfying community, the therapist described with enthusiasm how well people worked together. The actors in the narrative held shared beliefs and expectations, mutual views of the present, and hopes for the future—they were part of the same story, built together. A sense of collaboration and active engagement of the client and family in the therapy process also seemed to be sources of satisfaction in community: "We did a lot of neat adaptive equipment, and he actually helped to design some of his own equipment. We would work on things together that way." For the therapists, a sense of being appreciated, of feeling special, and of deeply caring and being cared about were themes of meaning. As one therapist said about the family of a patient, "They felt like and treated me as if I was some kind of miracle worker."

Community stories of dissatisfaction included themes of the therapist being thwarted by other characters in the story (e.g., being blocked or overruled by a person of authority), as well as not feeling valued by other health professionals, the patient or family, or the health care system: "What I'm finding is that as you work in OT, if you move beyond being a hands-on clinician and start into the management area, that level knows so little about what OT is, nor do they really care, and you end up hitting your head against the wall more and more." Therapists struggled with feelings of personal rejection when confronted with persistent discordance and disharmony in the therapy situation. One such narrative ended with the therapist's statement, "I felt like a failure as an OT."

Stories of Craft

The dimension of craft encompassed the skill and love for the task around which some respondents built their narratives. The focus of these stories was on the process of doing occupational therapy—carrying out tasks that the therapist found enjoyable, using skills and knowledge that were personally important, or, in the stories of dissatisfaction, sensing a lack of knowledge, skill deficits, or having committed treatment errors.

At the most elemental craft level, therapists spoke of enjoyment of a particular modality of their work: "I love making splints, especially dynamic splints, so anytime I have the opportunity to make a dynamic splint, I really enjoy that." The pleasures of learning new skills and of gaining recognition from other people were also part of this basic craft dimension. Alternatively, dissatisfaction accompanied feelings of being inadequately prepared, such as "not having the neurodevelopmental background" or "not being good enough to make it better." One therapist still remembered causing skin damage to a patient with a spinal cord injury while she was a student: "That was a humiliating experience. It was a small blister but it was always brought out in the team meeting—that it was still there."

At a deeper level, the dimension of craft was much broader and more complex. Therapists related stories of skillfully orchestrating a complex series of interventions, all leading to a successful outcome. In these complicated stories, the therapists demonstrated expertise in multiple contexts, while using a variety of abilities. The focus was on the process, or middle, rather than the beginning or ending of the experience. A sense of completeness characterized these narratives. For example, one such story focused on a man whose hand had been crushed in a work accident. The therapist described wound management, control of edema, use of a pressure glove and pneumatic device, débridement, and splinting during the early stages of treatment. This treatment was followed by work on hand function and a successful work-hardening program: "That was probably my most successful case because I was able to follow it from such an early onset and watch him return to work...and he returned full capacity, full-time to his previous employment."

Discussion

The dimensions of change, community, and craft are expressions of our way of being occupational therapists. Geertz (1973) proposed that one arrives at some understanding of the meaning of a situation by peeling back layer after layer of thick description. The cases we studied were often rich in description as therapists told detailed stories of satisfying and dissatisfying practice experiences. The dimension of change was perhaps the most predictable theme in the data; we had identified a similar theme—making a difference—in a pilot study (Hasselkus & Dickie, 1990). For community, we imagined that each person (therapist, client, family member) brings to therapy her or his own story, and, as therapy evolves, people's stories become superimposed on each other in such a way that a new story—a moiré—is created (Geertz, 1988). The success or failure of the therapist to create a mutually agreeable story with the other parties seems to be the essence of community. And late in our analysis, we realized that the dimension of craft encompasses not only the task-specific satisfactions of individual treatment programs but also the totality of the dynamic therapeutic processes of competently managed occupational therapy.

In terms of my own research program, this study of the meaning of doing occupational therapy complemented findings from the previous study of the meaning of family caregiving for the elderly. The craft dimension of doing occupational therapy has congruence with the theme of managing found in the family caregivers' experiences ("I wash everything up good, and I'm sure I kill germs, and then I'm satisfied") and with the sense of self as expressed in statements such as "Nobody knows her better than I do." For occupational therapists, the dimension of change was strongly linked to a hoped-for and worked-for positive outcome. Alternatively, the family caregivers seemed to worry about a future worsening of the care-receiver's condition, associating change with fearfulness and risk. The pervasive theme of discord between the family caregivers' and the health professionals' views of the caregiving situations was reflected in the dimension of community for the occupational therapists, especially in the disharmony of relationships represented in narratives of dissatisfaction.

The correspondence found between these two sets of data—that of the family caregivers and that of the occupational therapists—offers a beginning understanding of common threads that may exist across different contexts in the caregiving experience. The initial insights gained from these two studies point to the need for a continuing effort to seek more and enriched understandings of family and professional caregiving. The goal of ongoing research is to enable family and professional caregivers to work together in informed and sensitive ways, as both seek to provide high-quality care for others.

Study 3: Negotiations of Care: Older Patient, Family Caregiver, and Physician in the Medical Visit

The purpose of this study was to gain understandings of the meanings and patterns of interaction among older patients, their accompanying family members, and physicians in outpatient clinic visits (Hasselkus, 1992a, 1992b, 1994). Family caregiving tasks often include accompanying an older person to medical appointments. Adelman, Greene, and Charon (1987) estimated that 20% to 37% of internal medicine visits by elderly patients include a third person. The meaning of a third person's presence in the geriatric medical encounter has rarely been studied. The theme of discord between family caregivers and health professionals found in Study 1 and the dissatisfactions stemming from disharmony in relationships for occupational therapists in Study 2 led to Study 3's goal of exploring further the health care context of formal and informal systems working together.

Seeking a physician's help in a medical clinic visit is a form of self-care carried out by adult individuals (Levin, 1977; Orem, 1980). The scenario of an older person being accompanied into the medical examining room by a family member, for whatever reason, is likely to convey a strong signal of dependence. Further, the ambiguity of the three-way division of responsibilities in such a scenario may, in and of itself, contribute to the dependent status of the patient in the medical encounter. Coe and Prendergast (1985) viewed the three-person medical visit as an unstable triad of shifting coalitions, such as doctor and caregiver versus patient or caregiver and patient versus doctor. Adelman et al. (1987) described the third person-family caregiver in terms of roles—advocate, antagonist, and passive participant. These authors suggested the need to further examine the behaviors of third persons and to develop an overall conceptual framework for understanding their functions.

Method

The study took place in the general internal medicine and geriatric outpatient clinics of a university-affiliated hospital in the Midwest. Forty clinic visits—each with physician, family member, and older patient—were audiotaped and transcribed. Participants included 27 patients (60 years of age or older), 31 family caregivers, and 11 physicians.

With the assistance of the clinic physicians and nurses, I identified older patients with upcoming appointments who were highly likely to be accompanied to the clinic by a family member. I then contacted potential study participants by telephone to explain the study and seek tentative agreement to participate. Follow-up occurred at the appointment when signed consent was obtained from both the family member and the patient. Signed consent from participating physicians was obtained prior to the patient-caregiver contacts.

To collect the data, my research assistant or I placed an audiotape recorder in the examining room and turned it on at the start of an appointment. We were not present during the interview and simply returned to retrieve the recorder when the appointment was concluded. All audiotapes were then transcribed in preparation for analysis.

The typology of 26 problem situations generated in Study 1 (Hasselkus, 1988) was used to organize the transcribed data for analysis in Study 3. All transcribed data were first examined and then coded into problem situations. Using a computer software word-processing program, the coded data for each clinic visit were then reorganized by problem situation. For example, all narrative data for Clinic Visit #10 coded Eat were clumped together. With the data thus aggregated by problem situation, it was possible to qualitatively analyze the data within visits and then across visits for topical themes and exchanges of meaning.

This basic approach to analysis led to three pathways of thinking. Analysis for Pathway 1—the family caregiver as interpreter—generated three themes of meanings: Facilitator (prompting, clarifying, explaining, correcting); Intermediary (e.g., answering doctor's questions addressed to patient, questioning doctor for patient); and Direct Source (caregiver and physician shift into dyadic dialogue) (Hasselkus, 1992b). A major finding in Pathway 2 was the caregiver as a second practitioner in the medical visit context. In this pathway, the caregivers contributed extensively to traditional physician domains of care, such as making diagnoses, interpreting symptoms, and offering treatment recommendations (Hasselkus, 1992a).

In the analysis for Pathway 3, the three-person interactions in the clinic visit were examined as they related to the older patients' self-care dependence and independence in the clinic setting (Hasselkus, 1994). The following results and discussion are for Pathway 3. Included are concepts derived from Pathways 1 (caregiver as interpreter) and 2 (caregiver as second practitioner) as they contribute to the analytical thinking and negotiations regarding dependence and independence of the older patient in the clinic visit.

Results

In this study, interactive behaviors that support patient self-care capabilities and those that support dependency in medical encounters were identified and described. I also explored patterns of interaction related to the patients' cognitive or sensory impairments.

Ambiguous Capabilities

Clinical estimations of competency in older patients must occur "on the spot" in the clinical setting; "clues [regarding competency] may emerge from conversations with the patient, from observation of behavior, or from discussions with family members or others" (High, 1989, p. 84). In a way, physicians, family caregivers, and older patients must sort out capabilities as they engage in health care in the triadic medical visit.

In the clinical data in this study, clues about incapacity were conveyed in several ways. For instance, family caregivers' behaviors offered clues to the physician about the older patient's self-care capabilities in a number of ways. As an interpreter in the interview, the caregiver engaged in incidents of correcting, adding to, prompting, answering for, and paraphrasing—all potential signals to the physician that the patient needed assistance. As a second practitioner in the interview, the caregiver at times slipped into a direct two-way dialogue with the physician, discussing symptoms, medications, or other treatments—again, strong signals to the physician that the patient needed assistance. At times, the caregiver disclosed information to the physician against the wishes of the patient, questioned the truth of the patient's statements, or told the patient what to do or say.

Older patients themselves gave off signals of incapacity by talking to the doctor through the family member ("He'll [referring to the doctor] have to give me some new prescriptions") and by deferring to the caregiver regarding responsibility for instructions from the physician (Patient [to caregiver]: "You know how to do it now?"). At times, the patient would check with the caregiver about the accuracy of information he or she was giving to the physician ("That was right, wasn't it?").

Interactions also occurred that affirmed capacity of the patient, thus supporting the independent status of the older person in the triad. Physicians made efforts of support, such as interrupting the caregiver's dialogue to enable the patient to respond, deliberately turning back to the patient for information during an exchange with the caregiver, or turning to the patient to verify information. Patients themselves interrupted physician-caregiver dialogues to ask their own questions, to express their own opinions, or to remind the caregiver and doctor about other concerns. Caregivers, at times, exhibited frankly assertive behaviors on the patient's behalf. In the following exchange, the doctor was displaying new and old x-rays to the patient and caregiver. The physician starts by addressing the patient, but shifts almost immediately to addressing the caregiver instead and referring to the patient in the third-person pronoun "she":

Doctor: All right, let's compare it to when you were at your worst.... Okay, you can see this is when she was really sick [note shift to caregiver]. How...

Caregiver [interrupts, talking to her mother]: Why don't you get up? I don't know if you can see this.

Doctor [continuing]: So she's much better than she was before, they look pretty clear. I don't see any fluid on there. (Hasselkus, 1994)

Here, the caregiver's deliberate inclusion of her mother sends a message that the mother is cognitively capable of understanding such information, thus affirming her capabilities. The physician has seemingly not picked up on the clues offered by the caregiver.

Dependency and Impairment

In order to examine the relationship of patterns of interaction (supportive of dependence or independence in the clinic visit) to functional status of the patient, the transcripts were divided into three categories of patient impairment (marked impairment, moderate or questionable impairment, and no apparent impairment [see Hasselkus, 1994, for criteria]). As might be expected, in those interviews in which the patient had a marked impairment, direct involvement of the patient was largely limited to the physical examination phase of the visit. The physician and caregiver tended to interact as two practitioners in an extended dyadic exchange. This pattern of interaction was particularly evident when the patient's impairment was cognitive.

Alternatively, when the marked impairment was a hearing loss, physicians and caregivers tried various strategies to enhance the patient's ability to take part in the clinic process. Sometimes, the physician sought the advice of the caregiver ("Am I talking into the wrong ear, do you think?") or the caregiver volunteered suggestions to the physician ("When you're speaking to him, it's much easier if you look at him."). One exception to this pattern of very limited patient involvement was the hearing-impaired patient who, accompanied by her daughter, stated to the doctor early in the interview, "I have a hearing problem, you know...that's why I have to ask you to repeat things," conveying a strong signal of initiative and responsibility for self-disclosure, in spite of her marked impairment.

When a cognitive or sensory moderate impairment was present, the uncertainties of the situation became a pervasive force. In the presence of this uncertainty about capabilities, it was not uncommon for the physician to shift back and forth repeatedly, negotiating between the caregiver and the patient during history taking and explanations of diagnoses and treatments. Protective caregiving (when the caregiver attempts to protect the older person from being aware that he or she is being cared for) was represented in much of the discourse in these clinic visits. It seemed, too, that the uncertainty of capabilities in this clinic situation entailed a corollary uncertainty of responsibilities. The caregivers and patients with moderate impairment struggled to determine where their respective responsibilities began and ended in relation to each other and to the physician.

A small number of clinic visits in the marked and moderate impairment categories included more than one family caregiver. In one such situation, after a fairly lengthy exchange between the two family caregivers and the patient about "multiple vitamins," the physician interjected his agreement with their suggestion for daily vitamins ("I think that's a good idea"), although, in fact, no one had actually even asked for his opinion! It seems that additional people in the medical visit lead to increased complexity from competing roles and redefinitions of control and capability (Glasser, Rubin, & Dickover, 1990).

Finally, patients who were in the no impairment group, having no observable sensory or cognitive impairment, tended to be more equitably present in the three-way clinic discourse. Patient self-care behaviors were often (although not always) integral to these clinic visits. In this group, patients exhibited some control over the agenda of the visit by stating their concerns, redirecting conversation back to topics of their priority, and by bringing up new topics. Further, in some interviews, the patients offered opinions on diagnoses and treatments, asked questions about medications, and asked for clarification on points not understood. The family caregivers tended to be more secondary and supplemental in these visits, although in some interviews the caregivers and physicians continued inexplicably to dominate the interactions.

It appears that, in the three-person geriatric medical clinic visit, the ambiguities of capabilities and responsibilities and the awkwardness of the three-way discourse interacted to potentiate the context of uncertainty, especially in the moderate impairment group. Much of the dependency behavior of the older patients and the dependency supportive behaviors by physicians and caregivers in these triadic medical encounters took place in situations of moderate impairment. The presence of a family member at an older patient's medical visit may have triggered underestimations of capacity for independent and responsible behaviors by all three people in the medical encounter. The shift of influence and responsibility away from the patient does not always reflect true impairment.

The need for on-the-spot calculations and negotiations of each other's capabilities and responsibilities—by all three people in the triad throughout the medical visit—seems paramount. In occupational therapy, the three-person (or more) therapy visit is probably common in all areas of practice. In geriatric outpatient practice, the presence of a cognitive impairment seems to be an especially strong influence on the patterns of interaction in the triadic medical visit. The need to sensitively interpret the patient's and family member's capabilities and responsibilities seems vital to harmonious relationships and to successful therapeutic outcomes.

Study 4: Occupation and Well-Being in Dementia: The Experience of Day-Care Staff

The purpose of this study was to gain understanding of the staff experience of occupation in the context of day care for people with dementia (Coppola, 1998; Hasselkus, 1998). The themes of meaning in professional caregiving described in Study 2—Change, Community, and Craft—seem likely to present in a markedly different manner or even be absent in dementia day care. What is the nature of community, change, and craft in the context of dementia care?

Narratives of especially satisfying and dissatisfying experiences of caregiving were elicited from a random state-wide sample of day-care staff members in Wisconsin. Whereas in Study 2 this same data collection approach was used to elicit narratives from occupational therapists about practice more broadly, in Study 4, I focused specifically on adult day-care staff members and the meaning of occupation in their experiences while working with day-care participants with dementia.

Assumptions about the relationship of occupation to health and well-being form the basis and rationale for planned activity programming in care for people with dementia. Guidelines for therapeutic activities for this population have been proposed, such as using activities that are familiar, that incorporate repetition and rhythm, and that ensure some measure of success (Dowling, 1995; Griffin & Matthews, 1986; Hellen, 1992; Teri & Logsdon, 1991; Zgola, 1990). Previous examination of the meanings of occupation in dementia day-care settings has led to understandings of occupation as an enabler of social connectedness (Josephsson, 1994), as a help in preventing harm (Hasselkus, 1992c), and as an assist in keeping order and maintaining "crowd control" (Borell, Gustavsson, Sandman, & Kielhofner, 1994, p. 231). Kitwood and Bredin (1992) used the term "relative well-being" (p. 280) to describe the wellness state of a person with dementia. They proposed 12 indicators of relative well-being, such as evidence of humor, expressions of affection, initiation of social contacts, and helpfulness to others. Albert and colleagues (1996) used frequency of participation in activities as an indicator of well-being, and Borell and colleagues (1994) used levels of spontaneous behavior. All in all, the nature of well-being in the everyday life of a person with dementia is not yet well understood, nor is the relationship of occupation to health and well-being in this population.

We do not fully understand how occupational programming relates to participant well-being in a day-care situation or how occupation is experienced by staff members in terms of satisfying and dissatisfying caregiving practices. Greater understanding of occupation in this context of care will lead to more responsive and therapeutic activity programming, will enable us to better articulate the meaning of occupation in the care of people with dementia, and will contribute to our developing theory base of the relationship between occupation and health.

Method

A random sample of 50 day-care centers was generated from the membership list of the Wisconsin Adult Day Care Association. Letters were sent to the directors of all centers in the sample, explaining the study and inviting each to designate a staff member to participate in a telephone interview. Interviews were successfully completed with 40 centers (42 informants). Ages of informants ranged from 28 to 66 years; experience in caring for people with dementia ranged from less than 1 year to 36 years. Forty-one of the 42 informants were women.

Each staff informant provided narratives of a satisfying and a dissatisfying experience of providing care for their day-care participants. Probes were used by the interviewer (graduate student assistant) to keep each informant "in" the experience, thereby minimizing an interpretive approach to the storytelling (Van Manen, 1990). Second call-back interviews with 10 informants were conducted to serve as member checks and as opportunities for the informants to elaborate and give feedback on the understandings emerging from early analysis.

The analysis began with a search for the structures of the satisfying and dissatisfying experiences that constitute the phenomenon of providing day care to people with dementia. Using a process similar to that of Study 2, the graduate assistant and I carried out parallel reading and preliminary coding of the first six interviews, worked for beginning consensus, conducted the remaining interviews, continued to do parallel reading and consensus building, and used probes in the call-back interviews to further elucidate the emerging themes and interpretations. The iterative cycle of reflective analysis, consensus building, and data collection helped us stay as close as possible to the text and maximized the authenticity of the interpretations that were emerging (Lincoln & Guba, 1986; Van Manen, 1990).

Results

The core meaning of occupation to staff members in day care for people with dementia was Occupation as the Gateway to Relative Well-Being. The narratives were stories of the day-care staff trying first to bring about connections or the meeting of minds (Phase 1) with the day-care clients, engagement in occupation (Phase 2) could then take place, and a state of relative well-being (Phase 3) was the hoped-for outcome (Figure 3-1).

The Meeting of Minds

In Phase 1 of the model, and as a necessary first step, a meeting of minds takes place. That is, a cognitive connection is made between the staff person and the day-care participant. Staff members used a variety of skills and strategies to bring about this meeting of minds, such as redirecting a participant's attention and action toward an activity that is safer, more calming, and has more potential for success than what the participant is engaged in at the time. Enabling strategies were used such as signage and cuing to help with orientation in the day-care room, simplifying the environment, and relying on already familiar routines. Searching for the "key" was a strategy employed by staff, such as one incident of finding out that one very unresponsive participant had done flower arranging in her past and then using this knowledge to successfully engage her in opening her eyes, sitting forward in her wheelchair, and putting flowers in a vase; "It was very satisfying to have found the key that opened her up...and showed her that she could do something."

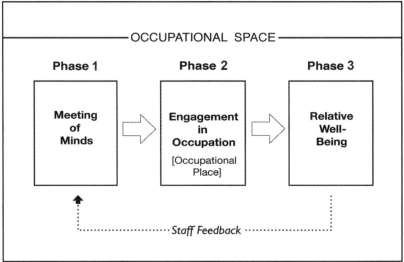

Figure 3-1. Occupation in day care for persons with dementia: The staff experience. (Republished with permission of *American Journal of Occupational Therapy*, from Occupation and well-being in dementia: The experience of day-care staff, Hasselkus, B. R., *52*, 1998; permission conveyed through Copyright Clearance Center, Inc.)

Engagement in Occupation

Phase 2 of the staff experience of occupation in dementia care is that of actual engagement of the client in occupation. Descriptions of occupational involvement were rich in detail, leading to a conceptualization of multiple levels of spontaneity, communication, capability, and affect. For example, one staff member described a bowling activity with one client, saying:

> He can negotiate the whole thing himself... You can tell he must have bowled in his time, he has the form, and he knows how to knock the pins down, and then he goes and he resets them up. To me, it is satisfying because he's doing this on his own. I'm not doing it for him, he's doing it. (Hasselkus, 1998)

Capability and spontaneity are evident in this narrative and are obviously satisfying to the staff member to observe. In another story, the staff informant described an incident with a client who had been persistently unresponsive to all attempts to bring about a meeting of minds, a connection:

> Then one day, I gave her a piece of paper and pencil. I just set it in front of her, I didn't even give her any instructions... And all of a sudden she just picked it up and started writing. She wrote her name! She did spell it wrong, but she wrote her name! (Hasselkus, 1998)

Again, the level of spontaneity in this day-care participant's occupation seemed especially satisfying to the staff person.

Relative Well-Being

Phase 3 of the model of occupation and dementia care is the phase of relative well-being for both day-care participants and staff members. Staff informants expressed their own well-being in statements of satisfaction, inspired by their observations and beliefs about the well-being brought about in the day-care clients. Indicators of well-being in the clients included affective behaviors such as smiles, looks of pleasure, socializing with others, singing with "gusto,"

being able to attend to tasks, eye contact and visual tracking, moments of remembering—both from the past and from the day to day of the present—laughter, and signs of independence in activities. For example, when one client was able to learn a medication regimen, the staff member called this newfound independence "absolutely wonderful." Staff spoke with pleasure and a sense of personal satisfaction derived from their own skills:

> I loved that woman. She could sit and laugh and talk, where at the beginning she was agitated, sullen; so, there was a real definite, good gain and a feeling that I had a little something to do with her being able to function the way she did. (Hasselkus, 1998)

When the meeting of minds was successfully brought about, when engagement in occupation occurred and indicators of client well-being were present, staff informants expressed their own well-being in phrases such as "I find that very rewarding" or "I was really pleased by that."

Discussion

The phases of the model of the staff experience of occupation in the care of people with dementia can be conceptualized as comprising a whole to which the term *occupational space* is applied (see Figure 3-1). The occupation itself, that is, the activity that takes place within that space, is the occupational place. The terms are borrowed from Tuan's (1977) writing on experiential space and place and from Josephsson's (1994) use of the term *meeting-places* to describe the social connectedness found through occupation by people with dementia. In dementia care, the occupational place is one of intimacy (i.e., an experience of the here and now—fleeting and momentary). In narrative terms, staff members are trying to create an occupational story to share with the day-care client—in the moment.

Buber (1958), a German philosopher, stated that "all real living is meeting" (p. 11). Findings from this study support the value of occupation in enabling people with dementia to continue to relate to and meet their worlds—to engage in "real living"—at whatever levels of engagement are within their capabilities. Occupational therapy practitioners are especially well qualified to use occupation therapeutically in the care of people with dementia. Bringing about indicators of client well-being through occupation is a primary source of satisfaction and reward for staff members in day care.

In fact, therapists in all contexts of care invest time and skills in an effort to establish a connection with the people with whom they work (Crepeau, 1991; Rosa & Hasselkus, 1997)—both for those with and those without cognitive impairment. The model of Occupation as a Gateway to Relative Well-Being represents a gestalt of the relationship between occupation and health as it is experienced in the lived world of occupational therapy. The concepts of occupational space and place are applicable to occupational therapy in all areas of practice.

CONTRIBUTIONS TO OCCUPATIONAL SCIENCE

The research program described previously represents a series of studies in which I investigated the nature of caregiving as an occupation, addressing the caregiving experiences in formal (health systems) and informal (family) care. The studies demonstrate ways to research occupation directly, focusing on one occupation—caregiving—in a variety of contexts in order to better understand this specific occupation but also occupation more broadly.

The first three studies offer new and enriching insights into the caregiving occupation of family members, occupational therapists, and physicians, drawing us closer to our world of care provision and enabling us to draw inferences about the similarities and the differences among these contexts of care. Perhaps the strongest contribution to occupational science in these studies is present in Study 4 (i.e., the study of staff experiences of occupation in the context of day care for people with dementia). The model of Occupation as a Gateway to Relative Well-Being that evolved from the analysis of these data is a theoretical representation of occupational engagement in the day-care setting. The model provides support for one of the basic tenets of our profession—our theoretical assumptions about the relationship between occupation and health and well-being. In Study 4, the model depicts the relationship between occupation and relative well-being in the day-care participants as perceived by the day-care staff, offering new theoretical insights related to the specific population of staff and participants in dementia day care. The three phases of the model—the meeting of minds, engagement in occupation, and relative well-being—represent an enriched conceptualization of the nature of occupation. Occupation becomes a phenomenon that is a process, and that process has both universal and context-specific defining characteristics. To work together

well with any client requires a meeting of minds before meaningful occupational engagement can take place; relative well-being is the hoped-for outcome. The meeting of minds, the occupational engagement, and the relative well-being can all take many forms and exist in varying strengths—all of which can be recognized and valued.

IMPLICATIONS FOR OCCUPATIONAL THERAPY

All four studies reported here are deeply embedded in the health care world and are examples of research that is occupation based and relevant to the practice of occupational therapy (Pierce et al., 2010). The conceptualization of the family caregiver as a second practitioner in home care and outpatient care, coupled with new insights into the reflective processes of formal and informal health care practices, can potentially enhance occupational therapists' abilities to work together with family in supporting the family as a caring unit. Understandings about satisfying and dissatisfying experiences of change, community, and craft in our practice of occupational therapy can help therapists maximize satisfying work experiences and career pathways. The subtleties and ambiguities that govern interactions in clinic visits involving more than the therapist and the patient are manifest in many occupational therapy treatment situations (parents, school staff members, adult son or daughter, spouse, other professionals). The need to sort out and be sensitive to the true capabilities and responsibilities of each person in the medical clinic data of Study 3 offers insights to occupational therapists in analogous clinic situations. And finally, the findings in Study 4 reveal clearly the staff members' views about the key role of occupation in bringing about relative well-being in day-care participants with dementia and a sense of satisfaction and reward for staff. These findings strongly underscore the importance of activity programming for people with dementia.

LEARNING SUPPORTS

The Structure of a Research Program

Purpose

The purpose of this learning support is to encourage the student to think about the ways that these four research studies are related to each other in method, focus, and research questions.

Primary Concepts

Concepts addressed are qualitative research design, occupation as related to health and well-being, and formal and informal health care coordination.

Instructions

1. Starting with Study 1, create a branching diagram or "tree" to portray the connections between the four studies described in this chapter.

2. Label the connecting links with themes or findings or questions raised that relate to occupational science and that lead from one study to the next.

Pathways of Analysis

Purpose

The goal of this Learning Support is to increase the student's awareness and understanding of and comfort with the multiple possible directions of interpretation and analysis that are embedded in the data of a qualitative research study.

Primary Concepts

Concepts addressed are subjective experience as authentic data, the many representations of occupation found in narrative data, and the process of moving from the data analysis to the findings to the clinical implications to the next possible research questions to ask.

Instructions

1. As stated in the chapter, the analysis of the data in Study 3 led to three pathways of deeper analysis: interpretation, clinical implications, and potential follow-up research. Studies 1, 2, and 4 also offer multiple pathways for analysis and future research. Choose one of these remaining three studies to examine for multiple pathways.

2. Think about the nature of the data in your chosen study (1, 2, or 4) and how the data differ from the data in Study 3.

3. What do the data offer in terms of other possible pathways for analysis and follow-up research?

4. How do these other possible pathways relate to occupational therapy practice?

The Dimensions of Doing Occupational Therapy

Purpose

The purpose of this Learning Support is to offer the student an opportunity to reflect on his or her own values, to recognize the different kinds of rewards found in different contexts of practice, and to acquire a sense of discernment about the diversity found in occupational therapy practice.

Primary Concepts

Concepts introduced in Study 2 include the lifeworld of doing occupational therapy, the nature of satisfying and dissatisfying practice, and clinical experience as narrative.

Instructions

1. Think about the three primary dimensions revealed in the experiential narrative data from occupational therapists in Study 2. As you consider your own approaching future as an occupational therapist, what aspects of the three dimensions stand out for you as important and as potentially most satisfying and rewarding?

2. Is there one dimension or one aspect of one dimension that seems less important to you personally?

3. What are your ideas at this point about which areas of practice best offer what is most meaningful to you and most valued?

Evidence of Relative Well-Being

Purpose

The purpose of this Learning Support is to increase the student's awareness of indicators of relative well-being in clients and to recognize the links between these indicators and occupational engagement.

Primary Concepts

Concepts introduced are the relationship of occupation to well-being; the concept of relative well-being, especially as applied to people with dementia; meeting of minds in client relationships; and occupational engagement as a multidimensional phenomenon.

Instructions

1. Go back to the brief narrative in Study 4 about the woman with dementia who had been a flower arranger in her earlier life. What evidence do you see here that engagement in occupation has brought about relative well-being?

2. How can this scenario serve as an example of evidence-based practice?

3. How does what the day-care staff person did to "connect" with this participant relate to the concept of reflective practice as discussed in the results of Study 1?

REFERENCES

Adelman, R. D., Greene, M. G., & Charon, R. (1987). The physician-elderly patient-companion triad in the medical encounter: The development of a conceptual framework and research agenda. *The Gerontologist, 27,* 729-734.

Albert, S. M., Del Castillo-Castaneda, C. D., Sano, M., Jacobs, D. M., Marder, K., Bell, K., . . . Stern, Y. (1996). Quality of life in patients with Alzheimer's disease as reported by patient proxies. *Journal of the American Geriatrics Society, 44,* 1342-1347.

Allen, D., Benner, P., & Diekelmann, N. (1986). Three paradigms for nursing research: Methodological implications. In P. E. Chinn (Ed.), *Nursing research methodology: Issues and implementation* (pp. 23-38). Rockville, MD: Aspen.

Borell, L., Gustavsson, A., Sandman, P. O., & Kielhofner, G. (1994). Occupational programming in a day hospital for patients with dementia. *Occupational Therapy Journal of Research, 14,* 219-238.

Bowers, B. J. (1987). Intergenerational caregiving: Adult caregivers and their aging parents. *Advanced Nursing Science, 9,* 20-31.

Bowyer, J. W. (1991). *Tally: A text analysis tool for the liberal arts.* Dubuque, IA: Wm. C. Brown.

Bruner, J. (1986). *Actual minds, possible worlds.* Cambridge, MA: Harvard University Press.

Buber, M. (1958). *I and thou.* (R. G. Smith, Trans.). New York, NY: Scribner.

Clark, N. M., & Rakowski, W. (1983). Family caregivers of older adults: Improving helping skills. *The Gerontologist, 23,* 637-642.

Coe, R., & Prendergast, C. G. (1985). The formation of coalitions: Interaction strategies in triads. *Sociology of Health & Illness, 7,* 236-247.

Coppola, S. (1998). Clinical interpretation of "Occupation and well-being in dementia: The experience of day-care staff." *American Journal of Occupational Therapy, 52,* 435-438.

Crepeau, E. B. (1991). Achieving intersubjective understanding: Examples from an occupational therapy treatment session. *American Journal of Occupational Therapy, 45,* 1016-1025.

Diekelmann, N. (1991). The emancipator power of the narrative. In National League for Nursing (Eds.), *Curriculum revolution: Community building and activism* (pp. 41-62). New York, NY: Author.

Dowling, J. R. (1995). *Keeping busy: A handbook of activities for persons with dementia.* Baltimore, MD: Johns Hopkins University Press.

Flanagan, J. C. (1954). The critical incident technique. *Psychological Bulletin, 51,* 327-358.

Frank, G., & Polkinghorne, D. (2010). Qualitative research in occupational therapy: From the first to the second generation. *OTJR: Occupation, Participation and Health, 30,* 51-57.

Geertz, C. (1973). *The interpretation of cultures.* New York, NY: Basic.

Geertz, C. (1988). *Works and lives: The anthropologist as author.* Stanford, CA: Stanford University Press.

Glasser, M. S., Rubin, S., & Dickover, M. (1990). The caregiver role: Review of family caregiver-physician relations and dementing disorders. In S. M. Stahl (Ed.), *The legacy of longevity* (pp. 321-337). Newbury Park, CA: Sage Publications.

Griffin, R. M., & Matthews, M. U. (1986). The selection of activities: A dual responsibility. *Physical and Occupational Therapy in Geriatrics, 4,* 105-112.

Guba, E. G. (1981). Criteria for assessing the trustworthiness of naturalistic inquiries. *Educational Communication & Technology: A Journal of Theory, Research, and Development, 29,* 75-91.

Hasselkus, B. R. (1988). Meaning in family caregiving: Perspectives on caregiver/professional relationships. *The Gerontologist, 28,* 686-691.

Hasselkus, B. R. (1989). The meaning of daily activity in family caregiving for the elderly. *American Journal of Occupational Therapy, 43,* 649-656.

Hasselkus, B. R. (1990). Ethnographic interviewing: A tool for practice with family caregivers for the elderly. *Occupational Therapy Practice, 2,* 9-16.

Hasselkus, B. R. (1992a). Physician and family caregiver in the medical setting: Negotiation of care? *Journal of Aging Studies, 6,* 67-80.

Hasselkus, B. R. (1992b). The family caregiver as interpreter in the geriatric medical interview. *Medical Anthropology Quarterly, 6,* 288-304.

Hasselkus, B. R. (1992c). The meaning of activity: Day care for persons with Alzheimer disease. *American Journal of Occupational Therapy, 46,* 199-206.

Hasselkus, B. R. (1994). Three-track care: Older patient, family member, and physician in the medical visit. *Journal of Aging Studies, 8,* 291-307.

Hasselkus, B. R. (1998). Occupation and well-being in dementia: The experience of day-care staff. *American Journal of Occupational Therapy, 52,* 423-434.

Hasselkus, B. R., & Dickie, V. A. (1990). Themes of meaning: Occupational therapists' perspectives on practice. *Occupational Therapy Journal of Research, 10,* 195-207.

Hasselkus, B. R., & Dickie, V. A. (1994). Doing occupational therapy: Dimensions of satisfaction and dissatisfaction. *American Journal of Occupational Therapy, 48,* 145-154.

Hasselkus, B. R., & Ray, R. O. (1988). Informal learning in family caregiving: A worm's eye view. *Adult Education Quarterly, 39,* 31-40.

Hellen, C. R. (1992). *Alzheimer's disease: Activity-focused care.* Boston, MA: Andover.

High, D. M. (1989). Caring for decisionally incapacitated elderly. *Theoretical Medicine, 10,* 83-96.

Hofer, A. (1985). *The caretaker family as the integrating agent.* (Available from A. Hofer, Consultant, Aging Programs, 1141 Loxford Terrace, Silver Spring, MD 20901.)

Josephsson, S. (1994). *Everyday activities and meeting-places in dementia* (Unpublished doctoral dissertation). Karolinska Institute, Stockholm, Sweden.

Kaye, L. (1985). Home care for the aged: A fragile partnership. *Social Work, 30,* 312-317.

Kermode, F. (1967). *The sense of an ending: Studies in the theory of fiction.* New York, NY: Oxford University Press.

Kitwood, T., & Bredin, K. (1992). Towards a theory of dementia care: Personhood and well-being. *Aging and Society, 12,* 269-287.

Kivitt, V. R. (1985). Consanguinity and kin level: Their relative importance to the helping network of older adults. *Journal of Gerontology, 40,* 228-234.

Levin, L. S. (1977). Forces and issues in the revival of interest in self-care: Impetus for redirection in health. *Health Education Monographs, 5,* 115-120.

Lincoln, Y. S., & Guba, E. G. (1986). But is it rigorous? Trustworthiness and authenticity in naturalistic evaluation. In D. D. Williams (Ed.), *Naturalistic evaluation: New directions for program evaluation* (pp. 73-84). San Francisco, CA: Jossey-Bass.

Litwak, E. (1985). *Helping the elderly: The complementary role of informal networks and formal systems.* New York, NY: Guilford.

Mattingly, C. (1991). The narrative nature of clinical reasoning. *American Journal of Occupational Therapy, 45,* 998-1005.

Notebook II [Computer software]. (1985). Walnut Creek, CA: ProTem Software, Inc.

Orem, D. C. (1980). Nursing and self-care. In *Nursing: Concepts of practice* (2nd ed.). New York, NY: McGraw-Hill.

Pierce, D., Atler, K., Baltisberger, J., Fehringer, E., Hunter, E., Malkawi, S., & Parr, T. (2010). Occupational science: A data-based American perspective. *Journal of Occupational Science, 17*(4), 204-215.

Rakowski, W., & Clark, N. M. (1985). Future outlook, caregiving, and care-receiving in the family context. *The Gerontologist, 25,* 618-623.

Ricoeur, P. (1984). *Time and narrative.* Chicago, IL: University of Chicago Press.

Rosa, S., & Hasselkus, B. R. (1997). Connecting with patients: The personal experience of professional helping. *Occupational Therapy Journal of Research, 16,* 245-260.

Schatzman, L. (1991). Dimensional analysis: Notes on an alternative approach to the grounding of theory in qualitative research. In D. R. Maines (Ed.), *Social organization and social process* (pp. 303-314). New York, NY: Aldine De Gruyter.

Schön, D. A. (1983). *The reflective practitioner.* New York, NY: Basic Books, Inc.

Shanas, E. (1979). The family as a social support system in old age. *The Gerontologist, 19,* 169-174.

Simmons, K. H., Ivry, J., & Seltzer, M. M. (1985). Agency-family collaboration. *The Gerontologist, 25,* 343-346.

Spradley, J. P. (1979). *The ethnographic interview.* Chicago, IL: Holt, Rinehart and Winston.

Teri, L., & Logsdon, R. G. (1991). Identifying pleasant activities for Alzheimer's disease patients: The pleasant events schedule-AD. *The Gerontologist, 31,* 124-127.

Tuan, Y.-F. (1977). *Space and place: The perspective of experience.* Minneapolis, MN: University of Minnesota Press.

Van Manen, M. (1990). *Researching lived experience.* London, Ontario, Canada: University of Western Ontario.

Waitzkin, J., & Stoeckle, J. D. (1976). Information control and the micropolitics of health care: Summary of an ongoing research project. *Social Science & Medicine, 10,* 263-276.

Zarit, S. H., Todd, P. A., & Zarit, J. M. (1986). Subjective burden of husbands and wives as caregivers: A longitudinal study. *The Gerontologist, 26,* 260-266.

Zgola, J. M. (1990). Therapeutic activity. In N. Mace (Ed.), *Dementia care: Patients, family and community* (pp. 148-172). Baltimore, MD: Johns Hopkins University Press.

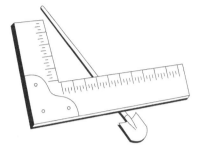

4

A Research Program on the Occupation of Mate Selection

Sheama Krishnagiri, PhD, OTR/L, FAOTA

Selection of another human being as a partner in marriage or as a companion is a universal human tendency. For the fruition of such an alliance, actions are taken, and decisions are made, usually by both parties. Whether it is a stroll in the village square with other young people and chaperones or a couple alone on the beach, there have always been prescribed and proscribed behaviors, the right way and the wrong, accepted and expected. Applying Clark and colleagues' (1991) definition of occupation as "chunks of culturally and personally meaningful activity in which humans engage that can be named in the lexicon of our culture" (p. 302), the process of mate selection is clearly an occupation. The fact that selection of a companion requires a series of activities and actions that engage an individual's time and affect one's life in innumerable ways indicates the importance of this occupation. I became interested in this occupation while in graduate school due to the inordinate amount of time I spent engaged in it. The sheer energy used in processing the day-to-day details with my friends and classmates made me curious about the impact of this occupation on everything I do. Additionally, the adapted version of the arranged marriage process that I was using (common among cultures in India) led to questions, discus-

sion, and reflections about my own process. There are many variations within and between different cultures as to what decisions need to be made, who makes them, and the process used in reaching those decisions. This decision-making process, generally considered the mate selection process, is also known as *courtship* (Hamon & Ingoldsby, 2003; Murstein, 1976). A study of mate selection as an occupation entails, at minimum, a description of the occupation, its boundaries, what actions and activities are parts of it, and an understanding of the meaning and motivation for its engagement.

LITERATURE

The predominant form of mate selection among humans in most Western societies is that of monogamy, most commonly uniting a female with a male and bound by the institution of marriage. The process encompasses the time from which one meets a potential mate to the point when one decides to make a long-term commitment. In the early years, theories about the mate selection process were mostly limited to social psychology, with a few explanations from

Pierce, D. (Ed.).
Occupational Science for Occupational Therapy (pp. 37-48).
© 2014 SLACK Incorporated.

biology (Schwartz & Scott, 2002). These theories envisioned the basis of pairing as a resource exchange: that is, mate selection was an exchange of food, access to property/territory, and/or social benefits (Klimek, 1979; Murstein, 1976; Nofz, 1984; Sabatelli, 1988). In other words, an individual was viewed as choosing a mate for an economic, political, or social benefit to one's family and/or to oneself. Choosing for love was also acknowledged in the classifications. Additionally, there were explications of gender-specific roles that guided behavior (Buss, Shackelford, Kirkpatrick, & Larsen, 2001). These, of course, vary by culture, as well as individually.

In recent years, mate selection theories have focused on the types of strategies and signals used in choosing a mate. Most of the described strategies are based on evolutionary concepts like parental investment, intrasexual competition, and intersexual competition (Buss, 2006; Eagly & Wood, 1999; Gangestad & Simpson, 2000; Hersch & Paul, 1996). That is, mate selection behaviors and preferences are explained in terms of the type of mate one is looking for and the corresponding evolutionary strategy. If one is looking for a long-term mate, the focus in preferences appears to be for someone who can best contribute to parenting. If the goal is a short-term mate, then the preferences are less specific. Strategies have also been described for mate poaching, extrapair mating, and mate guarding.

As one may discern, neither the socioculturally based mate selection theories nor evolution-based theories explain the process and experience of mate selection very thoroughly, nor do they examine the form, function, and meaning of engaging in these activities.

In addition to theories of mate selection, there is literature available on the types of characteristics (physical and psychological) sought in a mate (Buss et al., 2001; Davis, 1998; Liu, Campbell, & Condie, 1995); the effects of culture on emotions and on gender in selecting a mate (Geary, Vigil, & Byrd-Craven, 2004; Hamon & Ingoldsby, 2003; Miller & Todd, 1998; Shackelford, Schmitt, & Buss, 2005); intercultural dating patterns (Martin, Bradford, Drzewiecka, & Chitgopekar, 2003); and perceptions of potential mates (Buston & Emlen, 2003; Surra & Hughes, 1997). One study examined activity preferences by both members of the couple in the progression of premarital relationships (Surra, Cottle, Gray, Harmell, & Vandewater, 2000); however, this study was focused only on understanding the nature of participation in activities. Lastly, a study on routine love behaviors showed a short list of behaviors indicative of showing love (Lemieux, 1996). These are limited in scope and do not take into account engagement in the full occupation and its meaning to individuals.

As this condensed literature review shows, there are some theories that describe mate selection and the characteristics and preferences one may have for a mate, as well as some data on routine love behaviors. There is no definitive or satisfactory account of mate selection as an occupation.

Information is lacking on what activities make up this occupation and how they are integral to the occupation; when the processes begin and end; what stages, phases, or steps may occur and in what sequence; how much time each step takes; what the determining factor in selection is; how meaningful the occupation is to the individual; and how it affects the individual's daily life. Additionally, information is lacking on how engagement in the occupation is affected by individual internal factors such as physiological rhythms, past experiences such as failed relationships or marriages, future desires, maturity of the individual, personality, or by external factors such as social, financial, and spiritual circumstances.

Thus, the study of mate selection as an occupation calls for description of the boundaries of the occupation, what actions and activities are a part of it, how it varies with culture, what it means to the individual, what it means within the society and culture in which the individual participates, how the occupation has changed historically, and how changes over time have affected the current status of the occupation. Further, the neurological, biological, and physiological factors involved in mate selection, as well as how they affect or are affected by the occupation, need to be described. As may be apparent, exploring the many facets of an occupation can require a lifetime of work and study.

SEQUENCE OF STUDIES ON MATE SELECTION

In order to begin describing and defining this occupation, I felt it best to begin with typical adults representing the melting pot that is the United States. If one can understand what happens in the most common form of the occupation, then subpopulations can be studied to see what the variations are. Three studies of mate selection have been completed to date: of typical adults, of adults with an obvious physical disability, and of the elderly.

Study 1: Mate Selection in Typical Adults

The purpose of the first mate selection study was to describe this occupation as it was manifested in typical adults in a major urban center of the United States. Specifically, the activities and actions making up the occupation of mate selection, its time frames, and the way it affects the daily activities of the individual at each of the dating stages were focused upon as a beginning point. The stages referred to here are an adaptation of the five dating stages described by Roche (1986). They are Stage One, Early Dating, in which there is attraction but no love; Stage Two, Steady Dating, in which there is love developing; and Stage Three, Engaged or Committed, when the couple is in love. These elements were chosen to be studied initially, in order to provide a general description of the chunks of activities involved in the occupation to serve as a basis of a more in-depth description.

Methods

A total of 209 heterosexual subjects between the ages of 18 and 67 years from a major metropolitan area completed this study. After receiving approval from the institutional review board for ethical research, the researcher stood outside the Los Angeles County registrar's office every day for 3 months to recruit subjects for the survey portion of the study. A total of 1,600 people agreed to take the survey when approached. The self-selected subjects were obtaining marriage licenses and were recruited in this fashion so that all of them would be at the same point in the mate selection process and thus could be compared. Additionally, the intention was to gather a representative cross-section of the population in the county. The response rate of completed surveys was low for several reasons. First, because the county would not permit access to personal information, no follow-up was possible. Second, the majority of couples were getting married in the immediate future, and filling out a survey was most likely not high on their list of priorities. Ultimately, half of the 209 respondents completed the questionnaire in person, and the other half returned it by mail using the postage-paid envelope provided.

In part two of the study, in-depth interviews of 20 people were conducted. From the 40 subjects out of the survey sample who volunteered to participate, purposive sampling based on race, gender, and age was used to choose those who were interviewed. Whenever possible, both members of a couple were interviewed.

With respect to demographics, the sample was representative of racial, ethnic, and religious backgrounds found in Los Angeles. The sample consisted of 89 men and 120 women. The average age for the sample was 29 years.

Overall, 60% of the sample held professional jobs, as coded in the Occupational Information Network (U.S. Department of Labor, Employment and Training Administration, n.d.). More than 85% of the sample had at least some college, if not a bachelor's degree or higher. This is not representative of the general population but is a reflection of those who chose to return the surveys.

More than half of the group was at least a third-generation U.S. citizen, and 87% stated that English was their primary spoken language. More than 40%, however, were bilingual. About 89% of the sample was getting married for the first time, with an average of 10.47 years of dating experience and an average of 3.11 previous relationships.

The interview sample represented gender equally and had a large age distribution (21 to 68 years). Additionally, there were people with a history of previous marriages prior to the current one, some as many as four. Most subjects had married either interracially, interethnically, and/or across different religions, producing data from a broad spectrum

of perspectives. The survey was developed and piloted in several stages, using 10 subjects each time, to evaluate and refine its content and procedures. Consultation from survey experts and pilot testing resulted in the final version of the survey. In addition, two subjects were interviewed to evaluate the interview questions and time requirements. Questions on the survey included typical activities at each dating stage, who was involved in the activity, who decided on choice of activities, time spent at each stage of the dating process, and demographics. The majority of questions were open ended.

The interview content was an extension of the survey questions. For example, more detailed information on dating activities and their purpose, decision making, and the meaning of the occupation was sought. Each individual was interviewed twice for approximately 1.5 hours each time. In the second interview, the interviewee was usually more forthcoming. A rapport had been established, so information could be clarified to increase the depth and trustworthiness of the data.

The objective questions in the survey were converted and coded for statistical analysis (50 variables). The open-ended questions required reduction and classification of data prior to coding for analysis (59 variables). Specifically, the questions relating to the activities at different stages of courtship resulted in a list of 250 different descriptors. After repetitions were eliminated and synonyms were grouped, a reduced list of 175 activities resulted. This list of activities was then classified along two dimensions that naturally emerged from the data. Data were first classified by the types of activity and then by the socialization involved in doing the activity. Types of activities included dining, sports, arts/entertainment, home making, or physical/sexual/romance. Socialization referred to whether the activity involved just the two people who were dating or whether it included friends and/or family. Three graduate students and the researcher independently rated the list of 175 activities along these two dimensions. There was 100% agreement between the raters on type of activity and about 97% agreement on the social dimension. Each subject's answers were then coded along these two dimensions to be used for analysis. The interviews were transcribed verbatim and then subjected to content analysis (Grbich, 1999). Correlations between the interview and survey data were sought, along with an understanding of the purpose of these activities.

Results of Study 1

This was a large study, with results including a description of dating activities at each stage of mate selection, the average number of hours spent at each stage on dating and preparation activities, the purpose of activities at each stage of dating, decision-making processes involved in progression through stages, statistical associations between demographic variables and choices of activities, meanings

TABLE 4-1

PERCENTAGE OF ADULT SUBJECTS REPORTING ACTIVITIES AT EACH STAGE OF MATE SELECTION

ACTIVITIES	EARLY DATING	STEADY DATING	ENGAGED
Arts/entertainment	85%	70%	54%
Physical/sexual/romantic	76%	84%	80%
Dining	76%	50%	39%
Homemaking	25%	68%	87%
Sports	16%	15%	9%

Note. More than 50% is considered significant.

associated with finding a mate, and much more. While not all of it can be described here, some examples of results follow, along with a proposed model of the occupation of mate selection.

Dating Activities in Mate Selection

From the data collected, activities of mate selection were classified into two types: date activities and preparation activities. Date activities were those in which both members of the couple were present and participated but may have included others on occasion, such as family and friends (e.g., dinner together, bowling, and sex). Preparation activities were those in which the activities were performed individually by one member of the couple but were in some manner related to enhancing the process of courtship, such as making reservations, time spent on shopping and dressing for the date, daydreaming about the other, and composing and sending romantic messages.

Survey data on dating activities that were typical at each stage of the mate selection process were collected and analyzed as just described. Table 4-1 shows the frequency of activities reported (in percentages) at each of the three stages. If a category of activities was mentioned by at least 50% of the sample at any stage, then the category of activities was considered important for that stage. Using those criteria, arts/entertainment and physical/sexual/romantic types of activities occurred significantly in all three stages of the process. A larger proportion of the sample engaged in activities categorized as dining during the first two stages. Homemaking activities were reported by a majority of the sample during stages 2 and 3. Lastly, the percentage of sports-related activities was not significant during any of the three stages.

The interview data supported the survey data with respect to types of activities. In addition, the interview data contributed to an understanding of why certain activities were chosen and what they meant in the courtship process. For example, when interviewees were asked what activities they typically do on their first few dates, something related to dining was always the first response. Dining occupations included items such as meeting for lunch during the workday, dinner out, romantic dinner, dinner prepared at home, or coffee/dessert after enjoying an event. All of the subjects interviewed agreed that meal-oriented activities were a way to spend time together and have a chance to "talk and get to know each other." In addition to dining, arts/entertainment activities were mentioned most often. A majority of the interviewees suggested that doing an arts/entertainment type of activity gave them an opportunity to find out if they could enjoy some of the same "fun things" together and could gather more information about the other person than just dinner and conversation could provide. These opportunities to "check each other out" allowed individuals to sift through potential mates and decide whether to continue the courtship process.

These results provide information on the form and function of the activities within this occupation. When asked about the meaning of dating and selecting a mate, most subjects in the interview sample stated that finding a soul mate for life and getting married was of the utmost importance and took precedence in their lives. Please note, however, that these results reflect only this sample of self-selected subjects who were getting their marriage licenses.

Additional Results

Although the breadth of results from the complete analysis of the quantitative and qualitative data cannot be fully described here, suffice it to say that, similar to the examples just described, the interview data provided a much broader and deeper understanding of the types of activities included in this occupation, the reasons for engaging in the activities, the time spent on the relationship both during and in preparation for dates and what that meant, the reasoning involved in the decision as to whether or not to continue with the relationship, the influence of previous experiences on current behaviors and decisions, characteristics

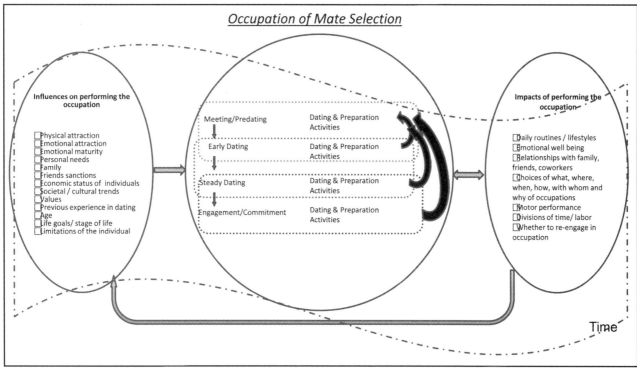

Figure 4-1. Model of the occupation of mate selection (Study 1).

preferred in a mate and why, and much more. In addition, the interviews provided data on the impact of engaging in this occupation: how courtship activities affected daily routines, physical space, and one's outlook on the opposite sex or on other relationships. All the subjects in this sample expressed a desire to be married and felt the time spent on mate selection activities was very meaningful to them. Using the survey results in combination with the content of the interviews, a model of this occupation was developed that reflects research findings (Figure 4-1).

Model of the Occupation of Mate Selection

The occupation consists of a repeated succession of four stages of activities, as portrayed in the middle circle of Figure 4-1. These stages have been labeled as meeting/pre-dating activities, early dating activities, steady dating activities, and engagement/commitment activities, based on the results and conclusions of this study (Krishnagiri, 1994). The activities at each stage can be further grouped into dating activities and preparation activities, as described previously. Meeting activities are those that are intended to lead to meeting potential dates/mates. Data were collected on where people meet but not on how they meet. However, from the survey and the interviews, it was determined that meeting activities constitute a separate group of activities, distinctive from early dating activities. Early dating activities are those that involve preparing for and actually spending time with the other individual, in order to get to know him or her. Steady dating activities are those that lead to an increase in involvement and time spent with one other, developing love,

and further exploring compatibility. Engagement/commitment activities are those that lead to an almost complete mixing of lives and routines and involve love.

Actions are a subdivision of the activities within this occupation. An example of this is the meeting activity of placing an advertisement on the Internet or in the newspaper. This activity may consist of several actions, such as choosing the Web site on which to advertise, writing the profile, and screening and corresponding with respondents, among others. Information at the level of actions within each activity was not collected systematically in this study, but the existence of this level was indicated by the interview data.

Engagement in this occupation was described as beginning as soon as one desires to find a mate and begins to search for mates and/or acts upon romantic feelings when faced with them. This may occur as early as pubescence, but, as the data in this study showed, for many individuals, meeting and subsequently dating appears to begin in high school.

The first chunks of activities engaged in during the occupation of choosing a mate are the meeting activities, followed by early dating activities, steady dating activities, and, finally, engaged/committed activities (see Figure 4-1). These groups of activities are not mutually exclusive, as the intersecting shapes indicate. As revealed in the interview data, activities and actions may belong to either of the adjacent stages, depending on the individual couple and the purpose the activity holds for them. The general sequencing from one stage to another indicates that this occupation of choosing a mate is a dynamic process.

Engagement in the occupation does not necessarily mean that the process is a steadily progressing sequence from meeting to commitment. As the results of the study showed, people begin dating in high school but do not get married for many years. Participants reported having had several serious relationships prior to the one in which they were currently engaged. Mate selection has many beginnings, reversions, and stalls. For example, if a meeting activity does not result in someone to date, then the meeting activities are repeated until someone is found. Another example is a couple engaging in steady dating activities: if one or both partners do not wish to, or are unable to, proceed to the next step of the process, they may linger in this stage of activities until they can move forward or disengage from the relationship. If they disengage, both individuals typically start the process all over again.

The intent with which one engages in the activities of mate selection at any given time also dictates the pace and stage of the occupation. For instance, if meeting activities are engaged in with the intent of exploring and learning about relationships (as they usually are when first beginning this occupation) or for being sexually satisfied for an evening, then the individual generally does not proceed further than early dating activities. On the other hand, if the individual is meeting to date with the intent of selecting a long-term mate and is using this opportunity to screen the individual as a prospective long-term partner, then the activities may continue to the next stage and at a rapid pace. This difference in intent is dependent upon the readiness of the individual to engage in a long-term relationship, which in turn is dependent upon many factors, such as emotional maturity and economic status.

Another factor affecting the temporality of this process is the individual nature and compatibility of each couple, resulting in possibly a short period of steady dating activities before a long period of engaged/committed activities. This is evident in the varying lengths of courtship reported. The varying nature of the pace of the occupation is indicated in the figure by the dashed wave encompassing the occupation.

During engagement in any of the activities in the sequence, the relationship may be terminated for a great many reasons, and the individual begins once again with meeting activities. The succession of activities then continues, contingent upon the success of the previous step of the process, as illustrated in the model by the arrows leading back to the meeting activities (see Figure 4-1). If an individual separates, divorces, becomes widowed, or for some other reason is no longer committed to the partner, engagement in mate selection may be renewed, as supported by the interview data.

An individual's overall performance in this occupation and the desire to be engaged in it are influenced by a host of variables. These variables include level of emotional maturity, emotional attraction, physical attraction, needs of the individual, families' perspectives, friends' sanctions,

societal/cultural trends, values, age, life goals, economic status, one's previous dating experience, and limitations of the individual. These variables manifest themselves as preferences in a mate, characteristics one likes or dislikes, and the influences one perceives as affecting the selection of a mate. These factors were gleaned from both the survey and interview data. They are indicated in the left oval of Figure 4-1.

Engagement in the occupation of mate selection, at any point and at any level, in turn affects the daily routines and lifestyles of those individuals involved. For example, the data indicated that engagement in this occupation impacted the relationships one had with one's family, friends, and coworkers. Additionally, it impacted choices of leisure, work, and rest occupations and when and how they were performed, emotional well-being, motor performance, division of time and labor, and the desire to engage in the occupation. These elements are indicated in the oval on the right side of Figure 4-1.

Each arrow in the model, besides indicating the direction of the succession of events, also indicates feedback influences. That is, if one is engaged in steady dating activities with another and something happens to terminate the process at this point, the experience of the relationship affects one's engagement in the occupation at all levels: the occupation, the activities, and the actions. Similarly, the effects of the occupation on daily routines provide feedback and influence engagement in the next group of mate selection activities at all levels. This was indicated by the overwhelming majority of the study sample that reported a high influence of previous relationships on current ones.

The nature of the sequence of activities in this occupation is dependent upon the cultural milieu to which an individual belongs. That is, the methods used to select a mate and the rules and rituals of a particular culture delineate the specific activities and their sequence, as has been reported in the literature (Geary et al., 2004; Hamon & Ingoldsby, 2003; Miller & Todd, 1998; Shackelford et al., 2005). In some cultures, there is a definite order to the activities with little room for variation. In others, there are very few rules and much flexibility. In Western culture and American society, the predominant method of choosing a mate is the love method described by many. In this method, there are no rules per se, but the process generally progresses from meeting to dating and then perhaps to engagement and marriage.

Challenges to participation in this occupation were mentioned. These mostly related to finding the "right one." That is, the challenge was in finding people who matched desired characteristics and traits, as well as reciprocating feelings. Several participants mentioned the number of years they have dated or described previous relationships to illustrate this difficulty.

In summary, the occupation of choosing a mate is actively engaged in from the time of adolescence to the point of actually being in a long-term committed relationship. It may be resumed at other stages of life when one is divorced, separated, widowed, not committed to an existing relationship, or even while engaging in other relationships simultaneously. The occupation consists of four stages of activities in sequence. Each of these consists of several activities and actions. The occupation, as well as its various components, are influenced by a host of variables and in turn influence many elements. The duration and pace of the occupation is dependent on a variety of factors. This model was developed from, and thus limited to, heterosexuals.

Study 2: Adults Who Have a Physical Disability

Given the description of the occupation based on typical adults, I became curious as to the nature of this occupation in adults who had an obvious physical disability and how it might be different. The literature on mate selection in those with disability primarily focused on the practical issues of how to engage in sex and sexual expression despite disability (Ducharme & Gill, 1997; Faulkner, 2008; Howland & Rintala, 2001; McCabe, Cummins, & Deeks, 2000) or on the psychosocial aspects of the dating process if one has a disability (Hwang, Johnston, & Smith, 2007; Lease, Cohen, & Dahlbeck, 2007; Taleporos & McCabe, 2003). There were no studies found on the activities, actions, or skills necessary for those with a physical disability to engage in mate selection. Therefore, the aim of the second study was to compare the activities, actions, processes, routines, contexts, preferences, and influence of the occupation on daily activities, meaning, and time use in mate selection in those with an obvious physical disability.

Methods

For the second study, pilot interviews were conducted to gather information that might have to be added to the survey to improve its fit to people with disabilities. Questions were added that solicited type and length of disability as well as barriers to dating. The survey was then revised and piloted to ensure the adequacy of the questions. The sample for the survey was obtained through Independent Living Centers in the state of Virginia, through personal recruitment at wheelchair basketball association events, and through veterans support groups. Through the local independent living center, the surveys were mailed out by the center to a list of addresses on their database. Those listed on the database who were age 21 or older and who had disclosed a physical disability were invited to participate in the study. Disabilities due to spinal cord injury, amputation, spina bifida, cerebral palsy, polio, arthritis, traumatic brain injury, and other such diagnoses resulting in possible physical limitations were selected from within the database. The final mailing was done by the center in order to protect individuals' privacy. A total of 65 people from across

the state returned the survey after two reminder postcards were sent. In addition, 21 people were interviewed in depth, 19 of whom had a disability and two who were nondisabled spouses. Some of the interviewees were chosen from the survey sample based on their affirmative response to being interviewed, and others were recruited via snowball sampling. That is, referrals from earlier participants were contacted and invited to be part of the study.

The survey sample in Study 2 included 21 women and 43 men, with a mean age of 39.79 years. The majority were single (63%). Almost all had completed high school, with 30% moving on to some college. All spoke English as their primary language. About 41% of participants held some sort of job, from professional employment to work within the service industry. Many (42%) were unemployed or retired, and 9% were students. The sample was representative in terms of race, ethnicity, and religion to the population of the state of Virginia, where the research originated. The average length of disability was 19 years, and the group had an average of 15 years of dating experience. The interview sample included 13 men and 8 women with 16 White and 5 Black subjects. The majority incurred a disability due to spinal cord injury (62%).

Analysis of the data followed a similar path to that of the first study. The objective questions in the survey were converted and coded for statistical analysis. The open-ended questions required reduction and classification of data prior to coding for analysis. After repetitions were eliminated and synonyms were grouped, the list of activities was classified along the two dimensions used in the first study. Data were first classified by the types of activity and then by the socialization involved in doing the activity. Two graduate students and the researcher independently rated the list of activities along these two dimensions. There was 100% agreement between the raters on type of activity and on the social dimension. Each subject's answers were then coded along these two dimensions to be used for analysis. The interviews were transcribed verbatim and then subjected to content analysis (Grbich, 1999). Correlations between the interview and survey data were sought along with an understanding of the purpose of these activities. Comparisons of data from this sample and the sample from the first study were also made.

Results From Study 2

After analysis of the survey and interview data, a comparison was made with the data on typical adults from Study 1. While the data acquired from this sample did not change the overall model of the occupation, there were several differences in what influenced the performance of activities and what impact engagement in the occupation had for this group. That is, the stages and processes of the occupation remained the same for people with a physical disability. Additionally, the types of activities at each stage and the categories were the same except for the addition of one category, that of educating the date. The education activities included providing information on one's disability, ability to perform sexually, physiological issues, adaptations needed, and disability awareness. This activity was reported to occur at various stages, depending on the comfort level and experience of the subject. That is, some subjects wanted to "lay out all the cards" at the beginning of the relationship, and others waited to see if the relationship progressed before they addressed this topic.

The average length of time spent increased as one moved through the stages of dating in both samples. The purpose and meaning of the performance of many of the activities were the same in the two groups. The desire to find a companion for life in a committed relationship was expressed similarly.

A second difference between the two samples was in the actual performance of the activities. That is, activities showed a distinct difference in the way they were performed. Subjects reported that dating and preparation activities typically required additional planning, preparation, and adaptation. For example, if the prospective mate wanted to go to a particular restaurant or entertainment venue, the person with the disability would first need to find out if the place was accessible and how to maneuver in that environment. Examples of barriers included limited access to tables or restrooms, historical places with no wheelchair access, and people's homes not being accessible. If the event was a long one and the individual had medical or physiological needs, extra planning and preparation was required to determine how these would be managed and who would assist if needed. In some instances, the whole activity might have to be adapted or not performed at all if the venue was not accessible or accommodations could not be made. In other instances, subjects reported that they were not physically capable of participating in some of the activities in which the date wanted to engage. While these instances were specifically related to the person's limitations, examples include not being able to go canoeing or dancing.

Not all participants indicated equal needs for adapting and planning. The older and more experienced subjects adapted more easily. Their interviews reflected less frustration and better problem solving. For example, an experienced man talked about setting up the lighting, music, wine, and access to the sofa before leaving home, so that when he and his date came home, he could slide right out of the chair and onto the sofa without losing the spontaneity of the moment. Data from the interviews indicated several factors that dictated a need for change in performance of activities. These were level of functioning with disability, date's expectations, resources available, experience in negotiating the environment, and experience in dating.

The last significant difference between the two samples was in the time spent for preparation activities while engaged in this occupation. While most preparation activities described were similar to the first sample, differences occurred in two areas. If a person had physiological or medical needs, he or she spent extra time adapting his or her routines to fit the needs of the date activity. Second, he or she spent more time in setting up the environment in preparation for the date.

Challenges to participation in this occupation were mentioned by most subjects. Interviewees complained about the difficulty of finding mates for the long term who were willing to live with their disability and accommodations. They also reported being disappointed very often when relationships did not progress. Their perceptions were that this was due to their disabilities and special needs.

Despite the differences just described in the performance of the activities within the occupation, overall, people with disabilities appeared to have similar concepts of the form and function and desire for the mate selection process. They engaged in similar types of activities as did the Study 1 sample, with the addition of the activity of educating about disability. The actions were adapted only when needed. Health was an added factor that influenced their engagement in the occupation. The subjects identified themselves as sexual beings and expressed in many ways the need to be as "normal" as possible with respect to the dating process. Spending time and energy on dating activities was valuable to them. These results did not significantly change the model of the occupation of mate selection, although it did add detail to some of the elements within the model.

Study 3: Mate Selection in Older Adults

Societal changes and trends lead to changes in the activities in which people engage. Aging of the population of the United States has led to a reoccurrence of some activities in later life as well as the development of new occupations. Dating and mate selection, an occupation typically associated with younger adults, is now recurring with increased frequency in older adults. Study 3 involved the dating and mating habits of older adults who are active and living independently in the community.

The literature on mate selection in older adults contains data on some aspects of the occupation but nothing to describe the typical process, the activities and routines involved, the time it takes, or the meaning it holds for this age group. Information available on the topic can be divided into a few distinct dimensions.

Beginning conceptualizations of the meaning and functions of dating in the elderly exist based on some older and newer qualitative studies (Bulcroft & Bulcroft, 1991; Bulcroft & O'Connor, 1986; Dickson, Hughes, & Walker, 2005). Sexuality among older adults is described more often (Howard, O'Neill, & Travers, 2006; Manderson, Bennett, & Sheldrake, 1999; Zeiss & Kasl-Godley, 2001). Cohabitation versus marriage in older adults has been minimally explored (Chevan, 1996; King & Scott, 2005; Moore & Stratton, 2002). Activities of dating in the elderly have been reported in some older literature, but more as secondary data rather than as the focus of research (Bulcroft & Bulcroft, 1985; Lopata, 1979). Courtship literature, while focused on adults and the mate selection process, is not based on older adult data and does not purport to apply to them (Hamon & Ingoldsby, 2003; Shackelford et al., 2005). Research on characteristics sought in a mate are primarily available for younger people, as described in the literature for Study 1. Study 3 was done because the literature on the form, function, and meaning of the occupation of mate selection in the elderly is meager. Additionally, I was curious about how the model of the occupation might change with the addition of data from the elderly population.

Methods

The sample for Study 3 was acquired using advertising and personal contact with older adults at senior centers, senior housing, and senior activity groups at hospitals in Florida. I volunteered to speak on topics of interest to the seniors in order to make additional contacts. In this study, because the age group was different and life experience is known to have a significant impact on engagement in this occupation, the decision was made to gather data through in-depth interviews, focus groups, and informal discussions with senior activity groups before proceeding to tailor a survey to this population. The following results are from interviews, focus groups, and informal discussions only. The data reflect not only the experiences of elders who were dating, but also those who have purposefully chosen not to date. Although examining why people may choose not to engage in this occupation is part of the long-term plan for this research program, in this case, it was the senior adults who raised the topic and insisted on discussing it. In general, most of the subjects were eager to tell their stories and spoke at length on the subject.

A total of 17 subjects were interviewed individually, and six people split into two focus groups. The majority were White, with only two Black and one Hispanic participants. Half of the sample belonged to the Jewish faith, and the other half were either Catholic or of some Christian denomination. Their income levels ranged from lower middle class (receiving only Social Security benefits) to independently wealthy individuals. All were very active in the community and kept themselves occupied through a variety of activities.

Results of Study 3

Based only on the qualitative data, it appears that the stages, process, and activities of this occupation remained the same with this group as in Study 1. There were, however, differences in the conceptualization of the occupation of mate selection in the elderly.

Subjects were asked to define and describe dating and mate selection, both currently and when they were young. In telling their story of marriages, relationships, and dating, it appeared that the subjects currently viewed dating as an activity that is engaged in for the purposes of finding companionship and not necessarily toward the goal of getting married. Although these subjects had experienced significant committed relationships in their lives, at the point that they had participated in the study, they were alone and doing well as independently functioning adults. They expressed no desire to enter into a marriage as a consequence of dating. Some reasons for this included financial challenges, health challenges, family challenges, and a lack of potential candidates. Participants also stated that they did not and could not have children, so they questioned why they should get married. They did state that finding a person to share meaningful activities with was their main purpose. If the relationship were to progress further, some said they would be open to a more committed relationship and would consider living together.

Comparing the subjects' notions of their current idea of dating to what they thought of it when they were younger, it was easy to note the shift of purpose, away from the purpose of procreation and making a life together and toward the purposes of companionship. Additionally, the criteria the potential date/mate needed to meet appeared to be different for an elder.

The characteristics desired in a date by an elder were more personality based, such as basic manners and having a sense of humor. The criteria these subjects used when younger included, not only the previous list, but also physical appearance, financial potential (job), education, religion, and other factors. Overall, the notion of dating appeared to be of a more carefree nature with no marriage-oriented goal, instead seeking someone with whom to share time.

Dating activities named in Study 3 were similar to those found in Studies 1 and 2. They can be classified into the five major groups from the earlier studies: dining, arts/entertainment, physical/sexual/romantic, homemaking, and sports (see Table 4-1). Essentially, the pace and level of participation was different in elders. Most go with the flow of whatever the other suggests. Women allow the man to suggest at the beginning because they are not sure what the man may be able to afford. If the man was expecting the woman to pay her half of dating expenses, or later even pay for them both once in a while, the female interviewees said that they would not continue in the relationship.

A significant difference in the form and function of the occupation in elders, as compared to Study 1, was in the details of the preparation activities. Two major activities were mentioned that were similar to Study 1. The first was dressing. The subjects stated that they would just dress normally for the occasion, as opposed to wearing something special for a date. Preparations for health-related activities were another item mentioned: these are special preparations for sexual activity, such as medications. Other preparation activities mentioned by participants in Studies 1 and 2, such as writing love notes, were not mentioned significantly by the elderly subjects.

Another difference between the responses of the older adults and those of participants in Studies 1 and 2 was the amount of time spent in the occupation. The older adults averaged one to four dates a week, with an average of 3 hours per date. While it appeared that the time spent with the person increased as the relationship progressed, most wanted to keep their daily routines intact and did not want dating to interfere with their desired activities. For example, subjects reported wanting to keep their bridge groups, exercise, and regular social meetings like senior singles groups as part of the weekly routines. The date activities were either outside of these routine activities or were included in them. This point further supports the apparent meaning of this occupation to the elderly population: it is for companionship rather than for a life-altering outcome. Specifically, dating is undertaken in order to have someone with whom to share an activity or hold hands.

Lastly, challenges to participation in this occupation were mentioned frequently by the older adults in Study 3. They were issues related to aging and not being able to always participate in some activities, as well as the difficulty in finding someone with compatible interests and characteristics. The significant ratio of more women to men and the perceived desire of men to find a "nurse with a purse" were also described. The majority of the subjects were comfortable with, and accepted, the possibility that they might not succeed in finding a mate, not only due to the challenges but also because of their previous relationship experiences.

Overall, the form of the occupation remained the same for most elderly research subjects. They participated in similar activities of dating as did those in Studies 1 and 2, although at a slower pace and with lower intensity, based on abilities. Health and resiliency were added factors that influenced engagement in this occupation. If they were unsuccessful in meeting compatible mates, they were comfortable with choosing not to engage in this occupation. The function of the occupation was significantly different for them, as was its meaning. Their life experiences, relationship histories, and economic status were major factors in their lack of desire to engage in this occupation in order to find a mate for marriage. In essence, if they chose to engage in this occupation, they were looking for an activity partner, a companion who fit into their daily life. Consequently, the average amount of time they spent on this occupation appeared to be significantly lower and was congruent with their "take it or leave it" attitude about prospective mates.

CONTRIBUTION TO OCCUPATIONAL SCIENCE

The primary contribution of this line of research is to begin describing the form, function, and meaning of this important occupation in a person's life. A basic understanding of the occupation of mate selection is provided by the results, describing the type of activities involved, their functions, and their impact on daily routines, occupations, and other relationships, as well as its meaningfulness. The differences in the way the activities and actions were performed by different populations, the challenges that can accompany engagement in this occupation, and the variations in its meaning at different stages of life supply further depth of understanding in regard to this important, and little studied, occupation.

IMPLICATIONS FOR PRACTICE

A greater understanding of the what, how, and why of an occupation in different populations allows a profession like occupational therapy to know what to expect, what is typical for a population. Supported by that knowledge, a practitioner can facilitate a client's successful engagement in this important occupation when the client identifies this as valued and meaningful. For example, knowing various ways that people with physical disabilities have problem solved issues relating to spontaneity of the moment or access to entertainment venues, a therapist can not only prepare the client to expect certain issues, but also have information ready to assist the client in having a personally satisfying dating and mate selection experience.

LEARNING SUPPORTS

Key Concepts for Strengthening Insight Into the Occupation of Mate Selection

- Mate selection as a universal human occupation
- Cultural variations on acceptable dating behaviors
- Purpose of occupation shifts with stage of life
- A process consisting of a series of actions/activities and decisions
- Time and energy involved in engaging in the occupation
- Influence on day-to-day routines
- Influence on other occupations
- Peer and family influences on mate selection activities and decisions
- Influence of experience on actions and decisions

Building Insight Into Your Personal Understanding of the Occupation of Mate Selection

Discuss the following topics in small groups.

- What is the purpose of dating for you at this time? Is it different than the purpose you had 5 years ago?

- List acceptable behaviors for dating at each stage of the dating process, and compare with others in the discussion group.

- How much time do you typically spend engaged in dating activities? Is the amount of time different as you get to know the person better? Does the quality of time you spend and the type of activities you choose shift the longer you have been with an individual?

- How do you feel when you have met someone you are interested in? What interests you about them? Where did the criteria for your interests come from? Your family, your friends, your personal interests?

- What criteria do you use to not date someone or to stop dating them? Where did these criteria stem from?

- Think about the energy and time you spend in preparing to go out with someone you find interesting. Does this change the longer you have known the person?

- Find an example in your life when you have shifted your typical routines or behaviors to meet someone or to make an impression on him or her. What does this say about the role of this occupation in your life? Its impact on one's life?

Understanding Clinical Implications

Discuss the following topics in small groups.

- How do you feel when you meet someone who has an obvious disability? What questions and concerns come to your mind? Given the desire to be as "normal" as possible, how would you prepare an individual with a disability to engage in this occupation? How would you prepare him or her to deal with possible rejection?

- Put yourself in the shoes of a person in a wheelchair. What would you have to do to plan a fun evening within your community with an able-bodied individual who likes Thai food, bowling, and cozy discussions on the couch with wine? The goal is to make things run as smoothly as possible and keep the mood for romance.

- In your experience, how are routine activities such as bathing, dressing, and grooming impacted when you are engaged in the mate selection process? Now, consider what happens when an individual with a disability performs these same activities differently or

slowly. What adaptations need to be made to the mate selection process for these individuals?

- Similarly, what is the impact of the disability on activities and instrumental activities of daily living and how might this influence typical dating activities? What adaptations need to be made with the elderly who have decreased stamina for activities?

Focus on Research

Discuss the following topics in small groups.

- Given the personal nature of this occupation, what methods beyond surveys and interviews are useful in gathering information? What kind of data will each method provide on the topic?

- Is the model of the occupation provided accurate with respect to your own experience? What seems to be missing? What needs to be researched further?

- What other research questions come to mind when you consider this topic? Questions may be clinically oriented as well as basic-science oriented.

REFERENCES

Bulcroft, K., & Bulcroft, R. (1985). Dating and courtship in later-life: An exploratory study. In W. A. Peterson & J. Quadagno (Eds.), *Social bonds in later-life: Aging and interdependence* (pp. 115-126). Beverly Hills, CA: Sage Publications.

Bulcroft, K., & O'Connor, M. (1986). The importance of dating relationships in quality of life for older persons. *Family Relations, 35*, 397-401. doi:10.2307/584367

Bulcroft, R. A., & Bulcroft, K. A. (1991). The nature and functions of dating in later life. *Research on Aging, 13*(2), 244-260. doi:10.1177/0164027591132007

Buss, D. M. (2006). Strategies of human mating. *Psychological Topics, 15*(2), 239-260.

Buss, D. M., Shackelford, T. K., Kirkpatrick, L. A., & Larsen, R. J. (2001). A half century of mate preferences: The cultural evolution of values. *Journal of Marriage & Family, 63*(2), 491-504. doi:10.1111/j.1741-3737.2001.00491.x

Buston, P. M., & Emlen, S. T. (2003). Cognitive processes underlying human mate choice: The relationship between self-perception and mate preference in Western society. *Proceedings of the National Academy of the Sciences, 3-6* (Early ed.), 1-6. doi:10.1073/pnas.1533220100

Chevan, A. (1996). As cheaply as one: Cohabitation in the older population. *Journal of Marriage and the Family, 58*(3), 656-667.

Clark, F. A., Parham, D., Carlson, M. E., Frank, G., Jackson, J., Pierce, D. ... Zemke, R. (1991). Occupational science: Academic innovation in the service of occupational therapy's future. *American Journal of Occupational Therapy, 45*(4), 300-310. doi:10.5014/ajot.45.4.300

Davis, A. (1998). Age differences in dating and marriage: Reproductive strategies or social preferences. *Current Anthropology, 39*(3), 374-380.

Dickson, F. C., Hughes, P. C., & Walker, K. L. (2005). An exploratory investigation into dating among later life women. *Western Journal of Communication, 69*(1), 67-82.

Ducharme, S. H., & Gill, K. M. (1997). *Sexuality after spinal cord injury.* Baltimore, MD: Brookes Publishing.

Eagly, A. H., & Wood, W. (1999). The origins of sex differences in human behavior: Evolved dispositions versus social roles. *American Psychologist, 54,* 408-423.

Faulkner, M. (2008). Easy does it. Dating in recovery: Pitfalls and possibilities. *Paradigm, 13*(1), 19.

Gangestad, S. W., & Simpson, J. A. (2000). The evolution of human mating: Trade-offs and strategic pluralism. *Behavioral and Brain Sciences, 23*(4), 573-587.

Geary, D. C., Vigil, J., & Byrd-Craven, J. (2004). Evolution of human mate choice. *Journal of Sex Research, 41*(1), 27-42. doi:10.1080/00224490409552211

Grbich, C. (1999). *Qualitative research in health.* Thousand Oaks, CA: Sage Publications.

Hamon, R. R., & Ingoldsby, B. B. (Ed.). (2003). *Mate selection across cultures.* Thousand Oaks, CA: Sage Publications.

Hersch, L. R., & Paul, L. (1996). Human male mating strategies: I. Courtship tactics of the "quality" and "quantity" alternatives. *Ethology and Sociobiology, 17,* 55-70. doi:10.1016/0162-3095(96)00128-8

Howard, J. R., O'Neill, S., & Travers, C. (2006). Factors affecting sexuality in older Australian women: Sexual interest, sexual arousal, relationships and sexual distress in older Australian women. *Climacteric, 9,* 355-367.

Howland, C. A., & Rintala, D. H. (2001). Dating behaviors of women with physical disabilities. *Sexuality & Disability, 19*(1), 41-70. doi:10.1023/A:1010768804747

Hwang, K., Johnston, M., & Smith, J. K. (2007). Romantic attachment in individuals with physical disabilities. *Rehabilitation Psychology. 52*(2), 184-195. doi:10.1037/0090-5550.52.2.184

King, V., & Scott, M. E. (2005). A comparison of cohabiting relationships among older and younger adults. *Journal of Marriage and Family, 67*(2), 271-285. doi:10.1111/j.0022-2445.2005.00115.x

Klimek, D. (1979). *Beneath mate selection and marriage: The unconscious motives in human pairing.* New York, NY: Van Nostrand Reinhold.

Krishnagiri, S. (1994). *The occupation of mate selection* (Unpublished doctoral dissertation). University of Southern California, Los Angeles, CA.

Lease, S. H., Cohen, J. E., & Dahlbeck, D. T. (2007). Body and sexual esteem as mediators of the physical disability-interpersonal competencies relation. *Rehabilitation Psychology, 52*(4), 399-408. doi:10.1037/0090-5550.52.4.399

Lemieux, R. (1996). Picnics, flowers, and moonlight strolls: An exploration of routine love behaviors. *Psychological Reports, 78,* 91-98.

Liu, J. H., Campbell, S. M., & Condie, H. (1995). Ethnocentrism in dating preferences for an American sample: The ingroup bias in social context. *European Journal of Social Psychology, 25,* 95-115. doi:10.1002/ejsp.2420250108

Lopata, H. Z. (1979). *Women as widows.* New York, NY: Elsevier.

Manderson, L., Bennett, L. R., & Sheldrake, M. (1999). Sex, social institutions, and social structure: Anthropological contributions to the study of sexuality. *Annual Review of Sex Research, 10,* 184-209.

Martin, J. N., Bradford, L. J., Drzewiecka, J. A., & Chitgopekar, A. S. (2003). Intercultural dating patterns among young white U.S. Americans: Have they changed in the past 20 years? *Howard Journal of Communications, 14,* 53-74.

McCabe, M. P., Cummins, R. A., & Deeks, A. A. (2000). Sexuality and quality of life among people with physical disability. *Sexuality and Disability, 18*(2), 115-123. doi:10.1023/A:1005562813603

Miller, G. F., & Todd, P. M. (1998). Mate choice turns cognitive. *Trends in Cognitive Sciences, 2*(5), 190-198. doi:10.1016/S1364-6613(98)01169-3

Moore, A. J., & Stratton, D. C. (2002). *Older men speak for themselves.* New York, NY: Springer Publishing.

Murstein, B. I. (1976). *Who will marry whom? Theories and research in marital choice.* New York, NY: Springer Publishing.

Nofz, M. P. (1984). Fantasy-testing assessment: A proposed model for the investigation of mate selection. *Family Relations, 33,* 273-281.

Roche, J. P. (1986). Premarital sex: Attitudes and behaviors by dating stages. *Adolescence, 21*(81), 107-121.

Sabatelli, R. M. (1988). Exploring relationship satisfaction: A social exchange perspective on the interdependence between theory, research and practice. *Family Relations, 37,* 217-222.

Schwartz, M. A., & Scott, B. M. (2002). *Marriages and families: Diversity and change* (4th ed.). Upper Saddle River, NJ: Prentice Hall.

Shackelford, T. K., Schmitt, D. P., & Buss, D. M. (2005). Universal dimensions of human mate preferences. *Personality and Individual Differences, 39*(2), 447-458. doi:10.1016/j.paid.2005.01.023

Surra, C. A., Cottle, N. R., Gray, C. R., Harmell, K., & Vandewater, E. A. (2000). Activity preferences, companionship, and progress in premarital relationships. *National Council on Family Relations Annual Conference Proceedings.* Retrieved from http://search.epnet.com/login.aspx?direct=true&db=sih&an=SN00126

Surra, C. A., & Hughes, D. K. (1997). Commitment processes in accounts of the development of premarital relationships. *Journal of Marriage & Family, 59,* 5-21. doi:10.2307/353658

Taleporos, G., & McCabe, M. P. (2003). Relationships, sexuality and adjustment among people with physical disability. *Sexual and Relationship Therapy, 18,* 25-43. doi:10.1080/1468199031000061245

U. S. Department of Labor Employment and Training Administration. (n.d.). 2006 O*NET Resource Center. Retrieved from http://www.onetcenter.org/taxonomy/2006/list.html

Zeiss, A. M., & Kasl-Godley, J. (2001). Sexuality in older adult's relationships. *Generations, 25*(2), 18-25.

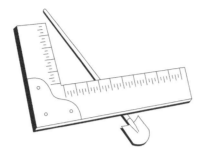

Environmental Influences on Daily Time Use and Well-Being

Wendy H. Wood, PhD, OTR, FAOTA

Research is autobiographical. By this, I mean that research careers often arise from personal interests and influential events, as well as from people with whom we have worked, mentors, and others who have touched our lives in poignant ways. Research careers likewise arise from irrepressible and often problematic puzzles that capture our imaginations. I once heard Elizabeth Yerxa, the founder of occupational science in the United States (Yerxa et al., 1989), refer to such attractions as *clinical irritations*. By a clinical irritation, Yerxa meant some irresistible hook that demands a practitioner's attention, like an itch that will not quit. It seems to me that the clinical irritations from which our research careers emerge are as much emotional as they are intellectual, as much personal as professional. They reveal their nature and power over us as they increasingly direct our time and attention toward this and away from that. In this way, we come to see that we actually like to do research. Furthermore, despite a near infinitude of possible topics, we find ourselves launched onto a very specific trajectory of inquiry. So launched, we persist. Why? Because we have been captured somehow by our research and hope, by pursuing it, to build new knowledge that supports a more occupationally just world.

Or, so has been true for me. When I graduated with a bachelor of science in occupational therapy from Tufts University, I never imagined that one day I would enjoy conducting research in the discipline of occupational science, let alone find this endeavor to be both meaningful and satisfying. Nor did I imagine that I would be interested in deriving theory from research to support the practice of occupational therapists in nursing homes. But years of immersion in practice, coupled with other influential experiences and people, worked on me, and I suddenly found myself embarking on a post-professional master's degree in occupational therapy at the University of Southern California (USC). I subsequently earned a PhD in Occupational Science from USC 20 years after first entering occupational therapy. While earning these degrees and since, I have studied the philosophical and historical foundations of occupational therapy, conducted research on the psychological well-being of zoo chimpanzees, and circled fully back to where I have been most at home: working on behalf of older adults in residential institutions, especially people with dementia.

I trace the roots of the clinical irritation that has compelled my research to a puzzle that drew my attention well

Pierce, D. (Ed.).
Occupational Science for Occupational Therapy (pp. 49-65).
© 2014 SLACK Incorporated.

before I knew occupational therapy existed. That puzzle was this: why do people often act one way in one context, including being so good at doing things and interacting with others, and yet act so differently in other contexts, including not being much good at much anything at all? For instance, when I was 12 years old, I was a popular star (or so it felt) during the summer when I won the outstanding camper award at my overnight camp. Yet, I was a dismal failure (or so it felt) later that year as I transitioned into a new high school. How did that happen, and so quickly? Surely I had not changed that much since the glory days of summer. Or had I? Later, as a camp counselor for children with autism, I was struck by how my campers settled down and into activities when given reliable routines and manageable tasks, yet became intensely agitated and unable to function in the absence of these things. What happened that such different personas and abilities were elicited?

Similar fascinations haunted me as an occupational therapy student. My first Level II fieldwork took place at a state psychiatric hospital in which two dueling philosophies of treatment were evident. One philosophy was based on a belief in the therapeutic power of activity; its practitioners, including several occupational and recreational therapists, sought to develop patients' interests and skills by offering activities that were fun, engaging, and likely to succeed. The key to this approach was taking patients to the bright and upbeat activity building, which afforded a host of appealing things to do from sensory activities to crafts, recreational games, and physical activities. The other philosophy was behaviorist in nature; its practitioners, including many psychiatrists and psychologists, sought to shape desirable behaviors through a system of rewards and punishments. Key to this approach was the view that pleasurable activity could be used as a reward for socially appropriate behavior. Similarly, withholding pleasurable activities could be used to negatively sanction problematic behaviors.

When I first visited a residential ward at this state hospital, what immediately caught my nose and eye were smells of urine and feces coupled with a swarm of patients pacing about muttering and yelling, seemingly miserable, in various states of undress. To my amazement, I had observed some of these same patients in the activity building; there at least some had looked and acted like reasonably functioning human beings while doing things. One Friday morning, a patient set his mattress on fire, prompting an emergency evacuation. Off-ward privileges were subsequently revoked for all other patients on the ward. Hence, no one could go outside for 3 days. Consistent with a behaviorist philosophy, it was reasoned that the fire-setter's peers, given how upset they were about their revoked outdoor privileges, would negatively sanction the fire-setting behavior themselves. I was horrified by this decision. After all, how would I feel if I were locked inside that ward for 3 days?

I came away from that fieldwork experience vowing that I would never again work in a residential institution. But what I could not appreciate then was that I had begun to develop a belief system that strongly aligned with Adolf Meyer's (1922) philosophy of occupational therapy, a philosophy that was originally implemented in psychiatric institutions. Subsequently, as a practitioner with older adults, I came to view my work through an environmental lens. This was because significant changes in behavior often appeared attributable to variations in the occupational opportunities and supports that a person's immediate social and physical contexts provided, or failed to provide. So compelling was this insight that I published a supporting account of a treatment session with a woman with dementia I called Betty (Wood, 1995). Betty was a former beautician who was known on the dementia unit as a screamer because she repeatedly yelled for her deceased husband to please come help her. In my article, I described how Betty had completely transformed, in little over 1 hour's time, from a so-called screamer into a competent beautician and wife and then back again. This striking transformation was simply due to the lack, then the presence, and then the lack again of opportunities to succeed in personally meaningful occupations.

Elizabeth Yerxa once proposed to my class of post-professional students that disability resides in the environment. I recall being struck by this idea given how parsimoniously it expressed what I had witnessed clinically. *Yes, disability resides in the environment*: this insight encapsulated my clinical irritation. It meant that the environment has the power to summon disability and distress just as it has the power to summon ability and well-being. Perennially intrigued by this irritation, I have sought to understand occupational engagement and its relationship to well-being in the context of people's social and physical environs. My overarching research question has consequently been: "How does the immediate social and physical environment influence time-use and well-being each day?"

Having received the Jane Goodall Fellowship for my doctoral studies in occupational science at USC (Wood, 1993, 1996, 1997), I initially pursued my question using a captive primate model. Jane Goodall (1981, 1990; Goodall & Berman, 2000), the renowned researcher of wild chimpanzees, humanitarian, and distinguished professor in occupational therapy at USC, believed that an occupational therapist was well suited to studying how best to enrich the lives of captive chimpanzees in order to optimize their activity patterns and psychological well-being. I once asked her opinion about how long in duration my observations of zoo chimpanzees should last. She replied, "Don't you have bad days?" Goodall, whose research of chimpanzees in Tanzania has been ongoing since 1960, went on to say that if observational research of either people or chimpanzees was to have any scientific validity at all, then sustained observations should be conducted for 2 full days at the very least and ideally much longer. In the following studies, I strove to heed Goodall's advice by insisting on persistent and prolonged observations and engagement.

A Research Program on Environmental Influences on Daily Time Use and Well-Being

Study 1: Environmental Influences on Daily Time Use and Well-Being of Zoo Chimpanzees

The purpose of Study 1 was to explore influences of the social and physical environment on the daily time-use patterns and psychological well-being of a group of zoo chimpanzees. Two theoretical concepts helped to define the study's view of environmental influences: total institutions and ecological microsystems. In his classic work, *Asylums,* Goffman (1961), a sociologist, defined a *total institution* as "a place of residence and work where a large number of like-situated individuals, cut off from the wider society for an appreciable period of time, together lead a formally administered round of life" (p. xiii). Zoos, prisons, and psychiatric institutions are good examples of total institutions. Many characteristics of total institutions are also evident in less restrictive settings, such as nursing homes. Bronfenbrenner, an environmental psychologist, defined *ecological microsystems* as face-to-face settings of daily life such as schools, homes, and workplaces (Bronfenbrenner, 1977; Bronfenbrenner & Crouter, 1993). Bronfenbrenner proposed that the unique physical, sensory, social, and symbolic features of microsystems constantly interact to influence the behavior of individuals and groups therein. Applying these concepts to Study 1, more distal environmental influences were viewed through the lens of a zoo as a total institution, whereas more proximal environmental influences were viewed at the level of the ecological microsystem of a specific enclosed zoo habitat for chimpanzees.

By studying the ecological microsystem of a chimpanzee habitat within a total institution, the study sought to shed light on the assumption of a biological need for occupation prevalent in the occupational therapy profession. In the animal literature, the term *ethological need* is used to describe innate motivations to engage in those behavioral patterns that characterize how members of a species typically live in the habitats to which their biological system and behavioral patterns became co-adapted over evolutionary time (Hughes & Duncan, 1988). Ethological needs are thus innate genetic factors that operate on the motivational systems of animals, whether they live in free-ranging or captive environments. The physical and psychological well-being of animals suffers when they live in environments that constrain their ability to satisfy ethological needs through performance of species-typical activities.

The idea that animal welfare hinges on meeting ethological needs parallels occupational therapy's assumption of a biological need for occupation and its relationship to well-being in people. This assumption dates to Meyer (1922) and remains prevalent today. For example, Reilly (1974) believed that human occupation was driven by biological needs to explore, create, achieve, exercise capacities, and satisfy curiosity. Christiansen and Baum (1991) asserted that "the human organism has an innate drive toward environmental mastery, which can only be met through occupation" (p. 19). Most recently, Wilcock (2006) posited in her occupational theory of human nature that occupation is the primary means through which people develop and sustain optimal health and well-being from birth through old age.

The design of Study 1 allowed systematic investigation of environmental influences on zoo chimpanzees' patterns of time use as well as their biological (ethological) needs for chimpanzee occupations, a dimension of psychological well-being. It asked this main question: What activities, if any, do the Los Angeles Zoo (LAZ) chimpanzees most value as gauged by how and with whom they spend time under different environmental conditions that range from occupational deprivation to relative occupational enrichment? To answer this question, a variety of materials that could be used in exploration and play, nesting, foraging, and tool using were introduced into the chimpanzees' otherwise barren (one might say boring) habitat, and their time-use patterns, or activity budgets, were compared across changing conditions.

Brief Description of Methods

Participants were 11 group-living chimpanzees (*Pan troglodytes*) at LAZ: seven females (ages 38, 26, 15, 10, 8, 6, and 3) and four males (ages 40, 15, 5, and 4). In addition to the two adult males, the group had two matrilineal families of three generations each. At the time of the study, the group's enclosure was quite outdated according to contemporary zoo standards, consisting of a barren concrete mountain, a tool-using device, two tree stumps, and a hammock, in addition to two indoor stalls.

Quantitative and qualitative methods were integrated in this instrumental case study. Yin (2003) defined the case study method as an empirical inquiry that investigates contemporary phenomena within their real-life contexts. Instrumental case studies are conducted when information-rich illustrations of the central phenomenon of interest are available for investigation (Stake, 2000). In this case study, extensive observations prior to formal data collection helped identify five environmental conditions that routinely occurred and differed considerably in opportunities for chimpanzee occupations. For the purpose of this chapter, three conditions pertaining specifically to environmental enrichment are described:

1. **New Enrichment (New ENR).** Materials and objects were introduced into the enclosure to enhance opportunities for participation in activities characteristic of free-ranging chimpanzees (Saturday, Monday) (Table 5-1).

TABLE 5-1

STUDY 1: INTRODUCED ENVIRONMENTAL ENRICHMENT AT THE LOS ANGELES ZOO

TYPE OF ENRICHMENT	DEFINITION
Browse	Sufficient browse was introduced to offer opportunities for exploring, foraging, nest building, object play, and as a source of natural tools. Browse included items such as dried corn stalks, dried bean vines, bamboo, honeysuckle, willow branches, or palm fronds.
Videotapes of wild chimpanzees	A 20-inch television monitor and a videocassette recorder were placed on a viewing stand next to the enclosure to offer opportunities for active orienting and visual exploration. Videotapes showed wild chimpanzees engaged in various activities.
Ice blocks with embedded foods	Foods such as sunflower seeds, peanuts, walnuts, dried fruits, bananas, apples, or pears were frozen in three layers within 9-gallon containers. Four frozen blocks offered opportunities for sustained foraging and tool using.
Tool-using device	A pipe feeder device was used to offer opportunities for tool using. The device consisted of a 5-foot section of PVC pipe with small holes drilled on top. It was mounted into the back stall of the chimpanzees' enclosure and filled with food.
Stuffed burlap sacks	Four burlap sacks were filled with novel objects such as dried grass, pine cones, rolls of adding paper, hard cardboard cylinders, colorful flowers, or socks to offer opportunities for exploring, playing, and nesting.
Full-length mirror	A full-length mirror was placed out of reach but in sight of the chimpanzees. The mirror offered opportunities for active orienting to a chimpanzee's own image and those of his or her peers.

Reprinted with permission from Wood, W. (1998). Environmental influences upon the social choices, occupational behaviors and adapt-edness of zoo chimpanzees: Relevance to occupational therapy. Scandinavian Journal of Occupational Therapy, 5(3), 119-131.

2. **Old Enrichment (Old ENR).** All enrichment materials remained after 1 day of use (Sunday, Tuesday).

3. **No Enrichment (No ENR).** Complete absence of enrichment materials owing to their removal for cleaning and health reasons (Wednesday).

To encompass these conditions, the group was videotaped on consecutive days, Monday through Wednesday, from 12:00 p.m. to 3:00 p.m., with repeated observations across 5 weeks. Researchers' real-time observations were audiorecorded. Altogether, 18 hours equally distributed across the three conditions were randomly selected for analysis.

Quantitatively, a three-by-one factorial design examined how the chimpanzees differently spent time and in what social context during New ENR, Old ENR, and No ENR. The chimpanzees' behaviors were coded using 12 mutually exclusive time-use categories: aggression, object-using, feeding, foraging, grooming, playing, care of nursing offspring, exploring, sexual activities, traveling, watching/idleness, and aberrant behaviors. Six mutually exclusive social contexts were also coded: solitary/nonsocial,

friendly, mother and child, agonistic, submissive, and public orientation. Frequencies of each code were computed to reveal the group's typical activity budgets in each condition, as well as in each social context. Logistical regression analyses and ANOVAs were conducted to identify significant differences in frequencies in the groups' activity budgets and social context across conditions in both the three-by-one and two-by-two factorial designs. Qualitatively, segments of videotape that corresponded with exploring, object using, playing, and aberrant behaviors were analyzed using the constant comparative method (Creswell, 2007).

Summary of Results

Diverse Occupational Choices During New Enrichment and Old Enrichment

During New ENR, the LAZ chimpanzees took advantage of new occupational opportunities as evident in significantly increased durations of time in object using (especially nest building), foraging, and feeding compared to both Old ENR and No ENR (Wood, 1998a, 1998b). The solitary/non-social context was most frequent during New ENR when the chimpanzees were so engaged. Thus, the chimpanzees chose to persist in solitary purposeful occupation when their environment supported this choice. The freshly introduced environmental enrichment appeared to give them a break both from social interaction and also from the long hours of likely boring empty time imposed by No ENR.

The chimpanzees socially reconvened during Old ENR, spending more time in social grooming, social play, and social travel, as well as simply being together when compared with either New ENR or No ENR (Wood, 1998a, 1998b). The species-typical occupations of grooming and playing were most frequent in Old ENR, as was the social context of friendly. Social play was observed to be especially creative during Old ENR, as the group found ways to sustain hour-long play sessions with up to four players. Though not as frequent as in New ENR, the group continued to use objects from day-old materials during Old ENR. Yet, as environmental opportunities for occupations waned during Old ENR, frequencies of aberrant behaviors (i.e., behaviors like mastication of feces or hair plucking that suggest psychological ill-being in captive chimpanzees) correspondingly increased.

To summarize, the chimpanzees' behaviors during New ENR and Old ENR illustrated what was important from their points of view. During these two enriched habitat conditions, the chimpanzees chose to readily exploit opportunities to forage, play, groom, build nests, or otherwise instrumentally use objects. These behavioral choices revealed the value that the chimpanzees placed on species-typical occupations over and above aberrant behaviors and prolonged idleness that, as reported below, predominated when their habitat was in its most barren state (Wood, 1998a). Furthermore, the chimpanzees employed flexibility and imaginativeness in context of exploratory behavior and social play when their habitat was comparatively more barren. This adaptive strategy enhanced their psychological well-being by constituting a resilient resistance to environmentally imposed occupational deprivation. Findings thus support the existence of ethological needs for occupation in chimpanzees—most especially, foraging, nest building, grooming, and playing—which, in turn, supports the assumption of a biological need for occupation in people as well (Wood, 1998a).

Idleness and Aberrant Behaviors, but Also Creativity, During No Enrichment

During No ENR, inactivity (watching and idleness) took almost half of the chimpanzees' time (43%), more so than any other condition (Wood, 1998a, 1998b). The emergence of increased frequencies of aberrant behaviors during Old ENR continued in No ENR as well. High frequencies of inactivity and aberrant behaviors also corresponded with significant increases in the solitary/nonsocial social context when compared to Old ENR. Interestingly, however, frequencies of the social context of mother-child, the third most prevalent social context overall, were highest in No ENR. Thus, the two chimpanzee mothers chose to engage with New ENR when it was freshly introduced, to reconnect mainly with other adults during Old ENR, and to pay more attention to their young offspring during No ENR.

Further analyses revealed that the group's occupational behaviors were significantly more flexible—one might say creative—when their habitat was in its most barren state during No ENR (Wood, 1998b). This creativity seemed to emerge when the chimpanzees appeared most bored and at loss for something to do. For example, of 11 episodes of sustained exploring, 10 episodes occurred during No ENR and sometimes resulted in the creation of new occupational opportunities. During one episode, the chimpanzees discovered a small hole in an inner wall of their concrete habitat. They broke this hole open wide enough so that the juveniles could climb inside and play a game that looked quite like hide-and-seek. In similar fashion, the chimpanzees occupied themselves during No ENR by dismantling branches from a dead tree that was cemented into the concrete floor. They also stripped away a plastic lining that had been on the wall of the enclosure.

Yet, while findings supported the existence of strong ethological needs for occupation in chimpanzees, they also revealed deleterious environmental influences on daily time use and psychological well-being. These deleterious effects seemed to be due to a dynamic called *environmental channeling*. Environmental channeling refers to the power of impoverished living environs to channel animal behavior into increasingly more rigid, truncated, and stereotypic forms (Rushen, Lawrence, & Terlouw, 1993). Whereas brief exposures to impoverished environs may have no channeling effects, longer exposures may have powerful lasting effects. Thus, as time wore on under No ENR, the chimpanzees' ethological needs to groom and manipulate objects were increasingly expressed in aberrant ways; for example, grooming gave way to plucking body hair and nearly all episodes of aberrant behaviors occurred as Old ENR transitioned into No ENR.

Ultimately, evidence of environmental channeling revealed how fleeting any state of adaptedness that the chimpanzees achieved was (Wood, 1998b). As posed by Porn (1993), for a state of adaptedness that supports health and well-being to persist, a dynamic equilibrium must be sustained between a living being's will for action, repertoire of abilities, and lived environment. In Study 1, the chimpanzees' strong motivations and capacities to engage in species-typical occupations were routinely thwarted by constraints imposed by an institutionalized habitat. Time acted as an omnipresent force in its own right that demanded a solution to the problem of how it would be filled. Though the chimpanzees creatively acted to solve this problem when their habitat was in its most barren state, they could, in effect, only keep up their solutions for so long. The chimpanzees' wills and capacities for action thus often existed in disequilibrium with the habitat in which they lived each day—a habitat that, unless deliberately enriched, imposed far too much empty time with far too few things to do.

Study 2: Environment, Time Use, and Adaptedness in Prosimians

Study 2 also used a primate model to advance knowledge pertaining to environmental influences on time use and adaptedness. In Study 2, however, participants consisted of a small family of Coquerel sifakas (*Propithecus verreauxi coquereli*) at the Duke University Primate Center ([DUPC] Wood, Towers, & Malchow, 2000). The study asked: How do different captive habitats influence the daily time-use patterns and state of adaptedness of captive sifakas?

Coquerel sifakas are in the prosimian suborder of primates and members of the superfamily of prosimians known as lemurs. Their natural habitats are in Madagascar, where they occupy home ranges of 5 to 21 acres and live in social groups of two to 12 members (Jolly, Gustafson, Oliver, & O'Connor, 1982; Richard, 1978). Environmental influences on the DUPC sifakas' time use and state of adaptedness were investigated by examining how they occupied time over summer, fall, and winter months in two outdoor enclosures and one indoor enclosure before and after a new infant was born. These enclosures were regarded as ecological microsystems, that is, face-to-face settings of daily life (Bronfenbrenner, 1977; Bronfenbrenner & Crouter, 1993). Once again drawing from Porn (1993), *adaptedness* was defined as a time-sensitive equilibrium among opportunities for action provided by ecological microsystems and an individual's capacities and motivations for action.

Brief Description of Methods

A case study of a family group of three Coquerel sifakas was undertaken at the DUPC using a naturalistic design in which no effort was made to control any aspect of the sifakas' day-to-day lives. Participants included Marcella, a 17-year-old adult female; Trajan, a 16-year-old adult male; and Neru, a 3-year-old adolescent. To the delight of caregivers as well as researchers (including two occupational therapy students), Alexianus, a male, was born to Marcella and Trajan during the study. As a result, three environmental conditions consisting of significantly different physical conditions were studied, in addition to a fourth condition due to change in the group's social composition. A total of 127 hours of observations were completed across four environmental conditions:

1. **Forested enclosure.** This 7-acre wooded enclosure approximated the size of sifakas' natural habitats in Madagascar and provided extensive opportunities for species-typical patterns of activity.

2. **Small outdoor enclosure.** This 21 x 18 x 8 foot enclosure located in the large forested enclosure was enclosed with wire and provided full visual, auditory, and olfactory access to the surrounding woods. The sifakas were housed in this enclosure for 2 months prior to moving inside for the colder winter months. Various materials and objects in this enclosure provided opportunities for species-typical activities.

3. **Small indoor room.** This enclosure consisted of a 9 x 16 foot room with a ceiling that angled upward from 12 to 16 feet. While this room had solid walls that precluded visual and auditory access to adjoining areas, materials and objects were available to provide opportunities for species-typical activities.

4. **Indoor room with baby.** The same physical environment as previously, however, with the addition of the infant, Alexianus.

Quantitatively, real-time direct observations were collected at 1-minute intervals between the hours of 9:00 a.m. and 4:00 p.m. using a scan sampling technique. When in the forested enclosure, this would require researchers to carefully follow the group through the woods so that accurate observations could be entered each minute on each of three adult sifakas, a delightful way to spend one's time, I might add. Eleven mutually exclusive and exhaustive time-use categories were recorded: aggression, comfort movement, foraging and feeding, hanging (suspension from a branch), inactivity, locomotion and traveling, marking, playing, scanning, self-grooming, and social grooming. Descriptive statistics were used to determine percentages of time in each time-use category under each environmental condition. Logistic regression analyses were used to reveal significant differences in these time-use frequencies under each condition. Qualitative data consisted of extensive written descriptions of how the sifakas engaged in foraging and feeding, grooming, and scanning activities, as well salient variations in their expressions of inactivity. Open and axial coding techniques were used to compare and contrast these behavioral expressions (Creswell, 2007).

Summary of Results

Sustained Adaptedness in the Large Forested Enclosure

The large forested enclosure offered the most plentiful and diverse environmental opportunities for action to the sifakas. When in this enclosure, the sifakas would travel as a group throughout the forest, leaping from tree to tree and also coming to the ground, where they would hop for short distances. Their traveling and locomotion took up 21% total time on average each day and was fluidly intertwined with other species-typical behaviors, especially foraging and feeding (29% total time) and scanning (40% total time). Locomotion and traveling, feeding and foraging, and scanning together occupied an average of 90% of the sifakas' time daily. In descending frequency, the group would pause their travels to rest, hang from branches, and sun in trees (2.46% total time); socially groom (2.35% total time); mark (2.25% total time); play (1.33% total time); and self-groom (1.09% total time). Altogether, systematic analyses of the sifakas' time-use patterns suggested that the group manifested, in the large forested habitat, a sustained state of adaptedness as defined by Porn (1993). That is, a stable equilibrium seemed to exist among the plethora of opportunities for action availed by the forested enclosure, the sifakas' motives for action, and their capacities for action. Supporting this conclusion, their observed daily time-use patterns approximated the range and prevalence of species-typical behaviors demonstrated by free-ranging sifakas in Madagascar (Richard, 1978).

Adaptedness Is Not Sustained in Other Environmental Conditions

In the small outdoor enclosure, opportunities for travel/locomotion were quite limited, and frequencies of this behavior significantly dropped from 21% to 3% total time on average each day. Scanning expanded to fill the time that the group would likely have otherwise spent traveling if provided the opportunity, increasing from a daily average of 40% total time in the forested enclosure to 62% in this enclosure. Indeed, scanning was more frequent than in any other condition. This finding was not surprising, because the sifakas were constantly exposed to visual, auditory, and olfactory stimuli from birds and other animals in the surrounding forest, falling leaves and branches, people, sounds from a highway, etc. While feeding and foraging was their second most prevalent way of spending time, frequencies significantly decreased compared to the forested enclosure. Social grooming and play were also at their lowest levels across all conditions. Corresponding to these decreases, the total time that the sifakas spent inactive significantly increased compared to the forested enclosure, from 1.6% to 3.3%, respectively.

In the indoor room, scanning was once again the sifakas' most frequent activity, occupying 56% of their time on average each day. Though still their most prominent behavior, scanning was significantly less frequent than in the small outdoor enclosure, presumably because the indoor room had solid walls, no outdoor access, and only one small window onto a corridor. Furthermore, in contrast to the keen responsiveness and attentiveness that characterized the sifakas' scanning in the small outdoor enclosure, their scanning indoors often appeared quite languid and unfocused. With eyelids slowly shifting among wide open, half drooping, and closed, scanning tended to precede long bouts of inactivity. While the sifakas second most frequent behavior was feeding and foraging (25% total time), its frequencies were significantly less than in the small outdoor enclosure. Conversely, play and grooming (1.3% total time each) significantly increased in comparison to the small outdoor enclosure. Grooming was 3.6 times more likely, and play was 40 times more likely, returning to levels observed in the large forested enclosure. Inactivity (9% total time) also significantly increased and was more frequently observed than in either preceding condition.

After Alexianus' birth (indoor room with baby), scanning significantly increased and again occupied the largest proportion of the sifakas' day (60% total time). Also, significantly increasing in frequency were traveling/locomotion (4.6% total time), social grooming (2.8% total time), and self-grooming (2% total time). Grooming activities were more frequent compared to any other condition; traveling/locomotion was more frequent compared to the indoor room before the infant and small outdoor enclosure. These increases in species-typical behaviors appeared attributable to Alexianus, who, as a novelty to Trajan and Neru and the focus of Marcella's maternal attention, sparked much more movement and grooming.

When Marcella, Trajan, and Neru were not focusing on Alexianus, their scanning often continued to evidence the vague unfocused quality first observed before the infant's birth. When scanning took on this quality, it sometimes lapsed into long bouts of inactivity of up to 40 minutes. As a result, inactivity grew to occupy 12% of the sifakas' total time, significantly more than in any other condition. As inactivity increased, the trend toward less time feeding and foraging continued. While the sifakas' caretakers reported that the group's actual daily food intake had not declined, feeding in both the small outdoor enclosure and small indoor room became progressively uncoupled from foraging. Hence, while the sifakas demonstrated some "empty foraging" (i.e., foraging directed toward nonedible items like wood chips or sticks), time spent eating was more and more compressed into brief periods immediately following the introduction of fresh foods.

Two concepts help to further explain changes in the group's daily time-use patterns across different environmental conditions. Environmental presses are created by the specific elements (social, physical, sensory, etc.) of immediate proximal environs; these elements together elicit, or press toward, expression of some behaviors while discouraging the expression of other behaviors (Lawton, 1989; Lawton & Nahemow, 1973). In Study 2, the small outdoor enclosure had a strong environmental press toward scanning. This press, coupled with environmentally imposed constraints on travel and locomotion, accounts for the near complete disappearance of play and social grooming as well as the doubling of inactivity in the small outdoor enclosure. Evidence of environmental channeling was suggested by progressive declines in the sifakas' foraging behaviors and increases in time spent inactive in the indoor room after the infant was born. Thus, though the sifakas demonstrated behavioral resilience in response to the infant by moving significantly more and reactivating play and grooming behaviors, the fabric of their natural daily living patterns, first observed in the forested enclosure, continued to unravel. Altogether, owing to environmentally imposed constraints on action, the power of specific environmental presses, and the influence of long durations of time in the small outdoor enclosure followed by the small indoor room, the group's state of adaptedness was not sustained over the fall and winter months. Happily, however, the sifakas' behavioral resilience after the infant was born suggested that they had maintained the capacities to reconstitute a state of adaptedness and would do just that once summer returned and they could again exploit the richly varied offerings for action availed by the forest.

Study 3: An Exploratory Case Study of Time Use, Apparent Affect, and Routine Activity Situations on Two Alzheimer's Special Care Units

Study 3 was a multiple instrumental case study that aimed to explore interrelationships among the social and physical environments of two Alzheimer's special care units (SCUs) and residents' quality of life. The study's keen attention to daily time use was based on the premise that a biological need for occupation persists in people in advanced stages of neurodegenerative dementias and thereby continues to function as an essential determinant of their health and well-being. This presumption is supported by Study 1 as well as by other research suggesting that how people with dementia occupy time each day influences their well-being (Hasselkus, 1998; Lawton, 1997; Lawton, Van Haitsma, & Klapper, 1996; Lawton, Van Haitsma, Perkinson, & Ruckdeschel, 2000; Moss, Lawton, Kleban, & Duhamel, 1993). Study 3 was also influenced by a prior multiple case study of two groups of zoo chimpanzees in which social interactions were found to influence the groups' respective time-use patterns and overall adaptedness far more than the design of their built habitats (Wood, 2002). Like zoo habitats, Alzheimer's SCUs were regarded as ecological microsystems situated in institutional contexts. Furthermore, how care partners provided environmental opportunities for meaningful time use and emotional well-being was viewed as a cornerstone of quality dementia care.

Given the above perspective, the present study investigated what transpired in specific activity situations within the microsystems of its two study sites (Wood, Harris, Snider, & Patchel, 2005; Wood, Womack, & Hooper, 2009). *Activity situations* refer to routinely occurring and observably different periods of time in long-term care settings that prevail from morning to night. Examples include time for activity groups, or for meals and snacks, television, and unstructured down time. Two quality of life indicators specific to people with dementia were used: daily time use and emotional well-being. The study presumed that the environmental press of specific activity situations would be revealed by how residents spent time and also their apparent affect. The primary research question was: What is the environmental press of each activity situation at both SCUs as gauged by participants' observed patterns of time use and apparent affect?

Brief Description of Methods

Study Sites and Participants

Two Alzheimer's SCUs were selected as study sites: a more home-like SCU with seven residents and a SCU with a more traditional nursing home environment with 28 residents. The more home-like SCU included a small kitchen, dining area, living room, activity room, and outdoor patio, garden, and walking path; it had a 7:1 resident-to-staff ratio. The SCU that looked like a more traditional nursing home setting had a large day room and central nursing station. At any given time, it had a resident-to-staff ratio of 8 or 9:1. Seven residents from each SCU participated for a total of 14 participants. Although not fully achieved, an effort was made to select seven participants from the more traditional setting who matched the age, gender, and functional status of the seven residents from the more home-like setting.

Data Collection and Analysis

Data were collected using the Activity in Context and Time (ACT), a computer-assisted observational tool (see Table 5-1) (Wood, 2005). The six mutually exclusive domains of the ACT allowed researchers to record each participant's immediate activity situation (environmental domain) and his or her corresponding way of occupying time and apparent affect. As shown in Table 5-2, in the ACT's time-use domains, specific codes were designated as optimal because of their associations with relative well-being; these codes constituted positive quality of life indicators when not associated with a negative emotional state. For example, with respect to gaze (the most elemental level of functional capacity), engaged gaze was viewed as an optimal time use code in contrast to both unengaged gaze and eyes closed. Drawing from observations of the sifakas in Study 2, simply being able to maintain an engaged gaze was viewed as a quality of life indicator because it conveyed positive qualities of intentionality and attention. The domain of Apparent Affect was borrowed from the work of Lawton and his colleagues (Lawton et al., 1996; Lawton et al., 2000). This domain included two codes for emotional well-being: interest and pleasure; it also included three codes for emotional ill-being: anger, anxiety/fear, and sadness/depression.

An instantaneous sampling method was used whereby one complete observational string was collected on each participant every 10 minutes from 8:00 a.m. to 8:00 p.m. for 4 days. Thus, every 10 minutes, a trained researcher would find each participant at the study site and enter a complete observational string using a hand-held computer. By complete observational string, it is meant that the researcher would enter into the computer a code from each domain of the ACT that best described the participant's prevailing activity situation as well as his or her time use and apparent affect. For example, a woman who was eating lunch in the dining room would be coded as being "in" meals and snacks (activity situation) and as spending time sitting (position and movement). If her time use was optimal, then these codes would also be entered: engaged

— TABLE 5-2 —

STUDY 3: DOMAINS AND CODES OF THE ACTIVITY IN CONTEXT AND TIME (ABRIDGED)

DOMAIN: ENVIRONMENTAL—ACTIVITY SITUATIONS

Codes

1. Activities of daily living: a staff intervention focused on direct assistance with mobility, toileting, dressing, hygiene, eating, and medications.

2. Activity groups: scheduled music groups; craft, game, or exercise groups; devotional services.

3. Background media: a staff-initiate enrichment that consists of playing the radio or music in the absence of any other enrichment, activity program, or staff intervention.

4. Downtime: absence of any other activity situation due to either no other situation occurring or because the resident left the situation that was occurring.

5. Meals and snacks: regularly scheduled meals and snacks throughout the day.

6. Television: a staff-initiated enrichment that consists of situating residents to watch movies or shows on television in the absence of any other enrichment, activity program, or staff intervention.

7. Other staff intervention: interventions related to medical care (e.g., passing medications) or social and emotional well-being (e.g., comforting).

DOMAIN: TIME USE

Codes: Gaze

1. Engaged gaze: an optimal time-use behavior indicated by some level of intentional involvement with, awareness or watching of, others or the physical environment. Code can be applied with eyes closed where active responsiveness to the environment is observable (e.g., tapping feet to music or engaging in conversation).

2. Unengaged gaze: a wakeful state yet no sustained intentional involvement with or attention to the environment.

3. Eyes closed: corresponds with dozing or sleeping.

Codes: Position and Movement

1. Standing/walking: an optimal time-use behavior indicated by upright exercise or walking in the absence of agitation or distress.

2. Sitting.

3. Lying/reclining.

Codes: Conversation

1. Participation in conversation: an optimal time-use behavior indicated by sustained efforts to communicate with someone whether coherent, incoherent, or in a nonverbal fashion.

2. No participation in conversation: absence of any observable conversational behavior.

Codes: Activity

1. Participation in activity: an optimal time-use behavior indicated by sustained engagement in some activity or task in the absence of agitation or distress. Simply being in an activity situation where activities are going on, but not participating in those activities, does not count as participating in activities.

2. No participation in activity: absence of any observable participation in activity beyond watching (engaged gaze), walking/standing, or participation in conversation.

DOMAIN: EMOTIONAL WELL-BEING

Codes

1. Interest and/or pleasure: optimal emotional well-being codes.

2. Absence of affect.

3. Anger, anxiety/fear, sadness/depression.

Republished with permission of American Journal of Occupational Therapy, from Dying of boredom: An exploratory case study of two Alzheimer's special care units, Wood, W., Womack, J., & Hooper, B. , 63, 2009; permission conveyed through Copyright Clearance Center, Inc.

gaze (gaze), participation in conversation (conversation), and participation in activity (activity). In addition, either interest or pleasure would be entered in the emotional well-being domain. Observational strings like this one would be completed on all participants in each 10-minute time period, after which the process would begin again. In this manner, a total of 4,032 observational strings on all participants at both sites were completed.

Data were analyzed by computing the mean proportion of time that each participant was observed in specific activity situations and each corresponding code in the domains of gaze, position and walking, conversation, activity, and apparent affect. These proportions were aggregated by facility and were divided by 4 to determine aggregated average daily proportions across all participants at each facility. The Goodman-Kruskal gamma correlation coefficient was derived from mean aggregated proportion of time and examined strength of associations between activity situations and codes in the time-use and apparent affect domains.

Summary of Results

Positive Quality of Life Associations

At both SCUs, the positive quality of life indicators of engaged gaze and participation in activity (specifically eating and drinking) in the time-use domain, plus interest in the emotional well-being domain, were significantly positively associated with the activity situation of meals and snacks. Although meals and snacks always occurred in social atmospheres, no associations with conversation or pleasure were found.

Like meal and snack times, the positive quality of life indicator of participation in activities was positively associated with the activity situation of formal activity groups at both SCUs. Thus, an environmental press toward the doing of things was evident in most activity groups. However, because activity groups were also associated with sitting, it appeared that upright physical activity and exercise, of which all participants were capable, was not promoted during activity groups at either SCU. Surprisingly, participation in conversation also was not significantly associated with the activity groups.

A number of interesting associations were found with the activity situation of downtime. At both SCUs, downtime was the sole situation significantly positively associated with the quality of life indicator of standing and walking (i.e., upright physical activity). Participants often initiated walking of their own accord during downtime, sometimes walking arm-in-arm with other residents and chatting. Thus, downtime was also associated with participation in conversation, another positive quality of life indicator, at the home-like facility. While downtime provided participants with the freedom to walk about and encounter and greet other residents and staff, it also was a time in which residents lacked opportunities to do much more. At both SCUs, therefore, downtime was significantly associated with spending time lying down without any activity participation.

No positive quality of life indicators were associated with two activity situations: television and background media. Each of these situations was associated with sitting, suggesting that they exerted an environmental press toward physical inactivity. Furthermore, being situated in front of a television was not significantly associated, as one might hope, with either an engaged gaze or expression of apparent interest. Worse, background media was strongly associated with no participation in activity, with eyes closed, and with an absence of any affect.

Setting Differences

Participants in the home-like facility experienced activity situations associated with quality of life indicators for less than half of their time each day (i.e., an average of 5 hours and 36 minutes from 8 a.m. to 8 p.m.). In comparison, participants in the more traditional setting averaged 9 hours and 25 minutes each day in activity situations that were associated with at least one quality of life indicator. These differences are explained by the fact that participants in the traditional SCU experienced more downtimes each day; hence, they walked about 1.5 hours more each day than those in the home-like SCU. Participants in the more traditional facility were also significantly more likely to have an engaged gaze (indicating intentionality) and to show pleasure, which mostly occurred while walking. Participants in the more home-like SCU spent, in contrast, significantly more time in physical inactivity sitting in front of the television and in the activity situation of background media, neither of which conferred quality of life benefits.

Limited Support for Daily Quality of Life

Altogether, daily aggregated portraits of time use and emotional well-being suggest that the prevailing activity situations at both SCUs failed to strongly support participants' quality of life. While the harsh reality of dementia is a major reason why participants were not more occupationally engaged and emotionally well each day, a solely disease-oriented explanation of findings is insufficient. As posited by Lawton (1989), older adults, including those with dementia, can express their maximum functional potential and experience positive emotions when their environs provide challenges and opportunities that slightly exceed their levels of competence. Older adults may also relax and be able to exercise and enjoy the use of their skills when environmental challenges and opportunities are slightly beneath their competency levels. Yet, extreme environmental presses in either direction lead to maladaptive behaviors and negative affect. If demands greatly exceed an older adult's capacities to respond, then high levels of stress and anxiety may result. Conversely, if demands are insufficiently challenging, interesting, or enabling, then boredom, withdrawal, and atrophy of skills ensue. Findings from Study 3 suggest that this scenario of insufficient support, opportunity, and challenge tended to prevail in most activity situations at both SCUs.

Enlivening and Deadening Activity Situations

The concept of occupational place suggests that some compromises in the daily quality of life of participants might have been prevented. As found by Hasselkus (1998), architectural spaces like activity areas or dining rooms can become "alive" occupational places if care partners of people with dementia support them doing things that tap their capacities and are congruent with their senses of self. This concept of occupational place suggests that any activity situation may exist on a continuum from occupationally deadening to occupationally enlivening. Zgola and Bordillon (2001), for instance, described mealtimes in nursing homes that are presented in ways that infuse residents' dining experiences with elements of prayer, fun, ritual, social connection, memories, community, and celebration. In this scenario, the architectural space of a dining room is effectively transformed into an enlivening occupational place. By way of contrast in Study 3, dining was often reduced to a concern with nutritional intake alone, and residents were discouraged from talking to each other, resulting in minimal social interaction and no expressions of pleasure. Because in this scenario dining rooms were not transformed into occupational places, mealtimes were far more occupationally deadening than enlivening.

A preponderance of more occupationally deadening activity situations are arguably strong environmental drivers of excess disability in people with dementia. *Excess disability* refers to disability that goes beyond that which is directly caused by a specific disease process such as Alzheimer's disease (Dawson, Kline, Wiancko, & Wells, 1986; Rogers et al., 2000). Notably, even in advanced stages of dementia, people with dementia can attend to their environs and experience interest and pleasure as expressed through smiling, laughter, affectionate touch, and more. They can participate appropriately in social exchanges, understand and enjoy humor, and perform many familiar activities. Yet, for these capacities to be expressed, the activity situations to which long-term care residents with dementia are routinely exposed each day must, on balance, be more occupationally enlivening than not.

Study 4: A Collaborative Education Program for Promoting Person-Centered and Ability-Focused Care of Nursing Home Residents

The experience of completing Study 3, in which I and other researchers functioned as outside observers, instilled a keen desire to become an inside player who could have real impact on the daily quality of care, hence, the daily quality of life, of nursing home residents with dementia,

who comprise an estimated 64% of all nursing home residents (Alzheimer's Association, 2012). Realization of this desire grew closer to reality when the director of a nursing home invited me to develop a comprehensive approach to staff training through a systematic research-based approach. With this opportunity, both the occupational therapist and occupational scientist in me were given expression in that I was able to fulfill roles of a consultant, educator, and researcher of a facility that was undergoing culture change reforms.

The culture change reform movement is dedicated to transforming nursing homes that have historically provided mainly only medical models of care into home-like communities that provide person-centered and abilities-focused care (Kane, 2001; Services, 2004). Person-centered care is individualized to the life history and current wants and needs of nursing home residents (Kitwood, 1997). Abilities-focused care seeks to provide opportunities for meaningful activities and social connections that help residents use their retained capacities (Rogers et al., 2000; Wells, Dawson, Sidani, Craig, & Pringle, 2000). Leading practitioners and researchers in long-term care (LTC) in general, and dementia care in particular, view person-centered and abilities-focused care approaches as a long over-due corrective to traditional pathology-oriented practices that have attended sufficiently neither to the quality of life of residents nor to the satisfaction of staff. This commitment is supported by evidence that when LTC residents can connect with others and participate in valued activities, they are more apt to maintain their functional capacities, experience continuity with their past lives, and derive meaning and satisfaction in their present lives (Hasselkus, 1998; Sifton, 2000; Zgola, 1999). Furthermore, culture change reforms have been associated with staff satisfaction (Services, 2004).

Despite their promise, however, culture change reforms have not been widely implemented (Kane, 2001). One reason for this gap has to do with insufficient or ineffective caregiver education and training. Educational content and approaches are often determined by managers or are shaped only by regulatory requirements, without being inclusive of the voices of frontline caregivers, service recipients, and support staff. Additionally, direct caregivers must not only be educated in how to provide person-centered and abilities-focused care across the day, they must also be organizationally rewarded and valued for provision of such care.

Accordingly, Study 4 responded to the need to develop caregiver educational programs, within supportive organizational cultures, that could simultaneously advance quality care on behalf of LTC residents while also increasing the satisfaction of staff in their work. Study 4 thus sought to develop a comprehensive empirically based approach to the education and training of staff that could be implemented in a LTC facility that was in the process

TABLE 5-3

STUDY 4: DESCRIPTION OF STUDY PARTICIPANTS

RESIDENTS AND FAMILY MEMBERS	*n*
Residents of the facility	5
Family members of residents	9
EMPLOYEES	***n***
Certified nursing assistants	9
Managers (executive director, nursing supervisors, the staff development coordinator, and directors of nursing and of rehabilitation)	11
Registered nurses and licensed practical nurses	6
Rehabilitation and activity therapists (occupational therapists, physical therapists, a speech and language pathologist, wellness and activity therapists, and restorative aides)	6

of implementing culture change reforms. This question was asked: As guided by the perceived needs, evaluations, and recommendations of key stakeholders, what content and instructional processes are needed to promote person-centered and ability-focused care through staff education? Secondary data analysis also examined the educational contributions of occupational therapists and other rehabilitation professionals to culture change reforms.

Brief Description of Methods

Consistent with the study's focus on person-centered and abilities-focused care, a democratic approach to program development and evaluation was adopted. This approach was based on the premise that, to be effective, educational programs must derive from a shared process of decision making among key stakeholders who are affected by the program (MacNeil, 2002; MacNeil & Mead, 2005). Given this premise, the research process involved dialogue among diverse members of the community (stakeholders) about their perceived needs, insights and suggestions pertaining to staff education, as well as barriers and enablers of person-centered and ability-focused care. In this highly participatory approach, a sincere effort was thus made to honor the voices of numerous stakeholders, especially those who lacked authority or high status in the setting.

Study Site and Participants

Site selection occurred as a function of a request by the executive director of a LTC facility that was committed to culture change. In addition to five residents and nine family members, 32 employees participated, representing 32% of all employees (Table 5-3).

Data Collection and Analysis

Table 5-4 provides an overview of the project's three phases, which together lasted 14 months. During Phase 1,

24 frontline caregivers attended and evaluated a 10-week curriculum on person-centered and ability-focused care through weekly surveys. Also, nine homogeneous forums, 60 to 90 minutes in length, were conducted with stakeholder groups (excluding residents). Homogenous forums were designed to provide a safe context for members of the same stakeholder group to explore their perceptions of (a) staff educational needs, (b) enablers and barriers to success in staff educational programs, and (c) specific suggestions for educational programming. Individual interviews were also completed with five residents and the facility's executive director.

During Phase 2, preliminary analyses of all data sources were completed, and an interim report was delivered to stakeholders. During Phase 3, 14 heterogeneous forums, each lasting 60 minutes, were conducted to finalize recommendations for a staff education program focused on person-centered and ability-focused care. The purpose of *heterogeneous forums* was to generate—across members of different stakeholder groups—shared understandings of staff educational needs, optimal educational content and processes, and factors that either enable or obstruct successful educational programming. Heterogeneous forums were audiotaped, and all data were qualitatively analyzed using a constant comparative method (Creswell, 2007).

Summary of Findings

Implement an Ongoing Comprehensive Approach to Staff Education and Training

Consensus emerged that staff education should include, but also go far beyond, trainings like the 10-week curriculum introduced at the start of the project. While this curriculum was quite favorably reviewed, it also was believed that day-to-day implementation of person-centered and ability-focused care required a more comprehensive

TABLE 5-4

STUDY 4: IMPLEMENTATION, DATA COLLECTION, AND ANALYSIS

PHASE 1 (7 MONTHS)	PHASE 2 (2 MONTHS)	PHASE 3 (5 MONTHS)
Development, Implementation, and Evaluation of 10-Week Curriculum • 10-week curriculum was implemented • Class feedback surveys	*Development of Interim Report* • Incorporate data analysis into interim report	*Data Collection: Deliberative Forums* • Four groups met biweekly for four meetings of 1-hour duration
Data Collection: Gathering Stakeholder Perspectives • Individual interviews with executive director and residents • Homogenous focus groups *Data Analysis* • Descriptive statistics of survey (mean, mode, range) • Qualitative analysis of data from focus groups, interviews, and participant observations	*Dissemination of Interim Report* • Executive director • Facility regional director • Employees of facility • Family members	*Data Analysis* • Qualitative analysis of data from deliberative forums *Dissemination of Final Report* • Executive director • Facility regional director • Employees of facility

approach to staff education. Four ongoing and complementary approaches to formal education programs were thus recommended: (a) initiate training during applicant interviews, (b) introduce new employees to person-centered and abilities-focused care during orientation, (c) develop a mentorship training program for certified nursing assistants (CNAs) and also assign responsibilities to CNAs for mentoring new CNAs, and (d) conduct monthly meetings on units to address various process and communication issues.

Empowerment and Respect as Foundational to Culture Change

In addition to these approaches, participants identified enablers of and barriers to the day-to-day implementation of person-centered and abilities-focused care. The most prominent enabler pertained to widespread support for the facility's commitment to culture change reforms (i.e., its vision for change was seen as the right thing to do). Barriers included breakdowns in communication, teamwork, and accountability (Knight, Wood, & Booth, 2013). Final educational recommendations reflected strong consensus around the need for staff to feel empowered and respected each day. Thus, maintenance of a respectful and empowering environment was viewed as just as vital to culture change as were staff education and training programs.

Minimal Involvement of Occupational Therapists and Other Skilled Rehabilitation Practitioners in Staff Education

For several reasons, occupational therapists and other rehabilitation therapists were only intermittently and distantly involved with staff education, hence, with the implementation of culture change reforms. These therapists indicated that they did not fully understand processes pertaining to staff education; they also expressed frustration at what they perceived to be poor follow-through by CNAs of therapy recommendations. Yet, this poor follow-through may have been due, in part, to the pull-out model of practice that predominated, which limited opportunities for engagement in staff education. In other words, for example, except for training in basic activities of daily living, occupational therapy practitioners mostly pulled residents from their living areas to provide one-to-one direct treatment in the designated rehabilitation area: a context that did not lend itself to training and building collaborative and empowering relationships with frontline caregivers. Formal maintenance programs also did not appear to be widespread. In such programs, which Medicare reimburses as a skilled service, therapists help frontline staff learn strategies that maximize function or prevent further decline of residents. Given how strongly the expertise of occupational therapists aligned with person-centered and ability-focused care, a more inclusive model of practice that encompassed frequent maintenance programs might have made their contributions as educators both more explicit and impactful. Yet, as things stood, residents, family members, and other employees rarely if ever mentioned occupational therapists or other rehabilitation professionals as important players in the implementation of culture change reforms.

IMPLICATIONS FOR OCCUPATIONAL SCIENCE AND OCCUPATIONAL THERAPY

I have shared the previous studies to emphasize how critical an environmental perspective is if occupational scientists, through their research, and occupational therapists, through their practices, are to enhance the everyday quality of life of institutionalized adults with dementia. Several implications of this work stand out as most important.

The Biological Need for Occupation

Empirical evidence of chimpanzees' ethological needs for occupation supports the difficult-to-examine assumption of a biological need for occupation in people as well. Findings from Study 1, when considered in context of other research on retained capacities in people with dementia, offer evidence that not even severe brain damage can completely eradicate a person's biological need for occupation. It matters that the biological need for occupation in people is tenacious. It matters because, with this knowledge, occupational therapists can be confident that their continued efforts to support and bring forth occupational engagement are well founded even in advanced stages of dementia. Stated differently, there is good reason to believe that the ravages of dementia cannot entirely nullify a biological endowment in which meaningful occupation functions as a gateway to well-being.

Environmental Impacts on Engagement and Well-Being

The program of research also identified specific environmental concepts and dynamics that influence occupational engagement and well-being for both better and worse. At a more macro level, identified concepts included total institutions and ecological microsystems. The complimentary ecological lenses afforded by these two concepts helped to illustrate the debilitating dynamic of environmental channeling, which elicited more simplistic behavioral patterns in captive primates and also excess disability in institutionalized people with dementia. States of adaptedness, including the functional capacities of people with dementia, were thus found to be quite environmentally vulnerable and time

sensitive. Because, however, functional capacities are not simply in a state of inexorable decline, they can be positively supported by one's immediate environs.

Occupation in Context: A More Subtle Understanding

Findings from Study 1 and Study 2 underscored the importance of adopting a nuanced, situation-specific approach to environmental dynamics, and, as a result, the concept of activity situations was introduced in Study 3. Findings from Study 3 showed that the environmental presses of activity situations on the two Alzheimer's SCUs were highly particularistic. Furthermore, the environmental press of most activity situations was found to suppress participants' optimal occupational engagement, hence, to push instead toward greater passivity, emotional flatness, and disuse of their retained capacities. The idea that activity situations could exist on a continuum from occupational enlivening to occupationally deadening was proposed and also directly tied to daily time use and emotional well-being, two dementia-specific gauges of quality of life.

Moving to Inclusive Models of Occupational Therapy Practice in Long-Term Care

How, then, might occupational therapy practitioners apply these findings, beginning with their approaches to evaluating LTC residents with dementia? Most basically, findings provide a compelling rationale for a highly fluid approach to assessment that is informed by multiple data points over time. The multiple data points would consist of brief snapshots of how LTC residents truly occupy time in the activity situations to which they are most often exposed. Snapshots could be mentally gathered while walking through a dining room, stepping into activity groups, or observing residents walking, wheeling, or sitting in front of a television. Snapshot taking would take note of activity situations that tend to evoke emotional well-being versus distress. More formally, practitioners could gather snapshots using the domains and codes specified in the ACT (Wood, 2005), including its specific quality of life indicators. Such a record would provide compelling evidence of how various activity situations influence a resident's occupational engagement and emotional well-being. Multiple fluid snapshots of time use could also be coupled with one-time assessments of, say, cognitive function or activities of daily living, in which optimal performance levels given various task and environmental modifications were ascertained.

Armed with such knowledge, practitioners would possess a wealth of intervention strategies. Yet, to be as useful as possible, these strategies would need to be integrated into an inclusive model of LTC practice. Consider the parallel to the evolution of school-based practice in occupational therapy. Removing students from classrooms to treat them in special therapy spaces, the pull-out model, has historically dominated school-based practice. Increasingly, though, inclusive models of practice whereby practitioners work with students and teachers in the settings in which school performance is desired or expected are viewed as best practices (Muhlenhaupt, 2003). My research supports a similar shift to inclusive models of occupational therapy in LTC settings.

Contrary to treating almost always in special rehabilitation spaces except for basic activities of daily living, inclusive practices would be predominantly situated where residents want and need to perform and participate in valued activities each day. Being so situated, practitioners could more easily build collaborative relationships with CNAs and other staff members who intimately care for residents from when they awake until they go to bed. In this inclusive context, occupational therapy practitioners could best coach, mentor, and educate frontline staff on time-efficient strategies that optimize performance. Moreover, armed with knowledge of what environmental features and dynamics bring out the best and the worst in residents, they could play a leadership role in creating and sustaining an abundance of activity situations each day that are as occupationally enlivening as possible.

LEARNING SUPPORTS

The Evolution of a Research Career

Purpose

The purpose of this exercise is to help students understand how research careers can unfold and also to prompt them to wonder if a nascent research career might be growing within them.

Primary Concepts

Key concepts include clinical irritation, research career, and program of research.

Instructions

1. Describe Dr. Wood's clinical irritation, and trace how that irritation grew into a program of research.

2. Create a graphic that portrays the progressive evolution of Dr. Wood's understandings of environmental influences on occupational engagement and well-being from the time of being a Level II fieldwork student to now.

3. Identify a clinical irritation of yours that relates to the concept of occupation in occupational science and occupational therapy. Draw at least two links between

your clinical irritation and a long-standing personal interest, puzzle, or fascination.

4. Create a research question that addresses your clinical irritation and at least one personal interest, puzzle, or fascination.

Evolutionary Basis of Human Occupational Behavior

Purpose

The purpose of this activity is to encourage students to think about the evolutionary basis of human occupational behavior and how institutional living affects behavior.

Primary Concepts

Key concepts include institutions, the primate order, and activity patterns of human and nonhuman primates.

Instructions

1. Find a nearby zoo that houses primates. Identify which branches of the primate order are represented at the zoo. Locate *Homo sapiens* in the primate order, and identify which of the zoo primates are most closely and least closely related to humans based on considerations of genetic (DNA) relatedness.

2. Observe members of one species of primates at your local zoo for at least 2 hours, recording how they spend time. If you have no local zoo, do this for a pet, farm animal, or any wildlife that you might watch over time.

3. Identify and describe at least four similarities that you have seen between the occupational behavior of people and animals.

Environmental Influences on Occupational Engagement and Well-Being

Purpose

The purpose of this learning support is to help students apply the concepts of institutions, activity situations, environmental presses, environmental channeling, and occupationally enlivening versus deadening activity situations to their own lives.

Instructions

1. Identify at least 10 activity situations that you encounter each week. Describe the environmental press of each situation as gauged by what you are most likely or least likely to do therein.

   ○ Do these activity situations vary on the continuum from occupationally enlivening to occupationally deadening? If so, describe how.

2. Imagine that you must live in an institution for the rest of your life—perhaps a prison, a nursing home, a board and care home, or some other highly restrictive setting—or think of someone you know who does.

   ○ Which of the activity situations under #1 would no longer be available in your imagined institutional setting?

   ○ What different activity situations might become most prominent?

   ○ How can you imagine the dynamic of environmental channeling playing out in this institutional setting?

Occupational Therapy in Long-Term Care Settings

Purpose

The purpose of this learning support is to prompt students to imagine new ways of delivering services to people with dementia in long-term care settings.

Primary Concepts

Key concepts include consultative models of care, dementia-specific quality of life indicators, occupational portraits, and adaptedness and well-being as time-sensitive and environmentally contingent phenomenon.

Instructions

The following questions are designed to prompt thinking on how practitioners might implement new models of intervention that benefit residents with dementia.

1. Identify two ways in which occupational therapy services for institutionalized people with dementia who lack rehabilitation potential can be funded.

2. Explain the limitations of one-time functional assessments for institutionalized people with dementia.

3. Develop two time-efficient strategies that an occupational therapy practitioner might use to create an occupational portrait of institutionalized people with dementia.

REFERENCES

Alzheimer's Association. (2012). 2012 Alzheimer's disease facts and figures. *Alzheimer's & Dementia, 8*(2), 131-168. doi:10.1016/j.jalz.2012.02.001

Bronfenbrenner, U. (1977). Toward an experimental ecology of human development. *American Psychologist, 32*(7), 513-531. doi:10.1037/0003-066X.32.7.513

Bronfenbrenner, U., & Crouter, A. C. (1993). The evolution of environmental models of developmental research. In P. H. Mussen (Ed.), *Handbook of child psychology: History, theory, methods* (Vol. 1, pp. 357-414). New York, NY: Wiley.

Christiansen, C., & Baum, C. (Eds.). (1991). *Occupational therapy: Intervention for life performance.* Thorofare, NJ: SLACK Incorporated.

Creswell, J. W. (2007). *Qualitative inquiry & research design: Choosing among five approaches* (2nd ed.). Thousand Oaks, CA: Sage Publications.

Dawson, P., Kline, K., Wiancko, D. C., & Wells, D. (1986). Preventing excess disability in patients with Alzheimer's disease. *Geriatric Nursing, 7*(6), 298-301.

Goffman, E. (1961). *Asylums: Essays on the social situation of mental patients and other inmates.* Garden City, NY: Anchor Books.

Goodall, J. (1981). *The chimpanzees of Gombe: Patterns of behavior.* Cambridge, MA: The Belknap Press of Harvard University.

Goodall, J. (1990). *Through a window: My 30 years with the chimpanzees of Gombe.* Boston, MA: Houghton Mifflin.

Goodall, J., & Berman, P. (2000). *Reason for hope: A spiritual journey.* New York, NY: Warner Books.

Hasselkus, B. R. (1998). Occupation and well-being in dementia: The experience of day-care staff. *American Journal of Occupational Therapy, 52*(6), 423-434. doi:10.5014/ajot.52.6.423

Hughes, B. O., & Duncan, J. H. (1988). The notion of "ethological need," models of motivation and animal welfare. *Animal Behavior, 36,* 1696-1707. doi:10.1016/S0003-3472(88)80110-6

Jolly, A., Gustafson, H., Oliver, W., & O'Connor, S. (1982). *Propithecus verreauxi* population and ranging at Berenty, Madagascar, 1975 and 1980. *Folio Primatologica, 39,* 124-144. doi:10.1159/000156071

Kane, R. (2001). Long term care and a good quality of life: Bringing them closer together. *The Gerontologist, 41,* 292-304.

Kitwood, T. (1997). *Dementia reconsidered: The person comes first.* Buckingham, United Kingdom: Open University Press.

Knight, K., Wood, W., & Booth, C. (2013). *Staff satisfactions and dissatisfactions in a long-term care facility undergoing culture change.* Manuscript submitted for publication.

Lawton, M. P. (1989). Environmental proactivity in older people. In S. Spacapan & S. Oskamp (Eds.), *The social psychology of aging.* Newbury Park, CA: Sage Publications.

Lawton, M. P. (1997). Quality of life in Alzheimer disease. *Alzheimer Disease & Associated Disorders, 8*(3), 138-150.

Lawton, M. P., & Nahemow, L. E. (1973). Ecology and the aging process. In C. Eisdorfer & M. P. Lawton (Eds.), *The psychology of adult development and aging* (pp. 619-674). Washington, DC: American Pschological Association.

Lawton, M. P., Van Haitsma, K., & Klapper, J. A. (1996). Observed affect in nursing home residents. *Journal of Gerontology: Psychological Sciences, 51B,* P3-P14.

Lawton, M. P., Van Haitsma, K., Perkinson, M., & Ruckdeschel, K. (2000). Observed affect and quality of life in dementia: Further affirmations and problems. In A. S. M. & R. G. Logsdon (Eds.), *Assessing quality of life in Alzheimer's disease* (1st ed., pp. 95-110). New York, NY: Springer Publishing.

MacNeil, C. (2002). Evaluator as steward of citizen deliberation. *American Journal of Evaluation, 23*(1), 45-54. doi:10.1177/109821400202300105

MacNeil, C., & Mead, S. (2005). A narrative approach to developing standards for trauma-informed peer support. *American Journal of Evaluation, 26,* 231-244. doi:10.1177/1098214005275633

Meyer, A. (1922). The philosophy of occupation therapy. *Archives of Occupational Therapy, 1*(1), 1-10.

Moss, M. S., Lawton, M. P., Kleban, M. H., & Duhamel, L. (1993). Time use of caregivers of impaired elders before and after institutionalization. *Journal of Gerontology, 48*(3), S102-S111.

Muhlenhaupt, M. (Ed.). (2003). *Enabling student participation through occupational therapy in the schools.* Thorofare, NJ: SLACK Incorporated.

Porn, I. (1993). Health and adaptedness. *Theoretical Medicine, 14*(4), 295-303. doi:10.1007/BF00996337

Reilly, M. (1974). *Play as exploratory learning.* Beverly Hills, CA: Sage Publications.

Richard, A. F. (1978). *Behavioral variation: Case study of a Malagasy lemur.* Lewisburg, PA: Bucknell University Press.

Rogers, J. C., Holm, M. B., Burgio, L. D., Hsu, C., Hardin, J. M., & McDowell, B. J. (2000). Excess disability during morning care in nursing home residents with dementia. *International Psychogeriatrics, 12*(2), 267-282. doi:10.1017/S1041610200006372

Rushen, J., Lawrence, A., & Terlouw, E. (1993). The motivational basis of stereotypies. In J. Rushen & A. Lawrence (Eds.), *Stereotypic animal behaviour: Fundamentals and applications to welfare* (pp. 41-64). Wallingford, United Kingdom: CAB International.

Services, C. f. M. a. M. (2004). *Action plan for further improvement of nursing home quality.* Retrieved from www.cms.hhs.gov/quality/nhqi/

Sifton, C. B. (2000). Activity (special issue). *Alzheimer's Care Quarterly, 1.*

Stake, R. E. (2000). Case studies. In N. K. Denzin & Y. S. Lincoln (Eds.), *Handbook of qualitative research* (2nd ed., pp. 435-454). Thousand Oaks, CA: Sage Publications.

Wells, D., Dawson, P., Sidani, S., Craig, D., & Pringle, D. (2000). The benefits of abilities-focused morning care for residents with dementia and their caregivers. *Perspectives, 24*(1), 17. doi:10.1111/j.1748-3743.2011.00273.x

Wilcock, A. A. (2006). *An occupational perspective of health* (2nd ed.). Thorofare, NJ: SLACK Incorporated.

Wood, W. (1993). Occupation and the relevance of primatology to occupational therapy. *American Journal of Occupational Therapy, 47,* 515-522. doi:10.5014/ajot.47.6.515

Wood, W. (1995). Weaving the warp and weft of occupational therapy: An art and science for all times. *American Journal of Occupational Therapy, 49*(1), 44-50. doi:10.5014/ajot.49.1.44

Wood, W. (1996). Delivering occupational therapy's fullest promise: Clinical interpretation of "life domains and adaptive strategies of a group of low-income, well older adults." *American Journal of Occupational Therapy, 50,* 109-112. doi:10.5014/ajot.50.2.109

Wood, W. (1997). Insights from the play of nonhuman primates. In B. Chandler (Ed.), *The essence of play: A child's occupation* (pp. 16-49). Bethesda, MD: American Occupational Therapy Association.

Wood, W. (1998a). Biological requirements for occupation in primates: An exploratory study and theoretical analysis. *Journal of Occupational Science, 5,* 66-81. doi:10.1080/14427591.1998.9686435

Wood, W. (1998b). Environmental influences upon the social choices, occupational behaviors and adaptedness of zoo chimpanzees: Relevance to occupational therapy. *Scandinavian Journal of Occupational Therapy, 5*(3), 119-131.

Wood, W. (2002). Ecological synergies in two groups of zoo chimpanzees: Divergent patterns of time use. *American Journal of Occupational Therapy, 56,* 160-170. doi:10.5014/ajot.56.2.160

Wood, W. (2005). Toward developing new occupational science measures: An example from dementia care research. *Journal of Occupational Science, 12,* 121-129. doi:10.1080/14427591.2005.9686555

Wood, W., Harris, S., Snider, M., & Patchel, S. (2005). Activity situations on an Alzheimer's disease special care unit and resident environmental interactions, time use and affect. *American Journal of Alzheimer's Disease and Other Dementias, 20*(2), 105-118. doi:10.1177/153331750502000210

Wood, W., Towers, L., & Malchow, J. (2000). Environment, time-use, and adaptedness in prosimians: Implications for discerning behavior that is occupational in nature. *Journal of Occupational Science, 7,* 14-27. doi:10.1080/14427591.2000.9686460

Wood, W., Womack, J., & Hooper, B. (2009). Dying of boredom: An exploratory case study of time use, apparent affect and routine activity situations on two Alzheimer's special care units. *American Journal of Occupational Therapy, 63*(3), 337-350.

Yerxa, E. J., Clark, F., Frank, G., Jackson, J., Parham, D., & Pierce, D. (1989). An introduction to occupational science: A foundation for occupational therapy in the 21st century. *Occupational Therapy in Health Care, 6,* 1-17.

Yin, K. (2003). *Case study research: Design and methods* (3rd ed.). Thousand Oaks, CA: Sage Publications.

Zgola, J. (1999). *Care that works: A relationship approach to persons with dementia.* Baltimore, MD: Johns Hopkins University Press.

Zgola, J., & Bordillon, G. (2001). *Bon appetit! The joy of dining in long-term care.* Baltimore, MD: Health Professions Press.

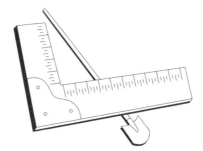

6

In Search of Graphical Methods to Describe Morning Routines in Occupational Science

Charlotte Brasic Royeen, PhD, OTR/L, FAOTA

As described by this book's editor, it is commonly accepted that there are four types of knowledge needed in disciplines that support practice professions. This chapter is devoted to looking at the most basic, or Level 1, research that is devoted to identifying and describing factors or key concepts within a discipline or profession. This may also be called *descriptive research* (Vogt, 1993). It is also commonly accepted that in order to do well-designed research at other levels, a discipline must have a critical mass of information in basic descriptive research. Otherwise, studies cannot be properly designed, and confounds of research are likely. It is, therefore, critical to attend to basic descriptive research on occupation in order to further develop the science.

After 20 years of the evolution of the discipline (Yerxa et al., 1989), the key constructs of what constitute occupational science are emerging. Thus, research into the key constructs has been challenging, because just what the key constructs are has continued in debate and dialogue among occupational science scholars. At this point in the development of the discipline, however, it does appear that a certain number of concepts have been commonly accepted as "key"

in the science. These are concepts such as context (Moyers & Dale, 2007), habit (Christiansen & Townsend, 2010), meaning (Wilcock, 2006), pleasure (Pierce, 2001), productivity (Pierce, 2001), routine (Christiansen & Townsend, 2010), occupation (Christiansen & Townsend, 2010), rest (Pierce, 2001), self-care (Creek, 2002), space (Bates, 1997), and temporality (Wilcock, 2006; Zemke, 2004). Continued research into these most basic of concepts pertinent to occupational science is critically important. Such a path of descriptive research deviates from the popularly prescribed plan for evidence-based practice and intervention research as currently called for by many in occupational therapy and other fields.

Based upon a series of Gordon-style conferences sponsored by the American Occupational Therapy Foundation in 1999, 2001, and 2007 at the Asilomar Conference Center in Monterey, CA, my interest in routines as a part of occupational science was aroused. More specifically, the presentations by speakers, as well as interactions with speakers and attendees at this conference, facilitated my quest into investigation of morning routines.

Pierce, D. (Ed.).
Occupational Science for Occupational Therapy (pp. 67-77).
© 2014 SLACK Incorporated.

THE NEED TO STUDY ROUTINES

Routines are critically important to occupational therapy practice and are foundational to occupational science. For purposes of this chapter, occupation is considered to be an all-encompassing process and not a product. Routines and habits are considered to be subcomponents of occupation. Fiese, Tomcho, Doublas, Josephs, Poltrock, and Baker (2002) define routine as a patterned interaction. Specifically, routines and habits are subsets of occupations and are considered to be the infrastructure, or support, for occupational engagement (Luebben & Royeen, 2007). In the American Occupational Therapy Association's (AOTA) *Occupational Therapy Practice Framework: Domain and Process, Second Edition* (2008), routines are considered under the rubric of performance patterns. The World Health Organization's *International Classification of Function of Functioning, Disability and Health* (2001) defines routines as "carrying out simple or complex coordinated actions to plan, manage, and complete the requirements of day-to-day procedures or duties, such as budgeting time and making plans for separate activities that construct the day" (p. 130).

In occupational therapy practice, we often talk of routines as a part of intervention. Yet, we actually know very little about routines. We assume we know what they are and how they support participation in occupation, but relatively little has been published in the area. This conundrum was clearly explicated by one of the Asilomar conference presentations by Gallimore and Lopez (2002), who identified that because of their commonplace occurrence, routines are transparent and invisible.

For most individuals in Western society, routines are assumed to be an important part of daily life. For purposes of this chapter, it is assumed that performance in daily life is, in part, related to the routines a person uses across the day. O'Leary, Quinn, and Turner (2008) support the notion that routines provide structure to the day. According to Dunn (1994), occupational therapy has a long heritage of considering routines in performance of daily life. In 1922, our esteemed founder, Eleanor Clarke Slagle, inferred much about what we recognize today as occupational science (National Society for the Promotion of Occupational Therapy, n.d.; Serrett, 1985).

Most often, when someone is referring to routines, he or she is doing so in reference to a particular individual. Yet, routines may also be parts of a group or of a culture as a whole. When routines become part of the group culture, they are often ascribed a special meaning and become rituals. Clearly, anthropology has studied groups' routines as rituals across cultures, but there is a dearth of study about individual routines across cultures or within cultures, particularly related to occupation.

What are practical examples of routines? Because habitual patterns of behavior are routines (behavior being the smaller unit of habits), consider the habitual patterns of behavior in which you engage on a daily basis. Examples may be how you prepare, organize, and eat your food; how you organize your music for listening on an iPod (Apple); the sequence of actions you undertake upon waking; the manner in which you dress and undress; or the steps you take in preparing for sleep.

There is probably no area of occupational therapy practice that does not use or integrate use of routines in some manner. The clearest example of use of routines in occupational therapy practice may be the Wilbarger Protocol, an intervention using brushing and compression integrated into the daily routines of an infant or toddler in order to facilitate appropriate sensory modulation (Segal & Beyer, 2006; Wilbarger & Wilbarger, 1991, 2004).

In addition to not being adequately addressed in our literature, the term *routine* is also employed in a confusing way. For example, Nelson (2006) pointed out how, in the first edition of the *Occupational Therapy Practice Framework: Domain and Process* (AOTA, 2002), the terms *habits* and *routines* were used interchangeably, like synonyms. Such confusion reflects the state of practice and scholarship in occupational therapy about habits and routines. This issue has been resolved in the second edition of the *Framework* (AOTA, 2008). But, confusion in our practice and in our literature persists.

LITERATURE

Considering the importance of routines in occupational science and occupational therapy, this chapter explores literature on the construct and a research strategy for investigating them. This literature review is organized into two sections. First, there is a review of the literature on routines. Based upon that review of the literature, it appeared that how routines were being studied might be a factor limiting research into routines. Second, therefore, is an exploration of the literature into alternative research methods, specifically, into graphical-based methods of inquiry.

Review of the Literature on Routines

A wide-ranging search of pertinent literature on routines was conducted. No profession or discipline appeared to dominate published scholarship about routines. The resulting array of literature was a challenge to synthesize, because it was not strongly referencing common theories or topics. To ease understanding, it was organized here into categories of temporality, planning, medication compliance, families and communities, disease states, learning, and outcomes.

Temporality

Studying visually and nonvisually impaired infants, Troster, Brambring, and Van der Burg (1996) concluded that there was a significant correlation between regularity of routines prior to bedtime and quality of sleep. Having staff members say goodbye, therefore making routines more explicit, assisted in the transitioning of clients from one set of staff to another (Pretti-Frontczak, Barr, Macy, & Carter, 2003). While studying schizophrenic clients, the regularity and sequence of routines influenced the subsequent occupation of sleep (Chuff & Craik, 2002). Thus, it is evident that temporality of routines, or how one action is linked in time to the next action, influences or affects subsequent occupational participation.

Planning

How teachers routinely plan the instruction day was studied by Earle (1996). How mothers create daily routines to promote self-care of young children with disabilities was studied by Kellegrew (2000). How mothers "designed their present" using daily routines was studied by Larson (2000), including how they planned, organized, balanced, anticipated, interpreted, forecasted, and created meaning. One could speculate that routines are prepackaged, or readymade, chunks of activity to be used in the manner that professionals, mothers, and families organize or plan for the day.

Medication Compliance

Prescription of intermittent medication (medication that is not taken at regular intervals) for elders living at home has been found to disrupt elders' routines (Bytheway, 2001). The consistency of daily routines for women who lived in rural settings allowed them more consistent use of contraceptive pills (Oakley et al., 1999). Based upon these studies, it can be surmised that routines affect medication compliance.

Families and Communities

Related to how complex occupation is, especially in a family setting, Primeau (2000) studied how routines were created and maintained in families. Burton and Graham (1998) studied how neighborhoods or communities of urban teen mothers shaped their daily activities around social routines. They found that the morning routine was courting behaviors, the parading of the babies was the afternoon routine, and drug hazing was the night routine. Access to transportation, child care, and social services was related to how low-income mothers structured their daily routines (Roy, Tubbs, & Burton, 2004). Routines and rituals in families with children who have autism were studied by Werner (2001), who found that families self-organize routines in order to optimize acquisition of social support and interactions.

Disease States

Caregivers' use of routines to facilitate exercise and physical therapy interventions among individuals with Alzheimer's disease was described by Cornman-Levy, Gitlin, Corcoran, and Schinfeld (2001). Considering disease management, Goldstein and Daly (1997) surmised that daily routines must match the drug-monitoring regimen. The effect of testicular cancer on daily routines of families was studied by Sanden and Huyden (2002). In people with HIV-AIDS, Bedell (2000) found that clients self-organized energy conservation adaptations. Based upon this literature, there appears to be an interdependent state between routines and disease: routines can improve health when disease is chronic, or routines can be disrupted by disease.

Learning

Fenichel (2002) found that, during the daily routines of children, learning occurs. Daily routines can facilitate children's development (Gonzales-Mena, 2002). Academic tasks can evolve from literacy routines for infants, toddlers, and preschoolers (Lawhon & Cobb, 2002). In a related manner, Grisham-Brown, Pretti-Frontczak, Hemmeter, and Ridgley (2002) speculated that integrating daily routines with the child's Individualized Education Program goals and objectives will facilitate reaching the goals. Integration of physical therapy services into classroom routines using teacher participation was studied by Sekerak, Kirkpatrick, Nelson, and Propoes (2003). An intervention based upon talking during daily routines was proposed as the Ecological Organizational model of communication (ECO Model) by MacDonald and Rabidoux (1997). Drawing from knowledge in neuroscience, Pretorius, Naude, and Pretorius (2005) postulated that selected types of activities during daily routines increased capacity for development of memory and reading ability by facilitating hippocampus and amygdala function. Others have proposed that routines promote social, emotional, and cognitive development of preschoolers (Administration for Children, Youth, and Families, 2002). In education, place-based education uses immersion of children into the routines of the community (Jaycox, 2001). This literature suggests a strong interaction, or co-effect, between routines and most forms of learning (social, cognitive, and emotional).

Outcomes

The literature also points to outcomes of routines in humans. It has been suggested that understanding of time is related to routines in children (Barclay, Benelli, & Wolf, 1997). According to Segal (2004), routines of families can organize the family and fosters meaning for the family unit. Accordingly, looking at the outcome of routines, this literature identifies learning, learning the concept of time, development of family bonds, and meaning making.

Synthesis of the Literature on Routines

Based upon this review of the literature, three conclusions may be drawn.

1. Some things are known about what routines can do and how they influence development.

2. Very little is known about what routines, in and of themselves, really are. The literature reviewed primarily

looked at the effects of routines or speculate upon how routines influenced something else. Level 1 research and understanding of what constitutes the construct of a routine was limited.

3. A collection of research methods that studied routines were identified from the literature review and included participant observation, interview, self-report (verbal and written), phenomenology, and case study. None of these research strategies allowed for investigation of routines in and of themselves.

Pieris and Craik (2004) suggest that many concepts in occupational therapy are based upon literature analysis and expert opinion, rather than research knowledge. In order to move occupational science and occupational therapy forward, primary constructs of interest must become the focus of descriptive research. Key variables of interest (such as routines) should be studied (Level 1 research) so that other levels of research (relational, predictive, and prescriptive) may be adequately designed.

The Search for Alternative Strategies for the Study of Routine: Graphical-Based Methods

Practicalities Produce Methods

Statistical and research methods are not static and unbending truths. In fact, they evolved in response to the need of a discipline, profession, or practical situation. For example, the *sign* test originated as a way to prove divine intervention for birth of a male (Bellhouse, 1989). And, a chemist in the Guinness brewery of Dublin, Ireland named William Sealy Gosset created the *t*-test so that small amounts of beer could be compared for quality control of the product (McMullen, 1939). As in these examples, occupational science and occupational therapy may require innovative methods of research design and analysis in order to examine questions important to the development of the science.

Graphical-Based Inquiry

Other fields use graphical-based inquiry, or art-based research, for their investigations. In such work, created objects may be considered to be a form of art (Eisner, 1991). Based upon the literature, the leading fields in this sort of research are art and education. Many occupational therapists of a certain age were well educated in art and crafts in a manner no longer done today. For us, there may be an intuitive link between art and expression of everyday life (Monet, Manet, and Degas did it best!). Even Dewey (1934/1980) acknowledged that many may be averse to considering art as a way of examining a subject in its environment, or what occupational scientists and occupational therapists would call occupational engagement in context. But Dewey did consider art a useful way to portray that engagement. Others do as well!

Stafstrom, Rostasy, and Minster (2002) discovered that children's self-drawings of a headache had a 90% correlation ($n = 266$) with clinical diagnosis of migraine compared to nonmigraine headaches. It was further discovered that pre-post self-drawings significantly correlated to improvement in the children's headaches (Stafstrom, Goldenholz, & Dulli, 2005). At the very least, there is some form of validity across drawings and medical conditions. It seems reasonable to assume such validity exists across drawings and routines. Denzin (1997) associates the pre-eminent forms of research of our current time as reflecting dominance of a male-gendered way of seeing and knowing. Conversely, a "pink collar" (Royeen, 2005) feminist call for adapted research methods may be in order to look at routines. The study reported here was based upon use of graphical, or arts-based, methods over the past decade (Findley, 2003). Ultimately, the goal is to expand research strategies in occupational science and occupational therapy. From a larger perspective, art-based occupations are coming back into vogue as therapeutic approaches and have been used in occupational therapy since 1917 (Hyde & Hunt, 2008). Perhaps they will also find a way into our research methods.

METHODS

This study, published elsewhere (Royeen, 2010), was informed by a constructivist model (Higgs, 2001; LeCompte & Schensul, 1999) and employed an interpretive strategy with the philosophy of verstehen (or understanding) as the goal. Data collection and analysis were completed using a four-phase cycle similar to that employed by Dublouoz, Laporte, Hall, Ashe, and Smith (2004) and initially delineated by Strauss and Corbin (1990).

The Approach

The language of frame and strip used in this study is standard terminology in discussion of comic strips, defined as juxtaposed pictorial and other images in a deliberate sequence (McCloud, 1993). These images are intended to transmit information, which can also be called *graphical presentations, diagrams* (McCloud, 1993), or *pictograms*. In this study, (a) the collection of frames is the strip, (b) each frame is an individual part or component of the strip, (c) the entire strip is assumed to be analogous to the routine, and (d) each frame is assumed to be analogous to an individual activity or habit within that routine.

Figure 6-1 illustrates what constitutes a frame and a strip. All of the pictograms for frames within the strips for one participant are presented in Figure 6-1. Collectively, these are assumed to constitute a routine. Within the routine or strip, one can easily discern individual frames or actions that are in a sequenced order. Look at Figure 6-1: go

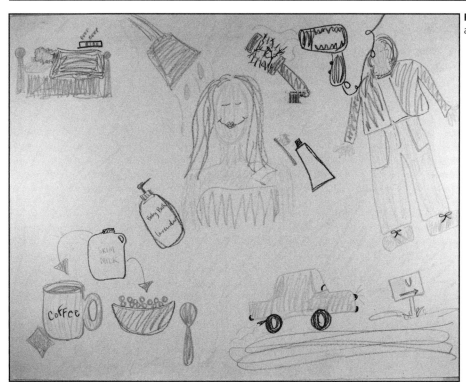

Figure 6-1. A sample graphical depiction of a morning routine.

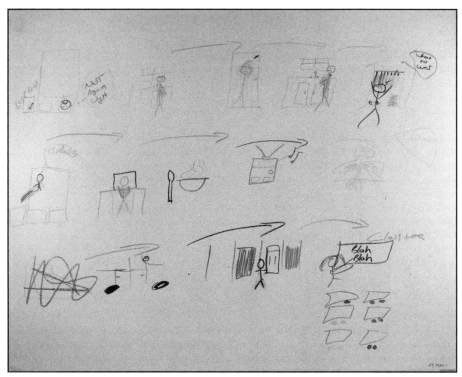

Figure 6-2. Another sample of a graphical depiction of a morning routine.

from the graphic of the bed, to the graphic of the smiling female, to the graphic of the hair dryer, to the graphic of the car. As pictorially presented, these data should provide the reader with a sense of how the morning routine unfolded. Figure 6-2 presents data that are even easier to discern, in that individual frames were separated by directional lines the participant spontaneously inserted. Figures 6-1 and 6-2 provide prototypical examples of the nature and extent of the data collected from all study participants.

TABLE 6-1

INFORMATION ON PARTICIPANTS (PARTICIPANT = P)

	FRAMES	PLACES	OBJECTS		FRAMES	PLACES	OBJECTS
P1	14	8	15	P24	11	3	9
P2	11	9	9	P25	9	0	13
P3	9	6	13	P26	14	4	13
P4	13	8	8	P27	7	3	10
P5	14	6	13	P28	6	4	13
P6	16	7	16	P29	15	5	15
P7	11	4	12	P30	10	4	12
P8	13	1	13	P31	14	3	14
P9	8	3	10	P32	15	2	9
P10	8	0	11	P33	13	4	19
P11	9	6	5	P34	12	2	7
P12	11	6	8	P35	5	2	6
P13	9	6	10	P36	8	2	9
P14	8	4	8	P37	10	0	10
P15	9	0	9	P38	6	4	4
P16	7	5	9	P39	7	4	4
P17	*	*	*	P40	14	5	14
P18	11	3	6	P41	7	4	11
P19	11	2	8	P42	11	5	13
P20	13	8	0	P43	7	5	15
P21	6	5	9	P44	11	0	4
P22	13	0	12	P45	15	6	17
P23	12	5	18	P46	7	2	9

Participants

For this investigation, participants (Table 6-1) were recruited through an on-site class for clinical doctoral students by another professor in the occupational therapy department of a comprehensive Midwestern university. Some of the participants were male ($n = 9$) but most were female ($n = 35$), while two failed to identify gender. Twelve of the 46 participants were enrolled in the professional occupational therapy program of the university. Participants recruited by occupational therapy students were regionally diverse. Ages ranged from 17 to 53 years, the mean being 29.5 years. Data collectors identified that it took approximately 10 to 30 minutes for each participant to draw his or her morning routine.

Data Collection

Data were obtained by asking a participant to draw his or her morning routine. Each of the six data collectors was instructed in soliciting an art-based pictograph. Data collectors were given a 3-month period for data collection. Directions to participants were: "Using pictures and on this page, tell the story of your morning routine." Data collectors were directed to use colored crayons and large pieces (91.4 x 61 inches) of manila paper with the participants.

The drawing activity occurred either (a) in a group setting (with classmates) with the instructor or (b) in the presence of an online clinical doctoral student at an off-site location. Data were mailed or hand delivered to the investigator.

Data Analysis

Using visual inspection, the strips were deconstructed into naturally occurring frames. Subsequently, each frame was numbered in a sequence. Accordingly, the frames in a strip could be counted, as could any of the objects or places within the frames of the strip. The ease of this was exceptional and evident.

The data were counted and analyzed frame by frame, or items were counted within each frame. This form of analysis may be considered to be an adaptation of occupational storytelling (Clark, 1993). Clark used narrative analysis (an interactive interpretation of words within a story sequence), whereas this study used interpretative analysis (an interactive interpretation of frames within the strips).

Data were interpreted by employing a constant-comparative process of thematic analysis, frequency counts, and descriptive statistics, yielding mixed-methods analysis of data, as consistent with Higgs (2001), Creswell (2003), and Miles and Huberman (1994). For quantitative analysis, frequency counts determined the number of frames in the strip, with each frame labeled as an activity. Frequency counts determined number of places depicted in the frames in each strip and the number of objects used in the frames in the strip. For qualitative analysis, interpretative analysis used constant comparisons (Denzin & Lincoln, 2000), using an iterative process that produced images, themes, and categories that were revealed by asking questions relating to "What is the meaning?" "What is the relationship?" and "What is the place, activity, or object?" Memoing during the data analysis was included.

Trustworthiness

In addition to memoing, expert review and conference presentation feedback were used to check trustworthiness of findings. In both cases, therapists confirmed overall clarity of action in the scripts, as well as the deployment of frames and the categorization of objects and places in reviewing the strips.

RESULTS

Initial Review of Data

Visual inspection of Figure 6-2 reveals that space on the paper was fully and nearly completely used as it was in almost all of the drawings. Review of all the strips revealed that, in some, a word is presented along with a depiction, such as the word "ouch" written to go along with the alarm clock ringing. In another case, a bar of soap is labeled as soap; Figure 6-2 features "not again" as labeled for waking up. Such word labeling appeared spontaneously. Figure 6-2

also clearly depicts the sense of sequence and order that most all of the strips presented.

The strips, collectively, were viewed as emotionally positive by the investigator. Somber tones were not seen. Rather, action and color were noted. Many strips had sunshine portrayed. No systematic differences were evident between the strips done in a group setting compared to those done individually.

Of the 46 strips, therefore, 45 provided useful scripts, depicting routines including activities. One participant's script consisted of words and was not, therefore, a strip. This left 45 strips for calculation of descriptive statistics on frames, objects, and place. Table 6-1 presents descriptive statistics on the number of frames in each strip.

Quantitative Descriptive Results

Table 6-1 summarizes the number of frames presented in each strip. The number of frames in each strip ranged from 5 to 16.

This is assumed to mean that 5 to 16 activities or actions were part of the morning routines. The mean numbers of frames in a strip were 10, with a median and mode of 11. For this group, it appears that there were 10 to 11 steps or sets of actions in a morning routine.

Table 6-1 also summarizes numbers of places that were identified in the morning routines. Places portrayed in the morning routines were primarily places in the home such as a kitchen, a bedroom, a bathroom, or a stairwell. Other places portrayed in the morning routines included space external to the home, such the outdoors, or the first place one arrives after a morning routine, such as a classroom. In six cases, no place or context for the activity could be discerned and was noted as "0." Ranges of places noted in the strips of morning routines were from 0 to 9, with 4 as mean, median, and mode. For this group of participants, four places were typically used in execution of the morning routine.

Qualitative Descriptive Results

Theme: Action in Space and Place

For this group of participants, morning routines consisted of an array of activities carried out within a limited number of places. The activities had practical purposes of preparing the participant in terms of eating, dressing, or cleansing of the body. Some activities (i.e., scanning computer e-mails or organizing backpacks) were interpreted to be methods of preparation for anticipated activities later in the day. This finding is congruent with Kellegrew (2000) and Larson (2000) regarding orchestration of the day through enactment of a routine.

It was assumed that every frame within the strip represented an activity or action. Given there were an average number of frames presented by participants, one may conclude that morning routines have a usual number of activities that are finite and specific. For this group of participants, 11 categories of activities in the morning routine were representative of their experience. It is notable that, for this group of individuals, most of the strips reflected activities inferred to be conducted in solitude. Among the strips, it was infrequent to have a frame presenting the participant as interacting with another, be it another adult or a child.

Theme: Clarity of Occupational Engagement

Among these participants, the morning routines presented in the strips were clear and evident. To illustrate, one could easily discern the collection of actions graphically presented as the morning routine (i.e., it was evident how they engaged in this chunk of daily activity). Such a degree of clarity in the sequence or amalgamation of activities was unexpected. The activities could collectively be categorized as activities of daily living, preparation for tasks later in the day, and reflection.

Theme: Using Objects in Space and Place

Humankind is distinguished from other mammals by the degree to which it uses material culture, including tools, clothing, books, shelters, crops, art, and many other categories of objects (Pierce, 2001). Use of objects during morning routines is clearly an example of this aspect of the occupational nature of humans. The data revealed that, for this group of participants, the use of nine categories of objects was typical. It could be that many of the objects used in the morning routines could be used again later in the day or at other times of the day and in other routines. It is likely that tools used in morning routines are not exclusively used in morning routines. The categories of tools or objects used include tools for activities of daily living, tools for work or study, and tools for home organization and cooking.

Theme: Dynamical Nature of the Pattern of Engagement

All of the scripts had a sequence of stages or settings portrayed: in none of them did the setting remain constant. Thus, nothing was static; the process was dynamic. For this group, morning routines were portrayed in four distinct environments. These four environments were home, outdoors, in some sort of transportation, or work or study site. Most of the routines started in a bed, and most of the morning routines ended up either in a car transporting the participant to another location or in presentation of a door. Finishing the morning routine by portraying a door may demark movement or egress from personal space to public space outside the home.

Theme: Routine Sequence

Pattern and order was clear in the scripts. Each script presented a story that could easily be discerned in a linear manner, revealing that, for this group of participants, multitasking did not appear to be an aspect of morning routines. Rather, all scripts presented a sequence in which a single activity was executed and then the next activity initiated. This finding was a surprise, given how much focus Western society has on multitasking. Further, there was intuitive logic manifested in the scripts, such as bathing or activities of daily living prior to organizing a backpack or eating breakfast.

Theme: Morning Routines Are Challenging

In the scripts, it was evident that arising or alerting in the morning was a very, very challenging task for many. What was inferred to be sleep deprivation was depicted in a variety of ways, such as portrayal of repeatedly hitting the snooze button on an alarm clock. Participants portrayed self-portraits of haggard eyes upon waking and a grumpy face upon waking. In spite of this, by the end of every script, the challenge of waking up seemed to be resolved.

Discussion

For these participants, the morning routine consisted of 11 categories of sequenced activities across four places, most typically carried out alone. Also for these participants, morning routines appeared to provide foundational organization for activities later in the day: many of the morning routines prepared the individual for what happens after the morning routine, such as going to school or work. The morning routine appeared to prepare the participant in some manner for entering the day. This finding is consistent with Segal (2004) who suggested that meaning was provided by family routine. The everyday, ordinary activities of morning routines could be the vehicle for support or preparation for the rest of the day or in general participation in life. Thus, this study generates a hypothesis that the morning routine prepares the individual for participation in life.

It is notable that multitasking was not evident in the strips. Is this an artifact of the method? Or, is unitasking more typical of morning routines? Is there something unique to morning routines that do not match with multitasking? Or, are we multitasking less than we assume? This is an area worthy of future study.

CONTRIBUTIONS TO OCCUPATIONAL SCIENCE

Understanding the Construct of the Morning Routine

For occupational science, an understanding of morning routines is important for several reasons. Morning routines are the start to the day's orchestration and hold potential for further developing theoretical understandings of the temporality of occupation. The morning routine is also the point of transition out of sleep, the most prevalent and health-impacting occupation of humans (Pierce, 2001, 2003). Lastly, morning routines are an important focus of intervention for occupational therapists. By contributing occupational science research on morning routines, this research supports the commitment of occupational science to provide basic knowledge of occupation that will support more effective practice.

Potential of Graphical Methods for Occupational Science

It might be that only in relatively modern times (or at least since the Guttenberg Bible) humans have relied solely, or primarily, upon the written or spoken word for communication. In a more ancient example, hieroglyphics were graphics that formed the Egyptian language. In this study, graphics represented the story of a morning routine. Because all participants except one were able to draw his or her morning routine, the study demonstrated the feasibility of a graphical method.

In order to expand the concept of morning routines, future work could use stratified samples across decades of life in order to look at morning routine across ages. Validation of provisional hypotheses and theory should be conducted by enlarging the participants to include those of diverse backgrounds, varied family status, and diverse culture and socioeconomic status.

IMPLICATIONS FOR PRACTICE

At this point, implications for practice are provisional. Yet, in everyday practice, many occupational therapists are already using routines in their interventions. The more we can learn about the construct of routines and varieties of routines (morning routine, lunchtime routine, bedtime routine, etc.), the better we can formulate theory to guide practice.

LEARNING SUPPORTS

Update Literature Search on Routines

Purpose

Conduct a literature review of 10 recent articles having to do with routines.

Primary Concepts

Applied research, searching the literature, and learning by doing.

Instructions

Using "routine" or "routines," locate research-based articles in the literature.

Replicate the Morning Routine Activity

Purpose

Replicate one aspect of the study of morning routines.

Primary Concepts

Applied research and exploring morning routines.

Instructions

Tell the story of your morning routine. Using crayons, draw your morning routine on a large piece of posterboard (27 x 22 inches).

REFERENCES

Administration for Children, Youth, and Families. (2002, November). *Helping children understand routines and classroom schedules.* (Issue Brief No. 3). Washington, DC: Ostrosky, Jung, Hemmeter, & Thomas.

American Occupational Therapy Association. (2002). Occupational therapy practice framework: Domain and process. *American Journal of Occupational Therapy, 56,* 609-639.

American Occupational Therapy Association. (2008). Occupational therapy practice framework: Domain and process (2nd ed.). *American Journal of Occupational Therapy, 62,* 625-283.

Barclay, K., Benelli, C., & Wolf, J. M. (1997). "Is it time yet?" Getting more out of daily routines. *Dimensions of Early Childhood, 25*(1), 22-26.

Bates, D. (1997). The role of the teacher: Visionary, vocationalist, or technogogue? *Irish Educational Studies, 16,* 19-17.

Bedell, G. (2000). Daily life for eight urban gay men with HIV/AIDS. *American Journal of Occupational Therapy, 54*(2), 197-206.

Bellhouse, D. R. (1989). A manuscript on chance written by John Arbuthnot. *International Statistical Review, 3,* 249-259.

Burton, L. M., & Graham, J. E. (1998). Neighborhood rhythms and the social activities of adolescent mothers. *New Directions for Child and Adolescent Development, 82,* 7-22.

Bytheway, B. (2001). Responsibility and routines: How older people manage their long-term medication. *Journal of Occupational Science, 8*(3), 5-13.

Christiansen, C., & Townsend, E. (2010). *Introduction to occupation: The art and science of living.* Upper Saddle River, NJ: Prentice Hall.

Chuff, A., & Craik, C. (2002). Some factors influencing occupational engagement for people with schizophrenia living in the community. *British Journal of Occupational Therapy, 65*(2), 67-74.

Clark, F. A. (1993). 1993 Eleanor Clarke Slagle Lecture. Occupation embedded in real life: Interweaving occupational science and occupational therapy. *American Journal of Occupational Therapy, 47,* 1067-1078.

Cornman-Levy, D., Gitlin, L., Corcoran, M., & Schinfeld, S. (2001). Caregiver aches and pains: The role of physical therapy in helping families provide daily care. *Alzheimer's Care Quarterly, 2*(1), 47-55.

Creek, J. (2002). *Occupational therapy and mental health* (3rd ed.). Edinburgh, Scotland: Churchill Livingston.

Creswell, J. W. (2003). *Research design: Qualitative, quantitative, and mixed methods approaches* (2nd ed.). Thousand Oaks, CA: Sage Publications.

Denzin, N. K. (1997). *The interpretive ethnography: Ethnographic practices for the 21st century.* Thousand Oaks: CA: Sage Publications.

Denzin, N. K., & Lincoln, Y. S. (2000). Strategies of inquiry. In N. K. Denzin & Y. S. Lincoln (Eds.), *Handbook of qualitative research* (2nd ed., pp. 367-378). Thousand Oaks, CA: Sage Publications.

Dewey, J. (1934/1980). *Art as experience.* New York, NY: Perigee.

Dublouoz, C., Laporte, D., Hall, M., Ashe, B., & Smith, C. D. (2004). Transformation of meaning perspectives in clients with rheumatoid arthritis. *American Journal of Occupational Therapy, 58*(4), 398-407.

Dunn, W. (1994). Getting ready for the day: A commentary in Chapter 10. Habits. In C. B. Royeen (Ed.), *AOTA's self study series: Putting occupation back into therapy.* Bethesda, MD: American Occupational Therapy Association.

Earle, R. S. (1996). *Instructional design fundamentals as elements of teacher planning routines: Perspectives and practices from two studies.* In Proceedings of Selected Research and Development Presentations at the 1996 National Convention of the Association for Educational Communications and Technology, Indianapolis, IN.

Eisner, E. W. (1991). *The enlightened eye: Qualitative inquiry and the enhancement of educational practice.* New York, NY: Macmillan.

Fenichel, E. (Ed.). (2002). Routines and rituals in the lives of infants, toddlers, and families. *Zero to Three, 22*(4), 57.

Fiese, B. H., Tomcho, T. J., Doublas, M., Josephs, K., Poltrock, S., & Baker, T. (2002). A review of 50 years of research on naturally occurring family routines and rituals: Cause for celebration? *Journal of Family Psychology, 16*(4), 381-390.

Findley, S. (2003). Arts-based inquiry in QI: Seven years from crisis to guerrilla warfare. *Qualitative Inquiry, 9*(2), 281-296.

Gallimore, R., & Lopez, E. (2002). Everyday routines, human agency, and ecocultural context: Construction and maintenance of individual habits. Proceedings of Habits 2 Conference. *Occupational Therapy Journal of Research, 22,* 70S-77S.

Goldstein, R., & Daly, H. (1997). Daily routines of elderly people with diabetes. *British Journal of Community Health Nursing, 2*(8), 392-395.

Gonzales-Mena, J. (2002). *Infant/toddler caregiving: A guide to routines* (2nd ed.). Sacramento, CA: California Department of Education Press.

Grisham-Brown, J., Pretti-Frontczak, K., Hemmeter, M., & Ridgley, R. (2002). Teaching IEP goals and objectives in the context of classroom routines and activities. *Young Exceptional Children, 6*(1), 18-27.

Higgs, J. (2001). Charting standpoints in qualitative research. In H. Bryne-Armstrong, J. Higgs, & D. Horsfall (Eds.), *Critical moments in qualitative research* (pp. 44-78). Oxford, United Kingdom: Butterworth-Heinemann.

Hyde, R., & Hunt, E. (2008). Exploring creativity in occupational therapy from a personal and professional perspective. *Irish Journal of Occupational Therapy, 36*(4).

Jaycox, R. (2001). Rural home schooling and place-based education. *Eric Digest.* Charleston, WV: ERIC Publications.

Kellegrew, D. H. (2000). Constructing daily routines: A qualitative examination of mothers with young children with disabilities. *American Journal of Occupational Therapy, 54*(3), 252-259.

Larson, E. A. (2000). The orchestration of occupation: The dance of mothers. *American Journal of Occupational Therapy, 54*(3), 269-280.

Lawhon, T., & Cobb, J. B. (2002). Routines that build emergent literacy skills in infants, toddlers, and preschoolers. *Early Childhood Education Journal, 30*(2), 113-118.

LeCompte, M. D., & Schensul, J. J. (1999). *Designing and conducting ethnographic research.* Thousand Oaks, CA: Sage Publications.

Luebben, A. J., & Royeen, C. B. (2007). Toward verstehen: An etymological and historical wave of the terms *habit, routine, occupation,* and *participation. OTJR: Occupation, Participation, and Health, 27*(S1), 86-87.

MacDonald, J. D., & Rabidoux, P. (1997). *Before your child talks: Practical guides for parents and professionals. A curriculum for building social habits that prepare children for language.* Tallmadge, OH: Family Child Learning Center.

McCloud, S. (1993). *Understanding comics: The invisible art.* New York, NY: Paradox Press.

McMullen, L. (1939). "Student" as a man. *Biometrika, 30*(3/4), 210-250.

Miles, M. B., & Huberman, A. M. (1994). *Qualitative data analysis* (2nd ed.). Thousand Oaks, CA: Sage Publications.

Moyers, P., & Dale, L. (2007). *The guide to occupational therapy practice* (2nd ed.). Bethesda, MD: American Occupational Therapy Association.

National Society for the Promotion of Occupational Therapy. (n.d.). Correspondence of W. R. Dutton and Eleanor Clarke Slagle (1929-1937). Archives of the American Occupational Therapy Foundation, Box 3, Folder 27.

Nelson, D. L. (2006). Critiquing the logic of the Domains section of the *Occupational Therapy Practice Framework: Domain and Process. American Journal of Occupational Therapy, 60*(5), 603-604.

Oakley, D., Yu, M. Y., Shang, Y. M., Zhu, X. L., Chen, W. H., & Yao, L. (1999). Combining qualitative with quantitative approaches to study contraceptive pill use. *Journal of Women's Health, 8*(2), 249-257.

O'Leary, T., Quinn, S., & Turner, N. (2008). Research article: The self-perceived community integration needs of adults with mental illness. *Irish Journal of Occupational Therapy, 32*(2), 14-23.

Pierce, D. (2001). Occupation by design: Dimension, creativity, and therapeutic power. *American Journal of Occupational Therapy, 55,* 249-259.

Pierce, D. (2003). *Occupation by design: Building therapeutic power.* Philadelphia, PA: F. A. Davis.

Pieris, Y., & Craik, C. (2004). Factors enabling and hindering participation in leisure for people with mental health problems. *British Journal of Occupational Therapy, 67*(6), 240-247.

Pretorius, E., Naude, H., & Pretorius, U. (2005). Training the hippocampus and amygdala of preschool children by means of priming tasks: Should parents focus on learning of facts more than reading fairy-tales? *Early Child Development and Care, 175*(4), 303-312.

Pretti-Frontczak, K. L., Barr, D. M., Macy, M., & Carter, A. (2003). Research and resources related to activity based intervention, embedded learning opportunities, and routines-based instruction. *Topics in Early Childhood Special Education, 23*(1), 29-39.

Primeau, L. (2000). Division of household work, routines, and child care occupations in families. *Journal of Occupational Science, 7*(1), 19-28.

Roy, K. M., Tubbs, C. Y., & Burton, C. M., (2004). Don't have no time: Daily rhythms and the organization of time for low-income families. *Family Relations, 53*(2), 168-178.

Royeen, C. B. (2005). Appendix F: Ongoing wisdom after the lecture: "Her-story": A polemic for action, or a pink-collar call for feminist development in occupational therapy. In Rene Padilla (Ed.), *A professional legacy: The Eleanor Clarke Slagle Lectures in occupational therapy, 1955-2004 (2nd ed.).* Bethesda: American Occupational Therapy Association.

Royeen, C. B. (2010). Towards an emerging understanding of morning routines: A preliminary study using developing methods in arts based inquiry. *Irish Journal of Occupational Therapy, 38*(1), 30-42.

Sanden, I., & Huyden, L. C. (2002). How everyday life is affected: An interview study of relatives of men suffering from testicular cancer. *Journal of Psychosocial Oncology, 20,* 27-44.

Segal, R. (2004). Family routines and rituals: A context for occupational therapy interventions. *American Journal of Occupational Therapy, 58*(5), 499-508.

Segal, R., & Beyer, C. (2006). Integration and application of a home treatment program: A study of parents and occupational therapists. *American Journal of Occupational Therapy, 60*(5), 500-510.

Sekerak, D. M., Kirkpatrick, D. B., Nelson, K. C., & Propoes, J. H. (2003). Physical therapy in preschool classrooms: Successful integration of therapy into classroom routines. *Pediatric Physical Therapy, 15*(2), 93-104.

Serrett, K. D. (1985). Eleanor Clarke Slagle: Founder and leader in occupational therapy. *Occupational Therapy in Health Care, 5*(3), 101-108.

Stafstrom, C. E., Goldenholz, S. R., & Dulli, D. A. (2005). Serial headache drawing by children with migraine: Correlation with clinical headache status. *Journal of Child Neurology, 20*(10), 809-813.

Stafstrom, C. E., Rostasy, K., & Minster, A. (2002). The usefulness of children's drawings in the diagnosis of headache. *Pediatrics, 109*(3), 460-472.

Strauss, A., & Corbin, J. (1990). *Basics of qualitative research.* San Francisco, CA: Sage Publications.

Troster, H., Brambring, M., & Van der Burg, J. (1996). Daily routines and sleep disorders in visually impaired children. *Early Child Development and Care, 119,* 1-14.

Vogt, W. P. (1993). *Dictionary of statistics and methodology: A nontechnical guide for the social sciences.* Thousand Oaks, CA: Sage Publications.

Werner, E. A. (2001). Families, children with autism and everyday occupations. *Dissertation Abstracts International: Section B: The Sciences and Engineering, 62*(4-B), 1835.

Wilbarger, J., & Wilbarger, P. (2004). The Wilbarger approach to tricking sensory defensiveness. In A. C. Bundy, S. J. Lane, & E. A. Murray (Eds.), *Sensory integration: therapy and practice* (2nd ed., pp. 335-338). Philadelphia, PA: F. A. Davis.

Wilbarger, P., & Wilbarger, J. (1991). *Sensory defensiveness in children aged 2-12: An intervention guide for parents and other caregivers.* Denver, CO: Avanti Educational Programs.

Wilcock, A. A. (2006) *An occupational perspective of health* (2nd ed.). Thorofare, NJ: SLACK Incorporated.

World Health Organization (2001). *International classification of functioning, disability and health.* Geneva, Switzerland: Author.

Yerxa, E. J., Clark, F., Frank, G., Jackson, J., Parham, D., Pierce, D., . . . Zemke, R. (1989). An introduction to occupational science: A foundation for occupational therapy in the 21st century. *Occupational Therapy in Health Care, 6*(7), 1-17.

Zemke, R. (2004). 2004 Eleanor Clarke Slagle Lecture. Time, space, and the kaleidoscope of occupation. *American Journal of Occupational Therapy, 58,* 608-620.

II

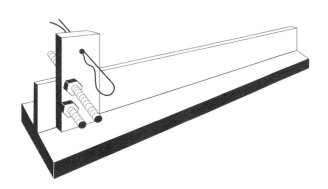

Level 2 Research

How Does Occupational Science Provide Knowledge of Relations Between Occupation and Other Phenomena?

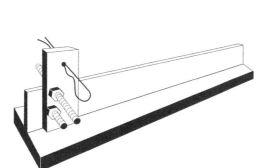

7

Relational Research in Occupational Science

Doris Pierce, PhD, OTR/L, FAOTA

THE EXPLOSION OF LEVEL 2, RELATIONAL RESEARCH IN OCCUPATIONAL SCIENCE

Within occupational science, Level 2 research examines the relations of occupation to a variety of primary concepts from other disciplines. In this sense, Level 2 occupational science is interdisciplinary. This is the level at which occupational science has grown the fastest, drawing on the developed research of established disciplines. It is also the level at which disciplines assess their value, according to the degree to which researchers from other disciplines make use of their work. Although this rapid growth at Level 2, where all research combines the perspectives of two different disciplines, has widened the scope of occupational science, it has also weakened its focus. Like a building with a small foundation and a wider first floor, the difference in productivity at Levels 1 and 2 of this young science threaten its balance.

Individualism: A Level 2 Issue

A more theoretical result of the strong interdisciplinarity of Level 2 is the recent concern that occupational science is too "individualistic" (Dickie, Cutchin, & Humphry, 2006). That is, occupational science is not close enough in its theories, epistemology, and disciplinary intent to that of established social sciences. Researchers who are trained in outside disciplines and whose primary concepts address population level concepts, such as those of community health or culture-wide dynamics, necessarily bring their knowledge to bear on occupation at these levels. And, of course, it is a key argument of all disciplines that their perspective is the most valuable perspective.

It is true that broader, cultural, or population-level interpretations are valuable. I emphatically disagree, however, that this logically implies that occupational science research that focuses on individual experiences and perspectives of participants is deeply flawed or less appropriate than a transactional, Deweyan perspective (Cutchin, Dickie, & Humphry, 2006, p. 99). Many have argued that the phenomenological, interpretive, or subjective perspective on occupation is critical to occupational science (Barber, 2006; Clark et al., 1991; Pierce, 2001; Yerxa, 1991).

Pierce, D. (Ed.).
Occupational Science for Occupational Therapy (pp. 81-89).
© 2014 SLACK Incorporated.

In fact, might not both views be equally valuable? Is it possible that some of the originality and uniqueness of occupational science as a distinct body of knowledge is the degree to which it illuminates individual experiences of occupation, rather than the broader levels of human action already addressed by other disciplines? In 1983, Janice Burke warned occupational therapy that the importation of extradisciplinary concepts required a critical inquiry into the match of the underlying premises of imported theories with the historical values and assumptions of occupational therapy. This outstanding advice should also be extended to the use of interdisciplinary knowledge by occupational scientists. Individualism honors the voices of research participants and clients. Producing research that addresses occupations as they are experienced by individuals also provides a strong match to the knowledge needs of occupational therapists, who primarily do their work within the lives of individuals, rather than with entire populations or at the juncture of individual and culture. Research that emphasizes personal experience makes an especially strong match with occupational therapy's concern for providing interventions that are client centered (Townsend & Wilcock, 2004; Wilkins, Pollock, Rochon, & Law, 2001).

A Level 2 Research Continuum

Because occupational science is still a young discipline, Level 2 studies usually combine highly developed research from an outside discipline with the less developed concept of occupation. These studies fall along a continuum, from results that contribute more to the theoretical focus of the outside discipline to those that are strategically and originally informing about occupation. The high volume of Level 2 research impacts occupational science. Some of these studies openly assert that the central concern of occupational science should not be occupation itself, but how occupation is related to, or interpreted by, the central concepts and theories of an outside discipline. To make the situation even more challenging, there is not just one brilliant outside discipline or theory being promoted as central to occupational science, there are many: anthropology, feminism, disability studies, critical theory, community medicine, rehabilitation medicine, and others. Stretched between them all, the science is certainly challenged to grow. But, it is also pulled thin. A focused body of research that is cumulative and evolving is difficult to produce in occupational science when so many studies use an extradisciplinary focus. Occupational science, without the historical solidity of a deeply developed science, is pulled in different directions and confused by a multidisciplinary set of values and assumptions about research that are often contradictory. In many ways, this multidisciplinary picture is highly reminiscent of occupational therapy's avid quest for useful imported theories in the latter 20th century.

PRECURSORS TO OCCUPATIONAL SCIENCE RESEARCH AT LEVEL 2

Occupation and Health

Since its inception, occupational therapy has expressed a deep faith in the connection of occupation and health. That is, a founding notion of occupational therapy was that engagement in desired activities was both indicative of health and curative to those in poor health. In 1905, Herbert Hall asserted that "a patient at work is a patient half cured" (Quiroga, 1995, p. 91). This holistic view of health was in synch with the arts and crafts movement of Hall's time, which emphasized the positive effects of a craftsman's lifestyle. His work-cure was carried out with invalids in occupational therapy workshops that were dedicated to developing a crafts approach.

In her Eleanor Clarke Slagle Lecture, Mary Reilly (1962) proposed that this foundational idea supporting practice should be investigated. She converted Hall's assumption into a famous hypothesis, "That man, through the use of his hands as they are energized by mind and will, can influence the state of his own health." She argued that an essential body of knowledge for occupational therapy was a full understanding of work and of how humans have evolved and developed to reach levels of skilled adult work. Reilly conceded the importance to occupational therapy of an understanding of neurology, physiology, psychology, sociology, and medical conditions, but asserted that the knowledge of outside disciplines was not sufficient to support practice. Essentially, she called for a science of occupation.

In 1985, the American Occupational Therapy Foundation and the American Occupational Therapy Association collaborated in funding focused reviews of literature on occupation and health. That project's results provide a window through which we can view the state of knowledge of the relation of occupation to health and quality of life in occupational therapy just prior to the emergence of occupational science. The Foundation and Association together called for reviews in the areas of rest/sleep, self-care/activities of daily living, work/productivity, and play/leisure (Gillette, 1990). Reviews were published in four areas: preschool play, elder cognition, adult productivity, and adolescent leisure. Play development was clearly tied to adult competence (Bundy, 1990). Cognitive capacity and life satisfaction with aging was presented as impacted by activity engagement and living environment (Prendergast, 1990). The productivity of adults in task groups was described as affected by their organization (Steffan, 1990). The leisure of adolescents was broadly described (Thorn, 1990). Perhaps even more interesting as we look through this window into the past are the areas that remained unaddressed in this effort: rest/sleep and self-care/activities of daily living. Not so long ago, this project was the peak of occupational therapy's knowledge of how occupation and health were related. It rested entirely on reviews of extradisciplinary research. Finding research that studied whole occupations, as opposed to research into components of occupation, such as motivation or role, was difficult.

Anthropology: The Sister Discipline of Occupational Science

The central disciplinary concept of anthropology is culture. Because culture is learned, expressed, and shaped by what we do every day, there is a match of disciplinary interests between occupational science and anthropology. Theories from anthropology have been widely used in occupational science research. Many active occupational science researchers have completed their doctorates in anthropology. It is not unusual to find an anthropologist holding a faculty appointment in an occupational therapy department. Yet, because culture and occupation are distinct concepts, each with unique histories and intents, these are clearly two separate disciplines. Much of relational, Level 2 occupational science occurs at the juncture of these two disciplines, exploring occupation in relation to culture, cultural meanings of activities, the cultural construction of identity, and the interaction of culture with disability. At times, in the early history of occupational science, this close match between the two disciplines led to confusion as to whether occupational science might be a subdiscipline of anthropology. There has been also been increased interest within applied anthropology in partnering with, and providing theoretical guidance to, occupational therapists. As occupational science has matured, developing its own unique disciplinary concepts and honoring its commitment to occupational therapy, the distinctions between the two disciplines have become clearer.

The Development of Occupational Science Relational Research

Dependence of Level 2 on Level 1

The adequacy and depth of Level 2 relational research is dependent on the degree to which it is built on concepts that are well described at Level 1. For example, at Level 2, it would be more strategic to do research into how caregiving is related to disability than into how sleep is related to disability, because the concept of caregiving as an occupation

is more deeply described in occupational science than is the occupation of sleep.

Occupation and Disability

The most developed area of relational occupational science is research into occupation and disability (Pierce, 2012; Pierce et al., 2010). Researchers have examined this theoretical crux in significantly different ways. Most straightforward, and possibly most helpful to the development of occupational science, are those balanced studies that produce significant findings in regard to both occupation and disability. Excellent examples are provided in the chapters of this section of the book. The work of Mary Law and Gillian King (Chapter 8) looks at degree of activity participation in children with disabilities. Similarly, Carolyn Baum's team (Chapter 9) details her research program on participation and engagement in occupation in adults with disabilities. Matthew Molineux and colleagues (Chapter 10) explore how living with HIV can be uniquely understood from an occupational perspective. Other examples of outstanding research that is strategically conceptualized to provide a balanced view of how the everyday lives of families are shaped by the disability of a child are the studies by Blanche (1996); Crowe and Florez (2006); Crowe, Vanleit, Berghmans, and Mann (1997); DeGrace (2004); Downs (2008); Larson (1996); and Segal (1999, 2000; Segal, Mandich, Polatajko, & Cook, 2002). A wide variety of specific disabilities and diagnoses are addressed in occupational science literature (Asaba, 2008; Baum, 1995; Crooks, Stone, & Owen, 2009; Heward, Molineux, & Gough, 2006; Hillman & Chapparo, 1995; Leufstadius, Erlandsson, Bjorkman, & Eklund, 2008; MacKinnon & Miller, 2003; MacKinnon, Noh, & Miller, 1998; Matuska & Erikson, 2008; Molyneaux-Smith, Townsend, & Guernsey, 2003; Nagle, Cook, & Polatajko, 2003; Pearson, 1996; Pentland et al., 2003; Pyatak, 2011; Spitzer, 2003; Wood, 2005; Wright-St Clair, 2003).

The Therapeutic Nature of Occupation for People With Disability

Some researchers have extended this focus on the relation of occupation and disability into a consideration of how occupation has a naturally positive effect that remedies or counters the effects of disability. These are not studies of the work of occupational therapists, but of occupation as it works within lives. Examples of those studies are Wright-St Clair's (2003) research into storymaking in women with multiple sclerosis; MacKinnon and Miller's (2003) study of how engagement in occupation affected self-esteem; MacKinnon, Noh, and Miller's (1998) study of how occupation mediated depression in people with arthritis; Unruh and Elvin's (2004) classic study of how dragon boat racing mediated women's experience of breast cancer; and

Ratcliff, Farnworth, and Lentin's (2002) research into the role of physical occupation in supporting women survivors of childhood sexual abuse to reconnect with their bodies and enrich their lives.

Occupation and Identity

In a secondary analysis of three qualitative studies, Debbie Laliberte Rudman (2002) concluded that there were five common themes in studies of occupation and identity: "demonstrating core characteristics; limiting and expanding possibilities; maintaining an acceptable self-identity; managing social identity; and control as an essential condition" (p. 12). As already described in the overview of Level 1 descriptive research (Chapter 2), occupational science has shown a distinct investment in the occupations of women and girls: mothering, caregiving, crafts, self-care, and others. In regard to research on the relation of occupation and identity, this also holds true. Some of the many occupational science studies of female gender identity and occupation include Primeau's milestone study of household work (2000a, 2000b), Taylor's research (2003) on women's leisure activities, and Goodman, Knotts, and Jackson's (2007) exploration of dress and the construction of women's gender identity.

A few studies of male identity and occupation have included Williamson's (2000) study of identity formation in a gay man through occupations at different stages of his life, Devine and Nolan's (2007) research on the role of occupation in the identity expression of gay men, and Beagan and Saunders (2005) study of occupations strongly associated with masculinity, such as body-building.

Disregarding a focus on gender identity by combining genders in a single study has been surprising. One such study examined men's and women's experiences of elite-level wheelchair basketball (Garci & Mandich, 2005). Christiansen (2000) explored personal projects, identity, and happiness. Dickie (2003) has studied how work shapes identity in craft workers, and Howie, Coulter, and Feldman (2004) have examined how creative occupations contribute to identity in retired people. Occupational identity is, and is likely to remain, a central interest in occupational science (Phelan & Kinsella, 2009).

Occupation, Disability, and Identity

Some occupational scientists have designed studies that triangulate the three concepts of occupation, disability, and identity. Thorn-Jonsson and Moller (1999) studied how the occupational self and choices of occupational strategies influenced sense of competence, goals, and values in people with polio. Braveman and Helfrich (2001) and Braveman, Helfrich, Kielhofner, and Albrecht (2003) studied the occupational identities of men living with AIDS in relation to return to work. Alsaker and Josephsson (2003) described how occupations were central to the expression of identity in people with chronic rheumatic disease.

The Therapeutic Nature of Occupation for the Identities of People With Disability

Just as researchers into occupation and disability discovered the therapeutic effect of occupation, occupational scientists have also found that occupation has a specific positive effect on identity in people with disability. Mee, Sumison, and Craik (2004) described the value to mental health clients of occupation to build competence, and thus personal identity. Stone (2003) studied the importance to injured workers of maintaining an identity as valued workers despite being unable to work. Similarly, Jakobsen (2001) examined the maintenance of self-esteem and identity in workers with chronic illnesses. Magnus (2001) described how women with debilitating diseases or injuries used occupational strategies to keep a disability identity at bay. The relation of occupation to worker identity is an emergent key concept in occupational science.

Research on Identity and Disability, but Not Occupation

Sometimes, the passions of occupational scientists for the concepts they frequently study in relation to occupation pull them into research that is unrelated, or only marginally related, to occupation. For example, Gelya Frank's (2000) well-known 20-year cultural biography of Diane DeVries, titled *Venus on Wheels,* focused on disability, female identity, and the construction of the self. It was an outstanding study, providing significant insight, and using an innovative methodology. And of course, such a highly detailed account of a life had in it occupations. Yet, occupation is not the focus of the study and was not meant to be. Because Gutman and Napier-Klemic (1996) studied gender identity in relation to traumatic brain injury and drew conclusions specifically tailored to inform occupational therapists, their study sounds somewhat like occupational science. But is it? Doubt and McColl (2003) completed a phenomenological study of mobility-impaired teens, finding they felt socially excluded in their schools. Fitzgerald and Patterson (1995) studied hidden disabilities and identity. Charmaz (2002) completed an interview study of 140 people with chronic illness, articulating the tensions between habitual and disability identities and drawing conclusions to guide occupational therapists. These are all excellent and interesting studies that touch on favorite research topics of occupational scientists: disability, identity, and research insights useful to occupational therapists. But, their primary intent was not to produce fresh, original knowledge to develop our understanding of occupation. Thus, they are not occupational science.

Occupation and Culture

There is a growing awareness in occupational science and occupational therapy of the degree to which the discipline and the profession spring from Western cultural roots (Frank & Zemke, 2008). This raises the question of epistemology, or how we know what we know. Do we internally construct our own unique understandings of the world with influences from our culture, or is there one reality out there for all of us to see and it is just a matter of interpreting it correctly? Unlike more mature disciplines, occupational science does not have a unified epistemological perspective. In fact, it can be quite entertaining at occupational science meetings to watch researchers with opposing epistemologies attempt to discuss their work together. They have real trouble connecting! They cannot get past the fact that they just cannot accept the other researcher's epistemology. Instead of understanding the differences as epistemological, they often view research based on an opposing epistemology as methodologically flawed.

Iwama (2003, 2005) has asserted that each culture should produce its own culturally based theories and models to guide interventions, his offering being the Kawa (River) Model. In essence, Iwama is advancing a constructivist view, asserting that each culture's perspective is unique and cannot be understood, studied, compared, or used in intervention by outsiders to that culture. This is not an uncommon view in anthropology. The opposite view, strongly offered in psychology and medicine, is positivism, which asserts that reality is outside us and can be dependably studied, quantified, and observed by anyone. Using this view, psychologists have done the bulk of cross-cultural research, using Western theories and translated instruments to study people of different cultures on characteristics such as intelligence, development, or specific skills. Post-positivists fall between these two opposing stances, asserting that reality is accessible, but imperfectly.

Some researchers have begun research into cross-cultural understandings of occupation (Darnell, 2009; Kondo, 2004; Odawara, 2005). In Chapter 11, we report our international team's research into elderly women's preparation of annual celebratory foods in rural eastern Kentucky, rural Chiangmai, Thailand, and urban Auckland, New Zealand. The team's epistemology is definitely post-positivist. We offer strong methods for how occupational scientists and others can do research that is grounded in subjective perceptions of people living within the cultures being studied, yet has the potential to look across the cultures studied to describe the unique meanings and shared dynamics in the occupation studied. It is my own dream that occupational science could, using strong methods, begin to look not only at how occupations differ over the globe, but also how they are similar. Too often, cross-cultural perspectives emphasize differences, leaving us feeling less connected to others. Research that showed how humans around the world share similar basic occupations, such as cooking, dressing, parenting, and working, could contribute to a global understanding of how we are also alike. In our research, we describe the similar and yet unique ways in which the older women of each culture were the leaders of this important food preparation, for Christmas in Kentucky and in New Zealand (in midsummer) and for Songkran (or Thai New Year), a day to honor the ancestors in Thailand.

In Chapter 12, Debbie Rudman describes the cultural construction of the meaning of retirement. As a constructivist, she asserts the importance to occupational science of understanding how cultures shape how people perceive and experience different occupations. Her approach is called *critical theory*, because it criticizes the lack of understanding of this macrolevel cultural construction of meaning, which can impede effective policy and just services. It is an excellent contribution to occupational science, although it may be an even greater contribution to critical theory, gerontology, and anthropology. Dr. Rudman is clearly aware of different research epistemologies. She acknowledges the value of views of occupation as they are subjectively experienced, as well as her own interest in how power and culture influence and reconstruct those experiences in ways not necessarily understood by individuals.

Because occupational science draws on different, and sometimes conflicting, epistemologies, being an occupational scientist requires remarkable levels of philosophical sophistication and open-mindedness. This is different from research training in many disciplines, where the science is done in an accepted way that has clear standards for epistemologies, methods, excellence, and pressing topics. Some occupational scientists fail to rise to this demanding philosophical level, especially those who have completed extradisciplinary doctorates. Their passion in regard to how obviously correct their own (extradisciplinary) perspectives are devolves into a simple rejection of all other perspectives as wrong, rather than recognizing that other works may be valuable even if they are based in a different epistemological foundation. A good example of this is the article by Dickie, Cutchin, and Humphry (2006), in which they assert that understandings of occupation as experiences of individuals must be wrong because occupation is culturally shaped and exists not at the individual level, but at the cultural level. This forced choice argument is a type of logical fallacy that is termed *the straw man*, asserting that an opposing argument is false and thus one's own argument must be true. This false logic disregards the possibility that both arguments may be right, or both wrong. Too often, I hear extradisciplinary-prepared occupational scientists say, "I am right, so you are wrong." It would be nice to hear them say, "I see what you are saying and what you value, here is my additional view."

Occupation and Justice

A strong focus at Level 2 of occupational science has been the relation of occupation and justice, mostly producing research that describes how different unjust societal conditions result in significant limitations to what occupational opportunities people may need or want in their lives (Blakeney & Marshall, 2009; Fiddler & Peerla, 2009; Shaw, Southcott, & Townsend, 2009; Steindl, Winding, & Runge, 2008; Wilcock, 2006). Interestingly, Townsend and Wilcock (2004) laid the groundwork for this Level 2 topic in a key article on the relation of occupational justice to client-centered practice. They described different types of occupational injustice: alienation, deprivation, marginalization, and imbalance. In Chapter 13, Diane Smith and Claudia Hilton present large database research on the relations of disability to intimate partner violence, which shows a societal pattern of occupational injustice.

Many theoretical and empirical articles have been published that describe occupational injustice as it exists within occupational therapy's service settings and populations (Galvin, Wilding, & Whiteford, 2011; Kronenberg, Algado, & Pollard, 2005; Paul-Ward, 2009; Riegel & Eglseder, 2009; Thomas, Gray, & McGinty, 2011). In Chapter 14, Gail Whiteford takes this dialogue to another level, using her research on occupational injustice within refugee populations to propose strategies though which occupational therapists might reduce occupational injustice. When occupational scientists begin to produce research that studies the outcomes and effectiveness of such processes of change, this exciting Level 2 research focus will further support occupational therapy with Level 4, prescriptive knowledge (Thibeault, 2012).

Level 2 Questions for Occupational Science

Will the Gap Regarding the Relation Between Occupation and Health or Quality of Life Be Filled?

A limited amount of research in regard to the relation of occupation to health or quality of life has been done (Piskur, Kinebanian, & Josephsson, 2002). This is the most critical gap in the body of work at Level 2 of occupational science. Describing the nature and importance of occupation to health, life satisfaction, and other related measures of life quality is essential to occupation therapy, which rests on the founding notion that engagement in occupation is essential to the well-lived human life, as well as being therapeutic to the restoration of health and life quality. To honor its promise to occupational therapy, occupation science must become more productive in this research area.

An area in which this tie could be very directly examined is in studies of the occupation of sleep, in both healthy and unhealthy individuals. Sleep affects cardiac, respiratory, cognitive, and immune functions. Manufacturing, driving, and flight accidents are increased by sleep loss. Clearly, sleep physicians impact health by improving the quality of sleep (Dement & Vaughn, 1999; Kryger, Roth, & Dement, 2005).

Will Occupational Science Test Its Primary Concepts Across Cultures?

As discussed under the heading "Occupation and Culture," it would be of great benefit to embark on further research that examines shared human occupations across cultures. This would be strategic for testing, refining, and growing emergent concepts in occupational science. It would also offer to the global future a science that might emphasize the degree to which we all engage in basic everyday occupations, although in unique cultural forms.

Will Occupation in Relation to Male Gender Identity Be Studied?

Lastly, and perhaps most obviously, occupational science needs to balance its strong interest in the occupations of women and girls with multiple insightful studies of the occupations of men and boys.

Section Chapters Illustrating Level 2 Relational Occupational Science Research

This section of *Occupational Science for Occupational Therapy* features Level 2 relational research. As just described, the chapters provided are the very best examples of the different foci that have emerged at this level. Research on occupation and disability include the following. Law and King (Chapter 8) describe occupation and participation in children with disabilities. Connor, Wolf, Foster, Hildebrand, and Baum (Chapter 9) study occupation and participation in adults with disabilities. Molineux, Strong, and Rickard (Chapter 10) examine the occupations of men living with HIV. Hocking, Shordike, Vittayakorn, Bunrayong, Rattakorn, Wright-St Clair, and Pierce (Chapter 11) describe the occupation of annual celebratory food preparation as it appears across three cultures. Rudman (Chapter 12) reflects on the cultural construction of the occupation of retirement. Smith and Hilton (Chapter 13) demonstrate a large-scale pattern of injustice in the association of disability and intimate partner violence against women with disability. Whiteford (Chapter 14) lights the way for research on occupational injustice to be transformed into the enactment of occupational justice through research and policy work.

Overall, Level 2 relational work in occupational science is growing explosively. Because this level of occupational science is built entirely from studies that relate key concepts from different disciplines, discerning where occupational science ends and another discipline begins requires philosophical sophistication. Despite the degree to which all this overlap may confound us, it is wonderful that occupational science has come so far in such a short time that it offers this volume of excellent relational research.

REFERENCES

Alsaker, S., & Josephsson, S. (2003). Negotiating occupational identities while living with chronic rheumatic disease. *Scandinavian Journal of Occupational Therapy, 10,* 167-176. doi:10.1080/11038120310017525

Asaba, E. (2008). Hashi-ire: Where occupation, chopsticks, and mental health intersect. *Journal of Occupational Science, 15*(2), 74-79. doi:1 0.1080/14427591.2008.9686612

Barber, M. D. (2006). Occupational science and the first-person perspective. *Journal of Occupational Science, 13,* 94-96. doi:10.1080/144275 91.2006.9686574

Baum, C. M. (1995). The contribution of occupation to function in persons with Alzheimer's disease. *Journal of Occupational Science, 2*(2), 50-67. doi:10.1080/14427591.1995.9686396

Beagan, B., & Saunders, S. (2005). Occupations of masculinity: Producing gender through what men do and don't do. *Journal of Occupational Science, 12*(3), 161-169. doi:10.1080/14427591.2005. 9686559

Blakeney, A. B., & Marshall, A. (2009). Water quality, health, and human occupations. *American Journal of Occupational Therapy, 63,* 46-57. doi:10.5014/ajot.63.1.46

Blanche, E. I. (1996). Alma: Coping with culture, poverty, and disability. *American Journal of Occupational Therapy, 50,* 265-276. doi:10.5014/ajot.50.4.265

Braveman, B., & Helfrich, C. (2001). Occupational identity: Exploring the narratives of three men living with AIDS. *Journal of Occupational Science, 8,* 25-31. doi:10.1080/14427591.2001.9686486

Braveman, B., Helfrich, C., Kielhofner, G., & Albrecht, G. (2003). The narratives of 12 men living with AIDS: Exploring return to work. *Journal of Occupational Rehabilitation, 13,* 143-157. doi:10.1023/A:1024949117344

Bundy, A. (1990). Free play of preschoolers. In A. Bundy, N. Prendergast, J. Steffan, & D. Thorn (Eds.), *Reviews of selected literature on occupation and health* (pp. 5-68). Rockville, MD: American Occupational Therapy Foundation and American Occupational Therapy Association.

Burke, J. (1983). Defining occupation: Importing and organizing interdisciplinary knowledge. In G. Kielhofner (Ed.), *Health through occupation: Theory and practice in occupational therapy* (pp. 125-138). Philadelphia, PA: F. A. Davis.

Charmaz, K. (2002). The self as habit: The reconstruction of self in chronic illness. *Occupational Therapy Journal of Research, 22*(Suppl.), 31S-41S.

Christiansen, C. (2000). Identity, personal projects and happiness: Self construction in everyday action. *Journal of Occupational Science, 7*(3), 98-107. doi:10.1080/14427591.2000.9686472

Clark, F. A., Parham, D., Carlson, M. E., Frank, G., Jackson, J., Pierce, D., . . . Zemke, R. (1991). Occupational science: Academic innovation in the service of occupational therapy's future. *American Journal of Occupational Therapy, 45,* 300-310. doi:10.5014/ajot.45.4.300

Crooks, V., Stone, S., & Owen, M. (2009). Multiple sclerosis and academic work: Socio-spatial strategies adopted to maintain employment. *Journal of Occupational Science, 16,* 25-31. doi:10.1080/1442 7591.2009.9686638

Crowe, T. K., & Florez, S. I. (2006). Time use of mothers with school-age children: A continuing impact of a child's disability. *American Journal of Occupational Therapy, 60*(2), 194-203. doi:10.5014/ajot.60.2.194

Crowe, T. K., Vanleit, B., Berghmans, K. K., & Mann, P. (1997). Role perceptions of mothers with young children: The impact of a child's disability. *American Journal of Occupational Therapy, 51*(8), 651-661. doi:10.5014/ajot.60.2.194

Cutchin, M. P., Dickie, V., & Humphry, R. (2006). Transaction versus interpretation, or transaction and interpretation? A response to Michael Barber. *Journal of Occupational Science, 13,* 97-99. doi:10.1 080/14427591.2006.9686575

Darnell, R. (2009). Cross-cultural constructions of work, leisure and community responsibility: Some first nations reflections. *Journal of Occupational Science, 16,* 4-9. doi:10.1080/14427591.2009.9686634

DeGrace, B. (2004). The everyday occupation of families with children with autism. *American Journal of Occupational Therapy, 58,* 543-550. doi:10.5014/ajot.58.5.543

Dement, W., & Vaughn, C. (1999). *The promise of sleep.* New York, NY: Dell Books Random House.

Devine, R., & Nolan, C. (2007). Sexual identity and human occupation: A qualitative exploration. *Journal of Occupational Science, 14*(3), 154-161. doi:10.1080/14427591.2007.9686596

Dickie, V. (2003). Establishing worker identity: A study of people in craft work. *American Journal of Occupational Therapy, 57,* 250-261. doi:10.5014/ajot.57.3.250

Dickie, V., Cutchin, M., & Humphry, R. (2006). Occupation as a transactional experience: A critique of individualism in occupational science. *Journal of Occupational Science, 13,* 83-93. doi:10.1080/144 27591.2006.9686573

Doubt, L., & McColl, M. (2003). A secondary guy: Physically disabled teenagers in secondary schools. *Canadian Journal of Occupational Therapy, 70,* 139-151.

Downs, M. L. (2008). Leisure routines: Parents and children with disability sharing occupation. *Journal of Occupational Science, 15*(2), 105-110. doi:10.1080/14427591.2008.9686616

Fiddler, A., & Peerla, A. (2009). The Kitchenuhmaykoosib Inninuwug and the struggle for the right to say no. *Journal of Occupational Science, 16,* 10-11. doi:10.1080/14427591.2009.9686635

Fitzgerald, M. H., & Patterson, K. A. (1995). The hidden disability dilemma for the preservation of self. *Journal of Occupational Science, 2,* 13-21. doi:10.1080/14427591.1995.9686392

Frank, G. (2000). *Venus on wheels.* Los Angeles, CA: University of California Press.

Frank, G., & Zemke, R. (2008). Occupational therapy foundations for political engagement and social transformation. In N. Pollard, D. Sakellariou, & F. Kronenberg (Eds.), *A political practice of occupational therapy* (pp. 111-136). Edinburgh, Scotland: Churchill Livingstone Elsevier.

Galvin, D., Wilding, C., & Whiteford, G. (2011). Utopian visions/dystopian realities: Exploring practice and taking action to enable human rights and occupational justice in a hospital context. *Australian Occupational Therapy Journal, 58,* 378-385. doi:10.1111/j.1440-1630.2011.00967.x

Garci, H., & Mandich, A. (2005). Going for gold: Understanding occupational engagement in elite-level wheelchair basketball athletes. *Journal of Occupational Science, 12*(3), 170-175. doi:10.1080/14427591.2005.9686560

Gillette, N. (1990). Introduction. In A. Bundy, N. Prendergast, J. Steffan, & D. Thorn (Eds.), *Reviews of selected literature on occupation and health* (pp. 1-3). Rockville, MD: American Occupational Therapy Foundation and American Occupational Therapy Association.

Goodman, J., Knotts, G., & Jackson, J. (2007). Doing dress and the construction of women's gender identity. *Journal of Occupational Science, 14*, 100-107. doi:10.1080/14427591.2007.9686590

Gutman, S., & Napier-Klemic, J. (1996). The experience of head injury on the impairment of gender identity and gender role. *American Journal of Occupational Therapy, 50*, 535-544. doi:10.5014/ajot.50.7.535

Heward, K., Molineux, M., & Gough, B. (2006). A grounded theory analysis of the occupational impact of caring for a partner who has multiple sclerosis. *Journal of Occupational Science, 13*(3), 188-197. doi:10.1080/14427591.2006.9726515

Hillman, A. M., & Chapparo, C. J. (1995). An intervention of occupational role performance in men over sixty years of age, following a stroke. *Journal of Occupational Science, 2*(3), 88-99. doi:10.1080/14427591.1995.9686399

Howie, L., Coulter, M., & Feldman, S. (2004). Crafting the self: Older person's narratives of occupational identity. *American Journal of Occupational Therapy, 58*, 446-454. doi:10.5014/ajot.58.4.446

Iwama, M. (2003). Toward culturally relevant epistemologies in occupational therapy. *American Journal of Occupational Therapy, 57*, 582-588. doi:10.5014/ajot.57.5.582

Iwama, M. (2005). The Kawa (River) model: Nature, life flow, and the power of culturally occupational therapy. In F. Kronenberg, S. S. Algado, & N. Pollard (Eds.), *Occupational therapy without borders: Learning from the spirit of survivors* (pp. 213-227). Edinburgh, Scotland: Elsevier Churchill Livingstone.

Jakobsen, K. (2001). Employment and reconstruction of the self: A model of space for maintenance of identity by occupation. *Scandinavian Journal of Occupational Therapy, 8*, 40-48. doi:10.1080/11038120120825

Kondo, T. (2004). Cultural tensions in occupational therapy practice: Considerations from a Japanese vantage point. *American Journal of Occupational Therapy, 58*(2), 174-184. doi:10.5014/ajot.58.2.174

Kronenberg, F., Algado, S., & Pollard, N. (2005). *Occupational therapy without borders: Learning from the spirit of survivors*. New York, NY: Elsevier.

Kryger, M., Roth, T., & Dement, W. (2005). *Principles and practice of sleep medicine* (4th ed.). Philadelphia, PA: Elsevier Saunders.

Laliberte Rudman, D. (2002). Linking occupation and identity: Lessons learned through qualitative exploration. *Journal of Occupational Science, 9*, 12-19. doi:10.1080/14427591.2002.9686489

Larson, E. A. (1996). The story of Maricela and Miguel: A narrative analysis of dimensions of adaptation. *Journal of Occupational Science, 50*(4), 286-298. doi:10.5014/ajot.50.4.286

Leufstadius, C., Erlandsson, L., Bjorkman, T., & Eklund, M. (2008). Meaningfulness in daily occupations among individuals with persistent mental illness. *Journal of Occupational Science, 15*, 27-35. doi:10.1080/14427591.2008.9686604

MacKinnon, J., & Miller, W. (2003). Rheumatoid arthritis and self-esteem: The impact of quality occupation. *Journal of Occupational Science, 10*, 90-98. doi:10.1080/14427591.2003.9686515

MacKinnon, J., Noh, S., & Miller, W. C. (1998). Occupations as a mediator of depression in people with rheumatoid arthritis. *Journal of Occupational Science, 5*(2), 82-92. doi:10.1080/14427591.1998.9686436

Magnus, E. (2001). Everyday occupations and the process of redefinition: A study of how meaning in occupation influences redefinition of identity in women with a disability. *Scandinavian Journal of Occupational Therapy, 8*, 115-124. doi:10.1080/110381201750464467

Matuska, K. M., & Erikson, B. (2008). Lifestyle balance: How it is described and experienced by women with multiple sclerosis. *Journal of Occupational Science, 15*, 20-26. doi:10.1080/14427591.2008.9686603

Mee, J., Sumison, T., & Craik, C. (2004). Mental health clients confirm the value of occupation in building competence and self-identity. *British Journal of Occupational Therapy, 67*, 225-233.

Molyneaux-Smith, L., Townsend, E., & Guernsey, J. R. (2003). Occupation disrupted: Impacts, challenges, and coping strategies for farmers with disabilities. *Journal of Occupational Science, 10*, 14-20. doi:10.1080/14427591.2003.9686506

Nagle, S., Cook, J. V., & Polatajko, H. J. (2003). I'm doing as much as I can: Occupational choices of persons with a severe and persistent mental illness. *Journal of Occupational Science, 9*(2), 72-81. doi:10.1080/14427591.2002.9686495

Odawara, E. (2005). Cultural competency in occupational therapy: Beyond a cross-cultural view of practice. *American Journal of Occupational Therapy, 59*(3), 325-334. doi:10.5014/ajot.59.3.325

Paul-Ward, A. (2009). Social and occupational justice barriers in the transition from foster care to independent adulthood. *American Journal of Occupational Therapy, 63*, 81-88. doi:10.5014/ajot.63.1.81

Pearson, S. (1996). An exploration of the effect of right homonymous hemianopia on engagement in occupation. *Journal of Occupational Science, 3*, 18-25. doi:10.1080/14427591.1996.9686404

Pentland, W., Walker, J., Minnes, P., Tremblay, M., Brouwer, B., & Gould, M. (2003). Occupational responses to mid-life and aging in women with disabilities. *Journal of Occupational Science, 10*, 21-30. doi:10.1080/14427591.2003.9686507

Phelan, S., & Kinsella, E. (2009). Occupational identity: Engaging socio-cultural perspectives. *Journal of Occupational Science, 16*, 85-91. doi:10.1080/14427591.2009.9686647

Pierce, D. (2001). Untangling occupation and activity. *American Journal of Occupational Therapy, 55*, 138-146.

Pierce, D. (2012). Promise. *Journal of Occupational Science, 19*(4), 298-311. doi:10.1080/14427591.2012.667778

Pierce, D., Atler, K., Baltisberger, J., Fehringer, E., Hunter, E., Malkawi, S., & Parr, T. (2010). Occupational science: A data-based American perspective. *Journal of Occupational Science, 17*(4), 204-215. doi:10.1080/14427591.2010.9686697

Piskur, B., Kinebanian, A., & Josephsson, S. (2002). Occupation and well-being: A study of some Slovenian people's experiences of engagement in occupation in relation to well-being. *Scandinavian Journal of Occupational Therapy, 9*, 63-70. doi:10.1080/110381202320000043

Prendergast, N. (1990). Cognitive functioning in the elderly and its implications for productivity. In: A. Bundy, N. Prendergast, J. Steffan, & D. Thorn (Eds.), *Reviews of selected literature on occupation and health* (pp. 69-174). Rockville, MD: American Occupational Therapy Foundation and American Occupational Therapy Association.

Primeau, L. (2000a). Divisions of household work, routines, and child care occupations in families. *Journal of Occupational Science, 7*, 19-28. doi:10.1080/14427591.2000.9686461

Primeau, L. (2000b). Household work: When gender ideologies and practices interact. *Journal of Occupational Science, 7*, 118-127. doi:10.1080/14427591.2000.9686474

Pyatak, E. (2011). Participation in occupation and diabetes self-management in emerging adulthood. *American Journal of Occupational Therapy, 65*, 462-469. doi:10.5014/ajot.2011.001453

Quiroga, V. (1995). *Occupational therapy: The first 30 years, 1900 to 1930.* Bethesda, MD: American Occupational Therapy Association.

Ratcliff, E., Farnworth, L., & Lentin, P. (2002). Journey into wholeness: The experience of engaging in physical occupation for women survivors of childhood abuse. *Journal of Occupational Science, 9,* 65-71. doi:10.1080/14427591.2002.9686494

Reilly, M. (1962). 1961 Eleanor Clarke Slagle Lecture: Occupational therapy can be one of the great ideas of 20th-century medicine. *American Journal of Occupational Therapy, 16,* 1-9.

Riegel, S., & Eglseder, K. (2009). Occupational justice as a quality indicator for occupational therapy services. *Occupational Therapy in Health Care, 23,* 288-301. doi:10.3109/07380570903236500

Segal, R. (1999). Doing for others: Occupations within families with children who have special needs. *Journal of Occupational Science, 6,* 53-60. doi:10.1080/14427591.1999.9686451

Segal, R. (2000). Adaptive strategies of mothers with children with attention deficit hyperactivity disorder: Enfolding and unfolding occupations. *American Journal of Occupational Therapy, 54*(3), 300-306. doi:10.5014/ajot.54.3.300

Segal, R., Mandich, A., Polatajko, H., & Cook, J. V. (2002). Stigma and its management: A pilot study of parental perceptions of the experiences of children with developmental coordination disorder. *American Journal of Occupational Therapy, 56,* 422-428. doi:10.5014/ajot.56.4.422

Shaw, L., Southcott, C., & Townswend, E. (2009). A community panel on occupations to consider economic opportunities outside major urban centres: Occupations in Thunder Bay, Canada. *Journal of Occupational Science, 16,* 12-17. doi:10.1080/14427591.2009.9686636

Spitzer, S. (2003). With and without words: Exploring occupation in relation to young children with autism. *Journal of Occupational Science, 10*(2), 67-79. doi:10.1080/14427591.2003.9686513

Steffan, J. (1990). Productive occupation in small task groups of adults. In A. Bundy, N. Prendergast, J. Steffan, & D. Thorn (Eds.), *Reviews of selected literature on occupation and health* (pp. 175-282). Rockville, MD: American Occupational Therapy Foundation and American Occupational Therapy Association.

Steindl, C., Winding, K., & Runge, U. (2008). Occupation and participation in everyday life: Women's experience of an Austrian refugee camp. *Journal of Occupational Science, 15,* 36-42. doi:10.1080/14427591.2008.9686605

Stone, S. (2003). Workers without work: Injured workers and well-being. *Journal of Occupational Science, 10,* 7-13. doi:10.1080/14427591.2003.9686505

Taylor, J. (2003). Women's leisure activities, their social stereotypes and some implications for identity. *British Journal of Occupational Therapy, 66,* 151-158.

Thibeault, R. (2012). Occupational justice's intents and impacts: From personal choices to community consequences. In M. Cutchin & V. Dickie (Eds.), *Transactional perspectives on occupation* (pp. 245-256). New York, NY: Springer.

Thomas, Y., Gray, M., & McGinty, S. (2011). Occupational therapy at the "cultural interface": Lessons from research with Aboriginal and Torres Strait Islander Australians. *Australian Occupational Therapy Journal, 58,* 11-16. doi:10.1111/j.1440-1630.2010.00917.x

Thorn, D. (1990). Psychosocial functions of leisure among adolescents. In A. Bundy, N. Prendergast, J. Steffan, & D. Thorn (Eds.), *Reviews of selected literature on occupation and health* (pp. 283-338). Rockville, MD: American Occupational Therapy Foundation and American Occupational Therapy Association.

Thorn-Jonsson, A., & Moller, A. (1999). How the conception of the occupational self influences everyday life strategies of people with poliomyelitis sequelae. *Scandinavian Journal of Occupational Therapy, 6,* 71-83. doi:10.1080/110381299443762

Townsend, E., & Wilcock, A. (2004). Occupational justice and client-centered practice: A dialogue in progress. *Canadian Journal of Occupational Therapy, 71,* 75-87.

Unruh, A., & Elvin, N. (2004). In the eye of the dragon: Women's experience of breast cancer and the occupation of dragon boat racing. *Canadian Journal of Occupational Therapy, 71,* 138-149.

Wilcock, A. (2006). *An occupational perspective of health* (2nd ed.). Thorofare, NJ: SLACK Incorporated.

Wilkins, S., Pollock, N., Rochon, S., & Law, M. (2001). Implementing client-centered practice: Why is it so difficult to do? *Canadian Journal of Occupational Therapy, 68,* 70-79.

Williamson, P. (2000). Football and tin cans: A model of identity formation based on sexual orientation expressed through engagement in occupations. *British Journal of Occupational Therapy, 3,* 432-439.

Wood, W. (2005). Toward developing new occupational science measures: An example from dementia care research. *Journal of Occupational Science, 12*(3), 121-129. doi:10.1080/14427591.2005.9686555

Wright-St Clair, V. (2003). Storymaking and storytelling: Making sense of living with multiple sclerosis. *Journal of Occupational Science, 10,* 46-51. doi:10.1080/14427591.2003.9686510

Yerxa, E. (1991). Seeking a relevant, ethical, and realistic way of knowing for occupational therapy. *American Journal of Occupational Therapy, 45,* 199-204. doi:10.5014/ajot.45.3.199.

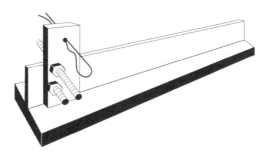

Participation of Children With Physical Disabilities in Everyday Occupations

Mary Law, PhD, FCAOT, FCAHS and Gillian King, PhD

This chapter describes a program of research over the past 20 years focused on understanding the participation of children with disabilities in everyday occupations. The research started from our curiosity about why participation might be different and has grown to include a focus on what could be changed to improve levels of participation. Participation has been defined by the World Health Organization ([WHO] 2001) as a person's involvement in life situations and includes the activities of personal maintenance, mobility, social relationships, education, leisure, spirituality, and community life. Coster and Khetani (2008) link the concepts inherent in occupational science in defining participation as "sets of organized sequences of activities directed toward a personally or socially meaningful goal" (p. 643).

Disability has the potential to impact children's occupations. Emerging evidence in the 1980s indicated that participation for children with disabilities differed from those of children without disabilities and reflected more time spent in self-care and passive activities within their home environment than in activities in the community (Brown & Gordon, 1987). This research, however, provided little evidence about the factors (child, family, environmental) that enable, promote, and reinforce the participation of children

with disabilities. In particular, knowledge about the interactions of children with disabilities, their occupations, and the influence of environmental supports and barriers was limited.

As this program of research began, our particular interest was the issue of environmental supports and barriers. There are significant environmental barriers in communities that prevent the development of satisfying daily occupations. While children who have no disability gradually assume more control, children with disabilities often have decisions made for them by parents, therapists, and teachers or influenced by environmental constraints. Environmental constraints include those physical, social, institutional, economic, and cultural factors in a child's home, neighborhood, or community that shape participation.

At that time, this point of view represented a challenge to see disability in a new way. If environments fostered dependency and poor resolution to the problems of disability, then solutions could exist predominantly in interventions aimed at the modification of the environment. However, the substantial effect that environments have on the occupations of a child with a disability is not well understood. Knowledge about the interactions between disability and the environment for children was scant. Disability, occupation, and

Pierce, D. (Ed.).
Occupational Science for Occupational Therapy (pp. 91-106).
© 2014 SLACK Incorporated.

environmental factors have rarely been examined together in the past. Rather, the practice has been to examine these factors independently.

Thus, at the beginning of this research program, we knew that the participation of children with disabilities in daily occupations was restricted. We did not know what factors were most important in leading to a participation restriction or in supporting participation. In order to plan interventions to enhance participation, research was needed about which factors were the most important in a potentially complex set of relationships between child, occupation, and environment.

LITERATURE

The WHO's *International Classification of Functioning, Disability and Health* defines participation as involvement in a life situation (2001). For children and youth, involvement in life situations includes participation in recreational and leisure activities as well as school and work activities. Recreational and leisure activities include artistic, creative, cultural, active physical, sports, play, social, and skill-based activities (Kalscheur, 1992; King et al., 2003; Sloper, Turner, Knussen, & Cunningham, 1990).

The Importance of Participation

Regular participation in day-to-day activities is an important aspect of children's health, well-being, and development. Participation in leisure and recreational activities has been shown to be of benefit to the development of children's skills and competencies, social relationships, and children's long-term mental and physical health (Caldwell & Gilbert, 1990; Forsyth & Jarvis, 2002; Larson & Verma, 1999; Lyons, 1993; Simeonsson, Carlson, Huntington, McMillen, & Brent, 2001; Werner, 1993).

For children, participation in day-to-day formal and informal activities is a vital part of their development. Participation enables children to understand societal expectations and acquire the physical and social competencies needed to function and flourish in their homes and communities (Brown & Gordon, 1987). Children with disabilities are clearly at risk for lower participation in ordinary daily activities (Brown & Gordon, 1987; Pless, Cripps, Davies, & Wadsworth, 1989). Because disability is manifested in the context of activity, it is of particular importance to examine how children with disabilities engage in activity (Brown & Gordon, 1987). The pattern of restricted participation starts in childhood, so this is the best time to understand the factors and processes at work. This is also the time to intervene—before patterns of lower participation are ingrained.

Participation Is Restricted for Children With Disabilities

People with disabilities are at risk for social isolation and lower life satisfaction due to lower participation (Rae-Grant, Thomas, Offord, & Boyle, 1989). There is strong evidence that children with disabilities often feel socially isolated (Anderson & Clarke, 1982; Blum, Resnick, Nelson, & St. Germaine, 1991; Cadman, Boyle, Szatmari, & Offord, 1987; LaGreca, 1990; Law & Dunn, 1993). In fact, social isolation and inactivity, fostered by a lack of leisure opportunities, are salient features of the lives of many people with a disability (Lyons, 1993). Furthermore, satisfaction with activities is an important predictor of life satisfaction among adults with physical disabilities (Kinney & Coyle, 1992) and is associated with adjustment and well-being (Brown & Gordon, 1987). Thus, participation has tremendous impact on people's lives and their quality of life.

The participation of children and youth with disabilities was known to decrease as children grew up (Brown & Gordon, 1987), and, by adulthood, participation was severely restricted (Crapps, Langone, & Swaim, 1985; Dempsey & Simmons, 1995). Rates of unemployment for these young people were staggering high, ranging from 27% to 68% (Clark & Hirst, 1989; Fuhrer, 1994; Hallum, 1995; LaPlante, Kennedy, Kaye, & Wenger, 1996), with the rates being higher for those with "severe" disability.

Children with physical disabilities were "2 to 3 times more likely to be unable to perform their usual activities than children with other conditions such as asthma" (Newacheck & Halfon, 1998, p. 612). Furthermore, there was evidence of significant differences in participation between children with and without disabilities—children with disabilities tend to be more restricted in their participation in daily activities (Brown & Gordon, 1987; Canadian Institute of Child Health, 1994; Hewett, Newson, & Newson, 1970; Margalit, 1981; Silanpaa, 1987; Statistics Canada, 1986; Stevenson, Pharoah, & Stevenson, 1997).

By the late 1990s, only four longitudinal studies had focused on research in this area (Crawford, Godbey, & Crouter, 1986; DiLorenzo, Stucky-Ropp, Vander Wal, & Gotham, 1998; Trost et al., 1997; Werner, 1993). None of these studies focused specifically on children with disabilities or focused on participation in its fullest sense. Werner (1993) took a broad look at the developmental courses of high-risk and resilient youth, not just children with disabilities (rather, she focused on children who experienced prenatal complications or adverse early rearing conditions). She also examined many outcomes in addition to participation (e.g., physical, cognitive, and psychosocial development). She concluded that participation in extracurricular activities plays an important part in the lives of resilient youth, especially activities that are cooperative enterprises. Crawford and colleagues (1986) looked at stability in adults' leisure preferences over time and found a lack of stability. Both DiLorenzo and colleagues (1998) and Trost and colleagues (1997) looked at the determinants of physical exercise in preadolescents without disabilities. They found variables such as social support, self-efficacy for physical activity, and preferences to be important determinants of physical activity. Both stated the need for further longitudinal studies employing larger sample sizes and examining additional familial and individual factors. It is evident, therefore, that a longitudinal study of the nature and determinants of children's participation will provide important and needed information.

In summary, we knew that the level of participation of children with disabilities in everyday activities (both formal and informal) was lower than that of their peers without disabilities and that the scope of their activities was limited. We also knew that these differences in level of participation increased in adolescence. We did not know (a) whether patterns of activity changed with age and (b) the relative importance of the various factors that could have potentially affected participation.

A RESEARCH PROGRAM CENTERED ON CHILDREN'S PARTICIPATION

The overall purpose of our program of research on children's participation was to understand and develop knowledge about the complexity of the participation of children with disabilities. Specifically, we were interested in developing methods to assess participation, describe patterns of participation, and determine the most important factors within the child, occupation, or environment that influenced participation. To focus the studies, we centered our research on children with physical disabilities.

Overview of the Research Program

In the mid to late 1980s, one of the authors (ML) began to question some observations she had made in her clinical practice with children with physical disabilities. She had observed that several children, although they had the same level of severity of disability, had a much different level of activity at home and in the community. Some of the children participated in more activities than others. While at the Health Sciences library, she found an article that studied the activity patterns of children with physical disabilities (Brown & Gordon, 1987). She was intrigued by the article and the fact that the researchers were unable to explain the differences in patterns. At that time, she had a developing interest in the environment and how environmental factors could influence children's daily activity patterns. These curiosities led her to apply for a PhD in the School of Urban and Regional Planning at the University of Waterloo, Canada.

Her PhD thesis was the first study in participation that she completed.

In the late 1980s, the two authors came together as members of CanChild Centre for Childhood Disability Research (www.canchild.ca) at McMaster University in Canada, discovering a common interest in children's participation. Over several years, they studied the literature and developed a theoretical model of children's participation in leisure activities and a grant proposal to study the outside-of-school participation of children with physical disabilities. This study was funded in 1999 by the National Institutes of Health in the United States. The PARTICIPATE study took place from 2000 to 2004 and collected longitudinal data from 427 children with physical disabilities and their families. The study has resulted in many dissemination materials and has led to the generation of participation research that is now being completed. The following sections describe our research on participation.

Identifying and Changing Disabling Environments Through Participatory Research

The first study in our research program was conducted by the first author (ML) as her dissertation research for her PhD. In this research, a broad range of environmental factors that affect the daily occupations, participation, and integration of children with physical disabilities were studied conjointly (Law et al., 1999). The study examined the process of bringing together participants who shared common concerns about childhood disability but did not know each other in a participatory research project. To that end, the process of the study and the community involvement of the participants during the project were as important as the research outcomes.

The primary goal in this research was to identify environmental factors that fundamentally affected the daily occupations of children with physical disabilities. Working together with parents of children with a disability, I wanted to discover the environmental situations that presented the most substantial challenges to their children. Focus groups and individual interviews were used to gain an understanding of the experiences and difficulties of parents who have a child with a disability. A second goal was to examine the use of participatory research in a community and disability context. The parents who participated in this research were the principal architects of the interview probes and the study's action process. A final aim of the research was to explore and make recommendations with parents about policy and planning strategies that could be used to enhance children's participation at a community level.

The research methodology chosen for this study was participatory research, which originated in the developing world. Participatory research is "an integrated activity that combines social investigation, educational work, and action" (Hall, 1981, p. 7). Its predominant characteristics include the active involvement of and control by citizens, empowerment of citizens, a commitment to action, and an obligation of the researchers to learn along with the participants. Participatory research is very action oriented, seeking always to empower the participants to make changes to improve their future. It is inherently political, often opposing the status quo, seeking changes in power and economic distribution (Brown, 1986).

The study took place in a city of 92,000 people in southwestern Ontario, Canada. Twenty-two families who had a child with a disability between the ages of 3 and 12 years participated. The study process included four stages: problem identification, data collection, data coding and analysis, and development of theoretical concepts. Qualitative methods were chosen as the most appropriate methodology to identify issues when little is known about the relative contribution of different factors to supporting or hindering children's participation. As in most qualitative research, the participatory research process used in this study was a cyclical, iterative process, establishing focus groups, exploring issues that affected activity patterns, determining how to study these, collecting data, discussing that data, determining actions based on the groups' perceptions and the data, performing actions, and evaluating results.

Through focus groups and individual interviews, participants identified factors that supported or hindered the daily activities of their children. Participants also made specific policy suggestions. Throughout the research, the action component of participatory research was emphasized. All interviews and focus groups were audiotaped and transcribed verbatim. The primary method of data analysis was the textual analysis of the investigator's field notes, interview records, and focus group proceedings, supplemented by the quantitative analysis of activity patterns data. A hermeneutic method of textual analysis was used to produce themes (Miller & Crabtree, 1992). In this method, significant units of text and thematic observations were independently identified and then compared. Discussion and comparison of observations were used to achieve consensus about emerging concepts. Observations were then sorted into concept categories from which themes were developed. The texts and interpretations were coded in a database for easy retrieval using Ethnograph software (Seidel & Clark, 1984). Textual analysis was completed by the research assistant and me. It took place throughout the study and was shared continually with the participants and other researchers so they could influence the analysis and act upon it.

Emerging themes reflecting the experiences of families included shattered dreams, personal growth, and doing it alone. The parents in the study loved their children, they had learned with them and from them, and they had no desire to change them. Most parents are not actively grieving the loss of a "normal" child. It is obvious that they want them to achieve and to develop to the best of their ability, but they do not want this to be accomplished simply by changes in their children so that they become more "normal." Certainly, parents did grieve when the disability was initially identified and did feel distress about specific situations and difficulties that they and their children faced. They wanted to change these difficulties so that they and their children were no longer confronted by them during their daily experiences.

The perception of the parents was that the major barriers to activity and participation were environmental, both structural and attitudinal, and not specifically related to disability severity or other factors in the child or family. Parents believed that the activities of their children could be enhanced by changing these environmental barriers. Generally, they were satisfied with the activities over which they have control, but they required changes in the community to increase their children's participation in many other activities. I was surprised by the degree of commonality about environmental barriers hindering participation.

Social and institutional barriers were identified as the most significant environmental barriers. Issues such as living in two worlds, labeling, competitiveness, institutional bureaucracy, and lack of parental power were important. Parents wanted their children to experience childhood, without disability always interfering with participation. Although many physical barriers were identified, participants believed that attitudes or lack of knowledge prevented these barriers from being changed. General themes for change included the parents' desire for more power and control over their situations, support of integration and inclusion as a means to change attitudes, a need for a more flexible bureaucracy in dealing with disability issues, and a profound concern about the societal view of normality. At the end of the interview phase of the study, participants came together to discuss the results of the study. They continued to meet and, in January 1992, formed an ongoing parent support and advocacy group. Through this group, participants continued to advocate for change to environmental constraints in their community.

We learned a great deal from the study. Participatory, qualitative methods, as used in this study, were particularly useful in chronicling the experiences of people and their interactions in a community context, as well as facilitating change. The children did not participate in a substantially different way from those of children of the same age without disabilities. This finding may have been influenced by the young age of the children. Parents indicated that the major barriers to participation were in the social and institutional environment. These barriers within the environment limited their children's participation. Removal or change of environmental barriers was a high priority for them. They believed that such actions would enhance their children's ability to participate. A surprising yet important finding of this research was that physical accessibility did not emerge as the most important barrier. Parents stated that whenever they encountered issues of physical accessibility, solutions were not typically pursued because of lack of information, bureaucratic inflexibility, or attitudes toward resource availability. Parents in the study wanted disabling environments to be changed rather than a focus on changing their children to fit the environment.

This study also highlighted the complexity of participation. There was a need to consider all factors (child, family, occupation, environment) that could potentially influence participation. This recognition led to the development of a conceptual model of participation.

Developing a Conceptual Model of Factors Influencing Participation

A conceptual model was developed to guide the selection of variables for a grant proposal examining factors affecting the recreation and leisure participation of children and youth with physical disabilities (King et al., 2003). Developing a comprehensive conceptual model of potential factors and their relationships is an important first step in identifying the most important causal factors and the pathways by which they influence children's participation (Mancini, Coster, Trombly, & Heeren, 2000; Sloper et al., 1990).

Our model was developed in 2001 and 2002 and was published in 2003 (King et al., 2003). It consists of 11 environmental, familial, and child factors thought to influence children's participation in recreation and leisure activities. The selection of these factors was based on the existing evidence at that time for the influence of these factors on one another and on children's participation. The review encompassed four bodies of literature: the participation of children or adults with disabilities, the risk and resilience of children facing adversity, the determinants of leisure and recreation activities, and the factors influencing physical activity and exercise. Although this review took a great deal of time, the development of the model was invaluable in defining further research.

Nature of Important Factors

The model includes environmental factors, family factors, and child factors. Review of the empirical literature available at that time indicated three major environmental factors relevant to participation: (a) supportive physical and institutional environments, (b) supportive relationships for the child, and (c) supportive relationships for the parents. Studies also indicated that four key family factors favored children's participation: (a) the absence of financial and time constraints caused by having a child with a disability, (b) a better family socioeconomic situation, (c) a supportive home environment, and (d) a strong family interest in recreational activities. Four key child factors were also identified: (a) children's own views of their competence; (b) their physical, cognitive, and communicative function; (c) their emotional, behavioral, and social function; and (d) their activity preferences.

Features of the Model

The major features of the proposed model were its (a) comprehensive nature, (b) socioecological scope, and (c) focus on the strengths of children, families, and communities. The model was comprehensive and transdisciplinary, incorporating notions of preferences, functioning, and perceived competencies, as well as the mechanisms of support and opportunity. It contained both distal variables, such as supportive relationships for the parents, and variables that are more proximal to the outcome of participation, such as the child's activity preferences.

Utility of the Model

A multivariate model of the broad range of factors influencing participation is important in guiding longitudinal research on the influence and interplay of these factors over time (Crawford, Jackson, & Godbey, 1991; Sloper et al., 1990). Such research will inform parents, service providers, managers, and policymakers about the nature of the environmental, interpersonal, and personal factors that are the most important determinants of children's participation, how these factors operate together to limit or enhance participation, and whether these factors change as children develop.

Development of a Measure of Outside-of-School Participation

One of the first tasks undertaken with the funding from the National Institutes of Health was to develop a measure to capture relevant dimensions of children's recreational and leisure participation. The Children's Assessment of Participation and Enjoyment (CAPE) and its companion measure Preferences for Activities of Children (PAC) (King et al., 2004; King, Law, King, et al., 2006) were developed because there were no appropriate child self-report measures that captured all the dimensions of participation of interest to us. In particular, existing measurement tools did not comprehensively measure contextual aspects of activity participation (with whom activities are done and where they are done). We set out to design a measure to capture five dimensions of participation discussed as important in the literature, namely diversity (a count of number of activities done in a 4-month period), frequency, location, companionship, and enjoyment.

A construct approach to test development was followed, in which items are generated to represent the domains of interest (Loevinger, 1957). The items in the CAPE were developed through a review of the literature, expert review, and pilot testing with children both with and without disabilities. Our objective was to develop a psychometrically sound measure appropriate for children/youth ages 6 to 21 years, with or without disabilities.

The CAPE provides information about participation in formal and informal domains, as well as five activity types (recreational, active physical, social, skill-based, self-improvement). The CAPE's conceptual strengths include its measurement of multiple dimensions of participation (Imms, 2008). CAPE test-retest reliability was evaluated by administering the test on two separate occasions to a group of 48 children with disabilities. The values for the CAPE activity-type intensity scores range from 0.72 to 0.81, indicating sufficient test-retest reliability. CAPE scores correlate in expected directions with environmental, family, and child variables, and hypotheses concerning differences in mean scores for boys versus girls have been supported, thus providing evidence of construct validity (King, Law, King, et al., 2006). The PAC has also demonstrated good internal consistency and construct validity (King, Law, Hanna, et al., 2006; King et al., 2004).

Longitudinal Study of Participation

The primary objective of this multisite project was to undertake a longitudinal study of children with physical disabilities aged 5 to 13 years (early childhood to adolescence) to determine the child, family, and environmental factors that enhance participation in the formal and informal activities of childhood. Innovative methodologies (structural equation modeling and a cross-sequential design) were used to evaluate the relative contribution of child, family, and environmental factors in determining participation of children with long-term, nonprogressive physical conditions associated with physical functional limitations in day-to-day activities (conditions such as cerebral palsy, traumatic brain injury, amputations, etc.). Conceptually, we subscribed to the notion of the "non-categorical" approach to childhood disability (Pless & Pinkerton, 1975), wherein specific diagnostic categories are less important than the presence of disability (from whatever cause) if the disability affects a child's development or function. Using a population-based sample of 427 children, we measured the quantity and quality of the participation of children in the formal and informal activities of childhood and delineated the relative influence of key child, family, and environmental factors on the level of their participation.

The broad goals of the study were as follows:

- To describe (a) the extent and nature of participation in everyday formal and informal activities of children with congenital or acquired nonprogressive conditions that cause long-term physical disabilities associated with limitations in day-to-day function, (b) how their participation changes as they grow older, and (c) their satisfaction with their participation. By "formal" activities, we meant those that were structured, involved

others (whether peers or adults), and required some degree of prior planning (examples would be music or art lessons, organized sports, youth groups, etc.). By "informal," we meant those activities that children choose to do for fun, either on their own (like reading or exercising) or with others (like playing outside at their own initiative) (after Sloper et al., 1990).

- To understand the factors within children, families, and environments that affect children's overall level of participation and how the influence of these factors may change over time.

Children in the study were recruited from publicly funded regional children's rehabilitation centers in Ontario, Canada. A list of all children at each center with physical disabilities born between October 1, 1985 and September 30, 1994, inclusive, was compiled. Children with the following primary diagnoses or conditions were included: amputation, cerebral palsy, cerebral vascular accident/stroke (vascular brain disorders), congenital anomalies, hydrocephalus, juvenile arthritis, muscular disorders (nonprogressive), neuropathy, orthopedic conditions (e.g., scoliosis), spinal cord injury, spina bifida, and traumatic brain injury. A developmental pediatrician reviewed the lists and determined the diagnostic category for each child as falling into either the "central nervous system-related disorders" group or "musculoskeletal disorders" group (structural and primary conditions of muscle tissue). Excluded diagnostic groups were progressive disorders, primary communication disorders of speech and/or language, hearing problems, cleft lip and palate, primary diagnosis of developmental delay, primary diagnosis of intellectual disability, fine motor difficulties, learning disability, behavioral/emotional disorders, autism, epilepsy, and anomalies of inner organs.

For the study, we recruited equal cohorts of boys and girls aged 6 to 8, 9 to 11, and 12+ years old and their families. Of 6,392 children identified, 2,444 were excluded because they did not fit the physical functional limitation criterion, were duplicate cases across two sites in one large city, had moved, did not fit the age range, or were already involved in a large research study. Families of these children were invited to participate in the study. A total of 509 families agreed to participate in the study. Of these 509, 40 did not meet all inclusion criteria, 28 withdrew prior to data collection, and 14 were unsuitable, leaving 427 children in the study. The study collected data three times, at approximately 9-month intervals. At Time 1, the participants were 427 parents and their children (229 boys and 198 girls). A total of 402 parents and children (216 boys and 186 girls) completed data collection at all three time points (dropout rate of 5.9%).

An additional study was conducted with 354 school-aged children without physical disabilities and their families. These families, all of whom lived in the London, Ontario area, were recruited through the assistance of the Thames Valley District School Board. The purpose of the study was to gather information about the leisure and recreational participation of children without physical disabilities.

Measures

Reflecting our conceptual model, a wide array of measures was used to assess child, family, and environmental variables likely to be contributors to the nature and extent of a child's participation in activities. These measures are listed in Table 8-1, in each of the categories to which they apply, along with information for constructs about which they will be providing indicators. A structural equation modeling analysis requires more than one indicator for each construct. These indicators were provided by several different measures or by one measure's subscales.

Analyses

Descriptive statistics (means, frequencies, etc.) were calculated to describe children's level of participation and enjoyment with participation in each of the CAPE scores. Using an analysis of variance, we examined the effects of age, gender, and family demographic variables on participation scores and enjoyment scores. The level of statistical significance was adjusted for the number of statistical comparisons within each analysis.

We used structural equation modeling (SEM) to examine the roles played by a wide range of factors in directly or indirectly predicting children's participation. The SEM approach enables one to examine simultaneously the relationships among predictor and outcome variables. Correlations among the variables were examined. The SEM was tested cross-sectionally at Time 1 of data collection using the hypothesized model developed for the project. Further analyses were completed to investigate specific questions of interest evolving from the study.

Results

Patterns of Participation

The 427 children and youth in the study were 6 to 14 years old at the time of enrollment in the study. Most of the children (41%) were between 9 and 11 years old. The percentages of study participants in the 6 to 8 years age range (29%) and 12+ years age range (30%) were similar. Slightly more boys (54%) than girls (46%) participated in the study. The participants had a wide range of physical disabilities (Table 8-2). The majority of the children and youth had cerebral palsy (51%), while the other children and youth in the study had a number of different types of health or developmental problems.

Study findings indicated that children with physical disabilities participated in a diverse range of activities. The most common activities, all of which were informal in nature, included watching television, listening to music, playing computer/video games, and crafts/drawing. In looking over the full range of activities, it was apparent that children were primarily involved in sedentary indoor activities. Importantly, we found no significant differences in participation intensity for children based on their diagnosis after we accounted for differences in age, gender, and functional ability (Law et al., 2004).

As expected, we found differences in participation based on children's gender and age. Girls tended to do more social and skill-based activities, while boys participated in more active physical activities. The range of activities was less diverse for youth 12 years or older, particularly within recreational activities. In terms of participation intensity, boys participated more intensely in active physical activities, whereas girls participated more intensely in both social and skill-based activities. Older children's overall participation and participation in informal activities was less intense than that of younger children. It is not surprising that participation patterns among the older group of children differed from the younger age group given that some of the activities, such as pretend play, are more appropriate for younger children.

We found significant differences in the diversity and intensity of children's overall participation between children with and without physical disabilities. Generally, children without physical disabilities reported more diverse participation than children with physical disabilities. We also found children without physical disabilities participated slightly more intensely in their overall activities as well as in their formal and informal activities than did children with physical disabilities. The differences in participation between these two groups of children were smaller than we expected but consistent across the five types of activities (recreational, social, active physical, skill-based, and self-improvement) measured in this study.

Predictors of Children's Participation Intensity

We examined the predictors of formal and informal participation intensity using structural equation modeling (King, Law, Hanna, et al., 2006) and the predictors of change over time in activity participation using latent growth curve modeling (King, McDougall, et al., 2009). There have been no previous studies of predictors of participation intensity at a given point in time and no previous studies of predictors of change in participation intensity for any population of children.

Cross-Sectional Predictors

In the cross-sectional study, structural equation modeling was used to test a theoretically based model of environmental, family, and child factors as determinants of the leisure and recreation participation of children with physical disabilities (King, Law, Hanna, et al., 2006). We developed a causal model to test, based on our conceptual model (King et al., 2003) and the literature on important determinants of children's development (Bronfenbrenner & Ceci, 1994). The causal model contained four categories of constructs (resources and barriers, supports, preferences, and child abilities), linked to one another in an ecological sequence from

TABLE 8-1

MODEL FOR **PARTICIPATE** STUDY INCLUDING NAMES OF SELECTED MEASURES/SCALES

	CONSTRUCT	INDICATORS	MEASURES
A	Environmental factors	Restrictions in environments Quality of environments Access to play space Parents' views of the attitudes of key others (in settings such as schools, recreational programs) Parents' perceptions of the availability of organized activities for children with disabilities Parents' awareness/satisfaction with policies and legislation	Craig Hospital Inventory of Environmental Factors
B	Supportive relationships	Social support from parents (e.g., mentoring/coaching) Social support from peers (e.g., mentoring/coaching) Social support from classmates Social support from adults (other than parents)	Social Support Scale for Children
C	Absence of instrumental limitations	Daily hassles	Child Health Questionnaire-50
D	Supportive family demographics	Mother's and father's level of education Mother's and father's employment Family income	Questionnaire developed and previously used by research group
E	Supportive home environment	Physical function of parents Mental/emotional function Social function General health	MOS Short-Form 36 Child Health Questionnaire-50
		General family functioning	Family Assessment Device
		Family cohesion Family adaptability	Family Environment Scale
F	Family preference for recreation	Recreational orientation Achievement orientation	Family Environment Scale
G	Child's self-perceptions of competence	Physical, social, behavioral, global self-worth	Self-Perception Profile for Children (Harter, 1985)
H	Child's physical, cognitive, and communicative function	Physical function	Activities Scale for Kids—Performance Version
		Cognitive function	Peabody Picture Vocabulary Test-Revised
		Receptive and expressive language function	Vineland Adaptive Behavior Scales
		Overall health/medical status	Child Health Questionnaire-50

(continued)

TABLE 8-1 (CONTINUED)

MODEL FOR PARTICIPATE STUDY INCLUDING NAMES OF SELECTED MEASURES/SCALES

	CONSTRUCT	INDICATORS	MEASURES
I	Child's emotional, behavioral, and social function	Emotional function	Child Health Questionnaire-50
		Behavioral function	Strengths and Difficulties Scale
		Social well-being (social competence)	Vineland Adaptive Behavior Scales
J	Child's participation	Number and extent of participation in organized activities	Children's Assessment of Participation and Enjoyment
		Number and extent of informal activities	
		Satisfaction with participation in organized activities	
		Satisfaction with participation in informal play activities	

TABLE 8-2

CHILDREN AND YOUTH INVOLVED IN THE STUDY

		# of Children and Youth	% of Children and Youth
Child's age	6 to 8 years	125	29.3
	9 to 11 years	176	41.2
	12+ years	126	29.5
Child's gender	Male	229	53.6
	Female	198	46.4
Child's health or development problem	Cerebral palsy	216	50.8
	Skeletal disorder	54	12.7
	Spina bifida	52	12.2
	Acquired brain injury	25	5.9
	Neuromuscular disorder	20	4.7
	Minor motor difficulties	18	4.2
	Developmental delay	12	2.8
	Other	30	6.7

more distal environmental and family variables to proximal child variables. The model outlined the mechanisms by which children's participation is thought to be enhanced, proposing that resources provide opportunities that, along with supportive contexts, influence both child and family preferences, as well as child abilities, which in turn are the more proximal predictors of children's participation in leisure and recreation activities.

As expected, the analysis indicated multiple interrelated determinants of children's participation. The significant direct predictors of children's participation intensity in both formal and informal activities were child functional ability, family participation in social and recreational activities, and child preferences for formal and informal activities. A unique and previously unreported finding was that, even after adjusting for functional ability, children's preferences and family preferences were important predictors of children's participation. Family cohesion, unsupportive environments, and supportive relationships for the child had significant indirect effects on participation. The direct and indirect paths indicate the importance of the mechanisms of opportunity, support, preference, and ability outlined in our theoretical model.

The findings indicated the vital role played by families and the importance of multifaceted approaches to supporting participation. Clinically speaking, the major role played by children's preferences suggests that children's participation can be encouraged by explicit consideration of children's motives for engaging in activities. The literature suggests that children are motivated to be involved in activities that supply them with meaningful experiences that satisfy basic psychological needs, including needs for control, self-esteem, and social relatedness (King et al., 2004; Sandler, Ayers, Suter, Schultz, & Twohey-Jacobs, 2004; Tinsley & Eldredge, 1995). Service providers can play an important role in helping children and families to recognize the multiple factors influencing participation. Service providers can assess participation and consider the supports that could be provided to influence a child's participation, because support from parents, close friends, and teachers plays an important role in promoting participation.

Predictors of Change in Participation Intensity Over Time

It is important to recognize that the predictors of participation intensity at a given point in time may be different from the predictors of rates of change. Our cross-sectional analysis indicated that children's preferences for particular types of activities are associated with their levels of participation intensity (King, Law, Hanna, et al., 2006), but preferences may be quite stable and, therefore, unlikely to be associated with change in activity intensity over time. Both cross-sectional and longitudinal approaches are required for a full understanding of the determinants of participation patterns and changes in these patterns.

We conducted a longitudinal analysis to investigate patterns and predictors of change, over a 3-year period, in the participation intensity of children/youth with physical disabilities. Latent growth curve modeling was used to determine the significant child, family, and community predictors of change in the intensity of children's participation in five types of activities (recreational, active physical,

social, skill-based, and self-improvement). Differences in predictors were examined for boys versus girls and older versus younger children.

We found that the intensity of children's participation in recreational, active physical, and social activities declined as children aged over the 3-year study period. The intensity of their involvement in skill-based and self-improvement activities did not show appreciable change, perhaps because these activities are more parent controlled, and parents are more likely to ensure that these activities continue. Significant predictors of change were found only for recreational and active physical activities. Overall, the findings indicated that factors associated with change in participation intensity are dependent on the type of activity and vary as a function of children's gender and age.

The findings indicated the importance of differentiating between cross-sectional determinants of status and longitudinal determinants of change in activity participation. Of note, children's physical functioning influenced initial levels of participation, but was not associated with change over time, indicating that physical functional limitations may affect where a child begins on a participation trajectory, but not the rate of change. Factors other than physical disability play more important roles with respect to change in participation levels over time. This is in line with models that portray an indirect rather than direct effect of physical functioning on children's outcomes (King et al., 2005). For more than 20 years, the literature has consistently indicated that chronic physical health status has little direct effect on adaptation (Lavigne & Faier-Routman, 1992), directing our attention to the psychosocial implications of reduced physical functioning, including the roles played by other factors and the indirect or mediating processes that lead to better or worse outcomes for children at risk (Wallander & Varni, 1998). Although our longitudinal study is quantitative in nature, it is interesting to note parallels with the qualitative findings of the PhD work of the first author, which also pointed to the importance of psychosocial and environmental variables.

Further Analyses

Our participation study dataset contains more than 2,500 child, parent, and family variables, providing a wealth of detailed information relevant to the antecedents, nature, and consequences of aspects of children's participation. We also collected a comparison dataset of 354 children without physical functional limitations. We conducted a number of comparative analyses involving this group of children without physical disabilities, including an investigation of the role of age, gender, and disability status as predictors of participation diversity, intensity, location, companionship, and enjoyment (King, Law, Hurley, Petrenchik, & Schwellnus, 2010), and a study examining the relative enjoyment of formal versus informal activities by children with and without disabilities (King, Petrenchik, et al., 2009).

Activity Participation as a Function of Age, Gender, and Disability Status

Previous studies have not examined the relative influence of age, gender, and disability on multiple dimensions of participation in a comprehensive set of out-of-school recreation and leisure activities. Controlling for income, we found important differences in the participation patterns of boys and girls with and without disabilities in three age groups representing early and middle childhood and early adolescence. The findings indicated that dimensions and types of activity participation are differentially influenced by age, gender, and disability and clarified what dimensions and types of activities are influenced more by age and gender than by disability.

Of particular interest, age cohort comparisons indicated that children without disabilities experienced a widening social world involving more intense social participation, greater participation with nonfamily members, and stable levels of enjoyment across the age groups. In contrast, children with disabilities in the various age groups were similar in their intensity of social participation and the nature of their companionship, with 12+ year olds reporting less enjoyment of social activities than those aged 6 to 8 or 9 to 11. This study, therefore, provided insight into the pattern of social isolation often reported by adolescents with disabilities. Their social participation does not decrease in actual terms, but they experience relative deprivation of social opportunities in comparison to their peers and their developmental needs.

Mechanisms Influencing Participation in Formal Versus Informal Activities

The literature on the benefits of participation in organized, out-of-school activities is just beginning to consider the processes by which formal activities bring about positive effects. To design programs that enable children to have optimal experiences, it is important to understand the mediating mechanisms underlying the positive developmental benefits of psychological engagement in organized activities (Eccles & Templeton, 2002; Simpkins, Ripke, Huston, & Eccles, 2005).

Based on our previous structural equation model outlining mechanisms thought to underlie participation (i.e., environmental opportunities, interpersonal resources and supports, and personal preferences and abilities) (King, Law, Hanna, et al., 2006), we developed a conceptual model of the sequence by which intrinsic motivation, opportunity, and support may lead to the experience of meaning and enjoyment in activity and, thus, to developmental benefits from activity, such as competency-related, social, or psychological benefits (King, Petrenchik, et al., 2009).

Although children who are typically developing enjoy formal activities (Vandell et al., 2005) and accrue a number of positive developmental benefits from their participation in structured activities (e.g., Eccles, Barber, Stone, & Hunt,

2003; Mahoney, Harris, & Eccles, 2006), this may not be the case for children with physical disabilities. We predicted that children without disabilities would report significantly greater enjoyment of formal than informal activities, whereas this would not be the case for children with disabilities. This prediction was confirmed. The lower average enjoyment of formal activities by children with disabilities may reflect a series of cascading processes underlying lack of psychological engagement in activity: lower activity choice and intrinsic motivation, lack of opportunities for meaningful experiences within the activity setting, and lack of physical and emotional support to encourage involvement.

Activity Participation Profiles

There is growing interest in determining the nature of children's activity profiles. Examining the determinants and consequences of membership in different leisure or school-based activity profiles may lead us to a deeper understanding of the factors influencing participation and the mechanisms by which participation influences development (Feldman & Matjasko, 2005). Practically speaking, children fitting different profiles may benefit from different types of interventions.

We examined the out-of-school activity participation profiles of children with disabilities by cluster analysis of their responses on multiple dimensions (intensity, location, companionship, enjoyment, preference) in five types of activity (King, Petrenchik, et al., 2010). Sociodemographic, child, parent, family, and environmental predictors of group membership were determined, along with child functioning, sociodemographic, self-concept, and social support variables significantly associated with group membership.

The cluster analysis revealed four groups, labeled Social Participators (a highly social and neighborhood-focused group), Broad Participators (a group of high participators who enjoy participation), Low Participators (a group with low enjoyment and weak preferences), and Recreational Participators (a group of younger children who participate in recreational activities with family members).

The findings indicate how children's activity profiles reflect differences in affective and motivational variables (enjoyment and preferences) and contextual features (companionship) and are associated with different sociodemographic, child, parent, family, and environmental variables. They also highlight the context-dependent nature of activity participation and the importance of recognizing roles played by multiple, activity-specific determinants, which was also shown in our previous work on predictors of change in participation intensity over time (King, McDougall, et al., 2009). Understanding how characteristics of children, families, and environments interact to influence engagement in activities throughout childhood is important for the development of appropriate and effective policies and programs.

Next Generation Research on Participation

Our research program continues to build and evolve. There are many intriguing and unanswered questions about the nature of children's recreational and leisure participation, including cross-geographical variation in patterns of participation, and how children's experiences of activity settings are related to the environmental qualities of these settings.

We are currently examining similarities and differences in the participation patterns of 1,000 children and youth with cerebral palsy in Australia, Canada, and the United States. As well, we are examining the extent to which children/youth take part in their most preferred activities in these countries. Both objectives may provide insights into geographical factors related to children's participation. These comparisons are made possible by the use of the CAPE by the four participating research projects.

One author (ML) has participated in studies led by Annette Majnemer from McGill University to examine factors influencing participation in children and adolescents with cerebral palsy. Funded by the Canadian Institutes of Health Research, study findings demonstrate that higher mastery motivation is associated with increased participation, fewer behavior problems, and less family burden (Majnemer et al., 2008). We also found that preferences for specific types of leisure participation are significantly influenced by personal factors (age, motivation, IQ) and functional abilities (prosocial behavior, motor abilities) (Majnemer et al., 2010).

In an emerging team grant led by GK (Canadian Institutes of Health Research Team in Optimal Environments for Severely Disabled Youth), we are in the process of developing measurement tools so that youth with little or no functional speech (users of augmentative and alternative communication systems) and youth with complex and continuing care needs can provide information about their experiences of activity settings. Understanding the home and community environments and experiences of these youth is a significant and largely neglected research issue. The ultimate aim is to examine causal patterns and relationships among qualities of environmental settings and activity experiences, in order to elucidate the optimal qualities of activity settings for children and youth with disabilities.

A research collaboration with researchers in Boston is leading to the development of a next-generation population-based participation measure (Coster, Law, & Bedell, 2010). The Participation and Environment Measure (PEM) is a population-based assessment of participation and environmental factors supporting or hindering participation. The PEM contains 24 items across three environmental settings (home, school, community). Psychometric testing is currently underway.

CONTRIBUTION TO OCCUPATIONAL SCIENCE

Through this research program, knowledge about the participation of children with physical disabilities has been generated. These findings highlight the importance of conducting larger and more longitudinal studies of occupation. We have learned that differences in participation between children with and without disabilities remain, although these differences are not as great as previously documented. There are more similarities in the participation of children with physical disabilities and typically developing children than previously thought. For example, participation among both groups reflects similar patterns of development across the child to adolescent age span. As well, patterns of participation are similar for boys and girls.

One of the most important findings across this research program is the recognition of the complexity of participation. Many factors influence outside-of-school participation, both initially and longitudinally. An understanding of these complex factors will help in the design of interventions to support the participation of children with disabilities. These findings emphasize the need for multipronged interventions to address inequities in participation.

We have learned that participation in occupations is not predicted by diagnosis, supporting a noncategorical approach to assessment and intervention. While a child's functional abilities predict initial participation, they do not significantly influence change in participation patterns over time. We have had many discussions about whether participation can be deemed to be "successful" or "optimal." While we know that participation influences health and development, is there a threshold effect for participation? Do children need at least a certain level of participation, but too much participation is counterproductive? This question remains to be answered.

IMPLICATIONS FOR PRACTICE

Key Findings From This Research

- Participation is complex and is influenced by many factors across the child, family, and environment. The main mechanisms influencing participation are opportunity, support, preference, and ability.

- Participation of children with physical disabilities is at a level that is now more similar to children without a disability. Differences still exist but they are smaller than 10 or 20 years ago.

- Children participate more intensely when their families are more engaged in social and recreational activities and value intellectual and cultural activities.

- Families provide and encourage supportive relationships and a feeling of togetherness, which are linked to children's preferences for activities. In turn, children's activity preferences directly influence their participation in out-of-school activities.

- Via indirect influences, children participate more intensely when environmental barriers are lower, when household income is higher, when social supports to children are higher, and when family members help and support one another.

On a broader level, the longitudinal study findings point to the utility of examining participation in types of activities rather than viewing participation as an undifferentiated conglomerate. They also point to a very complex set of determinants, which need to be examined holistically, contextually, and developmentally. The findings strongly support a socioecological conceptual framework that emphasizes the multiple, interrelated contexts within which children develop (Bronfenbrenner, 1979; Feldman & Matjasko, 2005). Understanding how the characteristics of children, families, and environments interact to influence engagement in activities throughout childhood and adolescence is important for the development of appropriate and effective policies and programs.

Research shows parents, communities, institutions, policies, and children's own choices mutually shape children's involvement in out-of-school activities. However, family-level influences are particularly powerful for young children and youth who are dependent upon their parents to help them meet their daily activity needs. In short, parents of children with complex needs play a particularly vital role in determining their child's participation in out-of-school activities. They are the child's primary source of social capital, and the resources available to parents affect the family's ability to make choices and to implement their goals and desires (Eccles, 2005).

Just as children are nested within a family system, families are situated within communities. The structure of community environments affects opportunities for sustained child and youth participation in organized recreational, social, cultural, and civic activities. As this research began, disability advocates stressed that disability is a problem in the relationship between the individual and the environment (Hahn, 1984; Jongbloed & Crichton, 1990). If our environments foster dependency and poor solutions to the problems of disability, then solutions would exist predominantly in planning and social policies aimed at the modification of the environment. The fundamental principle of this approach is the recognition of the ecological nature of disability, that the problems of disability are caused by the interactions of a child with a disability with the environment, not by the disability itself. Disability is seen as a collective problem, a problem caused by the inadequacies of the environments in which we live. Social policy would be used as the primary means to increase children's participation. The findings of our research program support this approach.

Policy Suggestions

Accordingly, and in keeping with current research, we developed the following policy suggestions as important for enhancing the participation of children and youth with complex needs:

- Focus on family-centered support and services.

  - Policy and intervention efforts to enhance the participation of children with complex needs should be ecological, integrated, and family-centered and should deliver practical, coordinated services and information.

- Build community infrastructure.

  - Build a base of high-quality, universally accessible community-based programs. Initiatives must include provisions to ensure program continuity, comprehensiveness, and integration of services into community settings.

  - Form strategic public-private alliances to develop strategic, long-term plans to renew recreation and culture infrastructures in municipalities and to identify and mobilize existing community-level resources.

- Reduce structural barriers.

  - Minimize structural barriers to child and youth participation in organized recreational, cultural, and civic activities, which includes addressing factors such as accessibility, costs, transportation, locations of activities, availability of necessary aides or support personnel, and organizational supports or accommodations. This is likely to be an especially pressing policy concern for children with complex needs in low-income families.

Recommendations for Practice

For practice, our research emphasizes the importance of opportunity; support from family, friends, and community; children's preferences for participation; and children's abilities to participate. These findings support an individualized approach to practice, in which a child's specific participation goals are identified as the basis for intervention. Therapists can play an important role in helping children and families to recognize the multiple factors influencing participation. They can formally assess children's functional abilities and activity preferences, family engagement in social and recreational activities, and family activity preferences and discuss these aspects with families—because these are the major factors influencing participation.

The major role played by children's preferences suggests that children's participation can be encouraged by explicit consideration of children's motives for engaging in activities. Building on child and family preferences for specific types of participation is an important starting point. Once participation goals have been set, intervention can address the factors that specifically support or hinder a child's participation, using an ecological approach. The child's abilities can be assessed and matched with their participation preferences. Intervention can focus on ensuring supports for participation and addressing environmental barriers.

This research also points to the importance of a child's age, gender, and the type of occupation. As children move into adolescence, their interests change and become more social in nature. Enabling social participation in the broader environment becomes increasingly important. Above all, a child's preferences for patterns of participation are important. As found in this research, some children are highly social while others participate in a broad cross-section of occupations. The ability of a therapist to discern these patterns and support children and families in taking part in preferred occupations is a key element to enabling successful participation.

LEARNING SUPPORTS

The Use of Different Research Methods

Purpose

The purpose of this learning activity is to explore the utility and impact of using different research methods to answer specific research questions.

Primary Concepts

Research methodology, quantitative methods, and qualitative methods.

Instructions

1. Choose two of the articles that are referenced in this chapter. When choosing, select one article that uses quantitative methods and one that uses qualitative methods.

2. Use the forms from this Web site—http://www.srs-mcmaster.ca/Default.aspx?tabid=630—to critically review these articles.

3. Write a one-page memo to your colleagues summarizing the results of your review and the implications for clinical practice. Describe what knowledge was generated from each study.

4. Classroom activity—Discuss how to link a research question with the most appropriate methods.

Expecting the Unexpected

Purpose

The purpose of this learning activity is to explore how research findings can often lead to surprising results.

Primary Concepts

Research findings, disability, diagnosis, and reflection.

Instructions

1. When reading over the research results in this chapter, choose a finding that appears surprising to you.

2. Write a one-half to one-page reflection on why you think this research result is surprising. To support your reflection, write down your assumptions about this result, and then read over an article from the chapter or other literature about this topic.

3. Classroom activity—Discuss the different perspectives of students regarding the results that were surprising. Reflect on how researchers may react to unexpected findings.

Intervention to Enhance Participation

Purpose

The research in this chapter has outlined findings that primarily focus on the measurement of participation and factors that support or hinder participation. The logical next step in this research program is to focus on the development and implementation of research to study interventions in this area. The purpose of this activity is to design a pilot study focused on enhancing participation.

Primary Concepts

Participation, measurement, intervention studies, and research design.

Instructions

1. Choose a specific client group and specify their age range (e.g., youth ages 13 to 15 years who have a physical disability).

2. Choose one or two participation goals that would be relevant for a client in this group (e.g., going to a concert with friends, text messaging, playing in a school band).

3. Develop an intervention plan to enhance the clients' participation in their chosen goal. Use information from the findings of this chapter to design the focus of your intervention.

4. Choose an appropriate outcome measure to evaluate the results of the intervention.

5. With this information, design a small pilot study to evaluate the feasibility and initial outcomes of your intervention to enhance participation.

6. Classroom activity—Discuss the most appropriate intervention methods, measurement of outcomes, and research design options for this pilot study.

REFERENCES

Anderson, E. M., & Clarke, L. (Eds.). (1982). *Disability and adolescence.* New York, NY: Methuen.

Blum, R. W., Resnick, M. D., Nelson, R., & St. Germaine, A. (1991). Family and peer issues among adolescents with spina bifida and cerebral palsy. *Pediatrics, 88*(22), 280-285.

Bronfenbrenner, U. (1979). *The ecology of human development.* Cambridge, MA: Harvard University Press.

Bronfenbrenner, U., & Ceci, S. (1994). Nature-nurture reconceptualized in developmental perspective: A bioecological model. *Psychological Review, 101*(4), 568-586.

Brown, L. D. (1986). Participatory research and community planning. In B. Checkoway (Ed.), *Strategic perspectives on planning practice.* Toronto, Canada: Lexington Books.

Brown, M., & Gordon, W. A. (1987). Impact of impairment on activity patterns of children. *Archives of Physical Medicine and Rehabilitation, 68,* 828-832.

Cadman, D., Boyle, M., Szatmari, P., & Offord, D. R. (1987). Chronic illness, disability, and mental and social well-being: Findings of the Ontario child health study. *Pediatrics, 79,* 805-813.

Caldwell, L. L., & Gilbert, A. A. (1990). Leisure, health, and disability: A review and discussion. *Canadian Journal of Community Mental Health, 9*(2), 111-122.

Canadian Institute of Child Health (1994). *The health of Canada's children: A CICH profile.* Ottawa, Ontario, Canada: Author.

Clark, A., & Hirst, M. (1989). Disability in adulthood: Ten year follow-up of young people with disabilities. *Disability, Handicap & Society, 4,* 271-283. doi:10.1080/02674648966780291

Coster, W., & Khetani, M. A. (2008). Measuring participation of children with disabilities: Issues and challenges. *Disability and Rehabilitation, 30,* 639-648. doi:10.1080/09638280701400375

Coster, W., Law, M., & Bedell, G. (2010). *Participation and Environment Measure—Child and Youth Version.* Boston, MA: Boston University.

Crapps, J., Langone, J., & Swaim, S. (1985). Quality and quantity of participation in community environments by mentally retarded adults. *Mental Retardation, 20,* 123-129.

Crawford, D., Godbey, G., & Crouter, A. (1986). The stability of leisure preferences. *Journal of Leisure Research, 18,* 96-115.

Crawford, D., Jackson, E. L., & Godbey, G. (1991). A hierarchical model of leisure constraints. *Leisure Sciences, 13,* 309-320. doi:10.1080/01490409109513147

Dempsey, I., & Simmons, B. (1995). National profile of away from home leisure activities of people with a disability. *Australian Leisure, 6,* 22-25.

DiLorenzo, T. M., Stucky-Ropp, R. C., Vander Wal, J. S., & Gotham, H. J. (1998). Determinants of exercise among children. II. A longitudinal analysis. *Preventive Medicine, 27,* 470-477. doi:10.1006/pmed.1998.0307

Eccles, J. S. (2005). Parental influences on children's achievement and engagement in academic and other skill-based domains. Invited address presented at the Society for Research in Child Development, Atlanta, GA.

Eccles, J. S., Barber, B. L., Stone, M., & Hunt, J. (2003). Extracurricular activities and adolescent development. *Journal of Social Issues, 59*(4), 865-889. doi:10.1046/j.0022-4537.2003.00095.x

Eccles, J. S., & Templeton, J. (2002). Extracurricular and other after-school activities for youth. *Review of Research in Education, 26,* 113-180.

Feldman, A. F., & Matjasko, J. L. (2005). The role of school-based extracurricular activities in adolescent development: A comprehensive review and future directions. *Review of Educational Research, 75*(2), 159-210. doi:10.3102/00346543075002159

Forsyth, R., & Jarvis, S. (2002). Editorial: Participation in childhood. *Child: Care, Health and Development, 28,* 277-279. doi:10.1046/j.1365-2214.2002.00272.x

Fuhrer, M. J. (1994). Subjective well-being: Implications for medical rehabilitation outcomes and models of disablement. *American Journal of Physical Medicine and Rehabilitation, 73*(5), 358-364.

Hahn, H. (1984). Reconceptualizing disability: A political science perspective. *Rehabilitation Literature, 45,* 362-365.

Hall, B. L. (1981). Participatory research, popular knowledge and power: A personal reflection. *Convergence, 14*(3), 6-17.

Hallum, A. (1995). Disability and the transition to adulthood: Issues for the disabled child, the family, and the pediatrician. *Current Problems in Pediatrics, 25,* 12-50.

Harter, S. (1985). *Social Support Scale for Children.* Denver, CO: University of Denver.

Hewett, S., Newson, J., & Newson, E. (1970). *The family and the handicapped child.* Chicago, IL: Aldine Publishing.

Imms, C. (2008). Review of the Children's Assessment of Participation and Enjoyment and the Preferences for Activity of Children. *Physical & Occupational Therapy in Pediatrics, 28*(4), 389-404.

Jongbloed, L., & Crichton, A. (1990). Difficulties in shifting from individualistic to sociopolitical policy regarding disability in Canada. *Disability, Handicap & Society, 5*(1), 25-36.

Kalscheur, J. A. (1992). Benefits of the Americans with Disabilities Act of 1990 for children and adolescents with disabilities. *American Journal of Occupational Therapy, 45*(5), 419-426. doi:10.5014/ajot.46.5.419

King, G., Law, M., Hanna, S., King, S., Hurley, P., Rosenbaum, P., . . . Petrenchik, T. (2006). Predictors of the leisure and recreation participation of children with physical disabilities: A structural equation modeling analysis. *Children's Health Care, 35*(3), 209-234. doi:10.1207/s15326888chc3503_2

King, G., Law, M., Hurley, P., Petrenchik, T., & Schwellnus, H. (2010). A developmental comparison of the out-of-school recreation and leisure activity participation of boys and girls with and without physical disabilities. *International Journal of Disability, Development and Education, 57*(1), 77-107. doi:10.1080/10349120903537988

King, G. A., Law, M., King, S., Hurley, P., Hanna, S., Kertoy, M., & Rosenbaum, P. (2006). Measuring children's participation in recreation and leisure activities: Construct validation of the CAPE and PAC. *Child: Care, Health and Development, 33*(1), 28-39. doi:10.1111/j.1365-2214.2006.00613.x

King, G., Law, M., King, S., Hurley, P., Rosenbaum, P., Hanna, S., . . . Young, N. (2004). *Children's Assessment of Participation and Enjoyment (CAPE) and Preferences for Activities of Children (PAC).* San Antonio, TX: Harcourt Assessment.

King, G., Law, M., King, S., Rosenbaum, P., Kertoy, M., & Young, N. L. (2003). A conceptual model of the factors affecting the recreation and leisure participation of children with disabilities. *Physical & Occupational Therapy in Pediatrics, 23*(1), 63-90. doi:10.1080/J006v23n01_05

King, G., McDougall, J., DeWit, D., Hong, S., Miller, L., Offord, D., . . . LaPorta, J. (2005). Pathways to children's academic performance and prosocial behaviour: Roles of physical health status, environmental, family, and child factors. *International Journal of Disability, Development and Education, 52*(4), 313-344. doi:10.1080/10349120500348680

King, G., McDougall, J., DeWit, D., Petrenchik, T., Hurley, P., & Law, M. (2009). Predictors of change over time in the activity participation of children and youth with physical disabilities. *Children's Health Care, 38*(4), 321-351. doi:10.1111/j.1469-8749.2011.04204.x

King, G., Petrenchik, T., DeWit, D., McDougall, J., Hurley, P., & Law, M. (2010). Out-of-school time activity participation profiles of children with physical disabilities: A cluster analysis. *Child: Care, Health and Development, 36*(5), 726-741. doi:10.1111/j.1365-2214.2010.01089.x

King, G., Petrenchik, T., Law, M., & Hurley, P. (2009). The enjoyment of formal and informal recreation and leisure activities: A comparison of school-aged children with and without physical disabilities. *International Journal of Disability, Development and Education, 56*(2), 109-130. doi:10.1080/10349120902868558

Kinney, V. B., & Coyle, C. P. (1992). Predicting life satisfaction among adults with physical disabilities. *Archives of Physical Medicine and Rehabilitation, 73*, 863-869.

LaGreca, A. M. (1990). Social consequences of pediatric conditions: Fertile area for future investigation and intervention? *Journal of Pediatric Psychology, 15*, 285-307. doi:10.1093/jpepsy/15.3.285

LaPlante, M. P., Kennedy, J., Kaye, H. S., & Wenger, B. L. (1996). *Disability and employment* (Report No. 11). Washington, DC: National Institute of Disability and Rehabilitation Research.

Larson, R. W., & Verma, S. (1999). How children and adolescents spend time across the world: Work, play and developmental opportunities. *Psychological Bulletin, 125*(6), 701-736. doi:10.1037/0033-2909.125.6.701

Lavigne, J. V., & Faier-Routman, J. (1992). Psychological adjustment to pediatric physical disorders: A meta-analytic review. *Journal of Pediatric Psychology, 17*(2), 133-157. doi:10.1093/jpepsy/17.2.133

Law, M., & Dunn, W. (1993). Perspectives on understanding and changing the environments of children with disabilities. *Physical and Occupational Therapy in Pediatrics, 13*(3), 1-17. doi:10.1080/J006v13n03_01

Law, M., Finkelman, S., Hurley, P., Rosenbaum, P., King, S., King, G., & Hanna, S. (2004). The participation of children with physical disabilities: Relationships with diagnosis, physical function, and demographic variables. *Scandinavian Journal of Occupational Therapy, 11*(4), 156-162.

Law, M., Haight, M., Milroy, B., Willms, D., Stewart, D., & Rosenbaum, P. (1999). Environmental factors affecting the occupations of children with physical disabilities. *Journal of Occupational Science, 6*(3), 102-110. doi:10.1080/14427591.1999.9686455

Loevinger, J. (1957). Objective tests as instruments of psychological theory [Monograph No. 9]. *Psychological Reports, 3*, 635-694.

Lyons, R. F. (1993). Meaningful activity and disability: Capitalizing upon the potential of outreach recreation networks in Canada. *Canadian Journal of Rehabilitation, 6*(4), 256-265.

Mahoney, J. L., Harris, A. L., & Eccles, J. S. (2006). Organized activity participation, positive youth development, and the over-scheduling hypothesis. *Social Policy Report, 20*(4), 1-31.

Majnemer, A., Shevell, M., Law, M., Birnbaum, R., Chilingaryan, G., Rosenbaum, P., & Poulin, C. (2008). Participation and enjoyment of leisure activities in school aged children with cerebral palsy. *Developmental Medicine and Child Neurology, 50*(10), 751-758.

Majnemer, A., Shikako-Thomas, K., Chokron, N., Law, M., Shevell, M., Chilingaryan, G., . . . Rosenbaum, P. (2010). Leisure activity preferences for 6-12 year old children with cerebral palsy. *Developmental Medicine and Child Neurology, 52*(2), 167-173.

Mancini, M. C., Coster, W. J., Trombly, C. A., & Heeren, T. C. (2000). Predicting elementary school participation in children with disabilities. *Archives of Physical Medicine and Rehabilitation, 81*, 339-347. doi:10.1016/S0003-9993(00)90081-9

Margalit, M. (1981). Leisure activities of cerebral palsied children. *Israel Journal of Psychiatry & Relational Science, 18*, 209-214.

Miller, W. L., & Crabtree, B. F. (1992). Primary care research: A multimethod typology and qualitative road map. In: B. F. Crabtree & W. L. Miller (Eds.), *Doing qualitative research* (pp. 3-28). Newbury Park, CA: Sage Publications.

Newacheck, P. W., & Halfon, N. (1998). Prevalence and impact of disabling chronic conditions in childhood. *American Journal of Public Health, 88*, 610-617.

Pless, I. B., Cripps, H. A., Davies, J. M. C., & Wadsworth, M. E. J. (1989). Chronic physical illness in childhood: Psychological and social effects in adolescence and adult life. *Developmental Medicine and Child Neurology, 31*, 746-755. doi:10.1111/j.1469-8749.1989.tb04070.x

Pless, I. B., & Pinkerton, P. (1975). *Chronic childhood disorder: Promoting patterns of adjustment.* London, England: Henry Kimpton.

Rae-Grant, N., Thomas, B. H., Offord, D. R., & Boyle, M. H. (1989). Risk, protective factors, and the prevalence of behavioral and emotional disorders in children and adolescents. *Journal of the American Academy of Child and Adolescent Psychiatry, 28*, 262-268. doi:10.1097/00004583-198903000-00019

Sandler, I. N., Ayers, T. S., Suter, J. C., Schultz, A., & Twohey-Jacobs, J. (2004). Adversities, strengths, and public policy. In K. I. Maton, C. J. Schellenbach, B. J. Leadbeater, & A. L. Solarz (Eds.), *Investing in children, youth, families, and communities: Strengths-based research and policy* (pp. 31-49). Washington, DC: American Psychological Association.

Seidel, J. V., & Clark, J. A. (1984). The Ethnograph: A computer program for the analysis of qualitative data. *Qualitative Sociology, 7*(1), 110-125. doi:10.1007/BF00987111

Silanpaa, M. (1987). Social adjustment and functioning of chronically ill and impaired children and adolescents. *Acta Paediatrica, 76*, Suppl. 340. doi:10.1111/j.16512227.1987.tb14938.x

Simeonsson, R. J., Carlson, D., Huntington, G. S., McMillen, J. S., & Brent, J. L. (2001). Students with disabilities: A national survey of participation in school activities. *Disability and Rehabilitation, 23*(2), 49-63. doi:10.1080/096382801750058134

Simpkins, S. D., Ripke, M., Huston, A. C., & Eccles, J. S. (2005). Predicting participation and outcomes in out-of-school activities: Similarities and differences across social ecologies. *New Directions for Youth Development, 105*, 51-69. doi:10.1002/yd.107

Sloper, P., Turner, S., Knussen, C., & Cunningham, C. (1990). Social life of school children with Down's syndrome. *Child: Care, Health & Development, 16*(4), 235-251. doi:10.1111/j.1365-2214.1990.tb00658.x

Statistics Canada. (1986). *The Canadian activity limitation survey.* Ottawa, Canada: Statistics Canada.

Stevenson, C. J., Pharoah, P. O. D., & Stevenson, R. (1997). Cerebral palsy—the transition from youth to adulthood. *Developmental Medicine and Child Neurology, 39*, 336-342. doi:10.1111/j.1469-8749.1997.tb07441.x

Tinsley, H. E. A., & Eldredge, B. D. (1995). Psychological benefits of leisure participation: A taxonomy of leisure activities based on their need-gratifying properties. *Journal of Consulting Psychology, 42*(2), 123-132. doi:10.1037/0022-0167.42.2.123

Trost, S. G., Pate, R. R., Saunders, R., Ward, D. S., Dowda, M., & Felton, G. (1997). A prospective study of the determinants of physical activity in rural fifth-grade children. *Preventative Medicine, 26*, 257-263. doi:10.1006/pmed.1996.0137

Vandell, D. L., Shernoff, D. J., Pierce, K. M., Bolt, D. M., Dadisman, K., & Brown, B. B. (2005). Activities, engagement, and emotion in after-school programs (and elsewhere). *New Directions for Youth Development, 105*, 121-129. doi:10.1002/yd.111

Wallander, J. L., & Varni, J. W. (1998). Effects of pediatric chronic physical disorders on child and family adjustment. *Journal of Child Psychology and Psychiatry, 39*(1), 29-46.

Werner, E. E. (1993). Risk, resilience, and recovery: Perspectives from the Kauai longitudinal study. *Development and Psychopathology, 5*, 503-515. doi:10.1017/S095457940000612X

World Health Organization. (2001). *International classification of functioning, disability and health.* Geneva, Switzerland: Author.

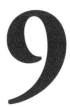

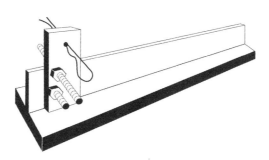

Participation and Engagement in Occupation in Adults With Disabilities

Lisa Tabor Connor, PhD; Timothy J. Wolf, OTD, MSCI, OTR/L;
Erin R. Foster, OTD, MSCI; Mary W. Hildebrand, OTD, OTR/L; and
Carolyn M. Baum, PhD, OTR/L, FAOTA

We are occupational scientists and occupational therapists. As scientists, we study occupation to understand its role in the everyday lives of those who experience restrictions, gaps, or dysfunction. As therapists, we help people overcome occupational restrictions; we do this by identifying barriers that limit their participation in occupations and by evaluating the process that supports engagement. Our interventions are designed to promote engagement, restore function, and address important activities, tasks, and roles. From both the scientific and clinical perspectives, we must have valid and reliable tools that assist in our inquiry and promote our unique roles as members of a team that is supporting a person's development or recovery.

We know that humans have a profound need to be active and that restricted engagement in activity leads to decreased competence in daily life. The basic assumption that underpins our profession is that people have a need and drive to be occupied. Meyer, in his "Philosophy of Occupation" speech delivered to the first meeting of the National Society for Occupational Therapy in 1921, said, "Our concept of man is that of an organism that maintains and balances itself in the world of reality and actuality by being in active life and active use" (p. 5, 1922). Since that time, leaders in our field have stressed that participation in occupation shapes our minds and bodies and is central to health and well-being (Law, 2002; Wilcock, 1993, 2001; Yerxa, 1998). Occupation is also a primary source of meaning (Christiansen, 1999; Hasselkus, 2002) and a determinant of life satisfaction (Eriksson, Kottorp, Borg, & Tham, 2009). A number of empirical studies have supported occupational engagement as a determinant of health and well-being (Clark et al., 1997; Glass, de Leon, Marottoli, & Berkman, 1999; Herzog, Franks, Markus, & Holmberg, 1998; Horgas, Wilms, & Baltes, 1998; Hultsch, Hertzog, Small, & Dixon, 1999).

Occupational therapists often bridge between a medical approach, under which people receive care for impairments, and a sociocultural context, in which people live their lives. Our goal is to maximize a person's performance and minimize disruption to his or her everyday life. Eriksson, Tham, and Borg (2006) describe the limitations to daily occupations caused by disruptions of health and social situation as "occupational gaps"—the gaps that occur between what

Pierce, D. (Ed.).
Occupational Science for Occupational Therapy (pp. 107-120).
© 2014 SLACK Incorporated.

the individual wants and needs to do and what he or she actually does.

A unique contribution that an occupational therapist or an occupational scientist can make is to understand the occupational needs and wants of a person, characterize the person's capacity to perform the occupation, and describe the gaps that can be filled by treatment to enable a person's performance. We are a team of scientists who believe strongly in the need to identify the occupations of the people who can benefit from our interventions. It was in response to this goal that we have developed and continue to use the Activity Card Sort (ACS) to examine participation in occupations by people with different types of disabilities.

A CLINICALLY USEFUL MEASURE OF OCCUPATION

The ACS (Baum & Edwards, 2001) was developed for a study of people with Alzheimer's disease (AD). The authors wanted a quantitative instrument to capture what people with AD were doing and what they had given up so that they could identify overlearned activities to use in building routines to sustain function. The ACS has proven to be a valuable clinical tool for collecting an occupational history and profile. It also offers the researcher a template to collect either quantitative or qualitative data, or both, depending on the questions the scientist wants to answer.

The ACS assesses the perceived level of activity participation at, or in relation to, various points in individuals' lives. It consists of photographic cards depicting activities that fall into four domains: instrumental activities (those necessary to maintain self and property), leisure activities that do not require high levels of physical strength or endurance, leisure activities that do require high levels of physical strength or endurance, and social activities. The activities in the ACS are validated as those most frequently performed by people over 55 years of age in the United States. (Versions have also been validated for use in Israel, Hong Kong, Australia, Singapore, South Korea, Puerto Rico, and the Netherlands.)

The ACS yields several quantitative scores that can be used in parametric analyses, and there are multiple versions, or forms, of the ACS that provide different perspectives on participation. Version A yields an activity count by simply asking whether or not the person performed each activity prior to a specific point in time (e.g., before entering the hospital, before beginning a new treatment, before turning a certain age). Version B measures the impact of a health or social condition (e.g., stroke, arthritis, an earthquake, job loss) on the person's participation by offering a range of responses: "Never done," "Continue to do with the 'condition,'" "Do less as a result of the 'condition,'" "Given up as a result of the 'condition,'" and "Began to do after the

'condition.'" Version B yields previous and current participation scores, which can then be used to calculate the percentage of activities retained (or given up) as a result of the condition. Version C directly assesses the person's perception of change in participation since a specific point in time (e.g., retirement, since turning a certain age). There are a number of ways to use the ACS to obtain qualitative data. The person is always asked to identify the five activities that he or she feels are most important to him or her. Those activities can be used as a starting point for more in-depth exploration of, for example, satisfaction with performance or participation or the meaning that the person ascribes to them. Specific questions can be asked to determine why activities have been abandoned (e.g., lost interest, lack of companions, limiting health conditions, environmental barriers, etc.).

The U.S. ACS has recently undergone revision. It has been 25 years since the original U.S. version was developed, and some activities of older adults have changed. The new (2008) version consists of 89 total activities: 20 instrumental activities, 35 low physical demand leisure activities, 17 high physical demand leisure activities, and 17 social activities.

A Clinical Example of the Use of the Activity Card Sort: A Therapist's Narrative
Mary W. Hildebrand, OTD, OTR/L

Mrs. S was a 78-year-old African American woman admitted to a skilled nursing facility 4 days after a total right knee arthroplasty. A chart review revealed that she had a medical history that included hypertension, cataracts, glaucoma, and osteoarthritis. She was oriented and alert and had no history of cognitive deficits or psychiatric diagnoses, such as depression. Occupational therapy evaluation took place 24 hours after admittance to the skilled nursing facility.

I began the occupational therapy evaluation of Mrs. S to determine if she had vision or hearing deficits for which I would need to adapt the assessments and my interaction. I began by asking her to perform the Near Acuity Vision Screening, the Simple Auditory Screening, and the Star Cancellation Test. Mrs. S wore her reading glasses and scored within the normal range on the vision screening. She stated that her cataracts had been surgically removed and she had gotten new prescription glasses 1 year ago. Mrs. S scored 5/5 on the Simple Auditory Screening, indicating that she had no significant hearing loss. She accurately completed the Star Cancellation Test with no indication of visuospatial neglect.

To build rapport, understand her prior level of function, and set goals, I had Mrs. S perform the ACS. I asked her to sort the 89 activity cards into two piles: done prior to illness/injury or admission and not done prior to illness/injury or admission. Mrs. S went through each card, making comments such as "Yes, I shop for groceries when my niece takes me to the store," "I cook dinner for myself most days," "I don't take care of children anymore—my three grandchildren are all grown now," "I read the newspaper every day," "I never did learn how to drive. My husband drove until he passed and now my children and other relatives take me where I need to go," "I love to go fishing! I haven't been in a year or so. I keep asking my kids to take me. They just don't have the time," "I love to garden and have flowers in my yard," and "I go to church every Sunday."

After sorting all the cards, I asked Mrs. S to choose five activities that she considers the most important to her. She chose going to church, visiting with friends and family, going fishing, cooking dinner, and gardening. We chose the first activity—going to church—to brainstorm what skills she would need to be able to perform this occupation, and we came up with the following list: getting out of bed, walking around the house, bathing, grooming, choosing clothing in the closet, dressing, getting in and out of her front door, going down her front steps, getting into and out of a car, walking from the car through the church entrance and into the sanctuary, and sitting and rising from the pew. I stated to Mrs. S that in occupational therapy we would be working with her on those tasks so that she would be able to go to church when she gets back home.

We continued the initial evaluation session by assessing transfers, dressing, and grooming. When I was ready to leave, I gathered the ACS cards. Mrs. S pointed to them and said, "I surely did enjoy that. Yes, I did. Thank you."

Examining Engagement in Occupations in the Presence of Disability Using the Activity Card Sort

The following section shows how the ACS has been used in four studies with participants who have common neurological conditions. Each study gives us insight to the importance of activity participation and thus gives guidance to practitioners in designing clinical programs to address the occupational needs of clients with these conditions.

The Impact of Activity Participation With Alzheimer's Disease *Carolyn M. Baum, PhD, OTR/L, FAOTA*

This study, originally published as "The Contribution of Occupation to Function in Persons with Alzheimer's Disease" in the *Journal of Occupational Science* (1995), used theory from ecological psychology (Csikszentmihalyi, 1988) and occupational science (Christiansen, 1991; Hasselkus, 1989; Kielhofner, 1992; Wilcock, 1993) to study the effect

of continued engagement in occupation on the behaviors of both the person with AD and the spouse.

The ACS was initially developed for use in this study. By using the ACS with the spouse reporting his or her loved one's activities, it was possible to calculate the impaired person's current level of engagement in activities compared with those performed prior to the onset of AD. The spouse's report was used, because we learned that people with AD were not always able to discriminate activities that were performed long ago from those currently performed. The scoring template used was Version C.

Brief Description of Methods

This study included 72 couples; one person in each couple was diagnosed with AD and had no other medical, neurological, or psychiatric disorders that could impair cognition. Participants were selected from the patient registry of the Washington University Alzheimer's Disease Research Center. All of the individuals were enrolled in a longitudinal study conducted by the Center; all were married couples living in the community; the mean age of the person with AD was 71.4 and the spouse was 66.4; and the educational level was 13.1 (person with AD) and 12.1 (spouse). Twelve participants were diagnosed with questionable AD, 29 with mild AD, 15 with moderate AD, and 16 with severe AD (AD determined with the Clinical Dementia Rating Scale; Berg, 1988); socioeconomic status measured with the Hollingshead Index (Hollingshead & Redlich, 1958) was 3.2, a score typical of middle class; and all had received the functional testing and the caregiver interviews that provided the data for this analysis.

Once informed consent was obtained, data were collected from the subject and the spouse by trained interviewers who were blind to the stage of AD. Subjects completed a measure of executive function (The Kitchen Task Assessment; Baum & Edwards, 1993) and an assessment of memory (The Short Portable Mental Status Questionnaire; Pfeiffer, 1975). The spouse completed a measure of observed behaviors (The Memory Behavior Problem Checklist; Zarit, Reever, & Bach-Peterson, 1980) and burden (The Zarit Burden Interview; Zarit, Todd, & Zarit, 1986), and completed the ACS to describe the activities their loved one continued to do, did less, and had given up since the onset of AD.

A Covariance Analysis of Linear Structural Equations procedure was used for the analysis (Loehlin, 1992). All of the variables were examined to determine if they were consistent with the assumptions of multivariate normality, and their correlations were reviewed prior to the covariance analysis of linear structural equations. This analysis builds on correlation and permits the construction of models that incorporate and correct for measurement error. The analysis allows the objective evaluation of the fit of a theoretical model to the data as indicated by the degree to which the relationships among the observed variables reproduced by the hypothesized model differ from the data in the sample.

Figure 9-1. Hypothesized model. (Reprinted with permission from Baum, C. M. [1995]. The contribution of occupation to function in person's with Alzheimer's disease. *Journal of Occupational Science: Australia, 2*[2], 59-67. Copyright Taylor & Francis Ltd. www.informaworld.com)

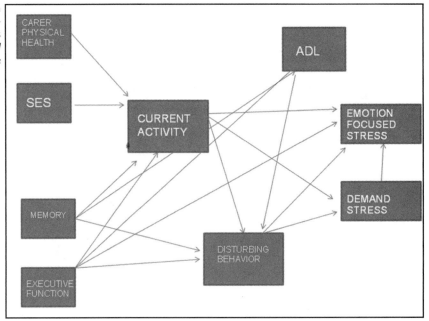

Figure 9-2. Best fit model. (Reprinted with permission from Baum, C. M. [1995]. The contribution of occupation to function in person's with Alzheimer's disease. *Journal of Occupational Science: Australia, 2*[2], 59-67. Copyright Taylor & Francis Ltd. www.informaworld.com)

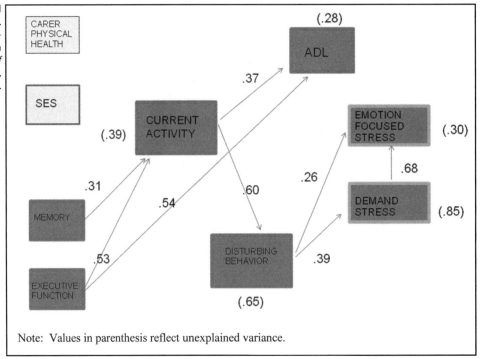

Note: Values in parenthesis reflect unexplained variance.

The analysis results in structural coefficients that express the degree of change in the outcome variables expected from a unit change in the causal variables in the model. The initial analysis tested the hypothesized model (Figure 9-1) and indicated that the model was restricted by a poor fit with 12 paths that did not have significant t-values. Further analysis removed the parameters that were not significant one by one until the model was determined to have the best fit (Figure 9-2).

Summary of Results

The analysis revealed the following. Higher executive performance corresponded to giving up fewer activities and less help needed to perform basic self-care. Better memory ability corresponded to giving up less activity. Current greater number of activities corresponded to fewer disturbing behaviors and less help in performing self-care. More disturbing behaviors resulted in greater demand stress and emotion-focused stress of the spouse, and more demand stress corresponded to greater emotion-focused stress. This model could be interpreted to mean that if cognitive support were used to bypass poor executive performance, the person with AD could remain engaged in occupation, would require less help with self-care, would demonstrate fewer disturbing behaviors, and the spouse would experience less stress as a result of the fewer disturbing behaviors. Such information can guide occupation-based interventions.

The Impact of Activity Participation With Parkinson Disease *Erin R. Foster, OTD, MSCI*

Parkinson disease (PD) is a progressive neurodegenerative disorder that affects approximately 1 million Americans (Tanner & Aston, 2000). In the later stages of the disease, motor impairments lead to significant difficulties in the performance of basic activities of daily living. At this point, physicians often refer individuals to occupational therapy to support safe functional mobility and self-care activity performance in the home. However, there are many subtle changes that occur in the initial stages of PD that have the potential to affect the occupations of those with the disease. Research in other populations has shown that instrumental, leisure, and social activities are essential for independent living, health, and well-being; yet, they are not typically assessed in research or clinical practice with individuals with PD. Therefore, the potential early effects of PD on occupation and quality of life may be underrecognized.

The purposes of this study were to investigate the effect of early PD on instrumental, leisure, and social activity participation and to explore relationships between participation and health-related quality of life (HR-QOL) in early PD. The ACS was chosen because it is a sensitive and comprehensive tool for measuring differences in complex activity participation between groups and over time.

Brief Description of Methods

Participants were 24 PD and 30 healthy control volunteers. The sample was 96% White and 52% male and had a mean age of 59.6 years ($SD = 7.7$) and a mean education of 15.1 years ($SD = 2.8$). The groups were equivalent in gender and race distributions, age, and years of education ($ps > .43$). PD participants were diagnosed with idiopathic PD according to accepted clinical criteria and were Hoehn and Yahr Stage I or II, indicating mild symptoms with no balance impairment (Hoehn & Yahr, 1967). Exclusionary criteria included global cognitive impairment (Mini-Mental Status Examination score < 27; Folstein, Folstein, & McHugh, 1975) and current significant psychiatric symptoms or diagnoses (as determined by a structured clinical interview; First, Spitzer, Gibbon, & Williams, 2002). Severity of motor dysfunction was measured using the Unified Parkinson's Disease Rating Scale Motor subscale (Fahn, Elton, Marsden, Goldstein, & Calne, 1987). PD participants had significantly lower motor scores (indicating better

motor functioning) while on, compared to off, their anti-Parkinsonian medications (on medications score: $M = 14.2$, $SD = 6.2$; off medications score: $M = 17.7$, $SD = 6.7$; $p = .01$).

Activity participation and HR-QOL were measured as part of a larger study battery. Participation in instrumental, leisure, and social activities was measured with the ACS (Version B). To rate current participation, respondents sorted the activity cards into the following categories with the corresponding numerical values: *Do not do/Given up* = 0, *Do now* = 1, *Do less* = 0.5. Participants in this study were instructed to rate their participation 5 years ago as their previous participation to ensure valid comparisons between groups (*Did 5 years ago* = 1). Activity retention over the previous 5 years was calculated by dividing each participant's current participation by his or her previous participation for each activity domain. The Medical Outcomes Study short-form health survey (SF-36; Ware & Sherbourne, 1992) was used to measure HR-QOL in PD and control participants. Scores ranged from 0 to 100, with higher scores indicating better perceived HR-QOL. PD participants also completed the Parkinson Disease Questionnaire (PDQ-39; Jenkinson, Fitzpatrick, Peto, Harris, & Saunders, 2008), a disease-specific HR-QOL measure. The PDQ-39 asks about the frequency of common symptoms or concerns of individuals with PD. Participants rate each item on a 5-point scale (0 = *Never*, 4 = *Always*). Scores range from 0 to 100, with higher scores indicating worse perceived HR-QOL. For parsimony, a calculated average of the SF-36 subscales and the PDQ-39 summary index were used in the analyses reported here.

Summary of Results

Descriptive statistics for current activity participation and HR-QOL showed no significant differences in previous activity participation between the PD and control groups, meaning that before they were diagnosed with PD the participants were active older adults. The PD group reported less current participation overall than the control group ($p = .008$) (Table 9-1). Comparisons of the separate activity domains revealed that people with PD participated in significantly fewer instrumental, low-demand leisure and social activities at the time of the study compared to controls ($ps < .03$).

In terms of activity retention, PD participants had given up on average 5% more of their total activities than the control group during the previous 5 years (*ns.*). Comparisons of the separate activity domains revealed that PD participants had given up significantly more social activities than control participants ($p = .03$). Specifically, control participants retained on average 87% of their social activities while PD participants retained only 79% of theirs.

Correlations between the ACS and HR-QOL measures were performed using total activity participation scores (versus correlations by activity domain). PD participants with higher current total activity participation had better

TABLE 9-1

CURRENT ACTIVITY PARTICIPATION AND HEALTH-RELATED QUALITY OF LIFE SCORES

VARIABLE	PD		CONTROL	
N	24		30	
ACS instrumental	14.0	(3.1)	15.7	(2.1)
ACS low-demand leisure	16.8	(3.9)	19.1	(3.3)
ACS high-demand leisure	6.4	(2.8)	7.7	(3.8)
ACS social	11.3	(2.3)	12.6	(1.6)
SF-36 average	63.5	(16.1)	82.7	(12.2)
PDQ-39 summary index	21.9	(9.9)	---	

Numbers represent means (standard deviation). PD=Parkinson's disease; ACS=Activity Card Sort; SF-36=Medical Outcomes Study Short-Form Health Survey; PDQ-39=Parkinson Disease Questionnnaire-39.

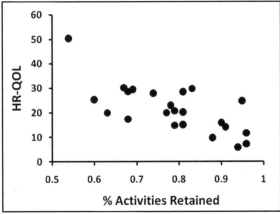

Figure 9-3. Relationship between activity retention and HR-QOL (PDQ-39 summary index) within PD (*n* = 24).

HR-QOL as measured by the SF-36 (*r* = .42, *p* = .04) and the PDQ-39 (*r* = -.44, *p* = .04). Similarly, those who retained a higher percentage of their total activities over the previous 5 years had better HR-QOL as measured by the SF-36 (*r* = .48, *p* = .02) and the PDQ-39 (*r* = -.65, *p* = .001; Figure 9-3). There were no significant correlations between ACS and SF-36 scores in the control group.

To summarize, we found that individuals with early and mild PD have reduced activity participation compared to healthy adults and that these reductions in activity participation are associated with worse HR-QOL. Social activities appear to be preferentially restricted in the initial stages of PD. This study encourages occupational therapists to focus on the occupational performance needs of the person at the time of diagnosis because PD presents challenges to activity participation.

Our results provide new insight into the effect of PD on the occupations of those with the disease. The prevailing view is that individuals with PD do not experience functional limitations until their motor impairments produce physical disability. The ACS allowed us to detect changes in participation early in disease progression and prior to physical disability that, although subtle, were significant determinants of HR-QOL. This highlights the importance of measuring complex activity participation in both research and clinical practice with this population.

Of particular concern is the apparent vulnerability of social activities to the onset of PD. Social engagement is thought to be protective against motor decline (Buchman et al., 2009), dementia (Wang, Karp, Winblad, & Fratiglioni, 2002), and death (Glass et al., 1999). Unnecessary reductions in social participation early in the course of PD could lead to a cycle of accelerated functional decline beyond the effects of the disease alone. These findings further stress the need to expand our focus from physical performance and disability in PD to consider the full effect of the disease on people's lives.

Our findings suggest an important role for occupational therapy early in the course of PD. Although the initial symptoms of PD are mild and individuals maintain their capacity to perform basic activities of daily living, they may still experience participation restrictions that disrupt their occupations and their overall quality of life. These individuals (and their families) may benefit from occupational therapy programs that provide strategies for maintaining participation in occupation and roles despite disease progression.

The Impact of Activity Participation

With Aphasia *Lisa Tabor Connor, PhD*

Aphasia is a disorder caused by damage to portions of the brain responsible for language. Aphasia produces difficulty in expressing oneself when speaking, trouble understanding speech, and difficulty with reading and writing. Approximately 1 million people in the United States are currently living with aphasia; the estimated prevalence of aphasia is 1 in 272 people. The prevalence is projected to double by 2020 due to the aging of the population and the rising incidence of stroke, the leading cause of aphasia (National Aphasia Association; National Institute of Neurologic Diseases and Stroke Aphasia; U.S. Census Bureau, 2007). Although people with aphasia receive rehabilitation services, they often return to the community with communication barriers that have an impact on quality of life (Cruice, Worrall, Hickson, & Murison, 2005) and participation in their most valued occupations (Connor, Tucker, Gotschall, Kauffman, & Baum, 2011). Moreover, people with aphasia do not generally receive occupational therapy services after their acute hospital stay, as they are thought to be able to resume activities if they receive services from speech-language pathologists for their communication problems. We believe, however, that most people with aphasia need assistance from occupational therapists to help them resume the occupations that they need and want to do. Currently, little is known about amount and quality of activity participation in people with aphasia.

In the current investigation, we used the ACS to explore the impact that aphasia has on activity participation beyond the effects that having a stroke exerts on activity participation. Our goal was to conduct a quantitative analysis of the degree to which people with aphasia give up activities and the nature of the activities that they report giving up.

Brief Description of Methods

The participants in this study originated from two sources. Individuals with aphasia were tested as part of a larger study conducted by members of our research team (Tucker, Edwards, Mathews, Baum, & Connor, 2012). The second group of participants included individuals post-stroke without aphasia. The data from the people without aphasia were obtained from the database of the Cognitive Rehabilitation Research Group located in the Program in Occupational Therapy at Washington University in St. Louis. Data from 136 individuals post-stroke without aphasia and 26 individuals post-stroke with aphasia were included. More men were found in the group without aphasia (51% vs. 42%) and more Whites were found in the group without aphasia (88% vs. 64%). A significant difference between groups was found for age (No Aphasia M = 61.6 years; Aphasia M = 56.1 years), education (No Aphasia M = 13.8 years; Aphasia M = 14.9 years), and chronicity (No Aphasia M = 6.1 months

post-stroke; Aphasia M = 44.1 months post-stroke), with individuals with aphasia being younger, more educated, and much more chronic than the individuals without aphasia.

Participants in both groups were administered the ACS, Form B as part of a larger assessment battery that included measures of stroke- and health-related quality of life, such as the Stroke Impact Scale (Lai, Studenski, Duncan, & Subashan, 2002), Reintegration to Normal Living Index (Wood-Dauphinée, Opzoomer, Williams, Marchand, & Spitzer, 1988), and the SF-36 (Ware, Snow, Kosinski, & Gandek, 1988). For individuals with aphasia, the physical format of the ACS was altered slightly to meet their specific communication demands. These alterations included fewer sorts presented to the participant at a time and additional, simplified explanation of the activity on each card, if required.

In addition to the traditional categories for the ACS, we wanted to classify the activities in terms of the amount of communication required to complete them. Both expressive and receptive communication was taken into account. Expressive communication is the ability of an individual to convey his or her thoughts, feelings, beliefs, and other ideas verbally or in writing. Receptive communication is the ability of an individual to receive and understand knowledge, ideas, and other information.

The 80 items on the ACS were compiled into a survey administered to seven occupational therapy students at Washington University. The amount of communication necessary to complete each activity was rated using a scale from 0 to 3. The survey revealed that 37 activities required minimal communication, such as doing dishes, sewing, using a computer, and swimming. Twenty-nine activities required moderate communication, such as shopping in a store, reading the newspaper, camping, and studying for personal advancement. Fourteen activities had maximal communication requirements, such as child care, table games, and maintaining a marriage/relationship.

Summary of Results

People with post-stroke aphasia retained fewer instrumental, low-, and high-demand leisure and social activities than their peers with stroke with no aphasia ($p < .01$) Participation levels in people with aphasia were correlated positively with scales on the Stroke Impact Scale, the Reintegration to Normal Living Index, and with scales on the SF-36 (all $ps < .05$).

To compare the percent of activities retained after stroke between those with aphasia and those without aphasia, a series of independent sample *t*-tests were performed (Table 9-2). In each domain of the ACS, individuals with aphasia gave up significantly more activities than their nonaphasic peers, revealing the existence of a greater loss of activities in the group of individuals with aphasia.

To address whether individuals with aphasia gave up more activities high in communication relative to their

TABLE 9-2

PERCENTAGE OF ACTIVITIES RETAINED BY ACTIVITY CARD SORT DOMAIN FOR INDIVIDUALS WITH AND WITHOUT APHASIA

	GROUP	MEAN	SD	t
Retained instrumental	No aphasia	80.67	2.04	2.90*
	Aphasia	65.81	4.86	
Retained low demand	No aphasia	88.86	1.29	7.13*
	Aphasia	65.09	3.54	
Retained high demand	No aphasia	73.63	2.77	2.87*
	Aphasia	54.36	5.18	
Retained social	No aphasia	87.60	1.46	5.52*
	Aphasia	67.57	3.36	

Note. *p < .01.

Figure 9-4. Group by communication level for percent retained of individuals with aphasia. Note. Group, $p < .001$; Communication Level, $p < .01$.

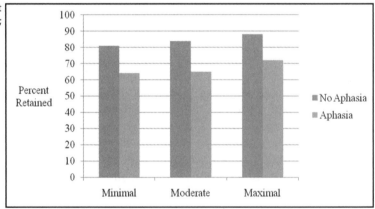

nonaphasic counterparts, a repeated-measures ANOVA was performed (Figure 9-4). Groups differed significantly in terms of their activities retained overall. In addition, percent of activities retained was influenced by level of communication. There was, however, no significant Group by Communication Level interaction. Therefore, individuals with aphasia did not give up more communication-intensive activities than their nonaphasic peers. Additionally, the direction of the Communication Level effect was not what we predicted. Instead, it appears that activities requiring maximal communication were retained more than those with minimal communication.

To determine specifically if people with aphasia gave up more activities that had high levels of communication, we conducted a one-way ANOVA and pairwise t-tests. Activities requiring minimal communication were retained less than activities requiring maximal communication

($p = .07$), which was opposite to our prediction. Additionally, significantly fewer activities requiring moderate communication were retained when compared to activities requiring maximal amounts of communication ($p < .05$).

Finally, we calculated Pearson correlations (r) between percent retained on the ACS and aphasia severity as measured by the Boston Diagnostic Aphasia Examination (Goodglass, Kaplan, & Barresi, 2001). Percent retained was higher for those with higher expressive language and auditory comprehension scores (rs from 0.43 to 0.57, all ps < .05). The same pattern held for instrumental activities, low-demand leisure activities, and overall percent retained. High-demand leisure and social activities were not related to expressive language (rs < .30). Percent of social activities retained, however, were related to comprehension ($r = .43$).

In this study, we found that people with stroke and aphasia retained fewer activities in each of the four ACS domains than people without aphasia; on average, 83% of activities were retained by the stroke, no aphasia group, but only 63% of activities were retained by people with aphasia. Interestingly, when we examined whether activities with a high communication demand were more likely to be given up by people with aphasia, we found that not to be true. By examining more thoroughly the activities comprising the high communication demand grouping, we found that many of these activities came from the social domain of the ACS. Although these activities were demanding of communication, they were reported retained by the majority of people with aphasia in our sample. We speculate that these activities were deemed central to their lives and remained high in importance (and plan to investigate this hypothesis in future studies).

Another finding from this study that is relevant to a more nuanced understanding of activity participation in people with aphasia is the degree of moderate correlation between ACS domain scores and aphasia severity. At first glance, this seems to affirm the notion that aphasia severity is the critical factor in determining activity participation. The average magnitude of the correlations, about 0.55, indicates, however, that a relatively modest amount of variance (only about 30%) in activity participation is accounted for by aphasia severity. Thus, language impairment alone is not the full explanation for the degree of activity participation that can be expected for someone with aphasia. Clinically, you may have known a client who had severe language impairment yet participated fully in life's activities; conversely, you may have known a client with mild language impairment who withdrew from social participation due to shyness or embarrassment. In this study, one aspect of aphasia, however, influenced the degree of social activities retained in our sample; if a person with aphasia had poor comprehension of spoken language, social activities were disproportionately affected. It is, therefore, important to work with people with aphasia and their families to develop skills and strategies to support occupational engagement.

The Impact of Stroke on
Participation *Timothy J. Wolf, OTD, MSCI, OTR/L*

According to recent research, the majority of strokes are classified as being mild to moderate in severity: meaning that the individuals may or may not have any outward signs of neurological impairment (Wolf, Conner, & Baum, 2009). Survivors of mild to moderate strokes are typically independent in activities of daily living and exhibit mild impairments on most assessments; therefore, approximately 70% are discharged directly home, discharged with home services only, or discharged with only limited outpatient services (Wolf et al., 2009). The services that people do receive have limited focus on their occupations in the community and at work, and often none at all. These practices reflect an assumption that an individual who

performs well on neurological assessments and measures of basic self-care tasks will likely be able to return to all other everyday life activities. However, many everyday life tasks like working, maintaining a home, community activities, leisure activities, and driving require capacities, such as higher level cognitive functioning, that are not captured by traditional stroke assessments. Assessments administered in the acute phase after mild to moderate stroke may be missing subtle deficits that could negatively affect individuals' longer term functioning and participation.

The purpose of this study was to challenge the assumption that limited to no visible impairment in the acute care setting following mild to moderate stroke corresponds to no problems in complex everyday life activities beyond self-care. We expected that, despite having minimal neurological impairment as indexed by the NIH Stroke Scale, people who were classified as having reduced participation based on ACS post-stroke would also demonstrate higher depressive symptomatology and would report less reintegration into the community.

Brief Description of Methods

Participants in this study ($N = 198$) were recruited from the Cognitive Rehabilitation Research Group Stroke Registry at the Program in Occupational Therapy at Washington University in St. Louis. This stroke registry maintains a record of everyone treated by the stroke service at Barnes-Jewish Hospital in St. Louis. For inclusion in this study, participants had to have a National Institute of Health Stroke Scale (NIHSS) score of less than 16, indicating a neurologically mild to moderate stroke. Stroke severity (NIHSS) and pre-morbid functional status (Barthel Index) were collected during the participant's acute hospital stay. Follow-up testing was completed 6 months post-stroke to determine the impact of the stroke on their occupations and included measures of activity participation (Baum & Edwards, 2008), depression (Center for Epidemiological Studies Depression Scale; Radloff, 1977), and community reintegration (Reintegration to Normal Living Index; Wood-Dauphinée et al., 1988).

The ACS percent of activities retained since having a stroke was chosen as the primary outcome measure for this study. This variable was calculated by averaging the percent retained values from the instrumental, low-demand leisure, and social activities domains. The high-demand leisure domain was excluded because the majority of participants reported participating in one or fewer of these activities before their stroke. We divided the cohort into two groups: those who had retained less than 80% of their pre-stroke activities (low retention, $n = 69$) and those who had retained 80% or more of their pre-stroke activities (high retention, $n = 129$) at 6 months post-stroke. We then compared these groups on baseline demographic and clinical characteristics and psychological adjustment and reintegration at 6 months post-stroke.

TABLE 9-3

COMPARISON OF LOW RETENTION (<80% ACTIVITIES RETAINED) AND HIGH RETENTION (>80% ACTIVITIES RETAINED) ON FOLLOW-UP (5 TO 8 MONTHS) MEASURES OF STROKE: REINTEGRATION TO NORMAL LIVING INDEX AND CENTER FOR EPIDEMIOLOGICAL STUDIES DEPRESSION SCALE

VARIABLE	GROUP	n	MEAN	SD	SIGNIFICANCE (p)
RNL—total score	Low retention	58	38.14	6.97	p<.944
	High retention	104	48.62	5.81	
CES-D—total score	Low retention	21	21.95	20.25	p<.000*
	High retention	38	7.55	9.478	

*Note. *p <.01. Higher scores on the RNL reflect better perceived reintegration. Higher scores on the CES-D reflect a greater number of depressive symptoms reported.*

Summary of Results

At the point of admission, there were no significant group differences in age ($p=.941$), years of education ($p=.120$), employment status ($p=.294$), or pre-morbid functioning ($p=.396$); however, the groups did differ in race ($p<.001$), gender ($p=.048$), discharge location ($p<.001$), and stroke severity ($p=.014$). Participants who had retained fewer than 80% of their activities since their stroke (low retention) had higher NIHSS scores at acute assessment (mean = 4.18) (indicating worse neurological impairment) than those who retained 80% or more of their activities since their stroke (high retention) (mean = 3.11). The correlation between the NIHSS scores and percent of activities retained on the ACS was small ($r = -.197$), but statistically reliable ($p < .01$).

Group comparisons of the follow-up data (Table 9-3) revealed that participants who had retained fewer activities since their stroke (low retention) reported significantly more depressive symptoms. There were no group differences in total Reintegration to Normal Living score, but an analysis of the individual items on the Reintegration to Normal Living revealed significant group differences for five of the 11 questions. Participants in the low retention group reported lower levels of reintegration related to home and community management, recreation and social activities, and work (Table 9-4), and higher scores on the Center for Epidemiological Studies Depression Scale indicate a higher level of depressive symptoms.

IMPLICATIONS FOR OCCUPATIONAL SCIENCE AND PRACTICE

In each of these studies, individuals with neurological conditions have limited activity participation compared to healthy adults. The limitations in their activity participation are related to other issues, such as quality of life, community participation, social interaction, and even the level of stress experienced by their caregivers. If we do not ask our patients or clients about their activities, their participation, and what has meaning to them, we will not have the necessary information to help them develop strategies to maintain their health and well-being.

In Dr. Baum's study, we saw that helping people remain active in their occupations results in the person with AD having fewer disturbing behaviors and requiring less help with self-care, which reduces the caregiver's burden. We know from Dr. Foster's study that activity participation declines early in people with PD, prior to the emergence of physical disability, and that this decline is associated with reduced HR-QOL. Dr. Connor's work challenges occupational therapists to remain involved in the care of a person with language problems. Through this study, we know that people with aphasia do not participate fully in their pre-stroke activities. Because severity of language impairment makes a relatively small contribution to participation in activities, occupational therapists should advocate for their role in assisting people with aphasia to resume their participation in everyday life.

TABLE 9-4

COMPARISON OF LOW RETENTION (< 80% ACTIVITIES RETAINED) AND HIGH RETENTION (> 80% ACTIVITIES RETAINED) ON INDIVIDUAL REINTEGRATION TO NORMAL LIVING ITEMS

RNL ITEM	GROUP	*n*	MEAN	*SD*	SIGNIFICANCE (*p*)
I move around my community as I feel necessary.	Low retention High retention	58 104	2.95 4.42	1.25 0.78	$p < .000$*
I spend most of my days occupied in work activity that is important to me.	Low retention High retention	58 104	2.88 4.28	1.10 0.91	$p < .001$*
I am able to participate in recreational activities.	Low retention High retention	58 104	3.07 4.17	1.14 0.86	$p < .000$*
I am able to participate in social activities with my family and friends.	Low retention High retention	58 104	3.03 4.42	1.14 0.62	$p < .000$*
I feel like I can deal with life events as they happen.	Low retention High retention	58 104	3.84 4.54	0.98 0.54	$p < .034$*

Note. *$p < .05$. SD = standard deviation. High scores indicate greater perceived reintegration.*

From Dr. Wolf's work, we see how easy it is to miss the person's occupational needs if we assess only people's ability to perform self-care and fail to evaluate all areas of participation that they are engaged in prior to their stroke. By using the ACS to measure changes in activity participation within the stroke population, we were able to discover that decreased ability to participate in activities post mild to moderate stroke is associated with decreased satisfaction with reintegrating back into community and work activities and increased feelings of depression.

Each of these studies demonstrates the power of occupation in recovery, in management of chronic health conditions, and in fostering health and well-being.

We shared these studies to show how important it is to measure activity participation when determining the impact of a disabling condition on the occupations of those we serve. Occupational therapy uses a client-centered approach to help people gain the skills, achieve the recovery, and design the environments that will support their ability to engage in the everyday occupations that bring meaning to their lives. We believe it is necessary to know what these occupations are, and we believe that the ACS is an important clinical tool that provides this information to the clinician. Rehabilitation is designed to help a person return to his or her prior level of function. The ACS provides a unique tool for occupational therapists to use to document the person's prior level of function and serves as a tool that helps the clinician identify the occupations that can become central to treatment plans and services.

LEARNING SUPPORTS

Learning Through Doing

Title

Identifying the role of occupations and conceptualizing their use in planning treatment.

Purpose

Introduce the student to the occupational interview process and explore how an individual's occupations could be integrated into treatment planning.

Primary Concepts

- Explore the concept of occupation from the perspective of the client.

- Introduction to using a tool. (For the purpose of this assignment, the modified ACS checklist will be used.)

- Explore how the occupational therapist can use an occupational science concept in a clinical application.

Instructions

1. Choose a person to interview (parent, roommate, friend, partner).

2. Use the Modified Activity Checklist in an interview format to determine current and past activities that are important to the person. Ask questions about

meaningfulness and frequency of participation (do they do it as much as they want or less). If they do not do it as much, ask them why (e.g., have they lost interest, have no one to do it with, etc.). Find out what activities are the most important to them.

3. Construct an occupational history of the person: what they do, what they are doing less, what they would like to do more. Just summarize who they are as an occupational being and whether they do things alone or with others.

4. If they were to need occupational therapy, how would you use what you have learned about them to plan treatment? What would be essential activities to address in occupational therapy?

Case Review

Title

Using an activity important to the person as a therapeutic tool.

Purpose

To help students learn to frame interventions using the occupations of choice of the individual.

Primary Concepts

- Explore the concept of occupation to frame treatment planning.
- Introduction to task analysis from an occupational perspective.

Instructions

1. Role play with a classmate using the case study in the chapter as a guide.

2. Pretend that your client said gardening was one of his favorite activities. In addition, you learned that the client grows many vegetables, which he and his wife can and freeze during the summer months to provide food for their table throughout the year.

3. How would you integrate his need to garden into your treatment planning? Ask the client to help you identify all the tasks associated with gardening that could be addressed in the occupational therapy intervention that would allow him to achieve the goal of returning to gardening. Talk about how gardening tasks could be used to achieve better physical, cognitive, and psychosocial performance.

Class Discussion

Title

Importance of using standard assessments in treatment.

Purpose

Ask the student to discuss the benefits of using a valid, reliable instrument in documenting a client's occupations.

Primary Concepts

- Use of valid instruments in occupational therapy assessment.
- Importance of a specific occupational therapy tool.
- Integration of measurement and client-centered information.

Instructions

1. Discuss the type of client information you obtained in the Learning Through Doing (first Learning Support) experience.

2. Why would it be important to get this using a valid standardized instrument?

3. Why is it important to document a client's occupational history in the medical record?

4. How could data collected from the ACS be used to guide practice? Review what you learned from the four studies about the occupational issues of people with AD, PD, aphasia, and stroke.

5. Why do you need to know a person's occupational history? (Discuss what you might learn about a child, a working-age adult, and an older adult that would enhance your occupational therapy practice).

REFERENCES

Baum, C. M. (1995). The contribution of occupation to function in persons with Alzheimer's disease. *Journal of Occupational Science, 2*(2), 59-67. doi:10.1080/14427591.1995.9686396

Baum, C. M., & Edwards, D. F. (1993). Cognitive performance in senile dementia of the Alzheimer's type: The Kitchen Task Assessment. *American Journal of Occupational Therapy, 47*(5), 431-436. doi:10.5014/ajot.47.5.431

Baum, C. M., & Edwards, D. F. (2001). *The Washington University Activity Card Sort.* St. Louis, MO: PenUltima Press.

Baum, C. M., & Edwards, D. F. (2008). Activity Card Sort. (2nd ed.). Bethesda, MD: AOTA Press.

Berg, L. (1988). Clinical dementia rating (CDR). *Psychopharmacology Bulletin, 24*(4), 637-638.

Buchman, A. S., Boyle, P. A., Wilson, R. S., Fleischman, D. A., Leurgans, S., & Bennett, D. A. (2009). Association between late-life social activity and motor decline in older adults. *Archives of Internal Medicine, 169*(12), 1139-1146. doi:10.1001/archinternmed.2009.135

Christiansen, C. (1991). Occupational therapy: Intervention for life performance. In C. Christiansen & C. Baum (Eds.), *Occupational therapy: Overcoming human performance deficits* (pp. 4-43). Thorofare, NJ: SLACK Incorporated.

Christiansen, C. (1999). Defining lives: Occupation as identity: An essay on competence, coherence, and the creation of meaning—The Eleanor Clarke Slagle Lecture. *American Journal of Occupational Therapy, 53*(6), 547-558. doi:10.5014/ajot.53.6.547

Clark, F., Azen, S. P., Zemke, R., Jackson, J., Carlson, M., Mandel, D., . . . Lipson, L. (1997). Occupational therapy for independent-living older adults: A randomized controlled trial. *Journal of American Medical Association, 278,* 1321-1326. doi:10.1001/jama.1997.03550160041036

Conner, L. T., Tucker, F. M., Gotschall, M., Kaufmann, A., & Baum, C. M. (2011). *Activity participation in people with aphasia: The surprising nature of what has been given up.* Manuscript in preparation.

Cruice, M., Worrall, L., Hickson, L., & Murison, R. (2005). Measuring quality of life: Comparing family members' and friends' rating with those of their aphasic partners. *Aphasiology, 19*(2), 111-129.

Csikszentmihalyi, M. (1988). A theoretical model for enjoyment. In M. Csikszentmihalyi (Ed.), *Beyond boredom and anxiety* (pp. 35-54). San Francisco, CA: Jossey-Bass.

Eriksson, G., Kottorp, A., Borg, J., & Tham, K. (2009). Relationship between occupational gaps in everyday life, depressive mood and life satisfaction after acquired brain injury. *Journal of Rehabilitation Medicine, 41,* 187-194. doi:10.2340/16501977-0307

Eriksson, G., Tham, K., & Borg, J. (2006). Occupational gaps in everyday life 1-4 years after acquired brain injury. *Journal of Rehabilitation Medicine, 38*(3), 159-165. doi:10.1080/16501970500415322

Fahn, S., Elton, R. L., Marsden, C. D., Goldstein, M., & Calne, D. B. (1987). Unified Parkinson's disease rating scale. In *Recent developments in Parkinson's disease* (pp. 153-163). New York, NY: Macmillan.

First, M. B., Spitzer, R. L., Gibbon, M., & Williams, J. B. W. (2002). *Structured clinical interview for DSM-IV-TR Axis I Disorders, research version, patient edition (SCID-I/P).* New York, NY: Biometrics Research, New York State Psychiatric Institute.

Folstein, M. F., Folstein, S. E., & McHugh, P. R. (1975). "Mini-mental state." A practical method for grading the cognitive state of patients for the clinician. *Journal of Psychiatry Research, 12*(3), 189-198.

Glass, T. A., de Leon, C. M., Marottoli, R. A., & Berkman, L. F. (1999). Population based study of social and productive activities as predictors of survival among elderly Americans. *British Medical Journal, 319*(7208), 478-483. doi:10.1136/bmj.319.7208.478

Goodglass, H., Kaplan, E., & Barresi, B. (2001). *Boston Diagnostic Aphasia Examination* (3rd ed.). Philadelphia, PA: Lippincott Williams & Wilkins.

Hasselkus, B. R. (1989). The meaning of daily activity in family caregiving for the elderly. *American Journal of Occupational Therapy, 43*(10), 649-656. doi:10.5014/ajot.43.10.649

Hasselkus, B. R. (2002). *The meaning of everyday occupation.* Thorofare, NJ: SLACK Incorporated.

Herzog, A. R., Franks, M. M., Markus, H. R., & Holmberg, D. (1998). Activities and well-being in older age: Effects of self-concept and educational attainment. *Psychology and Aging, 13,* 179-185. doi:10.1037/0882-7974.13

Hoehn, M. M., & Yahr, M. D. (1967). Parkinsonism: Onset, progression and mortality. *Neurology, 17*(5), 427-442.

Hollingshead, A. B., & Redlich, F. C. (1958). *Social class and mental illness: A community study.* New York, NY: John Wiley & Sons.

Horgas, A. L., Wilms, H., & Baltes, M. M. (1998). Daily life in very old age: Everyday activities as expression of successful living. *The Gerontologist, 38,* 556-568. doi:10.1093/geront/38.5.556

Hultsch, D. E., Hertzog, C., Small, B. J., & Dixon, R. A. (1999). Use it or lose it: Engaged lifestyle as a buffer of cognitive decline in old age? *Psychology and Aging, 14*(2), 245-263. doi:10.1037/0882-7974.14.2.245

Jenkinson, C., Fitzpatrick, R., Peto, V., Harris, R., & Saunders, P. (2008). *User Manual for the PDQ-39, PDQ-8 and PDQ Index* (2nd ed.). Oxford, United Kingdom: Health Services Research Unit.

Kielhofner, G. (1992). *Conceptual foundations of occupational therapy.* Philadelphia, PA: F. A. Davis.

Lai, S. M., Studenski, S., Duncan, P. W., & Subashan, P. (2002). Persisting consequences of stroke measured by the Stroke Impact Scale. *Stroke, 33,* 1840-1844.

Law, M. (2002). Participation in the occupations of everyday life. *American Journal of Occupational Therapy, 56,* 640-649. doi:10.1161/01.STR.0000019289.15440.F2

Loehlin, J. C. (1992). *Latent variable models: An introduction to factor, path, and structural analysis* (2nd ed.). Hillsdale, NJ: Erlbaum & Associates.

Meyer, A. (1922). The philosophy of occupational therapy. *Archives of Occupational Therapy, 1,* 1-10.

National Aphasia Association (n.d.). Retrieved from http://www.aphasia.org

National Institute of Neurologic Diseases and Stroke Aphasia Information page (n.d.). Retrieved from http://www.ninds.nih.gov/disorders/aphasia/aphasia.htm

Pfeiffer, E. (1975). A short portable mental status questionnaire for the assessment of organic brain deficit in elderly patients. *Journal of American Geriatric Society, 23,* 433-441.

Radloff, L. S. (1977). A self-report depression scale for research in the general population. *Applied Psychological Measurement, 1,* 385-401.

Tanner, C. M., & Aston, D. A. (2000). Epidemiology of Parkinson's disease and akinetic syndromes. *Current Opinion in Neurology, 13*(4), 427-430.

Tucker, F. M., Edwards, D. F., Mathews, L. K., Baum, C. M., & Connor, L. T. (2012). Modifying health outcome measures for people with aphasia. *American Journal of Occupational Therapy, 66,* 42-50.

U.S. Census Bureau. (2007). *American community survey.* Retrieved from http://www.census.gov/acs/www/index.html

Wang, H. X., Karp, A., Winblad, B., & Fratiglioni, L. (2002). Late-life engagement in social and leisure activities is associated with a decreased risk of dementia: A longitudinal study from the Kungsholmen project. *American Journal of Epidemiology, 155*(12), 1081-1087. doi:10.1093/aje/155.12.1081

Ware, J. E., Jr., & Sherbourne, C. D. (1992). The MOS 36-item short-form health survey (SF-36). I. Conceptual framework and item selection. *Medical Care, 30*(6), 473-483.

Ware, J. E., Snow, K. K., Kosinski, M., & Gandek, B. (1988). *SF-36 health survey manual and interpretation guide.* Boston, MA: The Health Institute.

Wilcock, A. (1993). A theory of the human need for occupation. *Journal of Occupational Science, 1*(1), 17-24. doi:10.1080/14427591.1993.9686375

Wilcock, A. (2001). *Occupation for health: Vol. 1. A journey from self health to prescription.* Southwark, London, England: British Association and College of Occupational Therapists.

Wolf, T., Conner, L., & Baum, C. (2009). Changing face of stroke: Implications for occupational therapy practice. *American Journal of Occupational Therapy, 63*(5), 621-625. doi:10.5014/ajot.63.5.621

Wood-Dauphinée, S. L., Opzoomer, M. A., Williams, J. I., Marchand, B., & Spitzer, W. O. (1988). Assessment of global function: The reintegration to normal living index. *Archives of Physical Medicine and Rehabilitation, 69,* 583-590.

Yerxa, E. (1998). Health and the human spirit for occupation. *American Journal of Occupational Therapy, 52*(6), 412-418. doi:10.5014/ajot.52.6.412

Zarit, S. H., Reever, K. E., & Bach-Peterson, J. (1980). Relatives of the impaired elderly, correlates of feeling of burden. *The Gerontologist, 20*(6), 649-655. doi:10.1093/geront/20.6.649

Zarit, S. H., Todd, P. A., & Zarit, J. M. (1986). Subjective burden of husbands and wives as caregivers: A longitudinal study. *The Gerontologist, 26*(3), 260-266. doi:10.1093/geront/26.3.260

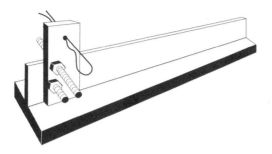

Living With HIV Infection
Insights Into Occupational Markers of Health and Occupational Adaptation

Matthew Molineux, BOccThy, MSc, PhD; Jenny Strong, BOccThy, MOccThy, PhD; and Wendy Rickard, PhD

Occupational therapy was founded on the belief that there was a link between occupational engagement and health. Although there is a growing evidence base to support that belief, more research is required to understand the complex relationship between occupation and health. This was one reason that we undertook the research reported in this chapter. It is clear in the literature, and from our clinical and research experiences, that living with a chronic and/or life-threatening illness provides an opportunity for examining how individuals respond to illness. This research provided us with an opportunity to bring both of these together in an exploration of the occupational experience of living with human immuno-deficiency virus (HIV) infection. For us, conducting this research was fascinating. It was also difficult at times, due to the challenges some participants had faced. Using a narrative approach resulted in a particularly deep and broad understanding of each man's life. Ultimately, this research provided useful insights into living with HIV and how this can be understood from an occupational perspective.

LITERATURE

HIV/AIDS and Occupational Therapy

In 1993, Yerxa warned that "chronic illness, disability, [and] the preservation of health" would be some of the greatest challenges of the 21st century (p. 3). This is attributable to advancements in science, technology, and medicine that result in people living longer and with ongoing health difficulties. HIV infection and acquired immune deficiency syndrome (AIDS) are examples of these changes. HIV was first discovered in the mid 1980s. At that time, infection generally led rapidly to poor health and ultimately death. Today, drug treatments have transformed HIV infection into a chronic, albeit potentially life-threatening, condition (Mitchell & Linsk, 2004). Despite medical advances, there are approximately 83,000 people living with HIV infection in the United Kingdom (Health Protection Agency, 2009) and approximately 580,371 people known to be infected in the United States in 2007 (This figure is only for the 33 states and dependent areas that

Pierce, D. (Ed.).
Occupational Science for Occupational Therapy (pp. 121-132).
© 2014 SLACK Incorporated.

have had confidential name-based reporting for a period of time, although all states and areas have now implemented confidential name-based reporting.) (Centers for Disease Control and Prevention, 2010). The result is a significant number of people living with a chronic and life-threatening condition.

Occupational therapists have been involved in providing services for people living with and affected by HIV infection for some time. It is notable that the occupational therapy literature generally takes one of three foci. One subset of published material focuses on legal, ethical, and moral issues and as such follows in the vein of Giles and Allen (1987). The second subset continues Denton's (1987) path of outlining the type of services occupational therapists might offer people living with HIV infection. This group of papers, which is in the majority, generally concentrates on occupational performance components, describing interventions that address symptoms such as fatigue and anxiety. In both of these groups of literature, the perspective adopted by occupational therapy authors is largely biomedical. In the medical paradigm, the presence and progression of HIV infection are labeled using biomedical markers, such as viral load and CD4 counts, and the mainstay of treatment is drugs that aim to reduce viral load and increase CD4 counts. As a result, the stages of HIV disease have been labeled as HIV positive but asymptomatic, HIV positive and symptomatic, and AIDS, and these have been adopted by occupational therapists (see for example Denton, 1987; Molineux, 1997).

Adopting a biomedical perspective in considering the experiences of people living with HIV infection is interesting for several reasons. First, HIV infection has for some time now been viewed as a chronic illness (Albert et al., 1994; Erlen, Mellors, Sereika, & Cook, 2001; Volberding, 2003), and a biomedical focus is not particularly well suited to understanding the complexities of a chronic illness with multifaceted determinants (Wade & Halligan, 2004). Second, it has been suggested that the profession of occupational therapy should focus its attention on people with chronic illness (Kidner, 1930; Yerxa, 2000). Despite the narrow focus of much of the occupational therapy literature on people with HIV/AIDS, there are some papers that do contribute to an occupational understanding of living with HIV infection (for example Bedell, 1998, 2000; Braveman & Helfrich, 2001; Pizzi, 1990; Yallop, 1999, 2004). Pizzi (1990) probably wrote the first such paper, arguing that occupational therapists must think beyond self-care occupations, and this challenge has been taken up by some practitioners and researchers. For example, the Positive Employment Service in Sydney, Australia, is an example of an occupational therapy intervention program that adopts an occupational perspective (Yallop, 1999, 2004).

Bedell (1998, 2000) explored the daily life of eight gay men living with HIV/AIDS in New York City. Bedell found that the daily lives of his participants were shaped by three themes: a reasonably stable base, finding and maintaining balance, and living by a tentative plan. The first theme, a reasonably stable base, recognized that all of the participants had either maintained or developed firm supports and resources, which comprised emotional, physical, and environmental aspects. The second theme encompassed "the act of orchestrating or developing strategies to manage daily and weekly activities, as well as the resultant experience of being able to perform one's necessary and desired activities without, with, or in spite of symptoms" (Bedell, 2000, p. 201). The third theme, living by a tentative plan, recognized that changes in participants' health required them to make changes to their occupations.

Other research within occupational therapy has sought to understand the experience of living with HIV infection using narrative methods. Braveman and Helfrich (2001) explored the concept of occupational identity of men living with HIV infection who participated in a vocational rehabilitation program. This research demonstrated that one way of understanding the varied experiences of living with HIV infection is to consider the entire life history of the individual. For example, HIV/AIDS did not come to the foreground of one participant's narrative. Instead, it was "woven within his life narrative with the many other positive and negative events that he colourfully described" (Braveman & Helfrich, 2001, p. 28).

The reasons for this small number of occupationally focused papers are likely to be numerous and might include the continuing paradigm quandary the occupational therapy profession has found itself in since the 1970s (Kielhofner, 2004). It is also likely that the changes in the ways in which society perceives HIV have impacted occupational therapy. For example, HIV is now less visible in traditional health and social care settings than it was earlier in the history of the condition. While these are largely valid reasons, the limited research into the occupational nature of living with HIV infection, and how this has changed over time, is surprising given the resurgence of interest in occupation. The research reported in this chapter aimed to contribute to the small body of literature within occupational therapy and occupational science, which brings occupation in chronic illness into sharp focus.

Occupational Adaptation

In order to better understand the occupational nature of living with HIV infection, it is necessary to conceptualize humans as occupational beings who live their lives through engaging in occupations. Furthermore, in seeking to understand humans as occupational beings, it is necessary to explore the temporal or ontogenetic perspective of occupational engagement. One construct that has been used within occupational therapy to link past, present, and future occupational engagement is occupational adaptation.

Occupational adaptation is an individualized process of change that enables humans to respond to the many challenges faced throughout life (Larson, 1996; Schkade & McClung, 2001). Occupational adaptation is usually viewed as a process that results in a positive outcome. For example, Llorens (1990, p. xi) suggested that occupational adaptation is the "functional adjustment of humans to environmental demands for productive performance." More specifically, adaptation through occupation occurs when an individual is able to perform the range of necessary occupations in order "to meet the physical, biopsychological and sociocultural environmental demands" (Reed, 1983, p. 495) and to perform those occupations in a way that is balanced and satisfying to the individual. It is a state of competence in occupational performance to which humans aspire, but also a dialectic between the individual and his or her environment and so can also be viewed as a process whereby humans respond occupationally to the challenges posed by the environment (Schkade & McClung, 2001; Schkade & Schultz, 1992; Spencer, Davidson, & White, 1996).

Kielhofner and colleagues (Kielhofner, 2002; Kielhofner, Mallinson, Forsyth, & Lai, 2001; Mallinson, Mahaffey, & Kielhofner, 1998) have also explored occupational adaptation, which they suggest is the "extent to which persons are able to develop, change in response to challenges, or otherwise achieve a state of well-being through what they do" (Kielhofner, 2002, p. 119). While this definition shares much in common with those discussed in the preceding paragraphs, Kielhofner and colleagues have explicated what they see as the components of occupational adaptation. This group has suggested that occupational adaptation comprises occupational identity and occupational competence (Kielhofner et al., 2001; Mallinson et al., 1998). Occupational identity is "a composite sense of who one is and wishes to become as an occupational being" (Kielhofner, 2002, p. 119) as influenced by the many experiences of occupational engagement throughout life. Occupational competence is "the degree to which one sustains a pattern of occupational participation that reflects one's identity" (Kielhofner, 2002, p. 120). Occupational adaptation, therefore, is "the construction of a positive occupational identity and achieving occupational competence over time in the context of one's environment" (Kielhofner, 2002, p. 121). Similar to the previously outlined perspectives on occupational adaptation, Kielhofner and colleagues view it as forming as a result of each individual participating in the array of occupations that makes up his or her life. For the purpose of this chapter, occupational adaptation is viewed as the ability to respond to environmental challenges through occupation, thereby maintaining health and well-being.

Because occupational adaptation is an ongoing process, Larson (1996) has argued that when considering the success, or otherwise, of occupational adaptation, it may be inappropriate to make judgments based on the short-term outcome and that a lifespan approach is imperative. Occupational adaptation must be judged in relation to how actions and decisions contribute "to the achievement of desired life goals within a temporal stream" (Larson, 1996, p. 297). By adopting occupational adaptation as the theoretical framework for understanding the experiences of individuals, it is possible to discern the theme of an individual's life. Such an approach portrays individuals' lives as "moving along a trajectory with a temporal horizon that integrates the past, present, and future" (Larson, 1996, p. 297).

METHODS

The purpose of this study was to explore the experiences of five men living with HIV infection in the United Kingdom. In particular, the study aimed to examine the trajectory of HIV infection from an occupational perspective, including understanding HIV infection in the context of the participants' lives. Given the constraints of chapter length, this chapter focuses on just one participant in the larger study.

This research sits within the qualitative paradigm and, more specifically, is an example of what Clark (1993) labeled interpretive occupational science, which is informed by a range of approaches such as life history ethnography, ethnomethodology, narrative analysis, and other naturalistic approaches. The strength of interpretive occupational science is that it provides thick descriptions that can capture an individual's occupational nature and experiences with all their richness (Clark, 1993). Using narrative/biographical research methods to understand humans as occupational beings is appropriate because occupational therapy practice requires the therapist to understand and work within the client's life story (Mattingly & Fleming, 1994). Furthermore, narrative/biographical methods connect with the philosophy of occupational therapy at a very rudimentary level (Duchek & Thessing, 1996; Larson & Fanchiang, 1996). The ability of these methods to fully contextualize life experiences has been recognized by occupational therapists given their need to understand occupational engagement as a situated phenomenon (Clark, 1993; Duchek & Thessing, 1996).

Participants

Five men participated in the larger study, and they all found out about the project through one of several avenues: personal networks, advertisements in the local and national HIV/AIDS and gay press, and letters to HIV/AIDS support groups and centers. The selection criterion was simply that each man had to be a good informant (Morse, 1994). Informed written consent was obtained from each participant prior to commencing his oral history interviews. To this end, each man was provided with a project information sheet and an opportunity to clarify any concerns he had before signing a consent form. Ethical approval for this study was given by the relevant university ethical review committee.

The findings presented in this paper are based on the analysis of data from all five men, but data from one participant, Fred, will be used to illustrate the findings. Fred found out about the research through an HIV organization in the city in northern England where he lived. Fred was 50 years of age when his oral history was recorded, and he had been diagnosed HIV positive for approximately 3 years. Fred was slightly less than 6 feet tall, with a slim build and receding dark grey hair. Fred was unemployed at the time of the interviews but had worked as a betting shop manager and a production line supervisor at a car manufacturing factory. (All names in this chapter are pseudonyms to protect the anonymity of the participant and others.)

Data Collection and Analysis

Extended oral history interviews were conducted (see Molineux & Rickard, 2003, for more detail), drawing on an interview guide previously developed for the British Library HIV/AIDS Testimonies Project. The guide was adapted to include probes and follow-up questions about occupation. The interviews covered the entire life of the participants from birth until the time of the final interview and included sections about the participant's grandparents, parents, and every stage of their life. The interview guide was piloted with a researcher familiar with narrative research. He provided verbal feedback, and the audio recording was reviewed and discussed by all authors. No significant changes were made to the interview schedule after the pilot, but it was useful in refining interview technique. After the pilot interview, the main interviews began.

The interviews were led by the participants, but were essentially co-constructions with the interviewer initiating the project, as well as prompting and guiding the interview. The number and frequency of interview sessions with each man varied and was determined by how long he was able to speak in one session and the length of the story he wished to tell. After four sessions at his home in as many months, Fred had completed 15.5 hours of recorded interview. Between each interview, the interviewer listened to the tapes of the previous session in order to re-engage with the material and ensure continuity of the oral history.

From the outset, it was acknowledged that, due to the subject of the research, it was possible that participants might become upset and distressed during the interviews. For this reason, it was vital to recognize that "interviews are interventions. They affect people" (Patton, 1990, p. 353). As such, it is possible that they can be affirming and/or distressing (Rickard, 1998). The interviewer informally assessed participants' behaviors during the entire inquiry to determine whether or not intervention was necessary (Kavanaugh & Ayres, 1998). Although

the interviews touched on sensitive topics, there was no evidence that they caused the participants undue distress. Not only did this research have the potential to be distressing for the men who told their stories, but given the first author's intense involvement with each man, there was a risk of the researcher being upset and distressed from hearing the stories (Lee, 1993). Measures were taken, however, to ensure sufficient formal and informal support was available: use of a research journal, discussions with supervisors, and informal support from friends, colleagues, and partner.

Each completed oral history was transcribed verbatim. The aim of the transcription process was to record as accurately as possible the content of the interviews, in a way that made the transcripts easily readable. Because the analysis relied primarily on the recorded tapes, there was no real need to document the nonverbal aspects of the interview situation. This approach was consistent with Portelli's (1981/1991) assertion that the actual "document" under consideration is the recorded interview on the tape.

The process of narrative analysis developed for this research was influenced by Clark (1993) in that the aim was to produce stories that were not only compelling, but also stories that made the occupational nature of the participants explicit. Our view of the narratives was also shaped by the work of authors such as Sacks (1985) and Frank (2000) who have presented stories that effectively incorporate both academic and personal perspectives. The analysis included six stages (Molineux & Rickard, 2003): define the boundaries of the story, order the events chronologically, establish the plot of the story to be told, determine what events and happenings are relevant to the story, write the narrative, and contextualize the narrative.

Trustworthiness

The methods employed in this research to ensure trustworthiness included providing a thick description of the research process and decisions made throughout (Creswell, 1997). The nature of the data collection allowed for prolonged exposure to the field/participants (Creswell, 1997; Jackson, 2000), and this also provided an opportunity for some member checking with the participants.

Analyst triangulation was used, drawing on existing models (Barnard, Towers, Boston, & Lambrinidou, 2000; Bedell, 1998, 2000; Creswell, 1997). This involved a formal review process of the initial analysis by an external expert reviewer. The aim was not to check that the analysis was correct, rather that it was cogent, persuasive, and grounded in the raw data (Angen, 2000). The conditions of the review process were respecting confidentiality, following a process similar to the initial analysis, and blinding to the produced narrative. The expert reviewer was asked to read the full oral history transcript of each man, consider key questions about plot, read the narrative, and answer questions about its cogency and relationship to the raw data. The written responses to the questions and general feedback provided were used to enrich the narratives. Instructions of each participant were sought and respected individually in this formal process.

RESULTS

This section will present the interpretation of Fred's story, highlighting the occupational aspects of the narrative, rather than presenting the full narrative and an interpretation. By making this distinction between the narrative and the interpretive discussion of the narrative, readers are reminded that the results of this research take multiple forms: the narratives, the interpretation of each narrative, and the final discussion in this chapter. Although only Fred's narrative is discussed in this section, the stories of all the participants informed the analysis process.

Fred's narrative comprised three phases. The first phase, labeled "developing an occupational identity," spans Fred's life up until the time he was diagnosed as being HIV positive. During this period, Fred was negotiating the challenges of his life with success and established himself as a skilled and effective occupational being. These experiences of occupational competence influenced the development of a positive occupational identity and allowed Fred to achieve and maintain occupational adaptation. The second phase, a period of "occupational rupture," began when Fred found out that he might be HIV positive and continued until he began seeing a psychiatrist for depression. This captures the way in which the impact of finding out he was HIV positive tore Fred apart from his previous way of life. Although Fred had dealt with some significant challenges in his life, his HIV diagnosis and what it meant for his family was so far outside his realm of experience that its impact was devastating and had significant negative occupational implications. The third phase of "occupational repair" was the stage Fred was negotiating at the time of the last interview. It was during this stage that Fred had begun to restore his occupational identity by resuming familiar occupations and contemplating new ones. Each of these three phases in Fred's life will be explored in greater depth to demonstrate the occupational plot of his life.

Developing an Occupational Identity

Fred's childhood was characterized by contradictions. On one hand, the family lived in a well-appointed house and had many happy times together. On the other hand, Fred remembers not eating well because the household money was being spent on the purchase of the furniture. Also, the family motto of "children should be seen and not heard" often meant that Fred and his siblings felt the force of their father's temper; "there were many times when my mother actually used to drag my dad off me because she thought he was going to kill me." Despite these challenging circumstances, Fred saw his childhood as a happy one. The key to this overall positive assessment of his childhood may be attributed to the influence of Fred's paternal grandparents. Many of the childhood occupations that stand out in Fred's memory were linked to his grandparents: attending the Saturday matinee with his brother, meals on the weekend, going to the shop for ice creams, and various fun occupations on family holidays. As a young boy, Fred did not enjoy the academic aspect of school, but it was at school that he became a runner and developed a role he valued greatly. It was also at school that Fred first became interested in fishing and he often missed school so that he could spend the day at the canal. During his early years, Fred participated in many of the usual occupations of childhood and did so with success, thereby sowing the seeds of a positive occupational identity. Given that the situation in which he grew up was at times challenging, it is likely that Fred's occupational identity was further enhanced because he not only mastered various occupations but did so despite potential threats to his success.

When Fred was 16 years of age, he left school and began working with his father. This was a positive milestone for Fred. He was finally out of school. He enjoyed work and fulfilled his duties effectively. Of particular influence was that, from the time he started working, Fred's relationship with his father improved greatly. "It was different at work. We could do anything together. We could talk together. We could say anything we wanted." The change in their relationship was strictly confined to the workplace, and they hardly spoke when at home together, although there was some carryover to home as his father was no longer violent toward Fred once he started work. This dramatic change in Fred's relationship with his father must have been confusing, but it seems that Fred interpreted it as another example of how he was able to meet the challenges he faced and master the occupations associated with being a teenage son and his father's work colleague.

It was not long, however, until Fred's security in his new roles was jeopardized when his mother asked him to leave the family home at 18 years of age for not contributing financially to the household. Once again, Fred's paternal grandparents stepped in, and it was at this time that Fred suggests his "life started." During this period of Fred's life, with the safety and support of his grandparents, Fred's participation in occupations flourished. In his new family unit, Fred was exposed to new occupations, such as gardening with his grandfather and gambling with his grandmother. As part of his peer network, Fred participated in a range of occupations, such as ice skating, nightclubbing, going to the movies, and 10-pin bowling. Through these occupations, Fred not only developed new interests, some of which continued throughout his life, but he also experienced himself as a valued and competent member of different social networks—his new family with his grandparents and his group of friends.

During his adult life, Fred continued to face many challenges to which he was able to respond positively. He, thus, continued to develop a sense of himself as a competent individual. One aspect of his adult life demonstrates this pattern of challenge followed by mastery, namely paid employment. Initially, Fred worked in the wood machining industry. The opportunity to become a betting shop manager provided Fred with the chance to incorporate his long-standing interest in horses and gambling, instilled in him by his grandmother, into his work. Although this was quite a change from the type of work with which he was familiar, Fred coped well with the training and probation period and soon became a respected shop manager. He experienced a potential threat to his occupational identity when he was passed over for promotion but soon found himself working in another large city in the south of England and eventually being recognized as a skilled and reliable manager. After leaving the city in the south and returning to the north of England, Fred's employment history was quite varied, but he always found work and was successful in his chosen positions, which have included jobs as diverse as wood machining, production line worker at a car manufacturing plant, and a construction worker/scaffolder.

The final aspect of Fred's life, which played a role in the development of his occupational identity, are his leisure occupations. Since he was a young boy, Fred had been active in his social networks and engaged in a range of leisure occupations. Although the exact occupations have changed according to his age and life stage, some leisure pursuits have been a constant part of his life. Running first appears in Fred's narrative when he was a child at school and was one of the few fond memories he had of being at school. He has continued to run as an adult, and it has played a significant part of his life. The other leisure pursuit in which Fred had a lifelong interest is fishing. He started as a child and remembers skipping school to spend the day fishing. Fishing is particularly interesting, as the enjoyment and meaning of it have changed over time for Fred. Initially, Fred attributed the attraction to fishing to simply a fascination with the water and fish. As he grew older, however, his interest changed, and the challenge of competition angling became enjoyable and satisfying.

Occupational Rupture and Repair

Finding out that he was HIV positive marked a period of immense disruption in Fred's life. It is conceived here as a period of rupture because his diagnosis disconnected Fred, in a fundamental way, from his previous life. So profound was this rupture that Fred was not able to verbalize his experience during the interviews: "It was unreal, my whole world was unreal... I can't describe it to you." Examination of Fred's narrative during this period illustrates that his rupture had occupational manifestations. First, Fred and

his partner Julia separated due to ongoing tensions in their relationship, and Fred moved back to his hometown in the north of England without Julia and his daughters. The physical distance between Fred and his daughters made enacting the occupations associated with being a father difficult for Fred, and this was compounded by Julia initially restricting Fred's access to his daughters. Given Fred's devotion to his children and his commitment to being a father, this has been the most difficult occupational change for Fred.

> I mean she's [Julia] ruined my life. As far as I'm concerned, she's ruined my relationship with my children, even if I do be able to carry on seeing them if you know what I mean, because we are still alienated. You know if you don't see your children for a month at a time, you're alienated from them. That's how I feel. So many things I miss, so many things I miss about them, them coming in and talking to me and telling me they love me, me tucking them in bed at night, all these things that I've missed, I'm missing now.

The second occupational change for Fred was that, in order to move back to his hometown, he took leave from his job at the car manufacturing plant and so was unemployed, a situation that was unfamiliar to him. He also participated less and less in his leisure occupations, so in many ways his life seemed empty. It was not long before these occupational changes impacted Fred's health, and he became depressed, turned to alcohol and sleeping tablets, and generally withdrew. It was not until after Fred contemplated and made some preparations to take his own life that an end to his period of occupational rupture became visible. After a visit from his social worker, Fred was referred to a psychiatrist. With support, he began to reconstruct his life and repair his occupational identity.

After sessions with his psychiatrist and a course of medication for his mental health, Fred was able to return to his previous round of occupations and thereby reconstruct this life and sense of self. Interestingly, the two occupations that figure prominently in Fred's period of occupational repair are two lifelong leisure pursuits rooted in his childhood: running and fishing. Just as these occupations had contributed to the development of Fred's positive occupational identity in the past, they were central in the process of reconstructing his occupational identity. Returning to running had immediate benefits for Fred: "I was having that feeling of euphoria when I came back from me runs and that feeling was continuing." Running also resonated with the image he had constructed of himself throughout his life but lost sight of during the period shortly after being diagnosed HIV positive. Since that time, running and maintaining his health and fitness have taken on new meaning in the context of HIV drug treatments. Returning to the valued occupation of fishing was another useful step in his process of repair. He first returned to fishing by himself at the local canal but it was there that he met Gary, with whom he became good friends. As a result, Fred joined an angling club and began to compete once again. This experience of fishing was beneficial for Fred on two levels. First, he has been able to re-engage with his former occupational identity and experience success and competence. Second, it also opened up new social networks that Fred can use for support as he continues his process of occupational repair.

At the time of the last interview, Fred was still engaged in the work needed to reconstruct his occupational identity. Unfortunately, he was still estranged from his two daughters, although he did have some contact with them, and this was a continuing source of concern for him. Furthermore, he remained unemployed and was beginning to feel the financial pressure as his savings dwindled. Fred had also realized that he wanted to return to work, given the routine and social identity associated with employment. While he could not see this happening immediately, he was considering an interim step of some voluntary work. Fred's process of occupational repair was, at the time of the last interview, still unfolding. While he felt he had made good progress, with real benefits, in terms of his leisure occupations, he was yet to return to all the occupations that were important to him.

CONTRIBUTION TO OCCUPATIONAL SCIENCE

The narrative analysis of Fred's oral history interview demonstrates how it is possible to view living with HIV from an occupational perspective, rather than that of the dominant biomedical paradigm. Furthermore, Fred's narrative shows how it can be useful to contextualize responses to, and experiences of, HIV infection within an individual's entire life. While both of these are useful simply by providing an alternative view of living with HIV infection, they also have implications for occupational therapy practice.

Occupational Markers of Living With HIV Infection

Using a perspective that examined occupational turning points, akin to the turnings described by Mandelbaum (1973) as major changes that circumscribe periods of a person's life, this study found that each man's life was structured around turning points that were occupational in nature and did not always correlate with medical markers. Fred's narrative provides clear examples in relation to his lifelong occupations of running, paid work, and fishing.

Fred's narrative records that it was at school that he first discovered he was a good runner and that he enjoyed long distance running. It was as a child that Fred also began fishing, often when skipping school. As an adult, he continued to fish and became a keen competition angler as a member of local teams. Fred first worked after leaving school when

he was 16 years old and continued to work until his HIV diagnosis. Fred took great pride in working hard and supporting his family. All these occupations came to the foreground at different times. In so doing, they demonstrate how they were potent markers of Fred's health and well-being. By exploring individual occupations in this way, it is possible to examine the careers of individual occupations (Russel, 2001).

The first re-emergence of running was when Fred and Julia were a couple, and she had developed a persistent cough. Fred noticed that he was not running as well as he usually did: his times were not as good, and he was eventually unable to complete his usual routes without walking. Fred's difficulty in completing a lifelong occupation meant, in his eyes at least, that there was something wrong with his health. More than that, however, Fred's inability to run threatened his sense of self because running was one of the key occupations that defined his identity (Christiansen, 1999). His changed occupational performance prompted Fred to speak to Julia, and as a result he eventually found out that she was HIV positive and so was he. This provides an example of the link between occupation and health. For Fred, his health, or lack thereof, was manifested in occupation. His suspicion about his health status was not triggered directly by an awareness of the reduced integrity of a body system, but by his difficulty in a particular occupation.

Another occupational marker, this one after diagnosis, was when Fred resigned from his job at the car manufacturing plant. Given the prominence of employment in Fred's narrative, the loss of this occupation was another significant event, and Fred recognized that he found himself in a very strange place psychologically. After resigning, Fred became further alienated from his usual occupations. He was not working, fishing, or running and was essentially doing "absolutely nothing at all." This period of Fred's occupational career provides a stark example of how HIV disrupted his everyday life, which is a common impact of illness (Kylma, Vehvilainen-Julkunen, & Lahdevirta, 2001; Rabkin, Remien, Katoff, & Williams, 1993; Sandstrom, 1990). Fred also began to engage in atypical occupations, such as drinking to excess and smoking marijuana. By engaging in this destructive behavior, he became even further removed from his secure and familiar ways of being. During this time following diagnosis, Fred would have been considered, from a medical perspective at least, HIV positive and asymptomatic. He would not have been expected to require much intervention, and yet he was at risk. This example provides a powerful illustration of the misalignment of the medical perspective of health and Fred's own occupational perspective.

The medical view of Fred at that time was that he was asymptomatic; he had no signs or symptoms of HIV infection. Fred's own, more occupational, perspective was very different. He no longer participated in most of the occupations that had filled his life, and he began to participate in occupations that were inconsistent with his view of himself. The result was a period of isolation when he experienced occupational disruption, occupational deprivation, and occupational alienation. Fred's response in this situation is consistent with other research, which has highlighted the way in which both the social and spatial worlds of people with chronic illness shrink (Charmaz, 1983). Fred's changed pattern of occupational engagement is also similar to that found in previous studies of men living with HIV infection (Albert et al., 1994; Takahashi, Wiebe, & Rodriguez, 2001). Given these alterations to Fred's occupations, it is no surprise that his health declined, as such changes are associated with an increase in stress, physiological changes, and a general reduction in health (Law, Steinwender, & Leclair, 1998). From an occupational perspective, he was not able to achieve or maintain a state of health and well-being. Although Fred was between two medical markers of HIV progression, of greater significance to him were the occupational markers of his reduced health status.

Conversely, Fred's narrative also documents how his lifelong occupations, particularly fishing and running, contributed to improvements in his health. The first instance was after he received support from the psychiatrist. At that time, Fred made a conscious effort to re-engage with his life. This re-engagement included resuming his familiar occupation of regular runs. He also returned to fishing at the local canal. Through engaging in his long-valued occupations of fishing and running, Fred was able to manage his occupational engagement so that he could mark and maintain his improved health and well-being. He was able to reinforce his occupational identity as a competent individual who could accomplish personal goals (Jackson, 1998; Laliberte Rudman, 2002; Magnus, 2001; Rebeiro, Day, Semeniuk, O'Brien, & Wilson, 2001; Unruh, Smith, & Scammell, 1999; Vrkljan & Miller-Polgar, 2001). Fishing in particular enabled Fred to address the isolation he experienced by reasserting his membership in valued social groups, namely anglers (Laliberte Rudman, Cook, & Polatajko, 1997; Rebeiro et al., 2001; Unruh et al., 1999). In doing so, Fred was able to use occupation to cope with his infection, in ways similar to participants in other studies. For Fred, the occupations were running and fishing. For the women in Unruh and colleagues' (1999) study, the occupation of choice was gardening, and for John Allen it was being a library volunteer (Rebeiro & Allen, 1998). Eventually, Fred joined a local fishing club and began to compete again. These occupations were not just coping mechanisms, however, but also the means by which Fred was able to improve his health (Barroso & Powell-Cope, 2000; Gaskins & Brown, 1997; Katz, 1996; Leenerts & Magilvy, 2000) and regain some control and mastery over his life (Bury, 1991; Taylor, 1983). For example, Fred used running to prepare for his second combination-therapy regimen. He went on holiday to Spain and ran regularly as well as spent time relaxing. Fred clearly articulated the ben-

efits of running at that time: "Well, it had seemed so long before I'd actually felt that way.... I was having that feeling of euphoria when I came back from me runs and that feeling was continuing."

A Contextualized Response to HIV Infection: Occupational Adaptation

Occupational adaptation is the ability to respond to challenges through occupation, in such a way as to achieve and maintain health and well-being (Larson, 1996; Llorens, 1990; Reed, 1983; Schkade & McClung, 2001). It is seen both as a state achieved and the process undertaken to achieve that state (Schkade & McClung, 2001; Schkade & Schultz, 1992; Spencer et al., 1996). Given that occupational adaptation is a lifelong process, it can be seen as a strand of continuity throughout people's lives. Indeed, in this study, the plot of each man's narrative revolved around occupational adaptation. For Fred's narrative, the plot was one of rupture and repair. By taking an occupational perspective, Fred's narrative captured the different ways he responded through occupation to the challenges he faced. Furthermore, his narrative shows how his occupational adaptation was shaped by opportunities for occupational engagement and the experience of varying degrees of occupational competence.

Fred's narrative records his multiple opportunities to respond occupationally to challenges. The challenges he faced included, for example, a violent family house as a child, frequently changing schools, being asked to leave home when he was 18 years old, being unemployed, and a complex relationship with his father. To all of these challenges, Fred was able to mount an adaptive response and so developed a positive occupational identity. At times, however, Fred struggled to respond adaptively, for example, in being a husband to his first wife, Suzanne, and father to his first daughter, Simone. In the short-term, Fred's dissatisfaction with his inability to achieve competence as a husband and father resulted in him leaving Suzanne and Simone on two occasions. Fred's response in these situations provides an interesting example of how occupational adaptation may not necessarily result from successful occupational engagement.

The literature on occupation tends to focus on individuals and/or groups engaging in occupation. That is, attention is generally focused on the level of the occupation. Restricting interpretation of the narratives to that level would not capture the way that Fred made an occupational response to the situation outlined in the preceding paragraph. Although not often acknowledged in the literature, it is important to recognize that humans not only engage in occupations, but they also manage or orchestrate that engagement (Yerxa et al., 1989). While he may not have achieved competence in fathering occupations at that time, by withdrawing from the situation, Fred modified the environmental demands and so greatly reduced the expectations he had of himself and others had of him. This illustrates the way in which occupations are contextualized and how individuals are not only influenced by their environments but can also alter their environments. It could be suggested then that Fred's response was not adaptive—it did not enable him to face the challenge in a way that was personally satisfying nor was it consistent with social norms (Reed, 1983). However, Reed's classification of adaptive, maladaptive, and nonadaptive responses centers on the actual occupation. The broader view suggested here, which is one of managing occupational engagement, shows that Fred's response permitted him to experience competence, not in individual occupations, but in the overall orchestration of his personal configuration of occupations.

Up until the time of Fred's HIV diagnosis, he developed a positive occupational identity through individual occupations or through managing his configuration of occupations. For Fred, HIV diagnosis marked a point of rupture. Diagnosis disconnected Fred, in a fundamental way, from his previous life. It would appear that the social and cultural contexts in which Fred had existed meant that the way Julia placed him at risk of contracting HIV, and indeed HIV infection itself, were completely beyond his realm of actual or possible experience. As such, finding out that he was HIV positive and that he was likely to have been infected by his partner wrenched Fred from his familiar world so dramatically that his existing adaptive strategies were rendered temporarily inadequate.

The preceding paragraphs demonstrate that the extent of perceived success experienced by an individual in responding to life's challenges will influence that person's occupational identity (Christiansen, 1999). However, Fred's narrative does not endorse the clear-cut picture of life intimated by Kielhofner and colleagues (2002). Further, the narratives do not demonstrate the linearity of the narrative slopes drawn by Braveman and Helfrich (2001). Using previously developed typologies to understand the narratives of men such as Fred is unlikely to capture the ever-changing and occupational nature of human life. Up until the time of his HIV diagnosis, the overall tone is generally positive. To use the narrative types of Gergen and Gergen (1986), Fred's narrative could be labeled as progressive. He was moving forward in fulfilling his valued roles of partner, father, and worker. However, in reading his narrative, it becomes clear that achieving those roles did not come easily for Fred. He had to contend with being rejected by his parents, a robbery and assault in London, a volatile relationship with Julia, and a brain hemorrhage. Labeling Fred's narrative as progressive would be accurate only up to the time of his HIV diagnosis. This highlights how occupational adaptation is an ongoing process. It is important to refrain from evaluating an individual's occupational adaptation based on a single instance that is not fully contextualized in the

individual's personal history. As Larson (1996) argued, short-term outcomes are not accurate indicators of occupational adaptation. In fact, it is possible that occupational adaptation can only be understood retrospectively.

IMPLICATIONS FOR PRACTICE

Although this research did not set out to investigate a practice issue per se, it contributes to the "generative discourse on occupation-based practice" (Pierce, 2003, p. 1). Acknowledging the difference between occupational and biomedical perspectives provides critical reflection on a dilemma inherent in much occupational therapy practice: between treating "the whole person and being credible within a medical world that pushes the therapist to redefine problems and treatment goals in biomedical terms" (Mattingly & Fleming, 1994, p. 296). In doing so, it contributes to discussions about returning to practice based on occupation. A return to paradigm-dependent practice will manifest in occupational therapists who are ever mindful of "where they come from," of their philosophical perspective, and who always "start where they mean to finish," engaging in therapy with an occupational goal in mind (Molineux, 2004, p. 7). Maintaining an occupational focus requires consideration at all stages of the occupational therapy process, but the assessment stage is particularly important as "therapists who focus their evaluations solely on performance components risk focusing treatment around those components, thus failing to address critical occupational issues" (Hocking, 2001, p. 463). Assessment should begin with a person's occupational performance areas and a treatment plan developed to improve or maintain occupational performance. This does not mean that occupational performance contexts and components are ignored, merely that they are secondary concerns.

Another implication for practice relates to the methods used in this research. Occupational therapy practice requires therapists to understand and work within the client's life story. As a result, biographic/narrative methods have become increasingly popular due to their congruence with the philosophy of occupational therapy (Duchek & Thessing, 1996; Larson & Fanchiang, 1996). The research reported here contributes to this literature by providing an example of how narrative methods make it possible to explore concepts such as occupational adaptation and occupational identity. While it may not be possible to spend 15 hours assessing a client by gathering his or her oral history, an increased awareness of the concept of a person's occupational career, within an approach to practice that is occupation based, is likely to impact positively on a therapist's work with a client.

LEARNING SUPPORTS

Adopting an Occupational Perspective

Purpose

The purpose of this learning support is for readers to consider the differences between occupational and biomedical perspectives on health.

Primary Concepts

An important message of this chapter is that occupational therapists must use an occupational perspective in their work with clients. Taking an occupational perspective can provide a unique insight into the experiences of people, which is different from a biomedical view. Occupational therapists must be able to both articulate what an occupational perspective is and use it in practice.

Instructions

1. Think of a health condition with which you are familiar, either through clinical or personal experience.

2. Make some notes about that condition that capture how it could be viewed from (a) a biomedical perspective and (b) an occupational perspective.

3. Once you have completed your notes, summarize the key similarities and differences between the two perspectives of that health condition.

Application to Self

Purpose

The purpose of this learning support is for readers to reflect on their own occupational responses to challenging situations.

Primary Concepts

Adopting an occupational perspective requires the ability to recognize and describe the occupational responses people make to situations in their lives. One way of refining this ability is to reflect on one's own experiences and describe them in occupational terms.

Instructions

1. Think of a situation in your life that has been challenging. It may be related to a health condition but could have been a difficulty at work, school, or in a relationship.

2. Make some notes about how you responded to that situation.

3. Review your notes, and try to classify your responses into (a) occupations you stopped, (b) occupations you continued but in different ways, or (c) new occupations

that you commenced. Were there any other ways you responded occupationally that are not captured by these three categories?

Biographical Methods

Purpose

The purpose of this learning support is for readers to reflect on the research design used in the work on which this chapter is based.

Primary Concepts

All research is subject to constraints, such as a finite amount of available finances and time. As a result, all research has limitations. As consumers and producers of research knowledge, it is important for occupational therapists to develop skills in appraising research papers.

Instructions

1. Review the methodology section of this chapter and make notes about the strengths and weaknesses of the research design.

2. For each weakness identified, suggest (a) a reason why this may have occurred in this instance and (b) a strategy to improve the design to address the weakness.

3. For each strength identified, make notes about how it added value to the research project.

REFERENCES

Albert, S., Todak, G., Elkin, E., Marder, K., Dooneief, G., & Stern, Y. (1994). Time allocation and disability in HIV infection: A correlational study. *Journal of Occupational Science: Australia, 1*(4), 21-30.

Angen, M. (2000). Evaluating interpretive inquiry: Reviewing the validity debate and opening the dialogue. *Qualitative Health Research, 10*(3), 378-395.

Barnard, D., Towers, A., Boston, P., & Lambrinidou, Y. (Eds.). (2000). *Crossing over: Narratives of palliative care*. New York, NY: Oxford University Press.

Barroso, J., & Powell-Cope, G. (2000). Metasynthesis of qualitative research on living with HIV infection. *Qualitative Health Research, 10*(3), 340-353.

Bedell, G. (1998). *Finding balance: The daily lives of eight urban gay men with HIV/AIDS*. Doctor of Philosophy Thesis, New York University, New York, NY.

Bedell, G. (2000). Daily life for eight urban gay men with HIV/AIDS. *American Journal of Occupational Therapy, 54*(2), 197-206.

Braveman, B., & Helfrich, C. (2001). Occupational identity: Exploring the narratives of three men living with AIDS. *Journal of Occupational Science, 8*(2), 25-31.

Bury, M. (1991). The sociology of chronic illness: A review of research and prospects. *Sociology of Health & Illness, 13*(4), 451-468.

Centers for Disease Control and Prevention. (2010). *HIV Surveillance Report 2008*. Retrieved September 18, 2010, from http://www.cdc.gov/hiv/topics/surveillance/resources/reports/.

Charmaz, K. (1983). Loss of self: A fundamental form of suffering in the chronically ill. *Sociology of Health & Illness, 5*(2), 168-195.

Christiansen, C. (1999). Defining lives: Occupation as identity: An essay on competence, coherence, and the creation of meaning. *American Journal of Occupational Therapy, 53*(6), 547-558.

Clark, F. (1993). Occupation embedded in a real life: Interweaving occupational science and occupational therapy. *American Journal of Occupational Therapy, 47*(12), 1067-1078.

Creswell, J. (1997). *Qualitative inquiry and research design: Choosing among five traditions.* Thousand Oaks, CA: Sage Publications.

Denton, R. (1987). AIDS: Guidelines for occupational therapy intervention. *American Journal of Occupational Therapy, 41*(7), 427-432.

Duchek, J., & Thessing, V. (1996). Is the use of life history and narrative in clinical practice fundable as research? *American Journal of Occupational Therapy, 50*(5), 393-396.

Erlen, J., Mellors, M., Sereika, S., & Cook, C. (2001). The use of life review to enhance quality of life of people living with AIDS: A feasibility study. *Quality of Life Research, 10*(5), 453-464.

Frank, G. (2000). *Venus on wheels: Two decades of dialogue on disability, biography, and being female.* Los Angeles, CA: University of California Press.

Gaskins, S., & Brown, K. (1997). Helping others: A response to HIV disease. *Journal of the Association of Nurses in AIDS Care, 8*(3), 35-39.

Gergen, K., & Gergen, M. (1986). Narrative form and the construction of psychological science. In T. Sarbin (Ed.), *Narrative psychology: The storied nature of human conduct* (pp. 22-44). Westport, CT: Praeger.

Giles, G., & Allen, M. (1987). AIDS, ARC and the occupational therapist. *British Journal of Occupational Therapy, 50*(4), 120-123.

Health Protection Agency. (2009). *HIV in the United Kingdom: 2009 Report.* London, England: Author.

Hocking, C. (2001). Implementing occupation-based assessment. *American Journal of Occupational Therapy, 55*(4), 463-469.

Jackson, J. (1998). The value of occupation as the core of treatment: Sandy's experience. *American Journal of Occupational Therapy, 52*(6), 466-473.

Jackson, J. (2000). Understanding the experience of noninclusive occupational therapy clinics: Lesbians' perspectives. *American Journal of Occupational Therapy, 54*(1), 26-35.

Katz, A. (1996). Gaining a new perspective on life as a consequence of uncertainty in HIV infection. *Journal of the Association of Nurses in AIDS Care, 7*(4), 51-60.

Kavanaugh, K., & Ayres, L. (1998). "Not as bad as it could have been": Assessing and mitigating harm during research on sensitive topics. *Research in Nursing and Health, 21*(1), 91-97.

Kidner, T. (1930). *Occupational therapy: The science of prescribed work for invalids.* Stuttgart, Germany: W. Kohlhammer.

Kielhofner, G. (2002). Dimensions of doing. In G. Kielhofner (Ed.), *A model of human occupation: Theory and application* (3rd ed., pp. 114-123). Baltimore, MD: Lippincott Williams & Wilkins.

Kielhofner, G. (2004). *Conceptual foundations of occupational therapy* (3rd ed.). Philadelphia, PA: F. A. Davis.

Kielhofner, G., Borell, L., Freidham, L., Goldstein, K., Helfrich, C., Jonsson, H., . . . Nygard, L. (2002). Crafting occupational life. In: G. Kielhofner (Ed.), *A model of human occupation: Theory and application* (3rd ed., pp. 124-144). Baltimore, MD: Lippincott Williams & Wilkins.

Kielhofner, G., Mallinson, T., Forsyth, K., & Lai, J.-S. (2001). Psychometric properties of the second version of the Occupational Performance History Interview. *American Journal of Occupational Therapy, 55*(3), 260-267.

Kylma, J., Vehvilainen-Julkunen, K., & Lahdevirta, J. (2001). Hope, despair and hopelessness in living with HIV/AIDS: A grounded theory study. *Journal of Advanced Nursing, 33*(6), 764-775.

Laliberte Rudman, D. (2002). Linking occupation and identity: Lessons learned through qualitative exploration. *Journal of Occupational Science, 9*(1), 12-19.

Laliberte Rudman, D., Cook, J., & Polatajko, H. (1997). Understanding the potential of occupation: A qualitative exploration of seniors' perspectives on activity. *American Journal of Occupational Therapy, 51*(8), 640-650.

Larson, E. (1996). The story of Maricela and Miguel: A narrative analysis of dimensions of adaptation. *American Journal of Occupational Therapy, 50*(4), 286-298.

Larson, E., & Fanchiang, S. (1996). Life history and narrative research: Generating a humanistic knowledge base for occupational therapy. *American Journal of Occupational Therapy, 50*(4), 247-250.

Law, M., Steinwender, S., & Leclair, L. (1998). Occupation, health and well-being. *Canadian Journal of Occupational Therapy, 65*(2), 81-91.

Lee, R. (1993). *Doing research on sensitive topics.* London, England: Sage Publications.

Leenerts, M., & Magilvy, J. (2000). Investing in self-care: A midrange theory of self-care grounded in the lived experience of low-income HIV-positive white women. *Advances in Nursing Science, 22*(3), 58-75.

Llorens, L. (1990). Foreword. In E. Gilfoyle, A. Grady, & J. Moore (Eds.), *Children adapt: A theory of sensorimotor-sensory development* (2nd ed., pp. xi-xii). Thorofare, NJ: SLACK Incorporated.

Magnus, E. (2001). Everyday occupations and the process of redefinition: A study of how meaning in occupation influences redefinition of identity in women with a disability. *Scandinavian Journal of Occupational Therapy, 8*(3), 115-124.

Mallinson, T., Mahaffey, L., & Kielhofner, G. (1998). The Occupational Performance History Interview: Evidence for three underlying constructs of occupational adaptation. *Canadian Journal of Occupational Therapy, 65*(4), 219-228.

Mandelbaum, D. (1973). The study of life history: Gandhi. *Current Anthropology, 14*(3), 177-196.

Mattingly, C., & Fleming, M. (1994). *Clinical reasoning: Forms of inquiry in a therapeutic practice.* Philadelphia, PA: F. A. Davis.

Mitchell, C., & Linsk, N. (2004). A multidimensional conceptual framework for understanding HIV/AIDS as a chronic long-term illness. *Social Work, 49*(3), 469-477.

Molineux, M. (1997). HIV/AIDS: A new service continuum for occupational therapy. *British Journal of Occupational Therapy, 60*(5), 194-198.

Molineux, M. (2004). Occupation in occupational therapy: A labour in vain? In M. Molineux (Ed.), *Occupation for occupational therapists* (pp. 1-14). Oxford, United Kingdom: Blackwell Publishing.

Molineux, M., & Rickard, W. (2003). Storied approaches to understanding occupation. *Journal of Occupational Science, 10*(1), 52-60.

Morse, J. (1994). "Emerging from the data": The cognitive processes of analysis in qualitative research. In J. Morse (Ed.), *Critical issues in qualitative research methods* (pp. 23-43). Thousand Oaks, CA: Sage Publications.

Patton, M. (1990). *Qualitative evaluation and research methods.* Newbury Park, CA: Sage Publications.

Pierce, D. (2003). How can the occupation base of occupational therapy be strengthened. *Australian Occupational Therapy Journal, 50*(1), 1-2.

Pizzi, M. (1990). The transformation of HIV infection and AIDS in occupational therapy: Beginning the conversation. *American Journal of Occupational Therapy, 44*(3), 199-203.

Portelli, A. (1981/1991). What makes oral history different. In A. Portelli (Ed.), *The death of Luigi Trastulli, and other stories: Form and meaning in oral history* (pp. 45-58). Albany, NY: State University of New York Press.

Rabkin, J., Remien, R., Katoff, L., & Williams, J. (1993). Resilience in adversity among long-term survivors of AIDS. *Hospital and Community Psychiatry, 44*(2), 162-167.

Rebeiro, K., & Allen, J. (1998). Voluntarism as occupation. *Canadian Journal of Occupational Therapy, 65*(5), 279-285.

Rebeiro, K., Day, D., Semeniuk, B., O'Brien, M., & Wilson, B. (2001). Northern Initiative for Social Action: An occupation-based mental health program. *American Journal of Occupational Therapy, 55*(5), 493-500.

Reed, K. (1983). *Models of practice in occupational therapy.* Baltimore, MD: Waverly Press.

Rickard, W. (1998). Oral history—"More dangerous than therapy?": Interviewees' reflections on recording traumatic or taboo issues. *Oral History, 26*(2), 34-48.

Russel, E. (2001). The occupational career revisited. *Journal of Occupational Science, 8*(2), 5-15.

Sacks, O. (1985). *The man who mistook his wife for a hat.* London, England: Picador.

Sandstrom, K. (1990). Confronting deadly disease: The drama of identity construction among gay men with AIDS. *Journal of Contemporary Ethnography, 19*(3), 271-295.

Schkade, J., & McClung, M. (2001). *Occupational adaptation in practice: Concepts and cases.* Thorofare, NJ: SLACK Incorporated.

Schkade, J., & Schultz, S. (1992). Occupational adaptation: Toward a holistic approach for contemporary practice, Part 1. *American Journal of Occupational Therapy, 46*(9), 829-837.

Spencer, J., Davidson, H., & White, V. (1996). Continuity and change: Past experience as adaptive repertoire in occupational adaptation. *American Journal of Occupational Therapy, 50*(7), 526-534.

Takahashi, L., Wiebe, D., & Rodriguez, R. (2001). Navigating the time-space context of HIV and AIDS: Daily routines and access to care. *Social Science & Medicine, 53*(7), 845-863.

Taylor, S. (1983). Adjustment to threatening events: A theory of cognitive adaptation. *American Psychologist, 38*(11), 1161-1173.

Unruh, A., Smith, N., & Scammell, C. (1999). The occupation of gardening in life-threatening illness: A qualitative pilot project. *Canadian Journal of Occupational Therapy, 67*(1), 70-77.

Volberding, P. (2003). HIV therapy in 2003: Consensus and controversy. *AIDS, 17*(Suppl. 1), S4-S11.

Vrkljan, B., & Miller-Polgar, J. (2001). Meaning of occupational engagement in life-threatening illness: A qualitative pilot project. *Canadian Journal of Occupational Therapy, 68*(4), 237-246.

Wade, D., & Halligan, P. (2004). Do biomedical models of illness make for good healthcare systems? *British Medical Journal, 329*(7479), 1398-1401.

Yallop, S. (1999). Positive employment service—facilitating employment for people living with HIV. *Work, 13*(3), 211-215.

Yallop, S. (2004). Occupational reconstruction for people living with HIV/AIDS. In M. Molineux (Ed.), *Occupation for occupational therapists* (pp. 137-154). Oxford, United Kingdom: Blackwell Publishing.

Yerxa, E. (1993). Occupational science: A new source of power for participants in occupational therapy. *Journal of Occupational Science: Australia, 1*(1), 3-9.

Yerxa, E. (2000). Confessions of an occupational therapist who became a detective. *British Journal of Occupational Therapy, 63*(5), 192-199.

Yerxa, E., Clark, F., Jackson, J., Parham, D., Pierce, D., Stein, C., & Zemke, R. (1989). An introduction to occupational science, a foundation for occupational therapy in the 21st century. *Occupational Therapy in Health Care, 6*(4), 1-17.

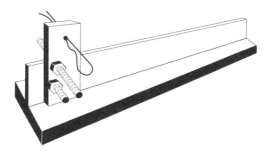

11

Different Ways of Doing Food
Cultural Influences on Food Preparation

Clare Hocking, PhD, NZROT; Anne Shordike, PhD, OTR/L;
Soisuda Vittayakorn, BS; Wannipa Bunrayong, PhD; Phuanjai Rattakorn, PhD;
Valerie A. Wright-St Clair, PhD, MPH, DipProfEthics, DipBusStudies, DipOccTherapy; and
Doris Pierce, PhD, OTR/L, FAOTA

If God had intended us to follow recipes,
He wouldn't have given us grandmothers.
                                    —Linda Henley
            (http://www.quotegarden.com/food.html)

The women who participated in our study, many of them grandmothers, knew a lot more about food than the recipe. They showed us that planning, preparing, cooking, serving, sharing, and offering food at Christmas or Songkran is about leadership, family, identity, tradition, and change. They taught us how these important aspects of food preparation are expressed differently in three regional cultures. To understand this, we worked together over 10 years on an international multisite study. It involved traveling between Auckland in New Zealand, Chiangmai in Thailand, and eastern Kentucky in the United States and weeks discussing the data and responding to where the data led us. By the time we finished, we had refined a useful research method for international research.

In this chapter, we describe how we went about exploring the meaning and experience of food preparation for older women, a major client group served by occupational therapists. Our discussion includes the theoretical background to our collaborative method and some of the cultural diversity we discovered in older women's food preparation at the three sites. To conclude, we consider what our study contributes to occupational science and occupational therapy.

LITERATURE

Food-Related Occupations

Occupational therapists' history of assisting women to cook dates from the 1950s, with the introduction of "gadgets" to enable women with disabilities to independently manage self-care and household tasks, including meal preparation (Hocking & Wilcock, 1997). The provision of assistive devices to support food preparation continues today, such as a providing a stove timer for people with cognitive impairment (Nygård, Starkhammar, & Lilja, 2008). Food-

Pierce, D. (Ed.).
Occupational Science for Occupational Therapy (pp. 133-142).
© 2014 SLACK Incorporated.

related occupations also feature in discussions of rehabilitation after stroke (Hartman-Maeir, Soroker, Ring, Avni, & Katz, 2007), caring for a family member with eating and swallowing difficulties (Johansson & Johansson, 2009), the activity limitations arising from specific health conditions (Poole, Willer, & Mendelson, 2009), and the occupational impact of environmental pollution (Blakeney & Marshall, 2009). Standardized tests to determine individuals' support needs incorporate food-related tasks (Baum et al., 2008). The optimal location for teaching people with a health condition to cook has been researched (Duncombe, 2004). Interventions to reduce obesity acknowledge the importance of the meaning of food preparation (Blanchard, 2009). Finally, an account of practice in Japan (Odawara, 2005) and a rationale for attending to the meaning of everyday occupation (Hasselkus, 2006) have both drawn on the findings of the study described here.

There are many other perspectives on food in the health literature. Nutritionists are concerned with the relationship between appetite and food intake (Parker, Ludher, Loon, Horowitz, & Chapman, 2004) and how cognitions influence people's involvement in food provisioning, preparation, and consumption (Blake, Bisogni, Sobal, Jastran, & Devine, 2008). Associations between family meals and adolescent obesity and depression (Fulkerson, Kubik, Story, Lytle, & Arcan, 2009) and between immigrants' adoption of fatty food and their age, degree of integration, and language mastery (Wandel, Råberg, Kumar, & Holmboe-Ottesen, 2008) have been established. The dietary patterns of households headed by men (Kroshus, 2008) have been examined. A screening tool for the activity limitations associated with peripheral neuropathy includes the question "Do you cook?" (Salsa Collaborative Study Group, 2007, p. 696). There is preliminary evidence that women's beliefs and food preparation techniques are highly consistent over time, but their self-efficacy about modifying their diet and the priority they place on food and nutrition alters in response to debilitating illness (Edstrom & Devine, 2001).

More than a decade ago, deVault (1994) studied how meals conform to cultural ideals and produce family life, and the complexity of ensuring family meals are acceptable to all members. More recently, psychologists examined how media stereotypes influence perceptions of food's healthfulness (Oakes, 2003), and cultural psychologists showed that different attitudes toward food and food intake exist in different contexts (Rozin, 2005). Historians have linked shifts in food customs with the changing self-identity of individuals who experienced that shift (Protschky, 2009). Economists are tracking changes in the food supply chain as Asian countries become more affluent and adopt energy-dense Western foods (Pingali, 2006). While each of these perspectives is informative, none identifies the similarities and differences in the meaning of food-related practices in different cultural contexts.

Culture and Occupation

It is increasingly accepted that, in order to address health disparities and provide effective health care, occupational therapists need to be culturally competent. This demanding aspiration requires openness to cultural diversity; awareness of the cultural basis of one's own beliefs, values, prejudices, and practices (Black & Wells, 2007); and skills to actively engage and respectfully communicate with people from diverse backgrounds. It requires knowledge of family structures and sociocultural roles, as well as the history, traditions and customs, language and pronunciation, religious beliefs, music and arts, values, and traditional medicines of other groups of people (Black & Wells, 2007). Such knowledge is the basis for getting to know individual clients, identifying their occupational goals, and ensuring that occupations used in therapy are culturally safe (Kinébanian & Stomph, 2010). Cultural competence also means critically evaluating knowledge transferred between cultural contexts and attending to issues of culture and diversity. With reference to the study reported here, responding to cultural diversity means using evidence "to better understand socioeconomic and cultural diversity in relation to occupation" (Kinébanian & Stomph, 2010, p. 1).

Cross-Cultural Research

To ensure that our study would generate trustworthy insights to inform practice, we searched for methodological advice about crossing cultural boundaries. We found that disciplines make different assumptions about cross-cultural research that shape the methods they adopt and the research questions they develop. Indigenous psychologists, for example, believe that only cultural insiders can fully interpret the concepts and values within a culture. Thus, they believe that transferring concepts between cultural contexts is difficult or impossible. They value emic (subjective) perspectives, such that each group is encouraged to develop its own concepts and theories, using culturally appropriate methods and relationships (Berry, Poortinga, Segall, & Dasen, 2002). Cultural psychologists, who focus on human development and cultural practices, hold that meanings are culturally relative. They allow that emic understandings can be compared to some extent, if those comparisons have interpretive, ecological, and theoretical validity (Kral, Burkhardt, & Kidd, 2002). At the other end of the spectrum, cross-cultural psychologists presume that psychological processes are universal and knowledge holds true irrespective of context. This is an etic (outsider and using a formal system) view that validates comparative studies that use accurately translated research instruments (van de Vijver, 2001).

Our perspective fell somewhere between the indigenous and cultural psychologists, anticipating that food occupations hold embedded meanings best interpreted by cultural insiders, yet feeling there is some equivalence in

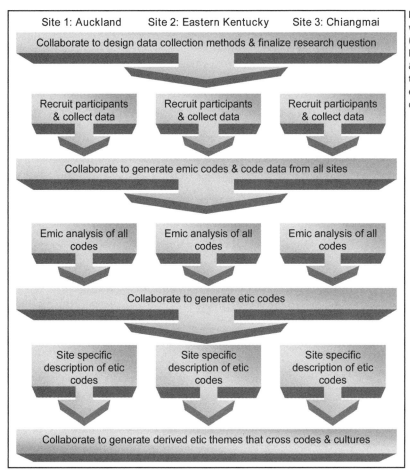

Figure 11-1. Schematic of derived etic steps with alternating immersion and collaboration. (Adapted from Shordike, A., Hocking, C., Pierce, D., Wright-St Clair, V., Vittayakorn, S., Rattakorn, P., & Bunrayong, W. [2010]. Respecting regional culture in an international multi-site study: A derived etic method. *Qualitative Research, 10*[3], 333-355. doi:10.1177/1468794109360145)

the importance, meaning, and function of such occupations that indicates a comparison is possible. To both honor local perspectives and look across cultures, we used Berry's (1989) derived etic research approach. This approach combines initial exploration of emic understandings by cultural insiders with subsequent collaborative comparison of findings to create "derived etics," or themes that explain things observed across the studied cultures. Accordingly, while we do not claim that our derived etic findings hold true in every culture, we think they reveal something important about the food occupations of older women in specific regions of New Zealand, Thailand, and the United States (Hocking et al., 2008). As this discussion reveals, we set out to develop new understandings of occupation that would be valuable to occupational therapists. Additionally, although some researchers would not agree, there is precedence in several disciplines for bringing the findings from culturally diverse participants together.

METHODS

Berry's (1989) derived etic approach proposes a five-step research design but does not prescribe the methods for analyzing the data. In this section, we describe the unique application of the derived etic approach and methods that we developed for our international study of food preparation. Our seven-step research process (Figure 11-1) has alternating phases of coming together in an international collaborative process of analysis and working with the data in our regional teams. Its development was hard won—one step at a time as we realized what was needed. At the beginning, we did not all know each other, and none of us had worked on a multisite study. As relationships, trust, and knowledge of each researcher's expertise developed, we were energized by our commitment to the project and each other, by our desire for cross-cultural insights into the food occupations of older women, and by the poignancy of the data offered to us by the older women of these three regions.

Working as a Team

Our team was initially composed of three researchers at each site who came together for face-to-face meetings between April 2000 and October 2008, funded by Asia 2000 Foundation New Zealand, a research award at Auckland University of Technology, and a grant from the Endowed Chair at Eastern Kentucky University. Despite the challenges of telephone and videoconferencing, our team and other large research teams generally have advantages in qualitative studies because multiple perspectives enrich the data analysis and findings are robustly debated (Pierce et al., 2010). A specific strength of our team was the inclusion of researchers from each region, who functioned both as insiders (in relation to their own data) and as outsiders, bringing critical insights to the findings from the other sites (Bartunek & Reis-Louis, 1996). Having a big team also meant that different people could take the lead on different parts of the process—development of the method, analysis, submitting abstracts, and writing for publication, while others completed PhDs, had children, and took on other responsibilities. A final advantage was that, being from the same discipline, we would occasionally meet at conferences where we discussed progress and plans. Shared presentations of the emerging methods and results also provided opportunities to crystallize our thoughts and focus our work.

Long exposure to working together and experiencing the social and culinary practices, history, and climate of each research region also developed our cultural competence (Black & Wells, 2007). We traveled internationally for five 1- to 2-week meetings during which we made kha nom jok (a traditional Northern Thailand dessert wrapped in banana leaf), went to the temple to offer Songkran food to the ancestors, ate Christmas dinner in New Zealand and Kentucky, shopped for groceries at all three sites, and visited museums and historic places. We discovered many differences not envisioned at the outset. Even our inclusion criteria reflected our cultures, with official definitions of "older" meaning 65 years of age and over in New Zealand and Kentucky, and 60 years and over in Thailand. Being competent team members meant, among other things, being vigilant about balancing and respecting cultural communication differences within the team, as well as acknowledging everyone's contributions by consistently attributing authorship to the whole team.

Alongside the rewards were the frustrations arising from lack of familiarity with aspects of the food occupations at each site, our different languages, and culturally embedded ways of working. Being together was expensive, and progress was slowed by needing to interpret almost every aspect of the data to each other and spend time promoting the study to students, colleagues, deans, vice chancellors, and university presidents. The Thai team had the additional burden of having to translate their data, analysis, and thoughts about how to proceed into English so that the other teams could understand. We spent a lot of time consulting dictionaries to find words with the right connotations to adequately express the Thai meanings. Developing our derived etic method took even more time. We talked and planned how to proceed; sent e-mail messages, schedules, and reminders; and searched the literature to understand the debate about researching across cultures.

We learned what was required as the analysis proceeded. The most dramatic rethinking occurred at Step 5 in the process described next. We had anticipated that we could move from the emic analyses that each team had completed to etic understandings of the food occupations of the older women that crossed the three cultures represented in the study. What transpired, however, was the realization that we had tried to move too fast, with some members feeling ill-informed to interpret others' summaries and some receiving feedback that their interpretation was not entirely accurate. This kind of re-evaluation, where researchers respond to the data and let go of what they thought would work is part of the rigorous development of methods. True to our intent to generate trustworthy findings, we engaged in another round of analysis.

We have previously documented our personal experiences of working in an international collaboration (Shordike et al., 2008), how our method might extend occupational therapy's knowledge base (Hocking et al., 2008), and the care we took to respect cultural differences (Shordike et al., 2010). In the account given here, we focus on describing the steps of our derived etic method and reporting selected findings.

Step 1: Finalizing the Research Question and Planning Data Collection

The first step involved teams working together to finalize the research question and design the data-gathering process. Ensuring that the method would work equally well at each site meant going back and forth between the question, recruitment strategies, the data-gathering strategy, and the schedule of questions for participants, as insights about the topic, the researchers and likely participants, institutional requirements, and the occupation emerged. Useful resources included research texts and information about each cultural context.

Questions of equivalence needed to be discussed, such as how the data might be influenced by participants at one site already knowing each other or rural versus urban differences. We assumed that older women would readily talk to us about cooking and that they would be comfortable in a group, despite participants at some sites not having previously met. Other questions about Christmas and Songkran took a lot of discussion: Was food an important part of both events? Was it everyday food or special dishes particularly associated with that celebration? Were family members involved in the cooking? Was there a lot of food, meaning that it was a demanding occupation? What we learned through this step was the need to stay as close as possible to the occupation itself, avoiding concepts like self-esteem, gender roles, or motivation because we did not know whether women in each country understood their food-related occupations in those terms. We took a full week to determine and document our data-gathering method and agree on the research question: For older women, what is the experience of gathering, preparing, and sharing food at Christmas/Songkran? See Table 11-1 for the fourth and final draft of our focus group questions.

TABLE 11-1

FOCUS GROUP QUESTIONS

KRUEGER'S (1994) STRUCTURE	OUR FOCUS QUESTION
Opening question (everyone answers around the group)	What is your name, and what food do you most associate with Christmas/Songkran?
Introductory question	What makes Christmas/Songkran food special or different?
Transition question	Thinking back to preparing the food for last Christmas/Songkran, what do you remember best?
Key questions	What jobs do you normally do in getting Christmas/Songkran food ready?
	What jobs come first (planning, purchasing, growing, cooking, storing)?
	When do the jobs start?
	How does it work on Christmas day/at Songkran?
	What's that like?
	Does it always go as planned?
	In some families, one person is responsible, in others the jobs are shared around. How does it happen for your Christmas/Songkran?
	How does each person know what to do? (Including you.)
	How does that work out?
	Sometimes, where we do things is as important as what we do. Where do you normally prepare and eat Christmas/Songkran food?
	What difference does it make to be in one place or another?
	How is it decided?
	For some people, the things they use to prepare, serve, and eat Christmas/Songkran food are important. What things do you use?
	What makes those things important?
	What happens once the food is ready?
	Is it different at Christmas/Songkran than at other times?
	How long does all of that take?
	What makes the event successful or not?
	What happens with leftovers?
	What do you do with the other special foods you make around Christmas time/for Songkran?
	Once Christmas dinner is over/the food for Songkran is ready, what happens?
	How does the cleanup get done?
	Who's involved?
	How long does it take?
	What's that like?
Closing questions	Thinking back to Christmases/Songkran in the past, what has changed?
	Do you like the changes that are happening?

Step 2: Data Collection

The next step was to collect the data, with each team acting independently to implement the planned method. Multiple human ethics board reviews were required. We did not gather the data simultaneously; indeed, that might have been a disadvantage, since Christmas is in December and Songkran is in April. Instead, all teams collected data just before or after the annual celebration, drawing participants from existing groups that broadly supported the members' well-being. In our case, the data were in different languages, so translation was necessary. Each team was responsible for meeting the costs associated with data gathering and transcription, but the New Zealand team provided funding to translate the Thai data from the Northern Thai dialect to Government Thai, and then to English.

An additional step undertaken by each team, but outside our derived etic method, was to present and publish site-specific findings (Hocking, Wright-St Clair, & Bunrayong, 2002; Rattakorn, Vittayakorn, Bunrayong, Hocking, & Wright-St Clair, 2003; Shordike & Pierce, 2005; Wright-St Clair & Hocking, 2005). Toward that, the New Zealanders also assisted the Thais to publish in English (Wright-St Clair, Bunrayong, Vittayakorn, Rattakorn, & Hocking, 2004). We remain undecided whether disseminating site-specific findings assisted the research process or not. It did mean that each team achieved deeper understanding of their data and got research outputs, which was important given the time invested in the study. However, publishing takes a lot of time and slowed down the collaboration regarding multisite methods and findings.

Step 3: Developing Emic Codes

With data collection completed, multisite collaborative teams face the challenge of bringing the findings together. The method we developed had three rounds of analysis, moving from emic codes informed by each team's understanding of its own data, to an initial attempt at developing derived etic codes informed by the collaboration's developing understanding of the whole data set and culminating in a final set of derived etic themes that capture more refined understandings of the occupation across all of the research sites. Accordingly, Step 3 brought members of the collaboration together to generate a set of emic codes. The process was for each research team to review the entire data set and to independently generate a list of codes that expressed commonalities across the data. The lists were then compared and discussed until a single set of collaboratively developed codes was agreed upon. Then, the entire data set was coded against the emic codes.

In our study, Step 3 involved three researchers from Kentucky and New Zealand meeting in Kentucky, supported by teleconferences and e-mail messages involving the whole team. The developed emic codes were activities and occupations, affect, change, congruence, food and objects, place, social, time, and tradition. Two members of the collaboration, one from Kentucky and one from New Zealand, then coded all nine transcripts against the codes, and their coded data were combined into one database. The resulting file was well over 300 pages in length.

Step 4: Emic Memos by Code

Step 4 prepared the team for the next round of collaborative analysis. It involved the regional (or emic) teams independently completing a detailed analysis of the data from their site that had been coded against each of the emic codes and writing a description of the meaning of the data in relation to that code. In our case, each researcher worked independently to analyze the coded data, then met with other members of their team to generate a site-specific description of each code. In preparation for the next step, the summaries were circulated by e-mail to all members of the research collaboration.

Step 5: Developing Understanding of the Data Across Cultures and Generating Etic Codes

This collaborative step involved reviewing the analyses of the emic codes produced in Step 4. This was achieved one code at a time, with each team in turn presenting its analysis. The challenge was to work together to ensure that all of the researchers understood each other's explanations of the data from a specific code, while resisting the urge to leap ahead and compare across cultures. After fully discussing the first code, the next code and the next were then similarly discussed.

Once all of the emic codes had been presented, the whole group worked cooperatively to generate initial etic codes. In this study, we found it useful to type the emerging etic codes into a document that was projected onto a screen that all researchers could see, so that we could collaboratively develop the exact wording of the codes and their descriptions. Our initial etic codes were regional identity as expressed through food and practices, collaborative food preparation, women's leadership, the symbolic meaning of the food, and flexibility and stability of food preparation practices.

Step 6: Etic Code Memos by Regional Teams

In Step 6, the researchers again worked in their separate teams to reanalyze their data in relation to the initial etic codes developed at Step 5 and to write site-specific descriptions of their data in relation to each of these codes. This phase of analysis generated new insights into the ways the initial derived etic code was expressed in each context. We began this work during a face-to-face meeting and, once familiar with the task, completed it through teleconferences and videoconferences.

Step 7: Deriving Etic Themes

In Step 7 we completed the analysis by bringing the site-specific memos together to discuss and define the themes that crossed the findings despite cultural differences in how they were expressed. The process of arriving at the final themes was similar to that described in Step 5. The intention was not to achieve consensus about what the derived etic meant, but rather to be assured that it had meaning at each of the research sites and to describe the similarities and differences in its presentation within each culture studied. Our derived etic themes captured the essence of the food-related occupations of older women to celebrate Christmas in New Zealand and Kentucky and Songkran in Thailand. The themes were older women's leadership in Christmas and Songkran food preparation (Wright-St Clair et al., 2013), complexity and diversity of the occupation across cultures, older women creating family over time, meaning of food preparation traditions, dealing with cultural change in and through valued food-centered occupations, and expressing regional identity.

RESULTS

Because the results of the study are multifaceted, we concentrate here on reporting results related to the derived etic theme that reveals most about what the women did: complexity and diversity across cultures.

Complexity of the Occupation Across Cultures

Planning and preparing food for Christmas or Songkran was a complex undertaking. Some of the things that made it complex run across all three sites, irrespective of cultural differences. Examples include the complicated recipes used and the amount and variety of food prepared, often involving the coordinated efforts of a number of women, and the women's preference for food prepared at home from scratch, even though that increased the workload. Other complexities were site specific. In Chiangmai, the recipes were familiar because the dishes have been cooked in the same way for generations and were cooked at other times as well. Nonetheless, in honor of Songkran, the food was more delicately made, in greater quantity, using the best ingredients the women could buy. Also, because the best of the food was to be taken to the temple to be offered to the ancestors and the monks, the women had to ensure that none was eaten before that special portion was separated off.

In Kentucky, older women were also very familiar with the recipes they used and the general routine for preparing food for Christmas. The food occupations were complicated, however, by the pressure of cooking for large numbers, cooking expensive meats, such as a whole ham or turkey, and needing to have all the dishes that make up the meal ready to serve at the same time. Additional complexity came from wanting to clean and adorn the house before visitors arrived, buying paperware or bringing out special tableware and serving dishes, and setting the table for a large group.

Many of the same complexities were experienced by older women in Auckland, although some participants made the point that New Zealanders typically did not decorate their houses to the same extent as North Americans. Added complexity came from Christmas falling in early summer. School children had started their long summer vacation at that time and might or might not have been available to share in the rituals associated with stirring the Christmas cake batter and cutting the cake after midnight mass. Because many workplaces shut down for several weeks starting just before Christmas, some family members might have already set off on holiday, which made it difficult to find a time when everyone was available. If the plan was to use home-grown produce, there was the additional complexity that the new season's potatoes, beans, and strawberries might not be ready in time, and, if a picnic or barbeque was planned, contingency plans could be needed in case of inclement weather.

Diversity of the Occupation Across Cultures

While the food occupations at all three research sites were complex, the diversity across households in Chiangmai, Kentucky, and Auckland varied enormously. A first point of difference was that, where women in Auckland and Kentucky might consult a recipe book, women in Chiangmai learned to cook by being shown what to do, and written recipes did not exist. There were also more specific differences. In Chiangmai, the participants agreed that the same food was cooked in each household, although some cook additional dishes that were particular favorites of an ancestor. Everyone started on the same day: April 14. In fact, "knowing and doing the same" was a frequently repeated phrase in the focus group transcripts. Participants affirmed other women's descriptions of what was done, by whom, when and where things happened, that the oldest woman in the household told the others what to do, and that all the women and girls in each household contributed willingly. There was enormous stability over time because each generation of women endeavored to respectfully carry out the occupations in the way they were taught and to teach their daughters and granddaughters to do the same. Accepted variations might be buying rice flour rather than pounding rice into flour themselves, or doing more of the work if the younger women of the household work outside the home.

In Kentucky, there was quite a high level of consistency from year to year and across families in the meat, desserts, and cookies the women cook. Yet, there were variations in the table settings, with "high-falutin" folks favoring china settings and cloth serviettes over paperware. There was some change in the side dishes from one year to the next, grudging acceptance of healthier food options, and changes to the date and time of the meal to accommodate the schedules of the various family members. There was also change over time, due to changes in the make up of the family and as older women felt the effects of aging and gradually handed the responsibility for preparing the primary foods and hosting the meal over to their daughters.

In New Zealand, there was enormous variation in the Christmas menu, and thus in the older women's occupations. Participants described a cultural shift that was brought about by celebrating Christmas in the heat of the southern hemisphere summer and by the country's strengthening economic ties to Asia taking precedence over its historic ties to Britain. Accordingly, as families "tried out" new traditions, the menu shifted from the more traditional roast dinner followed by Christmas pudding, to barbecued seafood or a picnic featuring an array of cold meats and salads. Also, and perhaps because of New Zealand's egalitarian values, older women sometimes had to adjust to younger members of the family deciding to host the Christmas meal at their homes.

As well as this diversity in older women's practices, the central purpose of preparing food for Songkran and Christmas differed. The primary focus for older women in Chiangmai was showing their respect and gratitude to their ancestors. They believed that by willingly doing the tasks expected of them, they would earn merit for themselves and their families, ensuring their good fortune in the next life. Accordingly, these women expected to continue to be involved in these valued food occupations until they were physically unable to do so. In contrast, when they plan, prepare, and offer food at Christmas time, older women in Kentucky and New Zealand primarily focus on catering to everyone's food preferences, including their own, and having all members of the family together, happy and healthy.

CONTRIBUTION TO OCCUPATIONAL SCIENCE

The international food study makes four significant contributions to occupational science. First, it is a partial response to concerns expressed about the predominance of Western perspectives in occupational science (Asaba, 2008) as well as doubts expressed in other disciplines about whether it is possible for Western researchers to transcend their own culture to understand and contribute to building knowledge of occupations in other cultures. While not discounting the considerable effort required, this study has been a successful collaboration of researchers who might be characterized as "Western" and "Eastern." Second, the study has demonstrated that there are commonalities in occupations that transcend diverse cultural contexts, despite marked differences in how they are done. Although that might be expected, given that occupations essential for human survival are present in some form in every culture, the nature of those commonalities has not previously been revealed. The third contribution is the question that arises from the study: Is there an essentially human aspect to occupations? That is, if all the cultural variations are stripped away, are there aspects of human occupation that hold true irrespective of their context? While derived etic methods cannot answer that question, this study is important in alerting occupational scientists to be attentive to similarities and differences in occupations across diverse settings. The final contribution of this study is the development of a method to look across cultures that has potential application to the study of other occupations. Indeed, we have frequently been asked which men's occupation we will study!

IMPLICATIONS FOR PRACTICE

Like other research reported in this book, this international study honors the intent of the founders of occupational science for the science itself to inform occupational therapy (Clark et al., 1991). The research has generated knowledge about the meaning of the food-related occupations of older women in three very different cultural contexts, giving new insights into what they value in preparing and sharing annual celebratory foods; the visible and invisible work that is done; the beliefs, hopes, and aspirations conveyed through the foods and foodways; and the women's intuitive responsiveness to the contexts in which the occupations are carried out. Beyond illuminating everyday understandings, this study's occupational science findings hold potential to inform occupational therapy practice. A fruitful way to approach an applied interpretation of the findings is to use the results to raise questions such as the following: What do these findings suggest for how I work with older women who want or need to continue cooking for their family or to prepare food for important events? What typical changes and adaptations in how older women work with others to prepare celebratory foods suggest acceptable strategies for my older clients, so that they can continue involvement in their valued occupations despite physical limitations? How well do the kitchen and cooking assessments I use in practice reveal the complex subtleties of meaning of the recipes, the foods, and the occupation itself? What am I not understanding about the deep relevance of continuing or relinquishing participation in food-related tasks when I design cooking interventions with older women? How can I draw on older women's deep understandings of family recipes, food traditions, and social changes in ways that engage them in food occupations within and beyond the therapy context? Other questions will come up for practitioners who reflect on the everyday relevance of these occupational science findings for occupational therapy practice. In this way, questioning gives practitioners a way of engaging with the findings in order to make sense of them in the practice context.

Importantly, the study provides new insights into cultural differences and similarities in an occupation performed and appreciated by many people. It makes otherwise hidden aspects of food-centered occupations visible. Information about other cultures and how they differ from one's own is the basis of developing cultural competence, which has been recognized nationally and internationally as a key concern for occupational therapists (Black & Wells, 2007; Kinébanian & Stomph, 2010). So, while occupational science knowledge offers implications for occupational therapy, practice holds many unanswered questions for occupational science to explore.

CONCLUSION

The food-related occupations study was an ambitious project that brought together researchers who did not previously know each other to collaborate on a shared project across very different cultural contexts and on a shoestring budget. The collaboration has been highly productive, with seven peer-reviewed articles, two chapters, and more than 20 conference presentations to date. Most importantly, it has influenced practice, having prompted Rachel Thibeault to use food occupations as a mechanism to enter communities in her work in Sierra Leone (R. Thibeault, personal communication, July, 2006) and informed scholarship (Hasselkus, 2006). We are confident that the results reported here will contribute to occupational therapists' competence to work with diverse older women and foster therapists' openness to cultural diversity. We are also hopeful that the method we developed will inform other occupational scientists' endeavors to uncover the complexity and similarities of occupations performed in very different places.

LEARNING SUPPORTS

1. Think of an important cultural event that you participate in that has special, homemade food associated with it—perhaps Christmas, Thanksgiving, or Passover. Describe the complexities of planning, preparing, and sharing the food for that occasion. Compare your description with our account of the occupation in Kentucky, Auckland, and Chiangmai.

2. Imagine you have funding to conduct an international multisite study of an occupation typical of men or children. What occupation and three research sites would you choose? Remember that you need the occupation and the research participants to be equivalent, so do not select an occupation that is considered to be work in one place but leisure at the other sites, is very popular in one place but relatively unknown at the others, or is performed by people of different ages at each of the sites.

3. Drawing on your knowledge of occupational therapy, outline a situation where the findings of this study would inform practice with an individual, group, or community.

4. If you could spend an hour with the researchers in the food study asking anything you want to know about the study's methods or findings, what would you ask us?

REFERENCES

Asaba, E. (2008). Hashi-ire: Where occupation, chopsticks, and mental health intersect. *Journal of Occupational Science, 15*(2), 74-79. doi: 10.1080/14427591.2008.9686612

Bartunek, J., & Reis-Louis, M. (1996). *Insider/outsider team research.* London, England: Sage Publications.

Baum, C. M., Connor, L. T., Morrison, T., Hahn, M., Dromerick, A. W., & Edwards, D. F. (2008). Reliability, validity, and clinical utility of the Executive Function Performance Test: A measure of executive function in a sample of people with stroke. *American Journal of Occupational Therapy, 62,* 446-455. doi:10.5014/ajot.62.4.446

Berry, J. W. (1989). Imposed etics-emics-derived etics: The operationalization of a compelling idea. *International Journal of Psychology, 24,* 721-735. doi:10.1080/00207598908246808

Berry, J. W., Poortinga, Y. H., Segall, M. H., & Dasen, P. R. (2002). *Cross-cultural psychology: Research and applications* (2nd ed.). New York, NY: Cambridge University Press.

Black, R. M., & Wells, S. A. (2007). *Culture and occupation: A model of empowerment in occupational therapy.* Bethesda, MD: American Occupational Therapy Association.

Blake, C. E., Bisogni, C. A., Sobal, J., Jastran, M., & Devine, C. M. (2008). How adults construct evening meals. Scripts for food choice. *Appetite, 51*(3), 654-662. doi:10.1016/j.appet.2008.05.062

Blakeney, A. B., & Marshall, A. (2009). Water quality, health, and human occupations. *American Journal of Occupational Therapy, 63,* 46-57. doi:10.5014/ajot.63.1.46

Blanchard, S. A. (2009). Variables associated with obesity among Africa-American women in Omaha. *American Journal of Occupational Therapy, 63,* 58-68. doi:10.5014/ajot.63.1.58

Clark, F. A., Parham, D., Carlson, M., Frank, G., Jackson, J., Pierce, D., . . . Zemke, R. (1991). Occupational science: Academic innovation in the service of occupational therapy's future. *American Journal of Occupational Therapy, 45,* 300-310. doi:10.5014/ajot.45.4.300

deVault, M. L. (1994). *Feeding the family: The social organization of caring as gendered work.* Chicago, IL: University of Chicago.

Duncombe, L. W. (2004). Comparing learning of cooking in home and clinic for people with schizophrenia. *American Journal of Occupational Therapy, 58,* 272-278. doi:10.5014/ajot.58.3.272

Edstrom, K. M., & Devine, C. M. (2001). Consistency in women's orientations to food and nutrition in midlife and older age: A 10-year qualitative follow-up. *Journal of Nutritional Education, 33*, 215-223. doi:10.1016/S1499-4046(06)60034-1

Fulkerson, J. A., Kubik, M. Y., Story, M., Lytle, L., & Arcan, C. (2009). Are there nutritional and other benefits associated with family meals among at-risk youth? *Journal of Adolescent Health, 45*, 389-395. doi:10.1016/j.jadohealth.2009.02.011

Hartman-Maeir, A., Soroker, N., Ring, H., Avni, N., & Katz, N. (2007). Activities, participation and satisfaction one-year post stroke. *Disability and Rehabilitation, 29*(7), 559-566. doi:10.1080/09638280600924996

Hasselkus, B. R. (2006). The world of everyday occupation: Real people, real lives. *American Journal of Occupational Therapy, 60*(6), 627-640. doi:10.5014/ajot.60.6.627

Hocking, C., Pierce, D., Shordike, A., Wright-St Clair, V., Bunrayong, W., Vittayakorn, S., & Rattakorn, P. (2008). The promise of internationally collaborative research for studying occupation: The example of the older women's food preparation study. *OTJR: Occupation, Participation and Health, 28*(4), 180-190. doi:10.3928/15394492-20080901-02

Hocking, C., & Wilcock, A. (1997). Occupational therapists as object users: A critique of Australian practice 1954-1995. *Australian Occupational Therapy Journal, 44*, 167-176. doi:10.1111/j.1440-1630.1997.tb00771.x

Hocking, C., Wright-St Clair, V., & Bunrayong, W. (2002). The meaning of cooking and recipe work for older Thai and New Zealand women. *Journal of Occupational Science, 9*(3), 117-127. doi:10.1080/14427591.2002.9686499

Johansson, A. E. M., & Johansson, U. (2009). Relatives' experiences of family members' eating difficulties. *Scandinavian Journal of Occupational Therapy, 16*, 25-32. doi:10.1080/11038120802257195

Kinébanian, A., & Stomph, M. (2010). *Draft position statement on diversity and culture*. Forrestfield, Australia: World Federation of Occupational Therapists.

Kral, M. J., Burkhardt, K. J., & Kidd, S. (2002). The new research agenda for a cultural psychology. *Canadian Psychology, 43*, 154-162. doi:10.1037/h0086912

Kroshus, E. (2008). Gender, marital status, and commercially prepared food expenditure. *Journal of Nutrition Education and Behavior, 40*, 355-360. doi:10.1016/j.jneb.2008.05.012

Krueger, R. (1994). *Focus groups: A practical guide for applied research* (2nd ed.). Thousand Oaks, CA: Sage Publications.

Nygård, L., Starkhammar, S., & Lilja, M. (2008). The provision of stove timers to individuals with cognitive impairment. *Scandinavian Journal of Occupational Therapy, 15*, 4-12. doi:10.1080/11038120601124240

Oakes, M. E. (2003). Difference in judgments of food healthfulness by young and elderly women. *Food Quality and Preference, 14*, 227-236.

Odawara, E. (2005). Cultural competency in occupational therapy: Beyond a cross-cultural view of practice. *American Journal of Occupational Therapy, 59*, 325-334. doi:10.5014/ajot.59.3.325

Parker, B. A., Ludher, A. K., Loon, T. K., Horowitz, M., & Chapman, I. M. (2004). Relationships of ratings of appetite to food intake in healthy older men and women. *Appetite, 43*, 227-233. doi:10.1016/j.appet.2004.05.004

Pierce, D., Atler, K., Baltisberger, J., Fehringer, E., Hunter, E., Malkawi, S., & Parr, T. (2010). Occupational science: A data-based American perspective. *Journal of Occupational Science, 17*(4), 204-215. doi:10.1080/14427591.2010.9686697

Pingali, P. (2006). Westernization of Asian diets and the transformation of food systems: Implications for research and policy. *Food Policy, 32*, 281-298. doi:10.1016/j.foodpol.2006.08.001

Poole, J. L., Willer, K., & Mendelson, C. (2009). Occupation of motherhood: Challenges for mothers with scleroderma. *American Journal of Occupational Therapy, 63*, 214-219. doi:10.5014/ajot.63.2.214

Protschky, S. (2009). The flavour of history: Food, family and subjectivity in two indo-European women's memoirs. *The History of Family, 14*, 369-385. doi:10.1016/j.hisfam.2009.08.006

Rattakorn, P., Vittayakorn, S., Bunrayong, W., Hocking, C., & Wright-St Clair, V. (2003). Cooking food for Songkran: Its meaning for the elderly women of Chiangmai. *Journal of Occupational Therapists Association of Thailand, 8*(1), 32-40.

Rozin, P. (2005). The meaning of food in our lives: A cross-cultural perspective on eating and well-being. *Journal of Nutritional Education and Behaviour, 37*, S107-S112. doi:10.1016/S1499-4046(06)60209-1

Salsa Collaborative Study Group. (2007). The development of a short questionnaire for screening of activity limitation and safety awareness (SALSA) in clients affected by leprosy or diabetes. *Disability and Rehabilitation, 29*(9), 689-700. doi:10.1080/09638280600926587

Shordike, A., Hocking, C., Pierce, D., Wright-St Clair, V., Vittayakorn, S., Rattakorn, P., & Bunrayong, W. (2010). Respecting regional culture in an international multi-site study: A derived etic method. *Qualitative Research, 10*(3), 333-355. doi:10.1177/1468794109360145

Shordike, A., Hocking, C., Vittayakorn, S., Bunrayong, W., Rattakorn, P., Wright-St Clair, V., & Pierce, D. (2008). Refining the occupation of research across cultures. In P. Liamputtong (Ed.), *Doing cross-cultural research: Ethical and methodological perspectives* (pp. 287-303). Dordrecht, The Netherlands: Springer.

Shordike, A., & Pierce, D. (2005). Cooking up Christmas in Kentucky: Occupation and tradition in the stream of time. *Journal of Occupational Science, 12*(3), 140-148. doi:10.1080/14427591.2005.9686557

van de Vijver, F. J. R. (2001). The evolution of cross-cultural research methods. In D. Matsumoto (Ed.), *The handbook of culture and psychology* (pp. 77-97). Oxford, United Kingdom: Oxford University Press.

Wandel, M., Råberg, M., Kumar, B., & Holmboe-Ottesen, G. (2008). Changes in food habits after migration among South Asians settled in Oslo: The effect of demographic, socio-economic and integration factors. *Appetite, 50*, 376-385. doi:10.1016/j.appet.2007.09.003

Wright-St Clair, V., Bunrayong, W., Vittayakorn, S., Rattakorn, P., & Hocking, C. (2004). Offerings: Food traditions of older Thai women at Songkran. *Journal of Occupational Science, 11*(3), 115-124. doi:10.1080/14427591.2004.9686539

Wright-St Clair, V., & Hocking, C. (2005). Older New Zealand women doing the work of Christmas: A recipe for identity formation. *Sociological Review, 53*(2), 332-350. doi:10.1111/j.1467-954X.2005.00517.x

Wright-St Clair, V. A., Pierce, D., Bunrayong, W., Rattakorn, P., Vittayakorn, S., Shordike, A., & Hocking, C. (2013). Cross-cultural understandings of festival food-related activities for older women in Chiang Mai, Thailand, Eastern Kentucky, USA and Auckland, New Zealand. *Journal of Cross Cultural Gerontology, 28*(2), 103-119. doi:10.1007/s10823-013-9194-5

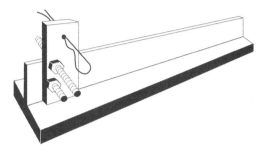

12

Reflecting on the Socially Situated and Constructed Nature of Occupation
A Research Program Addressing the Contemporary Restructuring of Retirement

---

Debbie Laliberte Rudman, PhD, OT Reg (ON)

This chapter describes a program of research investigating the contemporary social reconstruction of retirement, in order to illustrate one way forward in furthering our understanding of the socially situated and constructed nature of occupation. This program of research, grounded in occupational science, begins with the premise that the occupations that individuals and collectives do in everyday life are shaped by, and influence the shaping of, contextual features. Thus, understanding what clients do, and do not do, and enabling participation in occupations, requires consideration of the ways in which various layers of context influence what clients, as individuals and as members of collectives, come to view as possible, ideal, and ethical occupations for themselves and others. As such, this work addresses what Whiteford, Klomp, and Wright-St Clair (2005) have referred to as the situated nature of occupation:

> No human action is independent of the social, cultural, political and economic contexts in which it occurs. These contextual forces, to a greater or lesser extent, shape the form and performance of the occupation as well as the meaning ascribed to it by an individual or group. (p. 10)

Drawing on critical social theory perspectives that emphasize the need to consider how power operates to influence what societal members come to take for granted as real, including possible and ideal ways to be and do in everyday life (Rose, 1999), this work also addresses occupation as a socially constructed phenomenon intimately connected to issues of power.

LITERATURE

Why Focus on the Situated and Socially Constructed Nature of Occupation?

Attending to how occupation is socially situated and constructed requires consideration of macrolevel environmental elements, such as political, economic, and institutional elements. Despite the integration of macrolevel environmental elements in many models addressing occupation that inform contemporary practice, occupational

Pierce, D. (Ed.).
Occupational Science for Occupational Therapy (pp. 143-156).
© 2014 SLACK Incorporated.

therapy and occupational science have been critiqued for taking a primarily individualistic orientation to occupation (Dyck & Jongbloed, 2000; Hocking, 2000; O'Brien, Dyck, Caron, & Mortenson, 2002). For example, Dickie, Cutchin, and Humphry (2006) contend that occupational scientists often take on a position of individualism, involving a focus on individualized experience of and authority over occupation and "situating the individual in opposition to—in a dualism with—context" (p. 85). Frank and Zemke (2009) similarly note that occupational therapy practice in the United States, although rooted in reformist movements, became increasingly focused on addressing problems and solutions at the level of the individual following both World Wars.

Although attending to individual experiences does not preclude attending to context (Pierce et al., 2010), the emphasis on individualism in occupational science has also meant that when contexts are addressed, there is a focus on the most immediate micro, and sometimes meso, environmental aspects as they affect the occupations of individuals. There has been a growing recognition that this has limited research and practice (O'Brien et al., 2002; Whiteford, 2010). In relation to occupational therapy practice, Pollard, Kronenberg, and Sakellariou (2009) contend that the socially constructed nature of disability and marginalization necessitates deeper political awareness of social, economic, and political conditions, necessitating a greater theoretical and research focus on macroenvironmental features. This gap between theoretical understandings that articulate complex ways that occupation is interrelated with various layers of context and the tendency to address occupation as an individualistic phenomenon has been connected to the emphasis on particular methodological approaches within occupational science, as well as the pervasive influence of Western epidemiological, biomedical, and psychological frames of reference and particular political values and systems (Dickie et al., 2006; Jongbloed & Crichton, 1990; Molineux & Whiteford, 2006). In parallel, there has been a call for expansion of the methodologies and theories that inform occupational science to enable further exploration of issues such as social relations, power, justice, and marginalization (Laliberte Rudman et al., 2008; O'Brien et al., 2002; Phelan & Kinsella, 2009; Pollard et al., 2009).

The limited, but growing, body of research addressing macrolevel elements has begun to demonstrate their crucial role in shaping occupation (Dyck & Jongbloed, 2000; Suto, 2009). For example, Beagan and Etowa's (2009) mixed methods study involving 50 African Canadian women illustrated crucial impacts of everyday racism, itself embedded in larger structural relations, on the ways women chose, performed, and experienced leisure, caring, and productive occupations. Magasi and Hammel (2009) drew on a social justice perspective, disability studies, and Foucault's work on institutions to conduct an ethnographic study of women

with disabilities transitioning from a nursing home into the community. Several of their thematic findings point to intersections of occupation and macrolevel elements, such as how the nursing home's institutional rules restricted occupational opportunities and public policies limited support for transitioning. These authors challenged occupational therapists to question institutional ideologies and practices that shape forced dependency and perpetuate disability stereotypes. These examples draw on social theories and innovative methodologies to get at the complex ways macrolevel elements influence what occupations are framed as appropriate for particular types of people, how people perform occupations, and the meaning people attribute to occupations. They raise concerns related to how macrolevel elements set limits on occupation for particular groups of people and point to potential ways forward in addressing such issues through occupation-based research and practice.

Considering the identified need for further research addressing macrolevel contextual influences on occupation and the demonstrated value of existing work, the broad questions that inform my program of research are (a) How are the occupations of individuals and collectives situated within their social, political, economic, historical, and cultural contexts? and (b) How can we understand occupation as both socially and individually constructed? As highlighted by Whiteford (2010), the ways in which "contexts directly and indirectly influence the norms and forms of occupational engagement are not always immediately apparent" (p. 135). Furthering understanding of the ways in which occupation is situated and socially constructed demands getting at that which is not "immediately apparent," presenting both methodological and theoretical challenges. In this chapter, I illustrate another way forward in advancing understanding of how occupation is socially situated and constructed within particular contexts. To provide further background for my program of research, I provide an overview of the key ways retirement is being restructured in many parts of the Western world.

Why Focus on Retirement?

Consistent with key underlying assumptions of critical gerontological work, including that "age-related outcomes are... not mere consequences of organismic aging, but of complex interactions that combine social structural, cultural and interactional processes" (Baars, Dannefer, Phillipson, & Walker, 2006, p. 3), my program of research conceptualizes retirement as a socially constructed phenomena that shapes how individuals come to understand themselves and their occupations as they prepare for and move into retirement. Retirement, as an aspect of the life course socially constructed through various means, such as pension policies, employment practices, popular media, and the consumer market, provides a particularly interesting exemplar for the study of how context shapes occupational participation and experiences.

Retirement itself is being actively reconstructed via policy and discursive changes and is intricately tied to occupation (Jonsson, Josephsson, & Kielhofner, 2000; Phillipson, 2004). A number of countries belonging to the Organization for Economic Cooperation and Development ([OECD] 2006) have implemented policy changes over the past 2 decades to reverse early retirement trends, promote longer worker lives, and increasingly shift emphases toward individualized, as opposed to government-supported, pension plans (Mann, 2007; Shuey & O'Rand, 2006). OECD recommended policy changes, such as extending the age of eligibility for public pensions, banning mandatory retirement, and decreasing income replacement rates of state pensions, have been implemented to varying extents in countries in the West (Curl & Hokenstad, 2006). Although such policy changes have been justified in relation to economic and social changes, such as rising dependency ratios and the increasing health of aging people, critical gerontologists have critiqued how such changes obscure the differential abilities and resources of aging individuals to both financially prepare for retirement and continue work in later life. The increasing shift away from policies that shape retirement as a state-supported right toward those that shape it as an individualized responsibility has been linked to neoliberal aims of decreasing public expenditures, enhancing individual responsibility, and promoting consumerism (Polivka & Longino, 2006). My program of research raises concerns about the implications of these policy shifts as they relate to occupational possibilities for aging individuals (Laliberte Rudman, 2005).

Connected to concerns regarding the differential effects of policy changes and the rising influence of neoliberal political rationality in many Western nations, critical gerontologists have also focused on how retirement is being reconstructed through discourses. Discourses refer to ways a phenomenon is textually, visually, and verbally constructed within various kinds of texts and social institutions. Drawing on critical social perspectives, such gerontologists contend that discourses do not simply reflect the way phenomena are, but shape how particular phenomena come to be understood and what is done, by individuals and collectives, on the basis of the understandings shaped (Biggs, 2001; Katz, 2000). How retirement, and retirees, are discursively constructed, for example, in policy texts and popular media, comes to influence how those approaching retirement, as well as those already in retirement, think about and act in relation to retirement. These discursive constructions also

influence the types of programs and services made available to those planning for and in retirement (Ainsworth & Hardy, 2004). While acknowledging the existence of competing discourses about retirement, there is a general agreement that there has been a rise of so-called positive, healthy, or productive discourses of retirement in the Western world, with common emphases on the positivity and possibility of prolonging mid-life and avoiding old age through lifestyle and consumer choices; a shift away from collective responsibility for managing health, financial, and other risks associated with aging and retirement, toward individual responsibility for proactively dealing with such risks; and the promotion of an ethic of being busy and continued activity engagement. Although these discursive shifts have been celebrated within and outside occupational science and occupational therapy as enhancing opportunities for aging people, they have also been critiqued for their alliance with neoliberal emphases on consumerism, retrenchment of the welfare state, individualization of responsibility and risk, and the idealization of youthfulness (Biggs, 2001; Calasanti, 2002; Hugman, 1999; Katz, 2000; Martinson & Minkler, 2006).

As an occupational scientist and occupational therapist, a key question that arises as I experience this reconstruction of retirement within and through policies and discourses is: What are the implications of this restructuring for how individuals negotiate and experience occupation as they move toward their retirement years? To date, research examining the implications of this reconstruction has largely focused on the timing of retirement and how involvement in paid work is being altered in later life. For example, although there is some evidence that the average age of withdrawal from the formal labor force has been increasing since the late 1990s in several countries (Cooke, 2006), it is also clear that many individuals are reluctant to continue or return to employment past age 65 (Phillipson, 2004). Overall, it appears that the timing of retirement is becoming increasingly individualized and unpredictable, as well as dependent on individual characteristics and resources (Dannefer, 2000; Phillipson, 2004). Several authors have raised the concern that aging individuals who have the most financial, health, social, and other forms of resources will increasingly have greater choices regarding how to live in retirement, while those who lack such resources will have few choices not to continue active labor force involvement regardless of preferences or health (Mann, 2007; Polivka & Longino, 2006; Riach, 2007). However, there has been little investigation of the implications of such discourses for how aging people manage and experience occupation, as it is broadly conceived in occupational science and occupational therapy.

A Research Program Examining the Interaction Between the Contemporary Restructuring of Retirement and the Occupations of Aging Individuals

My ongoing program of research aims to examine interconnections between the ways retirement is being discursively reconstructed and how aging individuals manage, experience, and perform occupations as they prepare for and move into their retirement years. This focus initially stemmed from observing my own father's difficult transition into retirement following a sudden health issue and also from working with clients in occupational therapy who did not experience the ideals of positive aging espoused within government, media, research, and other types of texts. This program of research began with my doctoral research, which was a critical discourse analysis (CDA) of Canadian newspaper texts, and has evolved to include a CDA of a broader sample of newspaper texts and a narrative study. Prior to presenting an overview of the two main aspects of this program, key theoretical concepts informing how I am conceptualizing discourse and its interconnections with narrative are outlined.

Governmentality Concepts Key to the Research Program: Discourses as Technologies of Government, Political Rationalities, and Subjectivity

In addition to occupational science and critical social gerontology, governmentality theory is used to frame this program of research (Foucault, 1991; Rose, 1999). Drawing on governmentality theory, discourse is conceptualized as a productive technology of government, that is, a way that authorities and agents seek to guide the conduct of others toward certain political ends (Bennett, 2003; Foucault, 1991). As a technology of government, the production and circulation of discourses is intimately connected to power, such that particular types of authorities and agents (e.g., politicians, educators, and health care professionals), both within and outside the state, have more power to influence what truths are shaped within discourses and what discourses come to be pervasive. The truths that are created and promoted through discourses influence how people understand themselves and what they come to see as ideal, ethical, and moral ways to be and act (Allen, 1991;

Rose, 1999). How discourses come to be shaped and which discourses come to be most pervasive are linked to social, cultural, and political factors; for example, how retirement is written and talked about is influenced by demographic trends, consumer culture, and prevailing political schools of thought (Bratich, Packer, & McCarthy, 2003; Rose, 1999).

Governmentality theorists propose that, within a specific sociohistorical context, a broader system of thought, referred to as a *political rationality*, guides how various authorities and agencies seek to govern the conduct of others. The ideals and aims incorporated within a political rationality are drawn upon in the shaping of discourses. As noted previously, in relation to the contemporary restructuring of retirement, neoliberal political rationality is seen as the dominant rationality influencing both policy and discursive change in the West. As a political rationality, central aims of governing within neoliberalism are to decrease individual dependency on the state, support market mechanisms, and encourage privatization and consumerism. Concerns with equity and collective welfare tend to be de-emphasized, while issues related to individual responsibility, proactive risk management, and self-fulfillment are forefronted (Broad & Anthony, 1999; O'Rand, 2000; Polivka & Longino, 2006).

A key way in which contemporary discourses operate to shape conduct is through shaping subjectivity, defined as possibilities for organizing personhood. Power operates through the production and circulation of discourses that construct particular kinds of ideal subjects (tied to characteristics such as age, gender, or ability) who are to conduct themselves in ways consistent with the guiding ideals and aims of social and political authorities. Individuals, in turn, draw upon the subjectivities created and promoted through dominant discourses as they attempt to manage and perform their identities within everyday life in ethical and socially ideal ways (Ainsworth & Hardy, 2004; Dean, 1994). While the subjectivities constructed as ideal do not determine how individuals will act, and resistance is always possible, the taken-for-granted nature of these ideal subjects tends to limit possibilities for being in everyday life (Ainsworth & Hardy, 2004; Kemp & Denton, 2003). For example, discourses regarding retirement and aging construct particular types of aging subjects and associated sets of behaviors as ideal, such as the proactive body manager who engages in various types of physical and consumer activity to maintain a youthful-appearing body (Laliberte Rudman, 2006a).

Although several governmentality theorists frame discourse as a resource that individuals draw upon to negotiate subjectivity in everyday life (Dean, 1995; Rose, 1999), empirical work drawing on this theoretical perspective has been critiqued for its tendency to focus on how discourse is constructed and circulated within institutional realms, but not necessarily if and how it is taken up or resisted by individuals within everyday life (Kemp & Denton, 2003; Power,

2005). One way to address this critique is through linking individuals' narratives and discourses, in which discourses are viewed as a type of interpretive resource drawn upon by people when they construct narratives to make sense of their ways of being and doing. In other words, the individual stories people tell are bounded within the broader social and cultural stories available to them, such that narratives tell us not only about an individual's identities and occupations but also about how these are situated (Chase, 2005; Gubrium & Holstein, 1998, 2009).

Critical Discourse Analysis of Canadian Newspaper Texts Addressing Retirement

Methodology and Research Objectives for the Critical Discourse Analysis

CDA seeks to uncover how phenomenon have come to be constructed within particular contexts and how power is enacted through discourses in ways that "seek to shape the conduct, aspirations, needs, desires, capacities of specified categories of individuals, to enlist them in particular strategies and to seek defined goals" (Dean, 1994, p. 156). The use of the word *critical* expresses the intent to "'de-familiarize' and 'de-naturalize' taken for granted assumptions about social reality" (Ainsworth & Hardy, 2004, p. 238). Such critical work can enhance awareness of the subtle ways power influences what we come to take for granted regarding how we and others should be and act, and the underlying values and assumptions supporting these taken-for-granted ways of being and doing. In turn, raising such awareness can open up opportunities for other ways to be and do, tied to alternative values and assumptions (Ballinger & Cheek, 2006).

In relation to discourses of retirement, the objectives of my CDA work are to explore the ways of being (identity) and doing (occupation) shaped as ideal, moral, and ethical within contemporary media texts, and what is shaped as nonideal, immoral, and unethical. The analysis reported here aimed to consider the possibilities and boundaries for occupation established through such discourses and how these link with neoliberal political rationality. My work is also intended to promote critical awareness of what types of aging people benefit, and what types of aging people are marginalized, through such discourses.

Methods of the Critical Discourse Analysis

To date, the CDA study has focused on analyzing Canadian newspaper texts, because mass media plays a vital role in shaping subjectivity in the contemporary Western world (Rose, 1999). Full-text newspaper articles, focused on preparing for and living in retirement and published between 1999 and 2006, were electronically selected from the two largest Canadian newspapers. A database of more than 1,000 articles dealing with retirement was created;

these have been categorized in relation to year and broad topic area (work, housing, health and illness, finances, volunteer, general lifestyle, mixed, and other). Three specific substudies have drawn texts from this database: my doctoral dissertation, which drew on all texts published in one newspaper in 1999 and 2000 ($N = 138$) (Laliberte Rudman, 2005, 2006b); a substudy focused on work, which drew on texts from both newspapers published in 2006 ($N = 138$) (Laliberte Rudman & Molke, 2009); and a substudy focused on housing, which drew on texts from both newspapers published in 2006 ($N = 82$) (Laliberte Rudman, Huot, & Dennhardt, 2009). CDA, as a research methodology, enables a researcher to draw from a larger set of texts based on varying foci, as well as to expand one's set of texts to include various types of texts. Future studies in this program of research will extend into other topic areas addressed in the media, such as health and lifestyle, as well as include policy reports on retirement and aging.

Although specific research questions varied in these substudies, all employed an approach to CDA informed by governmentality theory as well as method guidelines provided by Cheek (2004), Fairclough (1992), and Potter and Wetherell (1987). Across these substudies, there has been an analytic focus on identifying the ways of being (identity) and doing (occupation) shaped within the texts, and values and aims highlighted as ideal and nonideal. In the first study, analysis was conducted by myself; in the second and third studies, it was conducted collaboratively with doctoral research trainees. The analysis approach involved several iterative steps. Questions derived from the governmentality perspective were used to develop an analysis sheet, on which analytic notes were inserted along with excerpts from texts. Texts were read several times, with each reading focusing on different aspects of the form, function, and content (e.g., what were presented as ideal and nonideal occupations for retirees, what were presented as problems and solutions, and who was held out as exemplars of successful retirees). Texts and analysis sheets were read iteratively and were compared to identify discursive emphases and patterns across texts. A final phase of analysis involved rereading all texts to confirm emphases and check for disconfirming aspects and elaborate discourse patterns.

Key Results of the Critical Discourse Analysis in Regard to Occupation

Specific results of the substudies have been previously published (Laliberte Rudman, 2005, 2006b; Laliberte Rudman & Molke, 2009; Laliberte Rudman et al., 2009), and raw data are not repeated in this chapter. Using the concept of occupational possibilities that has evolved out of these substudies (Laliberte Rudman, 2010), I overview here the key findings across the substudies in relation to the types of occupations, and their associated outcomes, that were shaped as possible, ideal, and ethical for people preparing for and living in retirement. To demonstrate how the findings relate to the situated and socially constructed nature of occupation, I present two analytical examples that address how ideal occupations are discursively shaped in ways that link with neoliberal rationality and critically consider the potentially marginalizing effects of these discourses.

Parallel to the contention of governmentality theorists that subjectivity is an essential object and target of contemporary discursive technologies of governing (Dean, 1995; Rose, 1999), I contend, based on these CDA studies, that occupation is also an essential object and target. Governing is intimately linked to occupation, such that power, operating through discourses, attempts to shape what people come to take for granted as the occupations they should do. Such discourses also align ideal occupations with desired outcomes, such as independence and productivity, that parallel broader political values and aims. I use the term *occupational possibilities* to refer to the ways and types of doing that come to be viewed as ideal, possible, and ethical within a specific context. While not deterministic, occupational possibilities that have been constructed through discourse demark acceptable possibilities for thought and action, for both individuals and the systems within which they act (Laliberte Rudman, 2010). For example, how various social agents, including occupational scientists and occupational therapists, come to write and talk about the occupational needs of aging individuals influences what comes to be seen as required occupational therapy services and what types of services are funded.

A consistent finding across the substudies was that retirement and the aging process, more broadly, were discursively framed as processes modern aging individuals can and should take on responsibility for managing, most often beginning in mid-life. This framing aligns well with neoliberal approaches to governing that seek to individualize responsibility and activate segments of the population who are at risk of becoming dependent on the state (Polivka & Longino, 2006). There was a pervasive message that choosing and enacting the right occupations is an essential part of becoming and being a "successful" retiree. Aging individuals were encouraged to defy or battle dependency, disability, and oldness through wise, proactive occupational choices. Problems previously framed as social, or that can be argued to be at least partially shaped by social, economic, and political conditions, such as ageism or later life poverty, were shaped as individual problems to be overcome through the right occupational choices. In relation to the so-called right occupations, texts promoted engagement in particular consumer-based, body management, and work-based occupations. Idealized consumer-based occupations involved seeking out and consuming products, services, and knowledge within the private marketplace, such as housing and travel options. Such occupations were framed as enabling one to stay youthful and active, as well as reduce risks of incurring negative outcomes associated

with oldness. Body management occupations, such as physically active leisure and cosmetic activities, often included consumerism and tied occupations to keeping one's body youthful, active, and healthy. Continued involvement in the formal labor market past the traditional retirement age was promoted as an option that can lead to age-defiance, self-reliance, and self-fulfillment, as well as reduced risks of negative outcomes, such as social isolation and poverty (Laliberte Rudman, 2005, 2006b; Laliberte & Molke, 2009; Laliberte Rudman et al., 2009).

While the overall message that engagement in occupation can support health and other positive outcomes in retirement appears consistent with the beliefs and values underlying occupational therapy, it is vitally important to critically reflect on the particular ways occupation is being shaped within contemporary discourses and for whom occupational possibilities are being created. Attending to how discourses are a means through which governing occurs leads to critical consideration of how occupational possibilities are being shaped for retirees and retirement in ways that align with broader political aims and desires, such as emphases on individual responsibility, and not necessarily in ways that promote equity or well-being.

For example, in the substudy focused on work, it was found that productivity was narrowly defined as participation in the paid labor market. Idealized work options were often part of the secondary or contingent job market, such as contract and part-time work, or involved drawing on personal finances to become an entrepreneur. Such options were portrayed as ideal for the older worker, who was depicted as more concerned with flexibility and stimulation than financial remuneration. Within occupational science and occupational therapy, there is a long-standing recognition that productive occupations extend beyond the formal labor force (Polatajko et al., 2007). However, in the texts analyzed, paid work was set apart, shaping a narrow definition of productive occupations that fit within a neoliberal emphasis on activating those who fail to make a contribution to the market or are at risk of state dependency. This narrow definition of productivity could, in turn, shape the types of productive occupations that are recognized, valued, and supported by social policy, workplaces, and health care services for aging individuals. For example, it may contribute to the continuing invisibility and lack of state support for informal caregiving work engaged in by many aging individuals, further removing discussion of ways to support such work from policy agendas and institutional practices. Moreover, by minimizing the need for financial remuneration, as well as individualizing any potential health and attitudinal barriers to work in later life, the productive aging discourse deflects attention away from those aging individuals whose social conditions and patterns of employment have led to lower lifetime earnings and limited opportunities for financial planning. In line with neoliberal political rationality, this deflection can support further state and business retreat from financial and other supports for later life, such as pensions or re-training programs. At the same time, it creates few positive occupational possibilities for those segments of the aging population who may have little choice but to remain in the labor force and are more likely to be relegated to unstable, contingent forms of employment in later life (Laliberte Rudman & Molke, 2009).

A second example is drawn from the substudy focused on housing. Within these texts, a key feature of the so-called right places for retirement living, which were often depicted as communities of active, youthful retirees, were that they provided access to consumer activities, physically active leisure options, and "cultured" occupations. Such communities, and the occupations they afforded, were presented as a means to achieve self-fulfillment, an active lifestyle, health, and, ultimately, the evasion of oldness itself. Both becoming part of these idealized retirement communities and participating in the occupations pro-moted requires aging individuals to have substantial health, financial, social, and other types of resources. In line with neoliberal rationality, these discourses of ideal housing promote options to be found in the private marketplace and either evade discussion of or present public housing options as undesirable places for those who have failed to take a responsible approach to aging. As such, discourses about ideal housing options for aging individuals sustain and promote the polarization of occupational possibilities between affluent and nonaffluent aging individuals, and between "youthful" and "old" retirees. Although occupa-tional possibilities are created for some aging individuals through these discourses, aging people who face financial, bodily, and social challenges to engagement in these com-munities and their associated menus of occupations are either excluded or are framed as vulnerable due to their own irresponsibility. In turn, this exclusion from dominant discourses about ideal housing options for later life, and the neoliberal emphases in these articles on the possibility of attaining such ideal options through proactive financial planning and wise lifestyle choices, may make the need for public support of housing options for later life and pro-grams to support meaningful occupational opportunities for aging individuals with varying resources less visible (Laliberte Rudman et al., 2009).

Research Linking Discourses and Individual Narratives

Methodology and Research Objectives for Linking Discourses and Narratives

The overall objective of the second aspect of this program of research is to explore the implications of contempo-rary discourses of retirement for how aging people convey how they negotiate, experience, and perform occupation in preparing for, and living in, retirement. This study draws on social constructionist approaches to narrative inquiry, conceptualizing people as both constructing and conveying meaning through the stories they tell. Narratives are not viewed as static representations of how life has been lived, but as active constructions in which individuals draw on various interpretive resources, including discourses, to make sense of whom they are and how they have lived life (Chase, 2005; Gubrium & Holstein, 2009). Narratives of preparing for and living in retirement have been elicited from 30 Canadians, aged 45 and older. At present, the analysis of these narratives is ongoing. Below, I outline the methods used and draw on two narratives to display the complex and varying ways that broader discourses regarding retirement were taken up and negotiated in relation to occupation.

Methods for Linking Discourses and Narratives

Ethics approval was obtained from the University of Western Ontario Research Ethics Board. Because media regarding retirement is increasingly aimed at those prepar-ing for retirement, as well as those living in retirement, the sample was stratified into two age groups: those aged 45 to 64 ($n = 15$) and those aged 65 and older ($n = 15$). Other inclu-sion criteria were that participants characterized them-selves as preparing for or living in their retirement years, had the ability to participate in an interview in English, and were exposed to Canadian print media.

Four trained interviewers and myself used a two-stage process based on Wengraf's (2001) framework for narrative elicitation. Methods of elicitation using visual prompts were also incorporated (Harrison, 2002). All interviews were audiorecorded and transcribed verbatim. The first stage was an open-ended narrative interview. For participants who defined themselves as preparing for, but not yet in, their retirement years, the main narrative prompt was "I would like you to tell me your story of how you are pre-paring for your retirement years, including all the events and experiences which are important for you. Start wher-ever you like." For participants who defined themselves as retired, a second main narrative prompt was "I would also like you to tell me your story of entering and living in your retirement years, including all the events and experi-ences which were important for you. Start wherever you like." Follow-up questions, aimed at eliciting further detail regarding topics raised in the open narrative interview, followed the responses to the narrative prompt(s). In the second stage, further follow-up questions were asked to elicit more narrative, and participants were asked to talk about their perceptions of media coverage of retirement. As well, images drawn from media sources to represent various discourse patterns regarding retirement were used to elicit participants' perceptions.

A two-step approach to narrative analysis is being used: (a) reconstruction of narratives from interview transcripts and (b) deconstruction of narratives to examine ways informants draw on discourses of retirement (Fraser, 2004; Polkinghorne, 1995). In the first step, following multiple readings of interview data, a condensed written story for each participant is developed from interview transcripts. This process involves placing information conveyed into chronological order and fleshing out key events and story threads (Polkinghorne, 1995). The second step, informed by a critical lens, focuses on how individuals "make sense of personal experience in relation to culturally and historically specific discourses, and how they draw on, resist, and/or transform these discourses as they narrate their selves, experiences, and realities" (Chase, 2005, p. 659). Drawing on the analyses conducted in the first stage of the research program, as well as other studies addressing discourses of retirement, I purposefully reread the reconstructed narratives and the original transcripts to look for sections in which informants refer to broader discourses about retirement. I then examined how they talk about these discourses and how they are linked to occupation.

Key Results Related to Occupation From Linking Discourses and Narratives

As narrative analysis is ongoing, this section focuses on displaying how this methodological approach provides a way forward in understanding the situated and socially constructed nature of occupation. An emerging finding is that broader discourses of retirement are taken up by informants in their narratives to make sense of how they have negotiated their occupations in moving toward retirement. Discourses appear to influence what informants convey as possible and ideal occupations for themselves and are narrated as impacting upon how they experience their occupations and selves in everyday life. Informants both took up and resisted so-called positive discourses of retirement, emphasizing autonomy, youthfulness, busyness, responsibility, and productivity. Many of the informants convey a desire to work toward ideal discursive constructions of retirement and the outcomes they portray. They also convey struggles in working toward these ideals. The complex, diverse ways discourses and occupation interrelate are illustrated next, through a critical, interpretive presentation of aspects of two narratives.

Narrative Example 1

Mrs. D. is a 58-year-old married woman who lives in a modest home in a middle-class neighborhood. She retired 3 years ago from a full-time management job in a large firm. Mrs. D. had thought, "I would probably work until I was 60," but took a "buy-out" package when "the writing kind of was on the wall." She perceived that this was the company's "way of nicely saying, you are not going to find anything else in this company and so it's probably in your interest to get out of it." Mrs. D. has not returned to paid employment, indicating she has "no desire to go back to work." Mrs. D. considers herself "partially retired" as her 59-year-old husband is still employed, largely for financial reasons, as a full-time janitor.

Mrs. D.'s narrative was characterized by a pervasive tension related to balancing social expectations regarding productivity for "young retirees" with her own resistance to paid work involvement. This resulted in expressions of guilt regarding not engaging in those occupations discursively defined as right. At the beginning of her narrative, Mrs. D. describes herself as "quite happy to sit at home and be a homemaker." She describes her typical day as follows.

> I get up in the morning, and I read the paper. Sometimes, I read the paper until 12 o'clock noon, and then I do what I have to do, go to Curves (an exercise club for women), I work out. I walk and do a little bit of housework, and watch a little bit of TV and talk to the cats, and it's kind of not a bad life at all. (Laliberte Rudman, 2009-2010)

Seemingly contradictory to the ethic of busyness that pervades contemporary discourses on retirement and the emphasis on productive activities, Mrs. D. indicates that she has chosen to not commit herself to many scheduled activities, particularly in the realms of work and volunteering. "I don't even want to volunteer because that to me is another commitment. I just don't want any commitments to deal with."

Although Mrs. D. sometimes confidently asserts she is content with her occupations, she also expresses an inner tension related to not living up to what she describes as the "norm." When asked to describe this norm, Mrs. D. drew on a media example that reflects the broader discursive emphasis on particular productive occupations.

> We get these books from X (previous company) on a monthly basis, and it's like for pensioners and... they'll target a pensioner and what this person is doing now. And, oh, she's started this home business or she's knitting afghans for the kids in Africa or, you know. And I think, ooh, please don't come see me because, I don't know whether it's an inner thing that I'm manifesting within myself because I'm not reconciling myself to accepting what I'm doing... The norm is that you're expected to do all this marvelous stuff after you retire, and it's just not easy. (Laliberte Rudman, 2009-2010)

Mrs. D. describes how dealing with this social expectation leads to "a constant inside fight you have... trying to not feel guilty about doing the things you want to do even though they're not what is the expected." She expresses feelings of guilt related to her occupations.

> There are times... that I had felt guilty. From the perspective of should I be more community-oriented? Should I be out volunteering? I have all this time, and I'm not giving back to the community. I'm not sharing all this free time that I have, because I think in a lot of cases expectations nowadays are, if you're retired then you should be pursuing something else. You should be starting a business yourself or you should be volunteering and sometimes I get guilt feelings over that... (Laliberte Rudman, 2009-2010)

Mrs. D. also appears to evaluate her days, and her occupations, in relation to the larger discursive message regarding productivity: "I have my bad days and my good days. Some days, I think at the end of the day, oh my God, what did you do today? You did nothing productive." She expresses frustration with the narrow definition of productivity conveyed through contemporary discourses and struggles to fit her current occupations into this definition: "I feel I've been very productive around here. I mean, since I was painting the other day and I'm trying to do some baking and other stuff like that but, just to someone else that's... not a productive thing."

Mrs. D. relates her feelings of guilt and lack of full acceptance of her current occupations to her identity as a responsible person. In line with contemporary discourses emphasizing the need for retirees to be responsible and productive, she questions if her current occupations convey that she is a responsible person. "It's hard for me. I think I've been very, what's the word I'm looking for...responsible. I've been a very, very responsible person, and if there's something I should be doing, then I should do it." After 2 years of retirement, Mrs. D. indicates she is "trying to figure out for myself, what do I do on a daily basis?" Mrs. D. ends her narrative talking about her uncertainty regarding her future occupations, musing that "maybe sometime within the next few years I will look for a job or I'll do volunteering, but right now it's more important for me to do what I want to do when I want to do it."

Narrative Example 2

Ms. S. is a 62-year-old woman who retired "very young" 10 years ago from a full-time job as an elementary school teacher. She received a retirement package and a private pension and felt "ready" to stop teaching. Her husband retired at the same time, and they subsequently separated. She considers herself partially retired, as she currently works part-time and volunteers as a musician in her "post-retirement job."

In many ways, Ms. S.'s narrative is different from that of Mrs. D. Ms. S. has readily taken on several ideal aspects of occupations promoted in contemporary discourses of retirement and identifies herself as an "active retiree." Indeed, Ms. S. draws on larger discourses of positive retirement to frame herself as a "young retiree" and to explain key decisions she has made. However, Ms. S's narrative also raises concerns about the marginalizing potential of such discourses, in that she actively works to distance herself from those she sees as "old."

Ms. S. describes her occupations in retirement in ways that draw on broader discursive messages regarding the importance of being proactive, stressing how retirees should take on responsibility for ensuring their health and security. "It's really important for retired people to do something with their life because they should be active as long as they can be." She explains that she is "extremely busy," interestingly highlighting the three types of occupations (body management, consumer-based, and productive) promoted within contemporary retirement discourses. She connects her engagement in exercise to living up to her responsibility to be self-reliant. "I feel it's important for us to keep ourselves as physically fit as we can, so that we can enjoy our retirement and not be a burden to others." She refers to consumption-based activities as a means to fulfill her obligation to remain youthful:

> You have an obligation to prolong... this healthy stage of your retirement... Do everything you can to stop it... I just heard... that you can buy, it's a video game… I think to help seniors have a better memory. It's on the market now, and I will look into it. (Laliberte Rudman, 2009-2010)

Indeed, Ms. S. frames her decision to return to performing music, which she put on hold when she became a teacher and mother, to the importance of being productive and youthful. "I have taken on another career. Because I'm a young retiree, I felt that I wanted to be an active retiree."

Although Ms. S. in many ways seems to have successfully taken on occupations that enable her to enact discursive messages regarding ideal ways to be and do, Ms. S. also appears to hold ageist attitudes toward those who she sees as "old." Consistent with concerns raised by critical gerontologists that contemporary discourses stressing the prolongation of youthfulness and the possibility of evading old age via responsible lifestyle choices may perpetuate ageist attitudes against those who are seen as having failed to evade oldness, Ms. S. actively engages in narrative work to distance herself from "old people."

> And there are a lot of seniors who do look senior. And senior means like overweight, not walking, walking with a... limp in their gait... Like I feel when I walk... I don't limp. I walk, I run... So I try not to portray that senior as much as I can. (Laliberte Rudman, 2009-2010)

Ms. S. indicates she is trying to avoid seeing herself and being seen as a "senior," pointing to the types of seniors she sees negatively.

> You see people... old, being overweight, can hardly walk, grey hair, etc. Those are not the seniors that I know. Seniors that I hang around with try to keep themselves looking as good as they can... they can watch their weight, they can be fairly trim, be fairly active. Most of my friends are very, very active, happy. (Laliberte Rudman, 2009-2010)

Indeed, while indicating that she and her husband "never had a really strong marriage," Ms. S. draws on the different approaches to occupations in retirement taken by herself and her former husband to provide a rationale for how they came to be separated.

> It turned out that I wanted to be active and going and enjoying and being positive and living each day. My husband... didn't want to be involved with volunteering so he tended to lead a very quiet, sedate life and wasn't very happy with maybe some of the things I was doing. I wanted to be active in that way so, as a result, we have separated, and I'm very happy about it. (Laliberte Rudman, 2009-2010)

Consistent with contemporary discourses that hold out the promise of the evasion of oldness, Ms. S. looks to the consumer market for various ways to defy becoming old, although she expresses that becoming "old" may be inevitable.

> I'm not lying to myself. I know that each year I'm getting closer and closer to that. I go to a hospital once a week to visit people, and I see, some of them a lot younger than me, the situation they're in. So I'm trying to keep as young at heart as I can be and do the very best I can be to be young and prolong that, as long as I can. (Laliberte Rudman, 2009-2010)

However, Ms. S. does not envision positive occupational possibilities if she becomes "old." Like broader discourses of retirement, she envisions this only as a time in which she will be a burden.

CONTRIBUTION TO OCCUPATIONAL SCIENCE

The key premise underpinning this program of research is that the occupations that individuals, and collectives, do in everyday life are shaped by, and influence the shaping of, contextual features. Integrating theoretical concepts from occupational science with critical social gerontology and governmentality theory, and drawing together CDA and narrative inquiry, this research raises concerns regarding how occupational possibilities come to be shaped for particular groups of people in ways that align with broader political aims and desires, particularly those emphasizing enhanced individual responsibility to proactively manage life course risks in the private market. It illustrates various ways that discursive constructions of retirement are shaping "the very nature of older age in a given society, and influence the conditions in which individuals materially and emotionally experience and live out their lives" (Kemp & Denton, 2003, p. 757). Both the CDA findings and the evolving narrative findings question increasingly taken-for-granted and ideal ways to be and do in retirement. This points to the need to critically analyze what forms of occupations are promoted or excluded and who can participate and not participate in those promoted occupations. Moreover, the narrative data point to various ways that discursive messages may be negotiated by individuals, influencing what they do, how they feel about what they do, and with whom they do things.

Of broader relevance to the research agenda in occupational science is the proposition that occupation itself is an essential aspect of how individuals and collectives are governed. Drawing on the broad notion of government advanced by governmentality theorists, which encompasses all actions designed to shape the conduct of others in ways

that align with political values and aims, it is argued that occupation and power have become intimately linked in many contemporary societies. Within the broader rise of the creation of the "active society," as it is informed by neoliberal rationality (Dannefer, 2000; Dean, 1995; Walters, 1997), various social authorities and agencies, such as formal governmental bodies, public media, health care institutions, workplaces, and educational institutions, seek to shape the occupations of collectives and individuals. Through various types of technologies of government, including discourses, these authorities and agencies mark out particular occupations as possible, ideal, and ethical and others as not possible, nonideal, and unethical. This research offers the concept of occupational possibilities as one way to think about how power shapes what comes to be taken for granted by individuals and collectivities, including occupational scientists and occupational therapists, as the right occupations for particular types of people. This research program demonstrates the critical role that occupational scientists can play, based upon their broad understanding of occupation, in examining the subtle ways in which occupational possibilities are shaped through discourse to create opportunities for some types of citizens while simultaneously marginalizing others.

In addition, if occupation is a key aspect of contemporary forms of government, then occupational scientists must continue to move forward in developing theoretical and methodological approaches to situating occupation. Within the field of social gerontology, Walker (2006) has argued that a primary focus on microsociological perspectives may mean that research will fail to address growing inequalities experienced by aging individuals arising from social and political conditions. While not negating the continued importance of work that seeks to highlight how individuals orchestrate occupations and the significance of occupations in the lives of individuals, a sole focus on occupation at the microlevel may mean that our work as occupational scientists will not enable us, and those who take up our work, to address vital contemporary issues related to occupational injustice, occupational apartheid, or occupational marginalization, on local, national, and global scales.

Within this program of research, merging concepts from occupational science with interdisciplinary concepts from governmentality and critical gerontology provided a theoretical basis that has enabled an innovative methodological approach to exploring interconnections between discourse and narrative (Clark, 2006; Yerxa, 2000). Based on my ongoing analysis of the narratives, I contend that focusing on how occupations are narrated in relation to discourses provides a useful lens through which one can analyze the ways in which macrolevel contextual features connect with how individuals negotiate and make sense of their occupations.

IMPLICATIONS FOR OCCUPATIONAL THERAPY

In relation to occupational therapy practice, this program of research seeks to raise awareness of the importance of attending to macrolevel contextual features and pressures in order to comprehensively understand how individuals negotiate and enact occupation in daily life. This work highlights the importance of considering how our own expectations of what clients should and should not do are themselves influenced by the contexts in which we live and practice. For example, funding mechanisms for home care services for aging clients may be based on taken-for-granted assumptions regarding the types of occupations in which they need to engage. In turn, these funding mechanisms set boundaries on the services that occupational therapists can provide, perhaps narrowing these to a range of occupations tied only to particular goals that support governmental aims, such as independence in self-care.

Moreover, as occupational therapists, the texts we construct and draw upon, in academia, in our professional organizations, in our teaching, and in our practices, influence how we think about particular types of clients and what we come to take for granted as the "right" occupations we should enable. This work challenges occupational therapists to critically reflect on what they have come to take for granted as what I have termed the *occupational possibilities for their clients*. We must understand how occupational therapists themselves may contribute to bounding what clients come to see as possible and ideal occupations. Consideration of the ways in which larger political, economic, and cultural contextual features shape occupational possibilities for particular client groups may also provide a foundation for the expansion of advocacy work in partnership with clients (Jongbloed & Crichton, 1990; O'Brien et al., 2002).

Within occupational therapy, there is a growing movement to expand professional objectives to include political critique and social transformation (Pollard et al., 2009). Incorporating a social transformation model within occupational therapy requires an extension in focus beyond the needs of individual clients (Frank & Zemke, 2009), based on a critical awareness of the ways in which problems, which are often individualized in current health and social systems, are rooted in economic, political, and social conditions. Occupational science research addressing the ways in which occupation is situated and socially constructed has much to offer to the development and enactment of occupational therapy's role in social transformation seeking to enhance the occupational participation of marginalized and disempowered groups.

LEARNING SUPPORTS

Reading Media Using a Critically Informed Occupational Perspective

Purpose

To apply a critically informed occupational perspective to popular media, thereby considering how messages in the media pertaining to occupation are connected with macrolevel elements and may shape occupational possibilities.

Primary Concepts

Macrolevel elements, occupational possibilities, and critical lens.

Instructions

1. Search for a popular media text (e.g., a newspaper article, an online article, an advertisement) that addresses some aspect of occupation (e.g., physical activity for youth, leisure in later life, becoming a university student).

2. Drawing on this chapter, develop a set of questions that will enable you to examine what occupations are framed as ideal or appropriate for what types of people (e.g., What types of occupations are people advised to participate in? What types of people are addressed in the text? What types of outcomes are people supposed to prioritize?).

3. Read the text and record responses to the questions on your analysis sheet.

4. Looking across your responses, write a four-page response to the following questions: What occupational possibilities are forefronted as ideal? Who can, and cannot, participate in these occupations? How might occupational possibilities framed as ideal be related to macrolevel elements, such as political and economic goals of enhancing individual responsibility or decreasing state dependency?

Self-Narrative Regarding Occupation

Purpose

To enhance sensitivity to macrolevel elements that shape occupational possibilities through examination of how one's own occupations are shaped within particular contexts.

Primary Concepts

Macrolevel elements, occupational possibilities, and reflexivity.

Instructions

1. Choose a key occupational transition you have experienced in your life, when you had to make an important choice related to occupation (e.g., becoming an occupational therapist, going to a particular college or university, becoming a parent).

2. Write a three-page reflective paper that considers contextual influences on your choice.

3. In your concluding paragraph, address these questions: In what ways are my occupations socially situated and constructed? How do I negotiate contextual influences on my occupations?

Group Critical Reflection on Texts Produced and Utilized by Occupational Therapists

Primary Concepts

Discourse, government, and role of occupational therapy in shaping occupational possibilities.

Instructions

1. Working with a group of students, select a text written by an occupational therapy author or organization that addresses the occupational therapy role with a particular client group (e.g., a professional association position paper on the role of occupational therapy with older adults or a book chapter outlining the occupational therapy scope of practice with children with physical disabilities).

2. Have each member of the group read the text individually and write notes regarding what the text conveys about what occupations are possible, right, and ideal for clients (and perhaps which are not possible, are inappropriate, or are nonideal).

3. As a group, discuss your notes addressing the questions: What key assumptions about occupations are conveyed in the text? What types of occupational therapy practice would be supported by this text? What types of practice, and what types of occupation, would not be supported by this text?

ACKNOWLEDGMENTS

Funding for the research program described in this chapter has been received from several sources, including the Social Sciences and Humanities Research Council of Canada, the Ontario Graduate Scholarship Program, the Royal Canadian Legion, and the Canadian Occupational Therapy Foundation. The following individuals were involved as graduate student research trainees and contributed to data collection and analysis activities: Silke Dennhardt, Suzanne Huot, and Daniel Molke. Kathy Ellis served as research coordinator for the narrative study.

REFERENCES

Ainsworth, S., & Hardy, C. (2004). Critical discourse analysis and identity: Why bother? *Critical Discourse Studies, 1*(2), 225-259. doi:10.1080/1740590042000302085

Allen, B. (1991). Government in Foucault. *Canadian Journal of Philosophy, 21*, 421-439.

Baars, J., Dannefer, D., Phillipson, C., & Walker, A. (2006). An introduction: Critical perspectives in social gerontology. In J. Baars, D. Dannefer, C. Phillipson, & A. Walker (Eds.), *Aging, globalization and inequality: The new critical gerontology* (pp. 1-14). Amityville, NY: Baywood Publishing.

Ballinger, C., & Cheek, J. (2006). Discourse analysis in action: The construction of risk in a community day hospital. In *Qualitative research for allied health professionals: Challenge choices* (pp. 200-217). Chichester, England: John Wiley and Sons.

Beagan, B. L., & Etowa, J. (2009). The impact of everyday racism on the occupations of African Canadian women. *Canadian Journal of Occupational Therapy, 76*(4), 285-293.

Bennett, T. (2003). Culture and governmentality. In J. Z. Bratich, J. Packer, & C. McCarthy (Eds.), *Foucault, cultural studies and governmentality* (pp. 47-66). Albany, NY: State University of New York Press.

Biggs, S. (2001). Towards critical narrativity: Stories of aging in contemporary social policy. *Journal of Aging Studies, 15*, 303-316. doi:10.1016/S0890-4065(01)00025-1

Bratich, J. Z., Packer, J., & McCarthy, C. (2003). Governing the present. In J. Z. Bratich, J. Packer & C. McCarthy (Eds.), *Foucault, cultural studies and governmentality* (pp. 3-22). Albany, NY: State University of New York Press.

Broad, D., & Anthony, W. (1999). Citizenship and social policy: Neoliberalism and beyond. In D. Broad & W. Anthony (Eds.), *Citizens or consumers? Social policy in a market society* (pp. 9-19). Halifax, Nova Scotia, Canada: Fernwood Publishing.

Calasanti, T. (2002). Work and retirement in the 21st century: Integrating issues of diversity and globalization. *Ageing International, 27*(3), 3-20.

Chase, S. E. (2005). Narrative inquiry: Multiple lenses, approaches, voices. In N. Denzin & Y. Lincoln (Eds.), *The Sage handbook of qualitative research* (3rd ed., pp. 651-679). Thousand Oaks, CA: Sage Publications.

Cheek, J. (2004). At the margins? Discourse analysis and qualitative research. *Qualitative Health Research, 14*, 1140-1150. doi:10.1177/1049732304266820

Clark, F. (2006). One person's thoughts on the future of occupational science. *Journal of Occupational Science, 13*(3), 167-179. doi:10.1080/14427591.2006.9726513

Cooke, M. (2006). Policy change and the labour force participation of older workers: Evidence from six countries. *Canadian Journal on Aging, 25*, 387-400. doi:10.1353/cja.2007.0015

Curl, A. L., & Hokenstad, M. C. (2006). Reshaping retirement policies in post-industrial nations: The need for flexibility. *Journal of Sociology and Social Welfare, 33*(2), 85-106.

Dannefer, D. (2000). Bringing risk back in: The regulation of the self in the postmodern state. In K. Warner Schaie & J. Hendricks (Eds.), *The evolution of the aging self: The societal impact of the aging process* (pp. 269-280). New York, NY: Springer.

Dean, M. (1994). 'A social structure of many souls': moral regulation, government and self-formation. *Canadian Journal of Sociology, 19,* 145-168. doi:10.2307/3341342

Dean, M. (1995). Governing the unemployed self in an active society. *Economy and Society, 24,* 559-583. doi:10.1080/03085149500000025

Dickie, V., Cutchin, M. P., & Humphry, R. (2006). Occupational as transactional experience: A critique of individualism in occupational science. *Journal of Occupational Science, 13,* 83-93. doi:10.1080/14427591.2006.9686573

Dyck, I., & Jongbloed, L. (2000). Women with multiple sclerosis and employment issues: A focus on social and institutional environments. *Canadian Journal of Occupational Therapy, 67,* 337-346.

Fairclough, N. (1992). *Discourse and social change.* Cambridge, United Kingdom: Polity Press.

Foucault, M. (1991). Governmentality (P. Pasquino, Trans.). In G. Burchell, C. Gordon, & P. Miller (Eds.), *The Foucault effect: Studies in governmentality* (pp. 87-104). Chicago, IL: University of Chicago Press.

Frank, G., & Zemke, R. (2009). Occupational therapy foundations for political engagement and social transformation. In N. Pollard, D. Sakellariou, & F. Kronenberg (Eds.), *A political practice of occupational therapy* (pp. 111-133). London, England: Churchill Livingstone, Elsevier.

Fraser, H. (2004). Doing narrative research. *Qualitative Social Work, 3*(2), 179-201. doi:10.1177/1473325004043383

Gubrium, J. F., & Holstein, J. A. (1998). Narrative practice and the coherence of personal stories. *The Sociological Quarterly, 39*(1), 163-187. doi:10.1111/j.1533-8525.1998.tb02354.x

Gubrium, J. F., & Holstein, J. A. (2009). *Analyzing narrative reality.* Thousand Oaks, CA: Sage Publications.

Harrison, B. (2002). Visual methodologies. *Sociology of Health and Illness, 24*(6), 856-872.

Hocking, C. (2000). Occupational science: A stock take of accumulated insights. *Journal of Occupational Science, 7*(2), 58-67. doi:10.1080/14427591.2000.9686466

Hugman, R. (1999). Ageing, occupation and social engagement: Towards a lively later life. *Journal of Occupational Science, 6,* 61-67. doi:10.1080/14427591.1999.9686452

Jongbloed, L., & Crichton, A. (1990). A new definition of disability: Implications for rehabilitation practice and social policy. *Canadian Journal of Occupational Therapy, 65,* 193-201.

Jonsson, H., Josephsson, S., & Kielhofner, G. (2000). Evolving narratives in the course of retirement: A longitudinal study. *American Journal of Occupational Therapy, 54,* 463-470. doi:10.5014/ajot.54.5.463

Katz, S. (2000). Busy bodies: Activity, aging and the management of everyday life. *Journal of Aging Studies, 14,* 135-162. doi:10.1016/S0890-4065(00)80008-0

Kemp, C. L., & Denton, M. (2003). The allocation of responsibility for later life: Canadian reflections on the roles of individuals, governments, employers and families. *Ageing & Society, 23,* 737-760. doi:10.1017/S0144686X03001363

Laliberte Rudman, D. (2005). Understanding political influences on occupational possibilities: An analysis of newspaper constructions of retirees. *Journal of Occupational Science, 12*(3), 149-160. doi:10.1080/14427591.2005.9686558

Laliberte Rudman, D. (2006a). "Positive aging" and its implications for occupational possibilities in later life. *Canadian Journal of Occupational Therapy, 73*(3), 188-192.

Laliberte Rudman, D. (2006b). Shaping the active, autonomous and responsible modern retiree: An analysis of discursive technologies and their connections with neoliberal political rationality. *Ageing and Society, 26,* 181-201. doi:10.1017/S0144686X05004253

Laliberte Rudman, D. (2009-2010). [Re-shaping the modern retiree]. Unpublished raw data.

Laliberte Rudman, D. (2010). Occupational possibilites. *Journal of Occupational Science, 17*(1), 55-59.

Laliberte Rudman, D., Dennhardt, S., Fok, D., Huot, S., Molke, D., Park, A., & Zur, B. (2008). A vision for occupational science: Reflecting on our disciplinary culture. *Journal of Occupational Science, 15*(3), 136-146. doi:10.1080/14427591.2008.9686623

Laliberte Rudman, D., Huot, S., & Dennhardt, S. (2009). Shaping ideal places for retirement: Occupational possibilities within contemporary media. *Journal of Occupational Science, 16*(1), 18-24. doi:10.1080/14427591.2009.9686637

Laliberte Rudman, D., & Molke, D. (2009). Forever productive: The discursive shaping of later life workers in contemporary Canadian newspapers. *WORK: A Journal of Prevention, Assessment & Rehabilitation, 32*(4), 377-390. doi:10.3233/WOR-2009-0850

Magasi, S., & Hammel, J. (2009). Women with disabilities' experiences in long-term care: A case for social justice. *American Journal of Occupational Therapy, 63*(1), 35-46. doi:10.5014/ajot.63.1.35

Mann, K. (2007). Activation, retirement planning and restraining the "third age." *Social Policy & Society, 6,* 279-292. doi:10.1017/S1474746407003624

Martinson, M., & Minkler, M. (2006). Civic engagement and older adults: A critical perspective. *The Gerontologist, 46*(3), 318-324. doi:10.1093/geront/46.3.318

Molineux, M., & Whiteford, G. (2006). Occupational science: Genesis, evolution and future contribution. In E. Duncan (Ed.), *Foundations for practice in occupational therapy* (pp. 297-312). Edinburgh, Scotland: Elsevier.

O'Brien, P., Dyck, I., Caron, S., & Mortenson, B. (2002). Environmental analysis: Insights from sociological and geographical perspectives. *Canadian Journal of Occupational Therapy, 69*(4), 229-238.

O'Rand, A. M. (2000). Risk, rationality and modernity: Social policy and the aging self. In K. Warner Schaie & J. Hendricks (Eds.), *The evolution of the aging self: The societal impact on the aging process* (pp. 225-249). New York, NY: Springer.

Organization for Economic Cooperation and Development (2006). *Live longer, work longer.* Paris: Author.

Phelan, S., & Kinsella, A. (2009). Occupational identity: Engaging sociocultural perspectives. *Journal of Occupational Science, 16*(2), 85-91. doi:10.1080/14427591.2009.9686647

Phillipson, C. (2004). Work and retirement transitions: Changing sociological and social policy contexts. *Social Policy & Society, 3,* 155-162. doi:10.1017/S1474746403001611

Pierce, D., Atler, K., Baltisberger, J., Fehringer, E., Hunter, E., Malkawi, S., & Parr, T. (2010). Occupational science: A data-based American perspective. *Journal of Occupational Science, 17*(3). doi:10.1080/14427591.2010.9686697

Polatajko, H., Molke, D., Baptiste, S., Doble, J., Caron Santha, B., Kirsh, B., . . . Stadnyk, R. (2007). Occupational science: Imperatives for occupational therapy. In E. A. Townsend & H. J. Polatajko (Eds.), *Enabling occupation II: Advancing an occupational therapy vision for health, well-being & justice through occupation* (pp. 63-82). Ottawa, Ontario, Canada: CAOT.

Polivka, L., & Longino, C. F. (2006). The emerging postmodern culture of aging and retirement society. In J. Baars, D. Dannefer, C. Phillipson, & A. Walker (Eds.), *Aging, globalization and inequality: The new critical gerontology* (pp. 183-204). Amityville, NY: Baywood Publishing.

Polkinghorne, D. E. (1995). Narrative configuration in qualitative analysis. In R. Miller (Ed.), *Biographical research methods* (pp. 69-89). Thousand Oaks, CA: Sage Publications.

Pollard, N., Kronenberg, F., & Sakellariou, D. (2009). A political practice of occupational therapy. In N. Pollard, D. Sakellariou, & F. Kronenberg (Eds.), *A political practice of occupational therapy* (pp. 3-17). London, England: Churchill Livingstone, Elsevier.

Potter, J., & Wetherell, M. (1987). *Discourse and social psychology: Beyond attitudes.* London, England: Sage Publications.

Power, E. (2005). The unfreedom of being other: Canadian lone mothers' experience of poverty and "life on the cheque." *Sociology, 39*(4), 643-660. doi:10.1177/0038038505056023

Riach, K. (2007). "Othering" older worker identity in recruitment. *Human Relations, 60*(11), 1701-1726. doi:10.1177/0018726707084305

Rose, N. (1999). *Powers of freedom: Reframing political thought.* Cambridge, United Kingdom: University of Cambridge Press.

Shuey, K., & O'Rand, A. (2006). Changing demographics and new pension risks. *Research on Aging, 28*(3), 317-340. doi:10.1177/0164027505285919

Suto, M. (2009). Compromised careers: The occupational transition of immigration and resettlement. *Work, 32*(4), 417-429. doi:10.3233/WOR-2009-0853

Townsend, E., & Wilcox, A. A. (2004). Occupational justice. In C. H. Christiansen & E. A. Townsend (Eds.), *Introduction to occupation: The art and science of living* (pp. 243-273). Thorofare, NJ: SLACK Incorporated.

Walker, A. (2006). Reexamining the political economy of aging: Understanding the structure/agency tension. In J. Baars, D. Dannefer, C. Phillipson, & A. Walker (Eds.), *Aging, globalization and inequality: The new critical gerontology* (pp. 59-80). Amityville, NY: Baywood Publishing.

Walters, W. (1997). The "active society": New designs for social policy. *Policy and Politics, 25*, 221-234.

Wengraf, T. (2001). *Qualitative research interviewing—Biographic narrative and semi-structured methods.* Thousand Oaks, CA: Sage Publications.

Whiteford, G. (2010). Occupation in context. In M. Curtin, M. Molineux, & J. Supyk-Mellson (Eds.), *Occupational therapy and physical dysfunction—Enabling occupation* (6th ed., pp. 135-149). London, England: Elsevier.

Whiteford, G., Klomp, N., & Wright-St Clair, V. (2005). Complexity theory: Understanding occupation, practice and context. In G. Whiteford & V. Wright-St Clair (Eds.), *Occupation and practice in context* (pp. 3-15). Sydney, Australia: Churchill Livingston.

Yerxa, E. J. (2000). Occupational science: A renaissance of service to humankind through knowledge. *Occupational Therapy International, 7*, 87-98. doi:10.1002/oti.109.

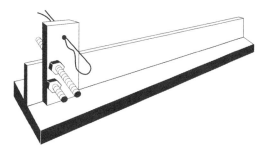

Intimate Partner Violence

Balancing Issues of Identity, Disability Culture, and Occupational Justice to Inform Occupational Therapy Practice

Diane L. Smith, PhD, OTR/L, FAOTA and Claudia List Hilton, PhD, OTR/L, FAOTA

This chapter will introduce the reader to the issue of abuse against women with disabilities as an example of occupational injustice. This particular area of research was explored because of the authors' mutual passion regarding the empowerment of women and the consideration of environmental influences that support or hinder the empowerment of women. Through personal knowledge and the experience of treating women and children with disabilities who have experienced abuse, these authors noted that the environmental influence of abuse hindered the ability of these clients to participate in meaningful and purposeful occupation of play, work, home care, and social engagement. However, the authors felt strongly that additional research and consideration of the influence of abuse on women with disabilities was necessary to fully inform themselves and occupational therapists of the issues and potential interventions.

Research shows that abuse is pervasive. National surveys to determine the prevalence of domestic violence reveal that between 25% and 31% of American women have been physically or sexually abused by a husband or boyfriend during their lifetimes (Collins, Schoen, Duchon, Simantor,

& Yellowitz, 1999; Tjaden & Thoennes, 2000). This number does not include those who experience nonphysical or nonsexual assaults, such as emotional abuse, intimidation, and controlling behaviors. Although some studies show that women without disabilities may be physically abused at a similar rate as women with disabilities, a significant difference was found in the duration of the violence, with women with disabilities experiencing multiple types of violence (sexual, physical, and emotional) for significantly longer periods of time (Nosek, Howland, & Young, 1997; Young, Nosek, Howland, Chanpong, & Rintala, 1997).

These research results confirm that women with disabilities experience all forms of abuse at a greater rate than women without disabilities, affecting their ability to participate in meaningful and purposeful activities—issues that the authors felt were examples of occupational justice. Therefore, using the occupational science components of occupational justice and injustice, this chapter will describe how research can conceptualize issues such as domestic abuse and further use this research to identify implications for occupational therapy practice in order to develop interventions to address the abuse.

Pierce, D. (Ed.).
Occupational Science for Occupational Therapy (pp. 157-167).
© 2014 SLACK Incorporated.

LITERATURE

Women With Disabilities Face Greater Risk

Due to the uniqueness of this issue, research addressing violence against women with disabilities has become more prevalent. One study conducted by the DisAbled Women's Network of Canada (Riddington, 1989) found that 40% of the 245 disabled women surveyed had experienced abuse, and 12% had been raped. However, although some studies have shown that women with disabilities were not significantly more likely than women without disabilities to have experienced any physical assault within the past year, as a woman with a disability, you could have four times the incidence of sexual assault (Martin et al., 2006).

Results from two focus groups at centers for independent living found that, although the reported violence experienced by women with disabilities is often identical to the violence experienced by women without disabilities, certain forms of violence are unique to women with disabilities (Gilson, Cramer, & DePoy, 2001). For example, a woman with a disability may need to depend on others to meet basic health or social needs, and actions that may not be considered abusive for women without disabilities may be extremely harmful for a woman with a disability (Curry, Hassouneh-Phillips, & Johnston-Silverberg, 2001). This may include behaviors such as removing a battery from her wheelchair, demanding a kiss before assisting her with a bath or transfer, or withholding medication that she needs.

Risk factors have been suggested to explain why a woman with a disability might experience increased vulnerability to violence. First, there is cultural devaluation of her gender as a female and her disability status. She may also be overprotected by her family with regard to exposing her to issues of sexuality, and there may be both internalized social stereotypes and reduced societal expectations with regard to sexuality (Belsky, 1980). Society often denies sexuality in women with disabilities, with women with disabilities often being considered asexual (Womendez & Schneiderman, 1991). In addition, if the woman has a certain type of disability that has associated cognitive limitations, such as traumatic brain injury, mental illness, and intellectual disability, she may have limited ability to recognize violence. Finally, a woman with disability may lack economic independence, increasing her risk of violence or abuse (Farmer & Tiefenthaler, 1996).

Brownridge (2006) examined the risk for partner violence against women with disabilities compared to women without disabilities. Women with disabilities reported 40% greater odds of violence in the 5 years preceding the interview, and those women appeared to be at particular risk for severe violence. There is also evidence that women with physical disabilities, who have higher levels of depression, are in a minority group, young, more educated, less mobile, and more socially isolated have a higher likelihood of experiencing abuse (Nosek, Hughes, Taylor, & Taylor, 2006).

Women with disabilities often have fewer resources to escape the violence than do women without disabilities. For example, as a woman with a disability who has been abused, you might face inaccessible shelter, home, or community environments or a lack of alternative attendant services (Hassouneh-Phillips & Curry, 2002). For many women, leaving an abusive relationship means a move toward greater independence. As a woman with disability, however, leaving may mean losing your independence and increasing your risk of moving to institutional care. You may not only be leaving a home environment that has been specifically modified to accommodate your disability, but you may be giving up the ability to care for your children as well. Thus, you may be faced with the dilemma of having to choose between giving up having essential health or personal needs met or experiencing violence. Even if you are able to seek help, you may not have access to information about existing services for victims of violence, you may not be able to contact these services if you do not have communication devices such as Text Telephones (TTYs), and you may be afraid of being misunderstood or not believed (Carlson, 1997; Furey, 1994; Womendez & Schneiderman, 1991).

Explanatory Models

Mays (2006) proposes feminist disability theory to explain violence against women with disabilities, which integrates traditional models articulated in criminology, law, medicine, psychology, and sociology (Dobash & Dobash, 1992; Finkelhor, 1988; Gelles, 1993; Gelles & Loseke, 1993a, 1993b; Rod, 1980) with disability and material feminist theory. With its emphasis on gender relations, disablism, and poverty, feminist disability theory can be used as a tool for exploring the nature and consequences of violence against women with disabilities. Feminist disability theory asserts the importance of recognizing the personal worth and dignity of women with disabilities, their collective identity, and their political organization. Therefore, this theory is a useful tool for interpreting individual experiences and how they link to broader societal conditions and arrangements. A weakness of this explanation, however, is its lack of attention to the relationship between domestic abuse of women with disabilities and the reduced opportunity for participation in meaningful occupations required for optimal health and quality of life.

Taking a more contextual approach, Sobsey (1994) proposes an ecological model for understanding the complex nature of the abuse of people with disabilities, which was expanded upon by Curry, Hassouneh-Phillips, and Johnston-Silverberg (2001). The model includes the environmental and cultural factors that contribute to the vulnerability of potential victims, the characteristics of potential victims that increase their vulnerability to abuse, and the characteristics of their potential offenders. Environmental and cultural factors include pervasive stigma and marginalization, which results in reduced status, increasing the risk for exploitation and abuse by those with higher status (Davis, 1997). This model suggests that factors such as negative stereotyping and failing to live up to the dominant standards of beauty may cause women with disabilities to have lower self-esteem, increasing their vulnerability to abuse (Asch & Fine, 1988; Blackwell-Stratton, Breslin, Mayerson, & Bailey, 1988; Thomas, 1998; Wendell, 1989). Finally, this model discusses rolelessness and lower income and how they can create a potential situation of dependency on the perpetrator for a woman with a disability, increasing the risk for abuse (Andrews & Veronen, 1993; Lonsdale, 1990).

The previous models have provided important conceptualizations regarding the abuse of women with and without disabilities. However, none explain how domestic abuse affects participation in meaningful and purposeful occupations by women with disabilities. As experienced occupational therapists and researchers, the authors considered it not only important for our profession to understand the enormity and impact of the issue of abuse for women with disabilities but also to consider how a uniquely "occupational" perspective, occupational science, frames this issue in order to provide the most effective intervention for clients with disabilities. Lack of understanding of the impact of abuse may hinder full engagement of the client in the therapeutic intervention and reduce outcomes. The remainder of this chapter will describe research that used secondary data analysis to determine the enormity of the issue, followed by a description of how components of occupational science, occupational justice, and injustice can be used to consider these issues for occupational therapy students and practitioners.

METHODS

Secondary Analysis of Existing Databases

To determine the importance of the issue of abuse against women with disabilities, the first author used secondary data analysis. Secondary analysis uses data that were gathered for previous research studies or other primary purposes but have not necessarily been used to examine issues relevant to occupational therapy. The main purpose of using this type of research is to describe or explore phenomena that may lead the researcher to ask more specific questions, to generate hypotheses, or to engage in prospective research (Classen, 2006). The first author frequently conducts secondary data analysis, finding it a useful method due to the ease of accessibility of the data. In addition, secondary analysis of existing data is receiving increased attention in health care due to shrinking grant dollars, pressure to produce replicable findings, and a

growing interest in outcomes investigation. It also reduces the amount of time and inconvenience to the participants, which is also referred to as *subject burden*.

Purpose

The purpose of the initial study conducted by the first author (Smith, 2008) was to determine the rate of sexual and physical violence experienced by women with disabilities compared to women without disabilities and men with disabilities using data previously collected in the 2005 Behavioral Risk Surveillance System (Centers for Disease Control and Prevention, 2010).

Data Source

In 2005, the Behavioral Risk Surveillance System, a state-wide telephone survey conducted by the Centers for Disease Control and Prevention included questions in an optional module regarding the experience of violence. The dataset also included variables that allowed the author to then stratify the data to examine the issues by gender and disability status.

Analysis

Chi square analyses were performed comparing demographics of women with and without disabilities who had been threatened with physical violence, had experienced attempted physical violence, and had been victims of physical violence or unwanted sex. This process was repeated, comparing the demographics of women and men with disabilities who had experienced these forms of violence.

Examination of the descriptive data revealed a consistent difference in the rates of abuse for women with disabilities compared to women without disabilities as well as in comparison to men with disabilities. To examine these relationships more fully, a series of logistic regression analyses were conducted using the four identified types of interpersonal violence. Potential confounding factors including age, race/ethnicity, education, employment, and relationship status were examined to determine if they increased the likelihood of abuse.

RESULTS

Risk Factors Increasing Likelihood of Interpersonal Violence: Being Female, Disabled, Younger, and Single

The relationship of risk factors to interpersonal violence indicated that those who are female are anywhere from one and a half (1.49) to almost nine times (8.79) more likely

TABLE 13-1

RELATIONSHIP OF RISK FACTORS TO INTERPERSONAL VIOLENCE

VARIABLE	THREATENED VIOLENCE		ATTEMPTED VIOLENCE		PHYSICALLY ABUSED (HIT, ETC.)		UNWANTED SEX	
	OR	95% CI	OR	95% CI	OR	95% CI	OR	95% CI
Gender								
1. Male (ref)	1.0		1.0		1.0		1.0	
2. Female	2.67	2.5-2.9	1.49	1.4-1.6	2.21	2.1-2.4	8.79	7.6-10.2
Disability								
1. Not disabled (ref)	1.0		1.0		1.0		1.0	
2. Disabled	2.04	1.9-2.2	1.88	1.7-2.0	1.99	1.9-2.1	2.3	2.1-2.6
Age								
1. 50 and above (ref)	1.0		1.0		1.0		1.0	
2. 18 to 49 years	1.46	1.4-1.6	1.52	1.4-1.6	1.44	1.4-1.5	1.23	1.1-1.4
Race/ethnicity								
1. Other race/ethnicity (ref)	1.0		1.0		1.0		1.0	
2. White	1.16	1.1-1.2	1.06	1.0-1.1	1.18	1.1-1.3	1.12	1.0-1.2
Education								
1. Some college and above (ref)	1.0		1.0		1.0		1.0	
2. No school/high school grad	0.91	0.9-1.0	1.03	1.0-1.1	0.90	0.9-1.0	0.80	0.7-0.9
Employment								
1. Employed (ref)	1.0		1.0		1.0		1.0	
2. Not employed	1.23	1.1-1.4	1.29	1.2-1.5	1.23	1.1-1.4	1.44	1.2-1.7
Relationship status								
1. Uncoupled (ref)	1.0		1.0		1.0		1.0	
2. Coupled	0.50	0.47-0.53	0.54	0.5-0.6	0.49	0.47-0.52	0.53	0.5-0.6

OR=odds ratio, CI=confidence interval.

to be victims of abuse (Table 13-1). Those who identified themselves as having a disability are approximately twice as likely to be victims of abuse (Table 13-2). Being younger (18 to 49 years) increases the likelihood for all types of abuse as does being unemployed. Those who are uncoupled are almost twice as likely to experience all forms of abuse as those who are in a relationship. However, the likelihood of abuse does not appear to be significantly affected by race/ethnicity or educational level.

When examining these relationships exclusively for women (Table 13-3), analysis shows that women who have a disability are twice as likely to be threatened with violence, to be a victim of attempted violence, to be physically abused, and to experience unwanted sex as women without a disability. Younger women consistently are more likely to experience abuse, as are White women, and those not employed. Those who are coupled are consistently almost half as likely to experience violence as those who are uncoupled.

DISCUSSION

The data supported the relationship between disability and gender and domestic physical and sexual abuse.

TABLE 13-2

RELATIONSHIP OF RISK FACTORS TO INTERPERSONAL VIOLENCE FOR PERSONS WITH DISABILITIES

VARIABLE	THREATENED VIOLENCE		ATTEMPTED VIOLENCE		PHYSICALLY ABUSED (HIT, ETC.)		UNWANTED SEX	
	OR	95% CI	OR	95% CI	OR	95% CI	OR	95% CI
Gender								
1. Male (ref)	1.0		1.0		1.0		1.0	
2. Female	2.68	2.3-3.1	1.58	1.4-1.8	2.52	2.2-2.9	12.22	8.8-16.9
Age								
1. 50 and above (ref)	1.0		1.0		1.0		1.0	
2. 18 to 49 years	1.54	1.3-1.8	1.56	1.4-1.8	1.51	1.3-1.7	1.24	1.0-1.5
Race/ethnicity								
1. Other race/ethnicity (ref)	1.0		1.0		1.0		1.0	
2. White	0.92	0.8-1.7	0.97	0.8-1.1	0.98	0.8-1.2	0.98	0.8-1.2
Education								
1. Some college and above (ref)	1.0		1.0		1.0		1.0	
2. No school/high school grad	0.88	0.8-1.0	1.06	0.9-1.2	0.88	0.8-1.0	0.82	0.7-1.0
Employment								
1. Employed (ref)	1.0		1.0		1.0		1.0	
2. Not employed	1.24	1.0-1.5	1.31	1.1-1.6	1.13	0.9-1.4	1.42	1.1-1.8
Relationship status								
1. Uncoupled (ref)	1.0		1.0		1.0		1.0	
2. Coupled	0.54	0.5-0.6	0.62	0.5-0.7	0.51	0.5-0.6	0.59	0.5-0.7

OR=odds ratio, CI=confidence interval.

Women with disabilities are at a higher risk of experiencing all forms of abuse than women without disabilities or men with disabilities. Gender and disability combine to increase the likelihood of all forms of abuse, especially unwanted sex. These results were consistent throughout the analyses and with previous studies (Curry et al., 2001; Hassouneh-Phillips & Curry, 2002; Mays, 2006; Nosek, Foley, Hughes, & Howland, 2001; Nosek, Howland, & Hughes, 2001). However, these results are unique because the data come from a large population-based database, with a national scope and rigorous and well-defined sampling and data collection methodology. Large databases allow subanalyses and multivariate analyses and give a more accurate estimate of conditions. Therefore, results are more descriptive, and

the examination of the effect of confounding factors is stronger than with smaller, more regional samples.

In addition, unlike other studies that show similar rates of violence for women with and without disabilities (Gilson et al., 2001; Martin et al., 2006), this study showed an increased likelihood for violence toward women with disabilities for all types of abuse. In chi square analyses, less significant differences were noted between women and men with disabilities with regard to experience of abuse, suggesting an "equalizing" effect of disability with regard to the experience of violence. In other words, disability was a stronger factor than gender. This study also does not show the strong influence of education or race/ethnicity that has been noted in other studies (Martin et al., 2006; Nosek et

TABLE 13-3

RELATIONSHIP OF RISK FACTORS TO INTERPERSONAL VIOLENCE FOR WOMEN

VARIABLE	THREATENED VIOLENCE		ATTEMPTED VIOLENCE		PHYSICALLY ABUSED (HIT, ETC.)		UNWANTED SEX	
	OR	*95% CI*	*OR*	*95% CI*	*OR*	*95% CI*	*OR*	*95% CI*
Disability								
1. Not disabled (ref)	1.0		1.0		1.0		1.0	
2. Disabled	1.99	1.8-2.2	1.89	1.7-2.1	2.05	1.9-2.2	2.38	2.1-2.7
Age								
1. 50 and above (ref)	1.0		1.0		1.0		1.0	
2. 18 to 49 years	1.39	1.3-1.5	1.43	1.3-1.6	1.34	1.2-1.4	1.22	1.1-1.3
Race/ethnicity								
1. Other race/ethnicity (ref)	1.0		1.0		1.0		1.0	
2. White	1.25	1.2-1.3	1.09	1.0-1.2	1.22	1.1-1.3	1.25	1.1-1.4
Education								
1. Some college and above (ref)	1.0		1.0		1.0		1.0	
2. No school/high school grad	0.90	0.8-1.0	1.07	1.0-1.2	0.94	0.9-1.0	0.78	0.7-0.9
Employment								
1. Employed (ref)	1.0		1.0		1.0		1.0	
2. Not employed	1.34	1.2-1.5	1.34	1.2-1.5	1.32	1.2-1.5	1.46	1.2-1.7
Relationship status								
1. Uncoupled (ref)	1.0		1.0		1.0		1.0	
2. Coupled	0.50	0.46-0.53	0.54	0.5-0.6	0.49	0.46-0.53	0.55	0.5-0.6

OR=odds ratio, CI=confidence interval.

al., 2006). Overall, in all analyses, gender and disability are the factors that overwhelmingly increase the likelihood of all forms of violence. The findings from this study and the supporting literature led the authors to consider abuse as an example of occupational justice and injustice and to consider occupational science as a framework for translating the results into guidance for intervention.

CONTRIBUTION TO OCCUPATIONAL SCIENCE

This study contributes to occupational science in several ways. First and foremost, it adds to our understanding of the multifaceted nature of occupational injustice. In addi-

tion, it adds a new perspective to how occupation is shaped by disability, which is a long-standing interest of occupational scientists. Finally, it opens the door for occupational science to grapple with less positive occupations, such as experiencing abuse, to expand the science's current overwhelmingly positive perspective on human occupation.

The Occupational Injustice of Abuse

Restriction From Participation

Occupational injustice occurs when "participation in occupations is barred, confined, restricted, segregated, prohibited, undeveloped, disrupted, alienated, marginalized, exploited, excluded, or otherwise restricted" (Townsend & Wilcock, 2004b, p. 77). A woman with a disability may not be able to play, work, or live without exploitation and violence and is, therefore, a victim of injustice. Furthermore, the restriction is often due to reasons that are not within her control, and, in case of abuse, participation may be under the control of her abuser.

Powerlessness and Abuse

Power, within the occupational justice framework, refers to equality, participation, and empowerment. Women with and without disabilities frequently have no power against their abusers; however, women with disabilities have even less power due to vulnerabilities to domestic abuse not experienced by women without disabilities. One example of vulnerability is a result of the social stereotype that assumes that as a woman with disability, you are asexual, passive, unaware and are, therefore, powerless and easy prey (Young et al., 1997).

Choice and Abuse

Basic to the idea of occupational justice is the assumption that humans ought to have choice about what to do with their lives. Choice is also the means by which humans prioritize their occupations and, more to the point, select those occupations that they consider most useful and most meaningful to them. As a person with a disability, male or female, abused or not, because you may be dependent on caregivers or personal assistants, you may have limited opportunity for choice in your life. These choices may include participation in home and community activities or employment. Occupational justice emphasizes the importance of individuals having choices in accepting opportunities and resources that are available to them.

Types of Occupational Injustice and Abuse

Occupational Imbalance and Abuse

Townsend and Wilcock (2004b) present four types of occupational injustice: occupational imbalance, occupational marginalization, occupational deprivation, and occupational alienation. The first, occupational imbalance, is a population-based term describing populations that do not share in the labor and benefits of economic production. Occupational segregation, which is associated with gender, disability, race, or other forms of difference, is actually a form of occupational imbalance (Townsend & Wilcock, 2004b). As a woman with a disability who has been abused, you are more likely to have higher levels of unemployment than a peer without disabilities who has been abused (Smith & Strauser, 2007). You are then more vulnerable to abuse through imbalance of participation in the workforce, as well as imbalance in access to education and society through segregated schooling or institutionalization. This vulnerability can be reversed if you experience improved economic opportunities.

Occupational Marginalization and Abuse

Occupational marginalization is the lack of opportunities for making everyday choices as people participate in occupations. If you are a woman with a disability, it occurs at the societal level by making your abuse less visible and making you less likely to be believed when you seek help, thus protecting your abusers (Townsend & Wilcock, 2004b). Occupational marginalization may also be attributed to lack of "the opportunity and resources (personal, environmental, societal) for individuals and communities to select and engage in a range of purposeful occupations that are culturally and personally meaningful" (Grainger, 1999). For example, as an employed woman with disability, it is more likely that you will participate in employment that does not reflect your skill levels. In addition, you are more likely to be in a lower paying, lower skilled service or domestic job (Baldwin, Johnson, & Watson, 1993).

Occupational Deprivation and Abuse

Occupational deprivation is a "state of prolonged preclusion from engagement in occupations of necessity and/or meaning due to factors that stand outside the control of the individual" (Whiteford, 2003, p. 222). Examples of incarceration, refugeeism, and the impact of technology and maldistributed labor have been cited as examples of occupational deprivation (Molineaux & Whiteford, 1999; Whiteford, 1997, 2000). As a woman with disability who has been abused, occupational deprivation could be experienced as limited access to education and social participation due to limited options allowed by your intimate partners. Occupational deprivation is magnified if you are physically confined or otherwise limited from participating in work, which contributes to your vulnerability to abuse due to lack of economic independence. Conversely, improved economic opportunities can decrease the level of violence in abusive relationships (Farmer & Tiefenthalter, 1996).

Occupational Alienation and Abuse

Occupational alienation is "the outcome when people experience daily life as meaningless or purposeless" (Townsend & Wilcock, 2004a, p. 252). Occupational alienation is the result of a social process in which the alienated person presents with prolonged experiences of disconnectedness, isolation, emptiness, lack of a sense of identity, a limited or confined expression of spirit, or a sense of meaninglessness. As a woman with a disability, you might experience occupational alienation as a result of being overprotected, which could increase your vulnerability to entering and staying in abusive relationships. The perpetrators' actions might lead to, or sustain, a sense of alienation from meaningful or purposeful occupations, such as social participation. Participation in occupation is a major force in shaping identity. For this reason, prolonged disconnectedness from occupations that are meaningful and purposeful can distort identity formation.

Abuse and Occupational Science

Examining the occupational patterns and experiences of women with disabilities who experience abuse provides an opportunity for occupational scientists to study a population with multiple vulnerabilities to injustice. In addition, this population is unique in the degree to which injustice is often hidden, not only by the perpetrator, but also by the victim who may tolerate the injustice by a perpetrator upon whom she depends. Women with disabilities who experience abuse may not self-disclose and may not be easily identified. Therefore, the occupational injustices are less easily identified, potentially resulting in even less opportunity for remediation.

Using occupational justice as a lens for the issue of violence against women with disabilities adds depth to the understanding of this issue because it examines a population who faces several layers of occupational injustice, due to their multiple challenges of being female and disabled and having suffered the indignity of abuse. In addition, the injustices faced by these women are often indiscernible by outsiders. The state of being female is obvious, but many disabilities are not apparent, and a situation of abuse is often concealed from outsiders. In many instances, these women spend little time outside of their homes, further marginalizing them through lack of exposure to potential supports. This combination of injustices, obvious and veiled, makes this group especially vulnerable and difficult to identify and support. This framework also points to empowerment as the mechanism that will most effectively address occupational justice for women with disabilities who have been abused.

Implications for Practice

Principles of occupational justice include empowerment through occupation, enablement of occupational potential and diversity, inclusion, and promoting the ability to participate in meaningful and purposeful activity. Empowerment through occupation supports equality in power sharing, defined as power exerted and accepted through collaboration and partnership (Townsend & Wilcock, 2004b). For example, as a therapist, this concept would include the establishment of client-centered practice, in which you would involve the client's participation in determination of her goals and strategies for intervention, including the performance of occupations related to her life such as work, community practice, and social engagement (Restall, Ripat, & Stern, 2003; Townsend, 1993).

The ultimate goal is to empower your patient who is being abused (a) to be able to live in an environment without abuse, (b) to have resources that provide respite from abuse or could support her in seeking nonabusive situations, (c) to participate in decision making, (d) to participate in occupations that are meaningful, and (e) to advocate changes in laws that would better support her toward these ends.

When planning interventions for a woman with a disability who exhibits obvious injuries, you, as an occupational therapist, should incorporate therapeutic use of self, including coaching, encouraging, facilitating, guiding, listening, prompting, or reflecting (Townsend & Landry, 2005). An example for a patient who wants to improve her employment skills might include having her focus on what she can do, what she wants to do but cannot, how she might get out of the abusive relationship, and how she can feel good about what she does. In addition, you are mandated to report suspected abuse. You may need to involve a social worker or other professional to support your client in making changes in her care provider, her living arrangement, or her child care arrangements.

Conclusion

Examination of the results from the secondary analysis of data not only confirmed that women with disabilities were indeed experiencing greater levels of abuse than their nondisabled counterparts, but also supported the authors' insights from practice. The authors were then able to use concepts of occupational justice to understand the dynamics of these findings to provide a framework for intervention. Beyond examining the statistical findings, the authors found that considering this issue within the context of occupational science provided valuable implications for intervention strategies. By combining knowledge gained through research findings, occupational science theoretical postulates, and clinical observations using a client-centered approach, it was possible to more effectively identify strategies to address the problems of abuse experienced by women with disabilities, thus completing the circle of research, theory, and practice.

Learning Supports

Understanding the Experience of Occupational Injustice

Purpose

This learning support provides the student with a personal example of occupational injustice.

Primary Concepts

Primary Concepts

- Occupational injustice
- Occupational deprivation
- Occupational justice

Instructions

Reflect on the following. Then discuss your responses in a group.

1. Make a list of times when someone coerced you into doing or not doing something because he or she was stronger than you or had another type of power over you (boss, sibling, spouse).

2. How did these experiences make you feel?

3. Do you think that you were experiencing occupational injustice? Explain.

4. Did you ever find a way to get around the person who was trying to control you?

5. What did you learn from the experience?

Understanding the Experience of Occupational Injustice as a Person With a Disability

Purpose

This learning support provides the student with an example of occupational injustice as a person with a disability.

Primary Concepts

- Occupational injustice
- Occupational deprivation
- Occupational justice
- Occupational alienation
- Occupational marginalization

Instructions

Reflect on the following, in discussion with others, as a journal entry or as a more formal paper:

1. List some commonly occurring occupations in your life that are very important to you, either because they are highly pleasurable or because they contribute to your concept of your identity. Imagine having a disability that limits your access to participation in those occupations but having the supports that allow you to continue participating in at least some of those important occupations.

2. Now, imagine that you are prevented from participation because your significant other or your care provider limits your ability to use the supports and limits your access to your friends and family and other

outside supports. Imagine further that your significant other or care provider regularly becomes violent toward you, causing you physical harm.

3. How do you think this would make you feel? How might you feel after a prolonged period of enduring this situation after your attempts to remedy the situation were not successful?

4. Discuss this situation from an occupational justice perspective. Include application of occupational deprivation and occupational marginalization.

Occupational Injustice Research

Purpose

This learning support helps the student understand how research can help use occupational justice principles to inform occupational therapy by developing a plan for research identifying the most valuable interventions that an occupational therapist might provide to support women with disabilities who are in abusive situations and experiencing occupational injustice.

Primary Concepts

- Occupational injustice
- Occupational deprivation
- Occupational justice
- Occupational alienation
- Occupational marginalization
- Qualitative and quantitative research methodologies

Instructions

Brainstorm supports that might be helpful to women with disabilities who are in abusive situations and experiencing occupational injustice to restore their occupational justice. Develop a research plan that would examine your hypotheses.

1. How might you use a qualitative methodology to better understand the most valuable interventions that an occupational therapist might provide to support women with disabilities who are in abusive situations and experiencing occupational injustice?

   - Identify your specific methodology (participatory action research, critical theory, ethnography, phenomenology, or grounded theory).

   - How many subjects would you pursue?

   - What qualifications would guide you in the selection of your subject(s)?

   - How might you recruit your subject(s)?

   - List questions that would guide your inquiries or experiences.

2. How might you use a quantitative methodology to better understand the most valuable interventions that an occupational therapist might provide to support women with disabilities who are in abusive situations and experiencing occupational injustice?

   ○ Identify your specific methodology (survey, secondary data analysis, etc.).

   ○ How many subjects would you pursue?

   ○ What qualifications would guide you in the selection of your subject?

   ○ How might you recruit your subject?

   ○ List questions that would guide your inquiries.

REFERENCES

Andrews, A. B., & Veronen, L. J. (1993). Sexual assault and people with disabilities. Special issue: Sexuality and disabilities: A guide for human service practitioners. *Journal of Social Work and Human Sexuality, 8*(2), 137-159. doi:10.1300/J291v08n02_08

Asch, A., & Fine, M. (1988). Introduction: Beyond pedestals. In M. Fine & A. Asch (Eds.), *Women with disabilities: Essays in psychology, culture and politics* (pp. 1-37). Philadelphia, PA: Temple University Press.

Baldwin, M., Johnson, W. G., & Watson, S. (1993). *A double burden of discrimination: Women with disabilities.* Washington, DC: Center for the Study of Social Policy.

Belsky, J. (1980). Child maltreatment: An ecological integration. *American Psychologist, 35,* 320-335. doi:10.1037/0003-066X.35.4.320

Blackwell-Stratton, M., Breslin, M., Mayerson, A., & Bailey, S. (1988). Smashing icons: Disabled women and the disability and women's movements. In M. Fine & A. Asch (Eds.), *Women with disabilities: Essays in psychology, culture and politics* (pp. 306-332). Philadelphia, PA: Temple University Press.

Brownridge, D. A. (2006). Partner violence against women with disabilities: Prevalence, risk, and explanations. *Violence Against Women, 12*(9), 805-822. doi:10.1177/1077801206292681

Carlson, B. E. (1997). Mental retardation and domestic violence: An ecological approach to intervention. *Social Work, 42,* 79-89. doi:10.1093/sw/42.1.79

Centers for Disease Control and Prevention. (2010). *Behavioral risk factor surveillance system: Frequently asked questions.* Retrieved from http://www.cdc.gov/brfss/faqs.htm

Classen, S. (2006). Study designs for secondary analysis of existing data. In G. Kielhofner (Ed.), *Research in occupational therapy: Methods of inquiry for enhancing practice* (pp. 110-126). Philadelphia, PA: F. A. Davis.

Collins, K. S., Schoen, S. J., Duchon, L., Simantor, E., & Yellowitz, M. (1999). *Health concerns across a woman's lifespan: The Commonwealth Fund 1998 survey of women's health.* New York, NY: Commonwealth Fund.

Curry, M. A., Hassouneh-Phillips, D. H., & Johnston-Silverberg, A. J. (2001). Abuse of women with disabilities: An ecological model and review. *Violence Against Women, 7*(1), 60-79. doi:10.1177/10778010122182307

Davis, L. (1997). The bell curve, the novel, and the invention of the disabled body in the nineteenth century. In L. Davis (Ed.), *The disability studies reader* (pp. 9-28). New York, NY: Routledge.

Dobash, R. E., & Dobash, R. P. (1992). *Women, violence, and social change.* New York, NY: Routledge.

Farmer, A., & Tiefenthaler, J. (1996). Domestic violence: The value of services as signals. *American Economic Review, 86*(2), 274-279.

Finkelhor, D. (1988). *Stopping family violence: Research priorities for the coming decade.* Newbury Park, CA: Sage Publications.

Furey, E. M. (1994). Sexual abuse of adults with mental retardation: Who and where. *Mental Retardation, 32*(13), 173-180.

Gelles, R. J. (1993). Through a sociological lens: Social structure and family violence. In R. J. Gelles & D. R. Loseke (Eds.), *Current controversies on family violence.* Newbury Park, CA: Sage Publications.

Gelles, R. J., & Loseke, D. R. (1993a). Introduction: Examining and evaluating controversies on family violence. In R. J. Gelles & D. R. Loseke (Eds.), *Current controversies on family violence.* Newbury Park, CA: Sage Publications.

Gelles, R. J., & Loseke, D. R. (1993b). Part 1: Issues in conceptualization. In R. J. Gelles & D. R. Loseke (Eds.), *Current controversies on family violence.* Newbury Park, CA: Sage Publications.

Gilson, S., Cramer, E., & DePoy, E. (2001). (Re)defining abuse of women with disabilities: A paradox of limitation and expansion. *AFFILIA: Journal of Women and Social Work, 16*(2), 220-235. doi:10.1177/08861090122094235

Grainger, C. (1999). Unpublished. Occupational Science Workshop. *Australian Association of Occupational Therapists Conference,* Canberra, Australia.

Hassouneh-Phillips, D., & Curry, M. A. (2002). Abuse of women with disabilities: State of the science. *Rehabilitation Counseling Bulletin, 45,* 96-104.

Lonsdale, S. (1990). *Women and disability: The experience of physical disability among women.* New York, NY: St. Martin's Press.

Martin, S. L., Ray, N., Sotres-Alvarez, D., Kupper, L. L., Moracco, K. E., & Dickens, P. A. (2006). Physical and sexual assault of women with disabilities. *Violence Against Women, 12*(9), 823-837. doi:10.1177/1077801206292672

Mays, J. M. (2006). Feminist disability theory: Domestic violence against women with a disability. *Disability & Society, 21*(2), 147-158. doi:10.1080/09687590500498077

Molineux, M. L., & Whiteford, G. E. (1999). Prisons: From occupational deprivation to occupational enrichment. *Journal of Occupational Science, 6*(3), 124-130. doi:10.1080/14427591.1999.9686457

Nosek, M. A., Foley, C. C., Hughes, R. B., & Howland, C. A. (2001). Vulnerabilities for abuse among women with disabilities. *Sexuality and Disability, 19,* 177-189.

Nosek, M. A., Howland, C. A., & Hughes, R. B. (2001). The investigation of abuse and women with disabilities: Going beyond assumptions. *Violence Against Women, 7,* 477-499. doi:10.1177/10778010122182569

Nosek, M. A., Howland, C. A., & Young, M. E. (1997). Abuse of women with disabilities: Policy implications. *Journal of Disability Policy Studies, 8,* 157-176. doi:10.1177/104420739700800208

Nosek, M. A., Hughes, R. B., Taylor, H. B., & Taylor, P. (2006). Disability, psychosocial, and demographic characteristics of abused women with physical disabilities. *Violence Against Women, 12*(9), 838-850. doi:10.1177/1077801206292671

Restall, G., Ripat, J., & Stern, M. (2003). A framework of strategies for client-centered practice. *Canadian Journal of Occupational Therapy, 70*(2), 103-112.

Riddington, J. (1989). *Beating the "odds:" Violence and women with disabilities.* (Position Paper 2). Vancouver, Canada: DisAbled Women's Network.

Rod, T. (1980). Marital murder. In J. A. Scott (Ed.), *Violence in the family.* Canberra, Australia: AIC.

Smith, D. L. (2008). Disability, gender and intimate partner violence: Relationships and risks from the behavioral risk factor surveillance system. *Sexuality and Disability, 26,* 15-28. doi:10.1007/s11195-007-9064-6

Smith, D. L., & Strauser, D. R. (2007). Examining the impact of physical and sexual abuse on the employment of women with disabilities: An exploratory analysis. *Disability and Rehabilitation, 30,* 1039-1046. doi:10.1080/09637480701539542

Sobsey, D. (1994). *Violence and abuse in the lives of people with disabilities.* Baltimore, MD: Paul Brookes.

Thomas, C. (1998). *Female forms: Experiencing and understanding disability.* Philadelphia, PA: Open University Press.

Tjaden, P., & Thoennes, N. (2000). *Extent, nature and consequence of intimate partner violence: Findings from the National Violence Against Women Survey* (Publication No. NCJ 18167). Washington, DC: U. S. Department of Justice. Retrieved October 20, 2006, from www.ojp.usdoj.gov/nij/pubs-sum/181867.htm

Townsend, E. (1993). 1993 Muriel Driver lecture: Occupational therapy's social vision. *Canadian Journal of Occupational Therapy, 60,* 174-184.

Townsend, E., & Landry, J. (2005). Interventions in a societal context: Enabling participation. In C. H. Christiansen & C. M. Baum (Eds.), *Occupational therapy performance, participation, and well-being.* Thorofare, NJ: SLACK Incorporated.

Townsend, E., & Wilcock, A. A. (2004a). Occupational justice. In C. Christiansen & E. Townsend (Eds.), *Introduction to occupation: The art and science of living* (pp. 243-273). Upper Saddle River, NJ: Prentice-Hall.

Townsend, E., & Wilcock, A. A. (2004b). Occupational justice and client centred practice: A dialogue in progress. *Canadian Journal of Occupational Therapy, 71,* 75-87.

Wendell, S. (1989). Toward a feminist theory of disability. *Hypatia, 4,* 104-124.

Whiteford, G. (1997). Occupational deprivation and incarceration. *Journal of Occupational Science, 4,* 126-130. doi:10.1080/14427591.1997.9686429

Whiteford, G. (2000). Occupational deprivation: Global challenges in the new millennium. *British Journal of Occupational Therapy, 63*(5), 200-204.

Whiteford, G. (2003). When people cannot participation: Occupational deprivation. In C. Christiansen & E. Townsend (Eds.), *An introduction to occupation: The art and science of living* (pp. 221-242). Upper Saddle River, NJ: Prentice Hall.

Womendez, C., & Schneiderman, K. (1991). Escaping from abuse: Unique issues for women with disabilities. *Sexuality & Disability, 9,* 273-280. doi:10.1007/BF01102397

Young, M. E., Nosek, M. A., Howland, C. A., Chanpong, G., & Rintala, D. H. (1997). Prevalence of abuse of women with physical disabilities. *Archives of Physical Medicine and Rehabilitation, 78*(12 Suppl.), S34-S38. doi:10.1016/S0003-9993(97)90219-7

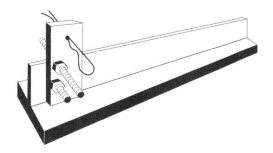

14

Enacting Occupational Justice in Research and Policy Development
Highlighting the Experience of Occupational Deprivation in Forced Migration

Gail Whiteford, BAppSc (Occ Therapy), MHSc (Occ Therapy), PhD

Research is a broad church. Through time and across cultural and political contexts, numerous distinct research traditions have developed, each with its own unique philosophical and theoretical underpinnings. Generally speaking, however, the purpose of research is more unified: ultimately, it is about generating new knowledge. However, as well as generating new knowledge, we need also to be able to apply it to the messy world of everyday life. In other words, we have to be able to translate insights generated from research into practice developments in the physical and social worlds. Thus, the ways in which knowledge is framed, undertaken, and communicated has a profound influence on how ultimately useful it is.

In this chapter, I describe a study undertaken with a group of people who had lived the experience of being a refugee. The chapter does not focus on the findings of the research. Rather, what I am presenting here is an account of the research, including my motivations for doing it, the experience of conducting it, and the ways in which I sought to politicize the findings so as to influence public opinion, policy directions, and everyday practices. In other words, I am recounting the story behind the research in a way that is not often done because researchers are usually focused on discussing the findings or results.

Overall, this chapter should be read as a rich narrative account of research as a practice. My aim is to be able to help shed light on aspects of research that are not often talked about in order to assist new occupational therapy and occupational science researchers in understanding how rich and complex the doing of research really is. Most importantly, my hope is that the chapter can inform practices that ultimately serve those marginalized populations whose everyday existence reflects situations of occupational deprivation, structural disadvantage, and occupational injustices.

NOT THE USUAL SUSPECTS

Imagination, empathy, moral obligation, and opportunity—these are not the usual suspects when we consider what motivates research. In the case of the research that I undertook with a group of people who had been through the refugee experience, however, these factors did indeed influence my decision to be involved.

- 169 -

Pierce, D. (Ed.).
Occupational Science for Occupational Therapy (pp. 169-178).
© 2014 SLACK Incorporated.

Let us start with imagination and empathy. Imagine the experience of violent conflict, terror, flight, hunger, uncertainty, and chaos. From an occupational perspective, imagine also the loss of most things you have had or done that are familiar. Your daily routine is gone and in its place is a sea of unstructured time outside of doing those things necessary for survival. Consistent with this state of occupational deprivation is a concomitant loss of identity. Despite the fact that you may have been a teacher, chef, or computer technician, your label is now refugee, and with that label comes a complete dependency on others: aid organizations, nongovernment organizations, refugee organizations, national governments, and bureaucratic machinery on a massive scale.

Imagining this certainly moved me. I struggled to comprehend the enormity of loss and dislocation felt by people who had been through this experience and then, in another major upheaval, were transported to another country for safe refuge and the chance to construct another life. Perhaps more importantly, however, I felt that, as someone privileged by history, geography, and education, I had a moral obligation. This obligation was about mobilizing not only the resources I had at hand but also the insights and understandings developed over many years as an occupational therapist and occupational science researcher. I have always had a strong belief that, ultimately, the ends of research should be to make the world a better place, what Patti Lather (1986) referred to as *research as praxis*.

What Lather meant in coining this term was that research should count; it should be oriented to social change and transformation. It should, in other words, make a difference. Of course, this is a utopian view. Not all research meets such lofty criteria. In fact, the motivations that fuel research activity around the globe represent a broad spectrum, including, for example, enhancing individual researchers' careers, increasing consumer consumption and corporate competitiveness, or, in the case of some military research, increasing the effectiveness of weapons. Clearly, such motivations are not consistent with an ultimate interest in social transformation and emancipation—far from it. Utopian or not, however, a perspective that enshrines a belief that research should be framed as a moral and ethical undertaking can still serve as a powerful societal aspiration.

Given this weave of values, knowledge, and skill sets, the arrival of the Kosovar refugees into the Australian community where I was living at the time provided me a unique opportunity. It was an opportunity to work with them and provide a vehicle through which they might have a collective voice with which to educate the broader community and counter fear or discrimination. It was also an opportunity to explore the concept of occupational deprivation on which I had been working for several years and

whether it had relevance to their experiences. Of course, it is important to note that these were indeed my objectives, and I was very conscious of that fact. Accordingly, I set about a process of community and stakeholder consultation to test these objectives and obtain feedback as to whether there was a shared perception of the value of such a research endeavor.

However, no research is undertaken a priori. In other words, theoretical orientations always influence the way research is valued and understood. So, before going on to describe the community consultations and other aspects of the research process, I will take a step back to share the theoretical and conceptual lenses that shaped the way I thought about and approached the research.

AN OCCUPATIONAL FRAMING

One of the most significant lenses through which I understand the world is an occupational one and, hopefully, through reading this book you will also be reinforced in such an occupational view of the world. You may say, "Hold on, don't all occupational therapists have an occupational perspective?" The answer is no, not necessarily. It is true that occupational therapy began historically with a deep concern with doing in society, with its meaning to people individually and collectively as well as the economic, transformative, and therapeutic value of occupation. Alongside this was an equal concern with the impacts of exclusion from doing everyday things like working, child rearing, socializing, or engaging in civic society because of personal, socioeconomic, or political factors (Wilcock, 2001). However, during the profession's journey of growth and development, there have been influences, such as that of biomedicine, that focused the profession's attention on individuals rather than families or groups and on impairments rather than capacities. This, in turn, influenced the way that occupational therapists thought about, talked about, and went about their work (Wilding & Whiteford, 2007).

In the past decade, an occupational perspective has again become more central in occupational therapy in what has been described as a *renaissance* that foregrounds what people do, how and why they do it, what the meanings and impacts are, and the conditions that either support or hinder individual and group engagement in different contexts. Occupational science, by advancing through research our understandings of the complexity and situated nature of human occupation, has contributed to the depth and sophistication with which this perspective can be articulated and applied. One of my early experiences with such application and articulation was in the development of the concept of occupational deprivation.

Kindling an Enduring Interest in Occupational Deprivation

While the mix of factors that may have led to an interest in occupational deprivation at a personal level are more complex (see Whiteford, 2005), at a professional level, it was a lot more straightforward for me. Basically, working with the corrective services in a prison in New Zealand was a powerful experience. It provided an opportunity to explore what happened to people when they were removed from society and all the occupations in which they routinely engage and have highly restricted access to other humans, materials, and equipment. Although I do not have the space here to reiterate the findings of the study that we did in the prison setting (Whiteford, 2007), it did kindle an enduring interest in occupational deprivation because I observed the impacts it can have, some of which are devastating. Because of this, I became increasingly concerned with the associated human rights issues and, as a corollary, the emergence of occupational justice.

Literature

Occupational Justice as an End of Occupational Therapy

Occupational justice could reasonably be described as an end of occupational therapy or, in other words, as what is hoped to be achieved by our collective efforts (Whiteford & Townsend, 2011). Occupational justice was conceptually developed by Townsend and Wilcock (2004) and has sparked a great deal of interest around the world, especially where occupational therapists practice in contexts in which overt oppression and inequality exist for historic and political reasons (Pollard, Sakellariou, & Kronenberg, 2009). However, it is important to remember that injustices occur everywhere and are sometimes less visible but still systemically entrenched, as Townsend (1998) pointed out in her investigations into mental services in Canada. One very important aspect of the discourse that has developed around occupational justice has been the requirement that those of us who work with people ask ourselves the hard questions. Do our own actions actually contribute to further oppression and marginalization? Are our practices ones that, even unintentionally, disempower vulnerable people? Although this may be a shocking notion, the professional lenses through which we understand or conceptualize people and the systems and structures within which we engage with them can reinforce power differentials through what has been referred to as *othering* (Arendt, 1963).

Enquiry and Knowledge Generation

As well as the theoretical and conceptual influences that have come from my disciplinary background, there are also those that have come from being involved in research over time. Primarily, these relate to the what and how of research.

When we think about doing research, one of the most important stages is the generation and subsequent clarification of the research question or questions. This is because it is the nature of the question that should guide the approach and methods used. Some research questions are deterministic. A medical researcher may seek to identify or determine the therapeutic dose of a particular medication for a particular condition (e.g., antihypertensives for older people with high blood pressure). Clearly, this is a question that involves quantification, or measurement. Alternately, a researcher may be seeking to find out how families cope with a young person who has a mental illness. This is a question concerned with understanding the interaction of complex social, cultural, psychological, and emotional processes. These are not things that can easily be measured (nor should be measured, one can argue), so a qualitative approach would be indicated, and rich narrative data would need to be obtained.

While this may seem basic, spending time on the research question itself is often overlooked by researchers. As you can imagine, if you get the question wrong and the approach, design, and methods along with it, you are probably going to end up doing research that has questionable value. More importantly, the stakeholders of the research may be left with their concerns and interests unaddressed.

Stakeholders and their relationships to the researcher raise another important dimension in the conduct of research—power relations. Power relations in research have come into sharper focus in recent times for a number of reasons, but, most significantly, probably as a response by those most vulnerable subgroups who have been subjected to research processes over which they had little power or control and certainly had no input into dissemination of findings. This has been especially true of indigenous peoples, who have suggested that they have enjoyed little benefit from being subject to enquiry over countless years (Rigney, 2006). Indeed, this history has led to a scenario in many countries where nonindigenous researchers are not able to obtain ethics approval for research without working in partnership with indigenous researchers. This is to ensure that research is conducted in a manner consistent with cultural values, norms, and traditions and also that the interests of the community are being served by the objectives and the predicted outcomes of the research.

The paradigm within which the research has been framed has historically influenced the ways in which research has been conducted and power relations in research have been constructed. Generally speaking, quantitative research frames people as research subjects. Aspects of them or their performance are measured and captured as numerical data. Within an interpretive, qualitative paradigm, people are framed as individuals, families, or community members in their own right. As such, their values, perspectives, experiences, and insights are sought and captured as narrative data.

As may be evident, the two different paradigms require different relationships between the researcher and the researched. In all research, ethical considerations must be addressed with respect to the treatment of research participants. In qualitative research, however, there is a greater likelihood that research participants are treated as partners. This means greater consultation and input on aspects of the research process, which may range from data checking by participants to recruiting field experts as co-researchers in collaborative, action-oriented processes (see, for example, Whiteford, Wilding, & Curtin's 2009 study with a group of therapists on enabling occupation in diverse contexts). The greater the degree to which power is shared and the research endeavor framed as a collaborative partnership, the more likely that the outcomes of the research are shared.

THE REFUGEE STUDY

Methods and Consultation

Before developing an ethics application, it was important to gain a sense of the value of the research from those people closer to the issues of the refugee community than I was. For this reason, I met with the local branch of the rural refugee action group, a group of individuals from a range of backgrounds concerned with the welfare of refugees collectively and highlighting their situation through direct and indirect means. I went to a meeting at an old church hall one evening to discuss the ideas behind my proposed study, and it was a powerful experience. The group was very positive and affirming of the purpose of the research. The deep ethic of care that was communicated by the group about the challenges and issues that the refugee community faced was energizing. There were former refugees present also, who expressed support and asked insightful questions about the orientation and conduct of the research. This was all very sobering and reinforced the importance of doing research with people who struggle to have a voice because of the multiple layers of disadvantage they face.

Ethics and Recruitment

One of the benefits of consulting with the broader refugee support community was that it gave me contacts for people in, or working with, refugee families. Thus, once ethical clearance was obtained, I had some points through which to disseminate information about the study. Although the ethics approval process was relatively straightforward, it did

highlight the need to address in advance how interpreters would be used in the study. I did use an interpreter, herself a former refugee and recommended by the consultative group, an aspect of this research that I will describe more fully.

Once the information sheets were distributed by volunteers to possible participants, the recruitment began when potentially interested people contacted me. From there on, a snowball sampling strategy swung into effect. As a researcher, I was comfortable with this organic process. It was based on normative patterns of social networking: someone tells someone else (with a shared background or similar experience) about the research and recommends making contact with the researcher, and thus the sample grows very naturally.

Data Collection and Analysis

I used an interpreter for half of the interviews. Using an interpreter is not easy in qualitative research, for several reasons. First and foremost, language is central to qualitative research, and language is inherently nuanced. So, when your words and questions are presented through an interpretive filter, it is hard to have any sense of how close they are to your intent. Similarly, when the participant responds, you have to trust that his or her words are likewise being treated with integrity.

Over time, I recruited more participants, including two families, and grew more used to working with an interpreter. What I did not get used to, however, was the content of the interviews. There were several long and detailed accounts of violence and degradation recounted by the participants that were quite shocking. Because of this and the impact that they had on me emotionally, I later sought debriefing counseling that was enormously beneficial.

As described elsewhere, the interviews were all transcribed and coded, and thematic analysis was undertaken in an iterative manner (see Whiteford, 2004). I also highlighted a single case from the data in order to illuminate the process of being and becoming a refugee over time (see Whiteford, 2005). Some of the themes and issues from the overall findings are presented briefly below, but a fuller reading of the published research is recommended for a more in-depth appreciation.

Results/Findings

The first year is the most difficult time, because you have left behind your family, your friends, your home and then you come here...into the unknown. You can't speak the language, you don't know the people, you don't know your place, that's very difficult. Despite the fact that the volunteer people that were around us were very good, it was difficult. I remember the first shopping trip we went to the supermarket, I didn't know any of the products and what they are.... After that first shopping they did for me, I felt like throwing everything in the rubbish because there was nothing I could use, nothing was familiar to me (Maria). (Whiteford, 2004)

Overview of the Findings

Maria (not her real name—all the research participants chose code names for themselves) was one of the participants in the research. I remember her vividly. I spent time with her and her children during the school holidays, which she described for her as being "a nightmare" because of a lack of resources with which to do anything with her children. Indeed, Maria had a number of stories that were provocative accounts of marginalization and exclusion, providing rich accounts of the sorts of everyday occupational struggles the refugee participants faced but remain poorly understood by the broader community. Based on a thematic analysis of all such accounts, a series of primary findings were generated, and most of these and the narrative extracts included next first appeared in 2004 (Whiteford). While I have not presented them here in great detail, hopefully, their inclusion will do three things: first, give you a sense of what can emerge from qualitative research; second, provide an understanding of the value of qualitative findings in informing policy and practice (more on this later in the chapter); and third, enhance your appreciation of the relationship between occupational science and occupational therapy.

Becoming a Refugee

What became evident during the research process was that none of the participants became a refugee overnight. Indeed, in narrating their experiences, all spoke about a process of exclusion and alienation that occurred over time due to political dynamics and shifting power relations. Mr. V., a middle-aged Albanian man with three children, for example, describes how he was forced into working in a factory despite being a qualified (and experienced) teacher:

> Discrimination politics started against normal Albanian people.... For Albanian teachers like me, I end up working in a Serbian program. The Serbian language is a different language.... I start working in a furniture factory for five years from '92. At this time there was a big difference in Kosovo—the politics of discrimination—some people had gone to live in other countries in Europe. By 1997 it was not a good situation. (Whiteford, 2004)

Analysis of such narrative accounts led me to theorize that occupational deprivation is best understood as a process occurring over time. Though this may seem self-evident from such descriptions, such an insight generated from research has very possibly changed the way that occupational deprivation is understood.

Refugee Camp Experiences Can Elicit Both Maladaptive and Adaptive/ Productive Occupational Responses

Like many people, before doing this research, I had made an assumption, probably based on media coverage, that refugee camps were places where people recovered from trauma in safe surroundings while awaiting either a return to their country or movement to another country for resettlement. This was not necessarily the case, however, as camps can be unsanitary, unstable, and particularly unsafe for women and children. What was interesting from an occupational perspective was that refugee camps seemed to be an environment that pressed for adaptive responses— or in the presence of post-traumatic stress, maladaptive responses. Although this is an area that requires much more investigation, consider here Mr. V.'s account:

> In our camp there were 40,000 people. There was no water, no way of washing, it was very bad, some people were sick and some died. There was no food and no eating...there was no sleeping...some people couldn't make it in to eat, the old or sick people, so we helped, very important to help...for me, I was up every morning at five trying to find out which country we would be going to. (Whiteford, 2004)

While this account reflects an agentic, or adaptive, response to the camp environment, not all camp residents responded to the extreme deprivations of the camp environment in this way. In the case study of Florim, presented and discussed in another publication (Whiteford, 2005), there are detailed descriptions of people acting "crazy" and in an aggressive and dangerous way. As previously suggested, there is much more work that needs to be done in both understanding and addressing this phenomenon more fully.

The Development of a New Routine Is One of the Most Challenging Aspects of Settling in a New Country

In 2002, Kielhofner suggested that routines "create the overall pattern by which we go about our various occupations" (p. 68). What was evident in the narratives of the refugee participants was that once they had gotten through the camp experience and were being resettled in a new country, they continued to experience a range of occupation-related issues. Establishing a new routine in a new environment was one of the biggest ones. Lack of familiarity with social mores, laws, facilities, currency, and social institutions were all reported as impacting the ability to recreate everyday life in the host country.

> (The volunteers) were older than me and I found their way of thinking different to mine. They had different routines than what I had and I felt they didn't really match, they were used to a different way of life (Maria). (Whiteford, 2004)

To me, this finding seemed like a very clear indicator of the need for an occupational therapy intervention.

Lack of Language Competence Delimits Most Forms of Occupational Participation in a New Country, Especially Work

If you have ever lived in a surrounding where everyone else is speaking another language, then you will know how tiring it is to constantly be learning that language and how alienated you can feel. All the participants spoke to this issue and the frustration it created as well as the division it created between parents and children when the children (who through schooling) became more competent in English very quickly. Though most countries require host country language attainment as part of resettlement processes, and all participants supported this requirement, there did seem to be a view that there was a low threshold of tolerance for refugees without good language skills.

Lack of Social Connectedness and Absence of Socially Oriented Occupations Contributes to Feelings of Isolation and Loneliness

This is, of course, linked to the issue of language proficiency as discussed previously. There were, however, reflections on the difference in lifestyles and social expectations about the extent to which people interacted. Many participants, like Maria, were used to high levels of connectivity in their previous lives and close relationships with extended family members:

> It's different there (Bosnia). You know there could be 10 villages…and when somebody comes for a visit everybody knows them and it's like a big family…the people in the neighborhoods know each other and help each other—but here you don't. (Whiteford, 2004)

Maria also asked me at some stage what people did when they arrived home from work. Her observation was that Australians just lived in their houses and backyards—rarely venturing out into shared or public spaces—and this contributed to her sense of isolation.

The Experience of Being a Refugee Impacts Identity

This last finding is one of the most complex. From what the participants said, being a refugee changed their life dramatically, but it was not an identity that they described as one they wanted to have as the most defining one in their new country. As Florim described it:

> When I hear the word "refugee," I don't take it as only refugees, it's "Remember me, I have a long story." I've had many times when people turn on the TV and look at the news, which I don't look at anymore, I just watch the sport, something which is normal. When it comes to refugees, war, and that stuff I just put it somewhere else, I change the channel, I don't watch it. Personally, I don't like to be called a refugee but in one way when I came as a refugee there was something that was really nice in being able to start a new life in a good way. But I just feel sometimes when somebody discusses refugees and I think of myself as a refugee, I am forced to remember, to face who I am. (Whiteford, 2005)

Communicating and Politicizing the Findings

One of the events that happened toward the end of my study was that one of the research participants who had been

through several terrifying and dangerous experiences as a refugee asked me to promise that I would tell his stories after the research concluded. The reason, he said, was that people generally did not understand the realities that refugees live through and that greater awareness and compassion would assist them at every stage of the refugee process. I took that promise seriously then, and still do today, which has been part of my motivation for writing this chapter!

Importantly though, it seemed to me that the usual process of publishing research in academic journals was not going to be adequate in order to raise community and political awareness of the occupational issues of refugees. There has been a lot of interest generated internationally through the publications, which seemed to act as a springboard through which other occupational therapists could begin to articulate their projects in camps, communities, and detention centers. What I did from the outset, however, was work with professional and university media expertise to generate some media releases highlighting key findings from the studies, timing this to coincide with a national occupational therapy conference. This, in turn, led to several radio interviews, one of which was nationally broadcast and the other offered in the neighboring country of New Zealand.

What followed next was quite extraordinary. As well as getting some very positive responses, I got some very negative responses in the form of hate mail! Getting hate mail was a very strange and disturbing thing, especially because I did not really feel that I had done anything to warrant such a response. However, on deeper inspection, the letters had extrapolated from my discussion on refugees (and asylum seekers) on radio that I was talking about an essentially Muslim community. Accordingly, the sentiments expressed were all anti-Muslim. I discussed what had happened with a friend, an experienced politician and former cabinet member of the Australian government, who suggested that such a response was really indicative of the fact that the issues of refugees and asylum seekers were very important (and sensitive) in the community.

Moving Into Policy Work

Using the impetus from these events and their media coverage, I worked with the refugee action group to pull together a national conference on refugee issues. To ensure national media interest, we invited two senators from different political parties, a former judge and human rights expert, and an activist from the Brotherhood of St. Lawrence. This conference was hosted at my university and achieved a lot. It enabled me to discuss further the findings of my research, it created a space in which refugee-related policies of the federal government could be discussed and challenged, and it also provided a forum through which refugee members of the community could have a voice and educate others. It was powerful and appropriate and a potent outcome of the research.

Professionally, there was also a lot of interest in the research and, following a meeting of occupational therapists at a national conference, Occupational Opportunities for Asylum Seekers was born. This is now an organization in its own right with an international reputation for lobbying as well as having more formal input to policy and service development. Its results include, for example, the development of community living skills program guidelines for refugee resettlement recently adopted by one of the state governments in Australia (A. Suleman, personal communication, 2011). Although service innovation and policy development are usually understood as very separate, in reality they are not—particularly at local and institutional levels. The development of the community living skills guidelines by occupational therapist Aakifah Suleman, as described above, is a good example. Adoption of the guidelines represented best practice, which then became co-opted into the policy framework at a state level, and resources were allocated accordingly. Occupational therapists, because of their unique occupational perspective, are ideally placed to contribute to the practice/policy nexus on pressing issues that include, not just the occupational needs of refugees and asylum seekers, but also, for example, populations living in poverty with attendant disabilities (Whiteford & Pereira, 2012).

Another outcome of the research has been what has now become a long-term commitment to opportunities to enhance the participation of, and inclusion into society for, refugee community groups. As I write this chapter, I have been involved in setting up a large mentoring project involving refugee students at six schools in a socioeconomically disadvantaged area in Sydney, Australia. The project, falling within my umbrella role of social inclusion, addresses many of the findings from the research I have described here. Most particularly, it focuses on building relationships and enhancing the connectedness of young people who have been through the refugee experience. Through them, we are hoping to reach their parents. Given that being a student is a significant occupation, one that has significant impacts on levels of representation and participation in society, this is an important area to focus on. This program, as well as another I have worked on with a dedicated team of educators, is commencing next year for adults as a foundation pathway into higher education. This will ensure that there will be a fuller economic participation of refugee and humanitarian entrants by gaining professional qualifications. From an occupational perspective, becoming a lawyer, teacher, or accountant is a life-changing process for all people. For people who have lived through refugee experiences, however, it represents a positive trajectory for individuals, families, and communities alike. In essence, a change in work status changes the destinies of whole groups of people. That is why what has become nationally and internationally known as a *Widening Participation Agenda* (DEEWR, 2011) has become a powerful vehicle for social transformation and one we as occupational therapists should see as highly relevant to our work.

CONTRIBUTION TO OCCUPATIONAL SCIENCE

Expanding Our Understandings of Occupational Justice

Although occupational therapists are fairly new at using the language of justice or rights, we know that injustice exists in everyday life when participation is barred, confined, segregated, prohibited, undeveloped, disrupted, alienated, marginalized, exploited, or otherwise devalued for some more than others. It follows that enabling occupational justice, as a matter of social inclusion, extends beyond enabling individual well-being to enabling more equitable opportunity, resources, privilege, and occupational rights. (Whiteford & Townsend, 2011, p. 69)

Given this description of how the research with the Kosovar refugees was conducted and the focus of that research on occupational deprivation, it is important to reflect on what contribution it has made to the growing body of knowledge of occupational science. Over time, the broad discourse surrounding occupational science has developed significantly. As theorists have added to the explanatory models through which we can understand the complexity of occupation, there has been a corresponding realignment of key concepts that underpin our constructions of occupation (Phillips & Kelk, 2010). One of the concepts that developed significantly over time is occupational justice. Occupational justice is a concept that has real utility when it comes to understanding how people either do or do not have opportunities to engage in occupations of necessity and meaning because it shifts our gaze away from individual causative factors to broader social, economic, and political forces. There are, however, two central concerns when we discuss occupational justice. One is how justice is constructed and understood, and the other is the framing of the right to engage in occupations as a human right. In this chapter, I focus on constructions of justice; however, I suggest strongly that interested readers consult the World Federation Guidelines, which specifically address occupation as a human right (World Federation of Occupational Therapists, 2006).

Occupational justice differs from other forms of justice and is concerned with

Inclusive embodied participation in the real life occupations that people decide are necessary or meaningful for them: and by the optimistic vision of possible societies in which all populations have equitable opportunities, resources, privilege, and occupational rights for meaningful occupational engagement. (Whiteford & Townsend, 2011, p. 70)

As may be evident from this description, occupational justice differs from social justice, restorative justice, and distributive justice (all of which are historically and

Figure 14-1. Three pillars of occupational therapy knowledge. (Adapted from Whiteford, G., & Townsend, E. [2011]. Participatory Occupational Justice Framework [POJF 2010]: Enabling occupational participation and inclusion. In F. Kronenberg, N. Pollard, & D. Sakellariou [Eds.], *Occupational therapies without borders. Volume 2: Towards an ecology of occupation based practices* [pp. 65-84]. London, England: Elsevier.)

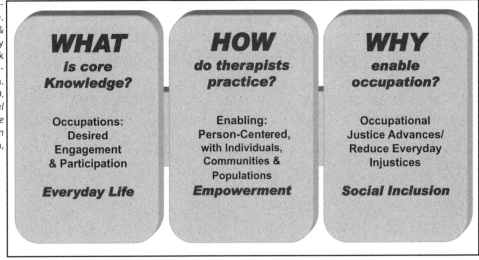

culturally located and understood) in several key ways. In essence, a justice of occupation allows for heterogeneity, or difference of doing, being, and having. This is best summed up in Figure 14-1.

If we return to the group of people at the center of the research described in this chapter, that is, refugees, we can begin to see how viewing their needs within an occupational justice framing requires us to address these through very specific sorts of processes and services. This will be the basis of the discussion in the next section. I do wish to close this section, however, by suggesting that occupational justice is but one element of what should be incorporated into a unified research agenda for occupational science into the future. Schematizing the levels at which the research could be conducted as being from the level of the individual through to that of whole populations (Molineux & Whiteford, 2011) can provide us with the means through which to also identify priorities as read against pressing social and occupational issues (e.g., chronic unemployment).

IMPLICATIONS FOR OCCUPATIONAL THERAPY

I have been optimistic about the future of occupational therapy for a long time, but my optimism these days is conditional. First, I believe we need to continue to be informed by a coherent body of knowledge generated through occupational science research. If occupation is our core domain and our purpose is to enable it across diverse and challenging contexts using a vast array of strategies, then we need to understand it as the rich and complex phenomenon it is.

Second, we need to locate ourselves more fully in those settings that are supportive of our unique focus on, and expertise in, occupation. I am unapologetic about the fact that I have always seen community as opposed to medical

institutions as being the most appropriate places for us to work for a variety of philosophical as well as practice-effectiveness reasons.

Third, we need to communicate what we do more strategically and powerfully (see Wilding & Whiteford, 2007). In this respect, we could learn from the discipline of marketing in which it is understood that you need to match your communication strategy to your intended audience. When working with community groups, the media, and people who have no knowledge of occupational therapy, I have often used the description of occupational therapists as *experts in doing*. People seem to get this, especially when you follow it with: *and we work with people so that they can participate fully in society*. In this way, we are claiming our domain of expertise and describing the ends of our input, rather than the means, which in my opinion has been a misguided focus for far too long. This description also allows us to claim our contribution to the broader discourse of social inclusion.

Fourth, and finally, we need to go about working with people in a different way. To this end, I have, along with Townsend, proposed the Participatory Occupational Justice Framework (Figure 14-2), which is a power-sharing approach based on a critical, reflexive basis. The six enablement skills profiled in the participatory occupational justice framework are raising consciousness, engaging collaboratively, mediating agreement, strategizing resources, supporting implementation, and inspiring advocacy. While Figure 14-2 provides a summary of these skills as an iterative process, a fuller discussion of this framework is provided in the Participatory Occupational Justice Framework 2010 (Whiteford & Townsend, 2011).

CONCLUSION

No research is politically innocent; it is being done for a purpose. As such there is always an element of taking

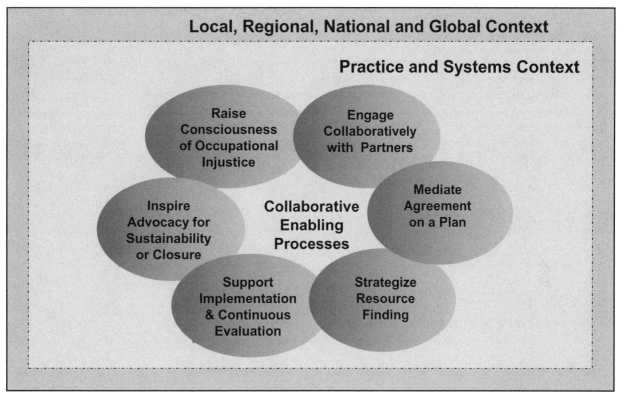

Figure 14-2. Participatory Occupational Justice Framework 2010. (Adapted from Whiteford, G., & Townsend, E. [2011]. Participatory Occupational Justice Framework [POJF 2010]: Enabling occupational participation and inclusion. In F. Kronenberg, N. Pollard, & D. Sakellariou [Eds.], *Occupational therapies without borders. Volume 2: Towards an ecology of occupation based practices* [pp. 65-84]. London, England: Elsevier.)

away people's words and some element of analysing the stories from the researcher's political, personal and intellectual perspectives. Denying this is being less than honest. Accepting and foregrounding it is an ethical way forwards. Making visible the political, personal, and intellectual perspectives of the researcher is, therefore, essential. (Higgs, Titchen, Horsfall, & Armstrong, 2007, p. 95)

What I have attempted to do in this chapter is what the above quote suggests is required of us when we engage in research—to present an account of who we are as researchers so that claims of omnipotence or objectivity cannot be made. Research, as Higgs and her colleagues suggested, is always a political undertaking and is always shaped by the belief system of the researcher.

As well as assisting you, the reader, to understand more fully those (often tacit) dimensions of research, I hope that I have also provided you with a basis to understand how strategic research, such as that which I undertook with members of the Kosovar refugee community, can have many powerful outcomes. In the case described here, these ranged from the broad outcomes of increasing community awareness and politicizing an issue of occupational deprivation and injustice to the very specific disciplinary outcomes of enhancing our understandings and conceptualizations of occupational justice within occupational science, as well as providing a basis for the

generation of new approaches to practice. Clearly, doing research is important, but ensuring that it makes a difference is even more so.

LEARNING SUPPORTS

- The United Nations High Commissioner for Refugees plays an important role internationally. In order to deepen your understandings of some of the issues covered in this chapter, visit their Web site at www.unhcr.org/cgi-bin/texis/vtx/home. When you are on the home page, what do you notice? Given that I was struck by the need of the people I interviewed (as described in the chapter) to tell their stories, I am impressed by the fact that individual stories are highlighted on the home page. What impact do you think this may have for first-time visitors to the site?

- Now, scroll down to the section labeled *Statistics*. There are numerous statistical reports available here. Of interest though is the fact that the banner for this site is "The Refugee Story in Data and Statistics." What are your thoughts on why they have given it this title? What is being communicated and represented here?

- Finally, using the menu at the top of the page, click on *Resources*. This will take you to a site that focuses on Policy Development and Evaluation. Imagine that you are an occupational therapist who has been approached to help develop a community program for newly settled refugees in your hometown. What on this site would be of interest to you? Why? Look back to the Participatory Occupational Justice Framework I discussed in this chapter. How would you follow these stages in planning your community program? Who would you meet with? Finally, referring back to the principles of evaluation identified on the RESOURCES site, think through the steps you would need to develop to plan an evaluation of your program at 12 months.

REFERENCES

Arendt, H. (1963). *Eichmann in Jerusalem: A report on the banality of evil.* London: Penguin.

Department of Education Employment and Workplace Relations. (2011). *Higher education participation and partnerships program.* Retrieved from http://www.deewr.gov.au/search/results.aspx?k=widening%20participation%20&s=All%20Sites&start1=1

Higgs, J., Titchen, A., Horsfall, D., & Armstrong, H. (2007). *Being critical and creative in qualitative research.* Sydney, Australia: Australian Hampden Press.

Kielhofner, G. (2002). Habituation: Patterns of daily occupation. In G. Kielhofner (Ed.). *A model of human occupation* (pp. 63-80). Baltimore, MD: Lippincott Williams & Wilkins.

Lather, P. (1986). Research as praxis. *Harvard Education Review, 56*(3), 257-275.

Molineux, M., & Whiteford, G. (2011). Occupational science: Genesis, evolution and future contribution. In E. Duncan (Ed.), *Foundations for practice in occupational therapy* (5th ed., pp. 262-278). London, England: Churchill Livingstone.

Phillips, P., & Kelk, N. (2010). A re-conceptualization of the person and the internal-external dichotomy present in theories that explain occupation. *Journal of Occupational Science, 17*(4), 246-255. doi:10.1080/14427591.2010.9686702

Pollard, N., Sakellariou, D., & Kronenberg, F. (2009). *A political practice of occupational therapy.* London, England: Churchill Livingstone.

Rigney, L. I. (2006). Indigenist research and Aboriginal Australia. In J. Kunnie & N. Goduka (Eds.), *Indigenous people's wisdom and power: Affirming our knowledge through narratives* (pp. 32-48). Burlington, VT: Ashgate.

Townsend, E. (1998). *Good intentions overruled: A critique of empowerment in the routine organisation of mental health services.* Toronto, Ontario, Canada: University of Toronto Press.

Townsend, E., & Wilcock, A. (2004). Occupational justice. In C. Christiansen & E. Townsend (Eds.), *Introduction to occupation* (pp. 243-273). Upper Saddle River, NJ: Prentice Hall.

Whiteford, G. (2004). Occupational issues of refugees. In M. Molineux (Ed.), *Occupation for occupational therapists* (pp. 183-199). Oxford, United Kingdom: Blackwell.

Whiteford, G. (2005). Understanding the occupational issues of refugees: A case study from Kosovo. *Canadian Journal of Occupational Therapy, 2*(2), 78-88.

Whiteford, G. (2007). Occupational deprivation and incarceration in New Zealand. *Journal of Occupational Science, 4*(3), 126-131.

Whiteford, G., & Pereira, R. (2012). Occupation, inclusion and participation. In G. Whiteford & C. Hocking (Eds.), *Occupational science: Society, inclusion and participation* (pp. 187-208). Oxford, United Kingdom: Wiley.

Whiteford, G., & Townsend, E. (2011). Participatory Occupational Justice Framework (POJF 2010): Enabling occupational participation and inclusion. In F. Kronenberg, N. Pollard, & D. Sakellariou (Eds.), *Occupational therapies without borders—Volume 2: Towards an ecology of occupation-based practices* (pp. 65-84). London, England: Elsevier.

Whiteford, G., Wilding, C., & Curtin, M. (2009). Writing as practice enquiry: Towards a scholarship of practice. In J. Higgs, D. Horsfall, & S. Grace (Eds.), *Writing qualitative research on practice* (pp. 27-36). Rotterdam, The Netherlands: Sense.

Wilcock, A. (2001). *Occupation for health. Volume 1: A journey from self health to prescription.* London, England: College of Occupational Therapists.

Wilding, C., & Whiteford, G. (2007). Language, identity and representation: Occupation and occupational therapy in acute settings. *Australian Journal of Occupational Therapy, 55*, 180-187. doi:10.1111/j.1440-1630.2007.00678.x

World Federation of Occupational Therapists. (2006). Position statement on human rights. Retrieved from http://www.wfot.org/office_files/Human%Rights%20Position%20Statement%20Final%20NLH.pdf

III

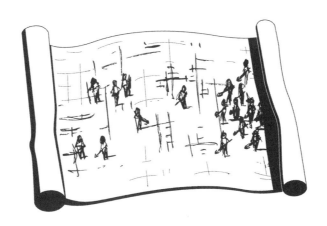

Level 3 Research

How Does Occupational Science Provide Predictive Knowledge to Support Occupational Therapy?

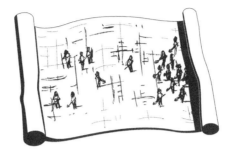

15

Predictive Research in Occupational Science

Doris Pierce, PhD, OTR/L, FAOTA

PREDICTIVE RESEARCH: SEARCHING FOR LARGER PATTERNS OF OCCUPATION

Level 3 is the least developed of the four levels of research in occupational science. Level 3 theories and studies attempt to reveal patterns of occupation across time and space, development, and usual life transitions. Level 3 provides insights into the broad patterns of occupation across large numbers of individuals. Being able to generally predict occupations is a knowledge need for occupational therapists when they first meet a client or support the movement of a client through a typical life transition. Level 3 theories are closely tied to Level 1, descriptive theories, because they attempt to expand the basic understanding of occupation that is developed at Level 1 to identify those same features across larger numbers of people, larger spaces, or longer periods of time.

PRECURSORS TO OCCUPATIONAL SCIENCE AT LEVEL 3

As was true for Level 1 occupational science, which focuses on descriptive research into occupation, predictive occupational science has been to some degree shaped by developmental theories. In the earliest conceptualizations of occupational science, when large-scale predictive potentials were considered at all, it was imagined that occupational science would describe typical development of occupational engagement. This vision was grounded in Mary Reilly's (1962, 1974) theory of occupational behavior, which described well before the emergence of occupational science a typical progression of occupational development from play exploration in childhood to adult competence and achievement. The example of Piaget's (1951) developmentally progressive play theory was influential. The dream of a predictive science was, however, only vaguely expressed in the beginnings of occupational science.

Pierce, D. (Ed.).
Occupational Science for Occupational Therapy (pp. 181-185).
© 2014 SLACK Incorporated.

Predictive Research in Occupational Science Thus Far

Typical Developmental Phases

In my own dissertation, I carried forward the vision of predictive developmental theories of occupation by completing a longitudinal study of naturalistic, in-home play in the first 18 months of life of 18 infants (Pierce, Myers, & Munier, 2009). I collected video, interview, and observation data in 313 home visits to nine boys and nine girls, each gender evenly distributed in an approximation of socioeconomic levels in the United States. Beyond the developmental description of their naturalistic play, a primary finding of that study was the degree to which the developmental patterns were shaped by and nested within the maternal management of the in-home play pattern (Pierce, 2000). Out of this work emerged an understanding not only of the developmental sequence of infant-object play, but also of the concept of co-occupation (Pierce, 2009).

Within occupational science, there has emerged an international grouping of studies into the common life transition of retirement from paid work. These researchers include Hans Jonsson and colleagues, who have primarily studied people in Sweden, and whose work is described in Chapter 18 (Jonsson & Andersson, 1999; Jonsson, Borell, & Sadlo, 2000; Jonsson, Josephsson, & Kielhofner, 2001; Jonsson, Kielhofner, & Borell, 1997). This group's research has looked at retirement as a passage, examining how it is anticipated, experienced, and viewed in retrospect by those who experience it. Although expectations and experiences of retirement most often matched, they also in some cases did not match. In related work, Vrkljan and Polgar (2007) studied the transition from driving to driving cessation in older adults, a key change in independence. Knight and colleagues (2007) examined older adults' engagement in productive occupations, such as homemaker, volunteer, or caregiver. Wiseman and Whiteford (2009) examined this transition in rural men, highlighting occupational adaptation as a theoretical framework for considering retirement. Bytheway (2003) studied elders' management of their medications. In Chapter 12, Debbie Rudman also described retirement using a critical theories perspective that emphasizes not the individual experience of retirement, but its social construction (Laliberte Rudman, 2005, 2006a, 2006b; Laliberte Rudman, Huot, & Dennhardt, 2009; Laliberte Rudman & Molke, 2009).

A few additional areas of typical development have received some research attention, attempting to move small-scale descriptive studies toward their potential for predictive patterns that may exist within common types of life transitions. For example, Horne, Corr, and Earle (2005) used mixed methods to examine the transition to first-time motherhood. Their primary finding was of a period of occupational disruption that existed between more balanced lives before motherhood versus strongly productive and obligatory patterns after motherhood.

Time Geography

A related, yet distinctly different approach to Level 3, predictive occupational science has unfolded in research into larger temporal patterns of occupation. Researchers have explored the fit of the concepts of occupation to time geography. The time-geographic approach was originally developed by Hargerstrand (1985) to use spatial and temporal context to describe large-scale patterns of activity in Sweden (Ellegaard, 1999; Kroksmark et al., 2006). It includes sophisticated methods and has been used across multiple disciplines. Occupational scientists have used time geography and other time-use methods to examine large patterns in caregiving (Ujimoto, 1998); daily occupational patterns of young Irish children (Lynch, 2009); the relationship between health, well-being, and time use in men with spinal cord injury (Pentland, Harvey, & Walker, 1998); the relation of psychological adjustment to activity patterns in people with arthritis (MacKinnon, Avison, & McCain, 1994); time allocation and HIV status (Albert et al., 1994); gender variations in weekly activity rhythms (Zuzanek & Mannell, 1993); and everyday activities of Scandinavian physiotherapy students (Alsaker, Moen, Nortvedt, & Baste, 2006).

Balance

A key concept in Level 3 predictive research in regard to large group patterns of occupation is balance (Christiansen & Matuska, 2006; Matuska, Christiansen, Polatajko, & Davis, 2009). Called either *occupational balance* or *lifestyle balance*, this research direction examines how different types of occupations exist in tension or complementarity with each other within the life patterns of individuals. Built on research into time use, studies of life balance hold potential insights into the effects on health and quality of life of imbalances in a person's occupations. Stress, burnout, circadian disruptions, and other negative health effects result from conditions of imbalance. In fact, this avenue of research has resulted in a most unusual product: an interdisciplinary edited collection titled, *Life Balance: Multidisciplinary Theories and Research* (Matuska, Christiansen, Polatajko, & Davis, 2009). This unique combination of perspectives from occupational scientists and time-use researchers provides a degree of in-depth theoretical, methodological, and empirical examination of a single area of research that is rare in such a young science. Other perspectives on occupational balance within occupational science have included Jonsson and Persson's (2006) use of flow theory and experience sampling method to examine balance, Erlandsson and Eklund's (2003) study of hassles and uplifts in women, and Hakansson, Dahlin-Ivanoff, and Sonn's (2006) study of balance in the lives of women with stress disorders.

Instruments

A critical factor in the emergence of Level 3, predictive occupational science, is the design and refinement of instruments to measure typical patterns of occupation. Although occupational therapists are quite familiar with evaluations of client function, most of those tools are not actually focused on occupations and would not be well fit to the needs of a study of large-scale patterns of occupation. To date, even instruments in occupational science that are appropriate to research that does not address disability or intervention remain strongly focused on subjective perceptions of experiences. In this section of the book, two assessments are described. Karen Atler (Chapter 16) describes the development of the Daily Experiences of Pleasure, Productivity and Restoration Profile, or PPR Profile, a time-use measure that examines the balance of three qualities of experience within a person's day. This instrument is well-grounded in time-use methods. Similarly, Phyllis Meltzer (Chapter 17) illustrates the process of designing the Self-Discovery Tapestry, a reflective instrument for examining continuities and adaptations over the personal life course that is strongly oriented toward understanding occupational change in one's life history.

QUESTIONS FOR OCCUPATIONAL SCIENCE AT LEVEL 3

Level 3, predictive occupational science, holds strong potential to make the case for the explanatory value of occupation in understanding large-scale patterns of human behavior, development, and quality of life. Of the four levels, however, it is the least developed. How will key questions in its unfolding be answered?

Why Is Predictive Occupational Science the Least Developed of the Four Levels?

There are three potential answers to the question of why Level 3 occupational science is the least developed. One is that, because large-scale prescriptive research extends basic descriptive concepts from Level 1 into patterns discernible across larger numbers, it may be that the development of Level 3 occupational science must await the deeper development of concepts within Level 1, descriptive occupational

science. Second, predictive occupational science requires quantitative, large participant number studies, but occupational science is largely qualitative (Glover, 2009). Third, it may be that occupational scientists are not particularly motivated to create predictive models of typical patterns of occupation. It is difficult to know how this challenge will be resolved. That answer can only be found in the future of occupational science research.

What Measures of Occupation Are Needed to Support Predictive Occupational Science?

The question of needed measures to better support the development of Level 3 occupational science is an interesting one. In the earliest years of occupational science, some of us envisioned descriptive work on age-related progressions of occupation that would eventually produce assessments of these typical patterns, in order to support developmental approaches to intervention. Certainly, any progress on research questions regarding occupational balance within intra-individual life patterns depends heavily on capacities of methods and instrumentation. Many imagined that time geography would provide occupational science with objective measures and methods for the portrayal of large-scale temporal and spatial patterns of occupation. Yet, not many researchers have followed this path. Instead, new measures, grounded in original Level 1 concepts, are being developed. It seems likely that this linking of Levels 1 and 3 will continue, with Level 1 producing new concepts and Level 3 producing instruments that can carry those concepts into large-scale studies.

How Is Occupation Similar and Different Across Populations?

This question speaks to the tie within occupational science of Level 2, relational theory and research, to that of Level 3, predictive research. Given Level 3 methods and instruments that are effective in examining patterns of occupation, interesting relational work can be extended from small within-population studies to lager, comparative studies. Examples might include the examination of occupational pattern differences across ability/disability, health/illness, wealth/poverty, gender difference, freedom/oppression, and many other key interdisciplinary concepts. The examination of occupations across cultures is methodologically challenging but possible, promising a harvest of critical insights into the ways that the Western roots of occupational science may be constraining (Hocking et al., 2008). Further, the potential of occupational science to identify not only what is different, but also what is alike, in global human occupations could be philosophically important to the way we view international human diversity.

Will Occupational Science Embrace an Understanding of Occupation Over a 24-Hour Cycle?

Because of my passionate interest in the human occupation of sleep, which is the temporally largest and most prevalent portion of our occupational pattern, I wonder if we will take our Western blinders off and begin to include sleep in our research? The effects of sleep quality on health, quality of life, stress, mood, and many other characteristics of human life are unquestioned. Yet, we continue to build this blind spot in regard to the "otherness" of the occupation of sleep into so many of our studies. Atler (Chapter 16) has transcended this limitation in her design of the PPR Profile. Hopefully others will follow, opening occupational science to a more honest and physiologically grounded understanding of large-scale occupational patterns, especially as they are related to health.

SECTION CHAPTERS ILLUSTRATING LEVEL 3, PREDICTIVE OCCUPATIONAL SCIENCE RESEARCH

In this section of the book, several chapters demonstrate the emergent state of Level 3, predictive work in occupational science. As just mentioned, Chapters 16 and 17 offer new instruments that measure occupational patterns on a larger scale than previously imagined. Hans Jonsson's work (Chapter 18) demonstrates the research potential of occupational science research in regard to important life transitions. In Chapter 19, Alison Wicks shares her research into the unfolding of occupational potential over lives through narratives, bringing our attention to the ways in which lives become increasingly unique in their occupational pattern as they choose one direction or another. Last in this section, Susan Corr and Alexandra Palombi (Chapter 20) explore the relation of occupations to quality of life through the innovation of Q methodology.

Level 3 predictive occupational science is a more recent and ambitious development within the discipline. Although initial visions of occupational science that were predictive on a larger scale have been expressed, they were largely limited to mapping out typical developmental progressions and grappling with the historical notion of occupational balance. At this level of the young science, Level 3 research is still in a stage of adventurous exploration of new theoretical and methodological territory. The potential of Level 3, predictive research, beckons us on. Only time and the passionate topical commitments of researchers will show what the future may hold for Level 3, predictive occupational science.

REFERENCES

Albert, S. M., Todak, G., Elkin, E., Marder, K., Dooneief, G., & Stern, Y. (1994). Time allocation and disability in HIV infection: A correlational study. *Journal of Occupational Science, 1*(4), 21-30. doi:10.1080/14427591.1994.9686389

Alsaker K., Moen B. E., Nortvedt, M. W., & Baste, V. (2006). Low health-related quality of life among abused women. *Quality of Life Research, 15*(6), 959-965. doi:10.1007/s11136-006-0046-4

Bytheway, B. (2003). Responsibility and routines: How older people manage their long-term medication. *Journal of Occupational Science, 8*(3), 5-13.

Christiansen, C., & Matuska, K. (2006). Lifestyle balance: A review of concepts and research. *Journal of Occupational Science, 13*, 49-61. doi:10.1080/14427591.2006.9686570

Ellegaard, K. (1999). A time-geographic approach to study everyday life of individuals: A challenge of complexity. *GeoJournal, 40*, 11-16.

Erlandsson, L., & Eklund, M. (2003). Women's experiences of hassles and uplifts in their everyday patterns of occupations. *Occupational Therapy International, 10*, 95-114. doi:10.1002/oti.179

Glover, J. (2009). The literature of occupational science: A systematic, quantitative examination of peer-reviewed publications from 1996 to 2006. *Journal of Occupational Science, 16*(2), 92-103. doi:10.1080/14427591.2009.9686648

Hakansson, C., Dahlin-Ivanoff, S., & Sonn, U. (2006). Achieving balance in everyday life. *Journal of Occupational Science, 13*, 74-82. doi:10.1080/14427591.2006.9686572

Hargerstrand, T. (1985). Time-geography: Focus on the corporeality of man, society and environment. Reprinted from *The science and praxis of complexity* (pp. 193-216). Tokyo, Japan: The United Nations University.

Hocking, C., Pierce, D., Shordike, A., Wright-St Clair, V., Bunrayong, W., Vittayakorn, S., & Rattakorn, P. (2008). The promise of internationally collaborative research for studying occupation: The example of the older women's food preparation study. *OTJR: Occupation, Participation, and Health, 28*, 180-190. doi:10.3928/15394492-20080901-02

Horne, J., Corr, S., & Earle, S. (2005). Becoming a mother: Occupational change in first time motherhood. *Journal of Occupational Science, 12*, 176-183. doi:10.1080/14427591.2005.9686561

Jonsson, H., & Andersson, L. (1999). Attitudes to work and retirement: Generalization or diversity? *Scandinavian Journal of Occupational Therapy, 6*(1), 29-35. doi:10.1080/110381299443825

Jonsson, H., Borell, L., & Sadlo, G. (2000). Retirement: An occupational transition with consequences on temporality, rhythm and balance. *Journal of Occupational Science, 7*, 5-13. doi:10.1080/14427591.2000.9686462

Jonsson, H., Josephsson, S., & Kielhofner, G. (2001). Narratives and experience in an occupational transition: A longitudinal study of the retirement process. *American Journal of Occupational Therapy, 55*, 424-432. doi:10.5014/ajot.55.4.424

Jonsson, H., Kielhofner, G., & Borell, L. (1997). Anticipating retirement: The formation of narratives concerning an occupational transition. *American Journal of Occupational Therapy, 51*(1), 49-56. doi:10.5014/ajot.51.1.49

Jonsson, H., & Persson, D. (2006). Towards an experiential model of occupational balance: An alternative perspective on flow theory analysis. *Journal of Occupational Science, 13*, 62-73. doi:10.1080/14427591.2006.9686571

Knight, J., Ball, V., Corr, S., Turner, A., Lowis, M., & Ekberg, M. (2007). An empirical study to identify older adults' engagement in productivity occupations. *Journal of Occupational Science, 14*(3), 145-153. doi:10.1080/14427591.2007.9686595

Kroksmark, U., Nordell, K., Bendixen, H., Magnus, E., Jakobsen, K., & Alsaker, S. (2006). Time geographic method: Application to studying patterns of occupation in different contexts. *Journal of Occupational Science, 13*, 11-16. doi:10.1080/14427591.2006.9686566

Laliberte Rudman, D. (2005). Understanding political influences on occupational possibilities: An analysis of newspaper constructions of retirees. *Journal of Occupational Science, 12*(3), 149-160. doi:10.1080/14427591.2005.9686558

Laliberte Rudman, D. (2006a). "Positive aging" and its implications for occupational possibilities in later life. *Canadian Journal of Occupational Therapy, 73*(3), 188-192.

Laliberte Rudman, D. (2006b). Shaping the active, autonomous and responsible modern retiree: An analysis of discursive technologies and their connections with neoliberal political rationality. *Ageing and Society, 26*, 181-201. doi:10.1017/S0144686X05004253

Laliberte Rudman, D., Huot, S., & Dennhardt, S. (2009). Shaping ideal places for retirement: Occupational possibilities within contemporary media. *Journal of Occupational Science, 16*(1), 18-24. doi:10.1080/14427591.2009.9686637

Laliberte Rudman, D., & Molke, D. (2009). Forever productive: The discursive shaping of later life workers in contemporary Canadian newspapers. *WORK: A Journal of Prevention, Assessment & Rehabilitation, 32*(4), 377-390. doi:10.3233/WOR-2009-0850

Lynch, H. (2009). Patterns of activity of Irish children aged five to eight years: City living in Ireland today. *Journal of Occupational Science, 16*, 44-49. doi:10.1080/14427591.2009.9686641

MacKinnon, J. R., Avison, W. R. & McCain, G. A. (1994). Rheumatoid arthritis, occupational profiles and psychological adjustment. *Journal of Occupational Science, 1*(4), 3-10. doi:10.1080/14427591.1994.9686387

Matuska, K., Christiansen, C., Polatajko, H., & Davis, J. (2009). *Life balance: Multidisciplinary theories and research*. Thorofare, NJ: SLACK Incorporated.

Pentland, W., Harvey, A. S., & Walker, J. (1998). The relationships between time use and health and well-being in men with spinal cord injury. *Journal of Occupational Science, 5*, 14-25. doi:10.1080/14427591.1998.9686431

Piaget, J. (1951). *Play, dreams, and imitation in childhood*. London, England: Routledge and Kegan Paul.

Pierce, D. (2000). Maternal management of the home as an infant/toddler developmental space. *American Journal of Occupational Therapy, 54*, 290-299. doi:10.5014/ajot.54.3.290

Pierce, D. (2009). Co-occupation: The challenges of defining concepts original to occupational science. *Journal of Occupational Science, 16*, 273-287. doi:10.1080/14427591.2009.9686663

Pierce, D., Myers, C., & Munier, V. (2009). Informing early intervention through an occupational science description of infant-toddler interactions with home space. *American Journal of Occupational Therapy, 63*, 273-287. doi:10.5014/ajot.63.3.273

Reilly, M. (1962). Occupational therapy can be one of the great ideas of 20th-century medicine. *American Journal of Occupational Therapy, 16*, 1-9.

Reilly, M. (1974). *Play as exploratory learning*. Beverly Hills, CA: Sage Publications.

Ujimoto, K. (1998). Frequency, duration, and social context of activities in daily living: Time-budget methodology for caregiving research. *Journal of Occupational Science, 5*, 6-13. doi:10.1080/14427591.1998.9686430

Vrkljan, B., & Polgar, J. (2007). Linking occupational participation and occupational identity: An exploratory study of the transition from driving to driving cessation in older adulthood. *Journal of Occupational Science, 14*, 30-39. doi:10.1080/14427591.2007.9686581

Wiseman, L., & Whiteford, G. (2009). Understanding occupational transitions: A study of older rural men's retirement experiences. *Journal of Occupational Science, 16*, 104-109. doi:10.1080/14427591.2009.9686649

Zuzanek, J., & Mannell, R. (1993). Gender variations in the weekly rhythms of daily behavior and experiences. *Journal of Occupational Science, 1*, 25-37. doi:10.1080/14427591.1993.9686376.

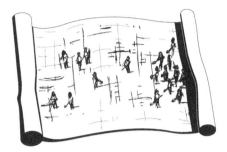

16

The Daily Experiences of Pleasure, Productivity and Restoration Profile
A Measure of Subjective Experiences

Karen Atler, PhD, OTR

My discovery of the limited number of occupation assessments that measure the effectiveness of occupation-based health education led my doctoral studies toward instrument development and validation. In fact, I learned in the late 1990s leading research demonstrating the effectiveness of activity-based interventions provided by occupational therapy practitioners to prevent health issues among older adults did not employ an occupation measure as an outcome (Clark et al., 1997; Eakman, 2007). Only in the past few years has the development of the Meaningful Activity Participation Assessment related to this work begun (Eakman, Carlson, & Clark, 2010).

While I recognized that measuring time spent in daily activities and the related subjective experiences were not new constructs, I wanted to design a measure that would attempt to quantify the subjective experiences of daily life and also provide an opportunity for individuals to reflect upon their occupational experiences. Creating an assessment that allowed personal reflection was influenced by my clinical and academic experiences that resonated with the results of the Well Elderly Study, which reported that enabling individuals to become aware of their occupations

was essential to promoting changes in daily occupations that support health and well-being (Clark, Jackson, & Carlson, 2004). These results substantiate the early tenets of occupational therapy. A detailed review of Meyer and colleagues' works illustrated that individuals experienced time and occupation differently (Christiansen, 2007). Therefore, assisting individuals in discovering their own balance of rest, pleasure, and accomplishment during daily occupations was what was important to balancing life and thus promoting health (Christiansen, 2007; Hall & Buck, 1915; Meyer, 1922; Quiroga, 1995; Slagle & Robeson, 1941).

The purpose of this chapter is to introduce the Daily Experiences of Pleasure, Productivity and Restoration Profile (PPR Profile) as a developing time-use measure designed to capture the objective and subjective dimensions of daily life (Atler, 2008). Initial steps in developing the measure are presented prior to reporting the results of the first two studies examining the reliability and validity of the PPR Profile. The chapter ends with a discussion on the contributions of this research to occupational science and the implications for occupational therapy practice.

Pierce, D. (Ed.).
Occupational Science for Occupational Therapy (pp. 187-199).
© 2014 SLACK Incorporated.

BACKGROUND

The development of the PPR Profile followed the four phases of instrument development outlined by Benson and Clark (1982): planning, designing, evaluating, and validating the assessment. In this section, I will highlight central steps taken during the first two phases with the intent to (a) illustrate the need for the PPR Profile, (b) highlight the literature supporting the major construct of the PPR Profile, and (c) describe the key characteristics of the PPR Profile.

Establishing the Need for the PPR Profile— A Review of Current Assessments

Planning for the development of the PPR Profile began with identifying its purpose. As mentioned earlier, there were few occupation measures that captured the subjective experiences of daily life in a detailed manner that allowed people to reflect on their daily experiences. Once I clarified this as the purpose of the PPR Profile, the literature was reviewed to ensure there were no current reliable and valid instruments available that addressed the identified purpose (Benson & Clark, 1982). Initially, I found evidence that there was a need to develop additional assessments that captured the complex process of engaging in daily occupations over time (Coster, 2006; Law, Dunn, & Baum, 2005). Three categories of assessments, participation, client-centered, and balance measures were reviewed in more detail. The review was limited to general assessments that represented a broad perspective of occupation (self-care, work, and leisure) and that could be used with adults and older adults with a wide range of abilities/disabilities.

The review showed that assessing and measuring participation can be challenging (Rochette, Korner-Bitensky, & Levasseur, 2006). Participation includes both basic human activities related to survival (i.e., eating, dressing, moving around in our environment), as well as self-development and health-promoting activities that are often unique to each individual (Rochette et al., 2006). My review of general participation measures resulted in the same conclusion as Law and colleagues (2005) who stated that the "majority of participation measures focus on the observable characteristics of participation" (p. 109). Several critiques of participation measures were also found that stated that participation measures focused on observable characteristics of doing were limiting, because they did not address the subjective experiences of participation (Hemmingsson & Jonsson, 2005; Perenboom & Chorus, 2003; Ueda & Okawa, 2003).

Five assessments were identified as client-centered assessments. These types of assessments are used to discover the subjective or personal experience of occupation (McColl & Pollock, 2001; Pollock, 1993). Four of the five assessments were developed from the same theoretical foundation. The procedures for two of these assessments

revealed that the therapist rates the client's performance, thus the client's perceptions may be altered through the perspective of the therapist. I concluded that client-centered assessments reviewed may not fully capture the complexity of occupations and their associated subjective experiences.

In the review of balance measures reported in the occupational therapy literature, there were two types of measures found: time diaries and social ecological approaches (Backman, 2005). Time-use diaries provide a contextual look at what people do (Harvey, 1999) and have been described as the most common method used (Christiansen & Matuska, 2006; Law, 2002). Yet, Christiansen (1996) suggested that time diaries that only examine the amount and type of activities may be too simplistic to identify occupational patterns and their relationship to health and well-being.

Experience sampling method, a social ecological approach, developed by Csikszentmihalyi, has advanced ways of measuring the quality of daily life experiences and balance, measuring the optimal experience called *flow* (Csikszentmihalyi, 1990; Jonsson & Persson, 2006; Persson, Eklund, & Isacsson, 1999; Seligman & Csikszentmihalyi, 2000). While some suggest optimal experience may measure balance at an activity level, others suggest optimal experience is not a measure of balance (Jonsson & Persson, 2006; Persson & Jonsson, 2009). Other critiques found suggested that experience sampling method involves high levels of participant burden, is not designed to gather activities across a full day, and is seen by some as impractical for clinical use (Backman, 2005; Kahneman, Krueger, Schkade, Schwarz, & Stone, 2004). Although the process of reviewing current assessments required extensive time, I gained a broader understanding of current assessments and was assured that there was a clear need for developing the PPR Profile.

Subjective Experiences of Pleasure, Productivity, and Restoration as the Main Construct of the PPR Profile

Once the need for developing the PPR Profile was confirmed, I began conceptualizing the measure. Designing the PPR Profile required establishment of instrument specifications including characteristics related to (a) item content and format, (b) scale and response formats, (c) instructions, (d) layout, and (e) intended audience (American Educational Research Association, 1999; DeVellis, 2003). Using principles from measurement theory, I chose the scale and response format to quantify the amount or levels of pleasure, productivity, and restoration experienced (Benson & Schelly, 1997). During this step of developing the PPR Profile, I went back to the literature to explicate the theoretical underpinnings of the major construct: the subjective experiences of pleasure, productivity, and restoration. The following section briefly introduces support for this conceptualization of subjective experience and provides two illustrations of the interrelated nature of pleasure, productivity, and restoration experiences in daily life.

Four foundational assumptions from occupational science on occupation and the occupational nature of humans provided support for the development of the PPR Profile (Clark et al., 1997; Wood, 1998; Yerxa et al., 1990):

1. Humans have an innate need or drive to engage in occupation.

2. Occupational engagement occurs within a sociocultural, physical, temporal, and historical context.

3. Occupation is a multidimensional and complex experience.

4. Occupation can be understood only by comprehending the personal experience, because individuals attach different meanings to engagement.

Recently, recognition of personal experiences related to occupation and occupational balance has increased due to the identified limitations of categorizing occupations into the categories of self-care, work, and leisure (Hammell, 2004, 2009a, 2009b; Jonsson, 2008). These three categories have come to be seen as unrealistically fixed, as well as "simplistic, value laden, decontextualized and insufficiently descriptive of subjective experience" (Pierce, 2003, p. 252). To replace the use of traditional typologies of occupation, Pierce (1997) proposed an alternative way of examining occupational patterns. In the early 1990s, Zemke and Pierce began to study "how occupation is individually experienced in terms of the degrees of pleasure (*commonly linked to leisure*), productivity (*commonly linked to work*), and restfulness during engagement (*commonly linked to self-care*)" (Pierce, 1997, p. 4). Wilcock (1993, 2006) not only identified satisfaction, fulfillment, and pleasure as innate needs, she also described sleep and relaxation as "natural mechanisms to prevent overuse and a time for repair" (2006).

My conceptualization of the three subjective experiences of pleasure, productivity, and restoration built upon the work of Pierce (1997, 2003) but expanded to emphasize the interrelated nature of these experiences. This conceptualization (a) allows for the examination of subjective experience with equal attention given to pleasure, productivity, and restoration; (b) highlights the interrelatedness of occupational experiences; and (c) brings restoration, an essential element of health, well-being, and balance, into a prominent place.

In the PPR Profile, pleasure was defined as enjoying the process. Little emphasis is placed on the outcome; the person is enjoying the moment. Participation in occupations producing a sense of productivity was defined as getting something done. Other descriptors include the following: met a goal, made a contribution, or learned something. Restoration was defined as being renewed by doing the

activity. In addition to the definitions, descriptors for each experience were provided on the rating scale to help people understand the concepts. An important feature of the PPR Profile is that people are encouraged to define their experiences as a blend of these three experiences. This allows for a greater understanding of how different occupations at various times, in various contexts, can lead to different levels of pleasure, productivity, and restoration. The following two illustrations provide a glimpse into the interrelated nature of these experiences.

The first illustration comes from the early writings in occupational therapy. Having opportunity to work, do, or learn was viewed as important because doing through the use of one's hands leads to a sense of achievement (Meyer, 1922). Engagement in doing used as a means to restore health was known as the work cure. The use of "work" was believed to be essential because, without experiencing tangible outcomes that led to a sense of satisfaction and accomplishment, people experienced a sense of mental unrest and delayed recovery (Hall & Buck, 1915; Slagle & Robeson, 1941). Although there was a large focus on ensuring that patients experienced a sense of accomplishment and satisfaction, the work cure expanded beyond the importance of doing. Paying particular attention to how patients experienced work was more important than specific types of activity. Occupational experiences leading to health emphasized the importance of experiencing both achievement and pleasure. The work cure was described as a "division of the twenty-four hours into changeable periods of work, rest and recreation..." (Hall, 1910, p. 13). Thus, there was a need to experience accomplishment, pleasure, and restoration within a day.

The second example illustrating the interrelated nature of pleasure, productivity, and restoration comes from a more recent framework designed to help understand the importance of restorative activities on work performance and health called the Effort-Recovery Model (Meijman & Mulder, 1998). Because people use physical and emotional resources to respond to work demands, this model proposes that a period of recovery is required to restore the body's resources. Without engagement in restorative activities that allows the body to return to its prestressor level of functioning, work productivity as well as well-being may be compromised (van Hooff, Geurts, Beckers, & Kompier, 2011). Because the growing body of research using this model has resulted in the discovery that a variety of activity types were found to allow recovery, Sonnentag and Fritz (2007) focused on understanding experiences during activities. They stated, "Going beyond the specific activities, and examining the underlying experiences is crucial for getting more insight into the psychological processes leading to recovery" (p. 204). Disengagement from work, mastery of new challenges, and connection with others were activity experiences associated with restoration.

COLUMN	INSTRUCTIONS
Time Activity Began	Record the time the activity began.
Time Activity Ended	Record the time the activity ended and you began the next activity.
What You Were Doing	Record what you did. Use one line per activity.
With Whom	Record who was present.
Where	Record where you were (e.g., home, car, work, grocery store).
Pleasure, Productivity, Restoration	Record the level (1 absent → 5 extremely high) of Pleasure, Productivity, and Restoration for each activity. Use the rating scale with definitions provided.
Comments	Record any thoughts you want to specifically remember about your experience during the activity.

TIME BEGAN	TIME ENDED	IDENTIFY WHAT YOU WERE DOING	WITH WHOM	WHERE	WHEN DOING THIS ACTIVITY MY LEVEL OF			COMMENTS
					Pleasure	Productivity	Restoration	
12:00 a.m.	6:00 a.m.	Sleeping	Self	Home	4	2	4	A good night
6:00 a.m.	6:45 a.m.	Got ready for the day	Self	Home	3	2	3	
6:45 a.m.	7:30 a.m.	Ate breakfast while reading newspaper	Self	Home	4	3	4	
7:30 a.m.	7:50 a.m.	Drove to work	Self	Car	2	3	1	Traffic crazy!

Figure 16-1. PPR Profile: Daily Experiences of Pleasure, Productivity and Restoration instructions and layout.

The Daily Experiences of the PPR Profile

The PPR Profile: Daily Experiences of Pleasure, Productivity and Restoration (Atler, 2008) is a measure being designed for use in occupational therapy practice and occupational science research with individuals from adolescence through older adulthood. It can be used with many individuals across the ability/disability continuum and with individuals challenged or potentially challenged by various life circumstances (e.g., stress, role changes, transitions).

Based on the identified purpose of the PPR Profile and the literature reviewed, the construction of the PPR Profile began by adapting the commonly used format of time-use surveys. Recording levels of pleasure, productivity, and restoration (as a measure of the subjective experience of daily life) was added to the common data points of time use, which are what a person does, when, where, and with whom (Harvey, 1999).

When completing the PPR Profile, individuals record their activities throughout a 24-hour period of time, begin-ning at midnight. Each line represents a chunk of time guided by what was done. Contextual factors are then recorded, including (a) the time the activity began and ended; (b) who was present; (c) where the activity occurred; and (d) the level of pleasure, productivity, and restoration experienced within each activity (Figure 16-1).

The current version of the PPR Profile is the result of many revisions, refinements, and testing. I used one of my doctoral classes to clarify and refine the conceptual development of the PPR Profile. This course only rein-forced my awareness of the importance and my experi-ence of research related to instrument development and validation as a collaborative process. My research advi-sors, colleagues, and peers have all played a part along the way. Even more clearly, I have begun to realize and experience instrument development and validation as an ongoing process. Through these early stages, the initial feedback from people using the PPR Profile provided posi-tive feedback. This was encouraging, exciting, and a bit mind boggling as I launched into a more formal validation process of examining the reliability and validity. The next section describes the first two studies completed with the PPR Profile.

Read all the instructions and example given before starting. Select a particular day to record. Using the booklet, recall and record your daily activities and experiences in sequence for a full 24 hours. Begin recording your activities at midnight, and continue through the last activity of the day ending at midnight the next day. Include the time you sleep. There should be no gaps in time. After recording your last activity and experience, complete the questions on the last pages of the booklet (see Figure 16-1).

INITIAL RESEARCH STUDIES OF THE PPR PROFILE

Study 1: Pretesting the PPR Profile

Validation of a developing assessment often begins with examination of its content and format to provide evidence of the intended purpose and use. In this first study, two sources of validity evidence were evaluated: evidence based on test content and evidence of the response process (American Educational Research Association, 1999). The two main purposes of this study were to evaluate if the structure of the wording and format generated the intended information and to gain insights into how individuals thought as they completed the PPR Profile.

Participants

Following approval from the institution's human subjects review committee, 19 participants (ranging from 18 to 89 years of age) were recruited from a variety of agencies including the local university, various community organizations, businesses, and churches through e-mail announcements, posted flyers, and in-person announcements. Fourteen participants were women and five were men. Inclusion criteria included the ability to (a) read and understand English, (b) recall and record one's activities and experiences, and (c) willingness to discuss and give feedback about the process of completing the PPR Profile. Individuals who had experienced a major illness or injury requiring hospitalization within the past 6 months were excluded because, for them, daily activities were likely to be disrupted.

Data Collection

Cognitive interviewing, a specific interviewing method designed to gain insights into how people perceive and think about information in order to respond to the information, was employed (Willis, 2005). Following Willis' (2005) guidelines, three rounds of interviews were completed to allow for modifications and retesting in smaller steps. Two interviewers, I and a graduate research assistant, completed the interviews using a pre-established interview

guide. We established consistency in our interviewing by completing the first seven interviews together. Following each interview, the interviewers made field notes capturing the main ideas and feedback gained. Additionally, all interviews were audiotaped to provide a way to review information gathered.

Round 1

During Round 1, seven diverse participants were selected using quota sampling (i.e., varying in age, education, and life roles). After consent to participate was obtained and demographic data were collected, participants were introduced to the PPR Profile and were scheduled for a 45- to 60-minute face-to-face interview. Participants were given the choice to either (a) fill out the PPR Profile 24 hours before the scheduled interview or (b) complete the PPR Profile during the interview. During the face-to-face interviews, participants were asked to think aloud, sharing their thoughts as they read and using the rating scales to identify their levels of pleasure, productivity, and restoration. The interview ended with questions designed to gather feedback on the instructions, wording, format, layout, and rating scale. The first round ended when there was general agreement as to what wording on the rating scale needed to be changed.

Rounds 2 and 3

Seven different participants were selected in Round 2 using the same sampling method as in Round 1 and oriented to the study. During Round 2, however, all participants took the PPR Profile home with them to read and complete for one 24-hour day. On the following day, a 1-hour interview was completed. Participants reflected on the process and thinking they used to complete the PPR Profile and gave feedback on the instructions, wording, format, layout, and rating scale. Following Round 2 interviews, the graduate research assistant and I met to examine the feedback gathered from all Round 1 and Round 2 interviews collectively. Five additional interviews (Round 3) were completed to gain feedback from more individuals 65 years of age or older and with more variation in levels of education.

Analysis

Content analysis (Creswell, 1998) and organized visual display strategies (Miles & Huberman, 1994) were used to analyze the data. Content analysis identified emerging themes that guided my decisions about how to make changes to the content and format of the PPR Profile. To increase trustworthiness, each interview was reviewed by both researchers (Krefting, 1991). We then met together to discuss and clarify emerging themes. The final themes identified were then compared to an organized visual display. The visual display was created by listening to each interview and placing all comments and feedback into the following categories: (a) instructions (including the example); (b) layout and format; (c) rating scale and identification of levels of pleasure, productivity, and restoration; and (d) constructs of pleasure, productivity, and restoration.

Findings

The information gained through cognitive interviewing led to several major changes being made, but also confirmed that the intent of the PPR Profile, which was to increase awareness of pleasure, productivity, and restoration experiences associated with daily activities, was met without high levels of participant burden. The feedback leading to the changes and the actual changes are summarized before reporting on the PPR Profile's intended purpose.

Changes to the Rating Scale

During Round 1 interviews, participants frequently commented on the word *lacking* when trying to rate their levels of subjective experiences. Until the word on the rating scale was changed from *lacking* to *absent*, participants' comments during the interview focused more on their confusion with the wording than explaining how they differentiated low and high levels of pleasure, productivity, and restoration. Once the wording was changed, participants' comments in Round 2 and Round 3 interviews began to reflect the process they used to choose a level. Participants, however, recommended adding clearer instructions on how to use the rating scale. In the next version of the PPR Profile, an example was provided to help participants learn how to determine different levels of pleasure, productivity, and restoration.

Analysis of participants' descriptions of the three subjective experiences obtained during Round 2 and Round 3 interviews revealed common themes in how participants talked about their experiences of pleasure, productivity, and restoration. Comparison of participants' examples and explanations of highly pleasurable, productive, and restorative experiences (one of the interview questions) to the definitions and descriptions on the rating scale also demonstrated consistent use of the three concepts. Important to note though was that the majority of the participants stated that they understood the concepts of productivity and pleasure, but found restoration to be a more difficult or unfamiliar concept. Commonly used descriptors related to pleasure, productivity, and restoration from the interviews were added to the next version of the rating scale.

As participants talked aloud about how and why they rated certain activities high in each characteristic, their explanations for the three experiences—pleasure, productivity, and restoration—at times overlapped. The most prominent theme was that participants frequently stated an activity was high in pleasure because they enjoyed getting something done. It was unclear whether participants enjoyed the process of completing the activity or if they were satisfied because the activity was done. Combining these findings with participant feedback on wording of the definitions led to simplifying the definitions of the

constructs to reflect more common everyday language. Clarifications in the instructions and examples were also added to assist in rating levels of pleasure, productivity, and restoration.

Did the Content and Format of the PPR Profile Support the Intended Purpose?

Data from the interviews were examined to explore whether the purpose of the PPR Profile (to increase awareness of one's experiences of pleasure, productivity, and restoration associated with one's daily activities) was realized by participants given the format and content. Several participants shared insights gained about themselves and their daily activities and patterns. For example, some participants reported that through completing the PPR Profile they became aware of their enjoyment in everyday activities, such as riding a bike or working. Other participants noticed the interrelationship between pleasure and productivity; when they enjoyed work, they also experienced a greater sense of productivity. One participant who did not think she had gotten much done recognized after filling out the PPR Profile that she was truly satisfied with what she did, and she was also surprised to realize she did experience pleasure throughout her day.

Discussion

The results of this study led to important clarifications and enhancements in the PPR Profile's rating scale and instructions, while also providing initial validity evidence of its content. Making refinements in the content and clarity of how to use the PPR Profile was essential to ensuring that participants were interpreting and using the PPR Profile as it was intended. Although in the early stages of development, the initial results appear to support the PPR Profile's ability to provide a mechanism that allowed participants to reflect on their daily experiences in a way that increased awareness. In addition, preliminary evidence suggests the PPR Profile may offer a way to capture and examine the interrelated experiences of pleasure, productivity, and restoration as innate needs met through engagement in occupations. Continued evidence, however, needs to be gathered to support the validity of the PPR Profile as a time-use survey that captures the objective and subjective aspects of daily occupational experiences.

The process of completing Study 1 allowed me to experience firsthand the importance of starting with an assessment of the basic features of a developing measure. In reflecting on the differences between the content of Round 1 and Round 2 interviews, I was struck by the significance of the words we use. Without having examined participants' thinking processes and interpretations of the rating scale, I would not have known how the word *lacking* created such confusion, which distracted participants and made the task of rating experiences even harder, leading to additional measurement error.

Study 2: Pilot Testing the PPR Profile

The purpose of the second study was to explore internal reliability of the rating scale and validity of the PPR Profile. The main research questions were the following:

- What is the internal reliability of the PPR Profile?

- What are the occupational patterns of pleasure, productivity, and restoration across participants of varying ages (18 to 80+ years)?

- What is the relationship between occupational patterns of pleasure, productivity, and restoration and (a) levels of health, (b) satisfaction, and (c) well-being?

- What is the utility of the PPR Profile?

Participants

Forty-seven individuals, ranging in age from 20 to 92 years of age, were selected using a nonprobability quota sampling procedure (Portney & Watkins, 2009). Following institutional review board approval, volunteers were recruited using the same inclusion and exclusion criteria as in Study 1: 18 years of age or older (a person who has primary control over how he or she plans and carries out activities), able to speak and read English at a 9th grade level, sufficient cognitive ability to record what he or she did and rate his or her experiences in a chosen day, and willing to participate in a discussion of his or her experiences the following day. Judgment about the potential participants' cognitive capacity was made based on the ability of the participant to understand the purpose of the study and the consent form.

Thirty-eight percent of the sample were young adults (20 to 35 years of age), 30% were middle-aged adults (36 to 59 years of age), and 32% were 60 years of age or older. Sixty-two percent of the sample was women (29 women, 17 men, and one transgender). Participants were highly educated, with 96% having some college education. Forty percent of the sample were married/partnered (the other 60% were single, divorced, or widowed). Employment status varied: 28% were employed full-time, 36% part-time, 8% unemployed, and 28% retired. Self-reported health status ranged from fair to excellent, with 74% of the sample reporting health as very good or excellent.

Data Collection

After consent to participate was obtained and demographic data collected, participants completed two health and well-being surveys (not reported in this chapter), were introduced to the PPR Profile, and were scheduled for a 45- to 60-minute interview following completion of the PPR Profile at home. Once data from 30 participants were collected, preliminary data analysis was initiated, which uncovered challenges in data management because participants started their day at different times. In addition, feedback collected through the follow-up interviews revealed some confusion with the instructions. Changes were made and approved through the institutional review board to have all participants begin recording their day at midnight and complete the PPR Profile twice to further examine issues of burden. Seventeen additional participants completed the PPR Profile for 2 days (1 weekday and 1 weekend day), along with a follow-up interview.

Analysis

Data were inputted initially into an episode file, in which each line correlates with each line or segment of activity recorded in the PPR Profile (Harvey, 1999). Descriptives were run to examine the use of scale. Each participant used all five options of the scale, indicating good use of the scale. Cronbach alphas were computed to examine internal consistency reliability for pleasure ($\alpha = .77$), productivity ($\alpha = .79$), and restoration ($\alpha = .80$). Reliability coefficients were obtained using 15 entries of all 47 participants. Because reliability increases as the number of items increases, a conservative number of entries was chosen to run reliability coefficients (Vaske, 2008).

Once reliability was established, average pleasure, productivity, and restoration scores were computed by summing the percentage of time spent in daily activities multiplied by the rating given for the activity. To examine differences between average pleasure, productivity, and restoration scores and activity categories, demographic variable ANOVAs and Scheffe post hoc tests were run. To examine the utility of the PPR Profile from the participants' perspectives, audiotaped interviews of the 17 participants who completed the PPR Profile for 2 days were analyzed using content analysis to explicate benefits and challenges from completing the PPR Profile.

Preliminary Findings

Because this portion of the development of the PPR Profile is underway as this chapter is being prepared, only initial findings supporting evidence of construct and consequential validity are reported.

Evidence of Construct Validity

Tables 16-1 and 16-2 report differences in means among age groups and various types of activities by average pleasure, productivity, and restoration scores.

Evidence of Consequential Validity

Each of the 17 participants completing the PPR Profile twice reported little to no burden, as well as increased awareness of how he or she spent time during the day and his or her resulting experiences. Ten of the 17 participants began to critique their experiences without prompting (e.g., "in my job I enjoy being with people, but realized it is not restorative").

TABLE 16-1

AVERAGE PLEASURE, PRODUCTIVITY, AND RESTORATION BY AGE GROUPINGS AND MAJOR ACTIVITIES

	EXPERIENCES REPORTED DURING ACTIVITIES IN A 24-HOUR PERIOD[1]			EXPERIENCES REPORTED ACCORDING TO MAJOR ACTIVITY CATEGORIES[1]		
	Young n = 14	*Middle* n = 18	*Older* n = 15	*Sleep* n = 47	*Self-Care* n = 47	*Work* n = 21
Avg. pleasure	3.41	3.23[a]	4.03[b]	3.89	2.89	2.67
Avg. productivity	2.97	3.03	3.26	2.38	3.26	3.69
Avg. restoration	3.21	2.89[a]	3.79[b]	4.44	2.84	2.02

Note. [1]Cell entries are mean scores coded on a 5-point scale from 1 "absent" to 5 "extremely high." Means with different superscripts across each row are significantly different at p < .01 using Scheffe post hoc tests.

TABLE 16-2

AVERAGE EXPERIENCES OF PLEASURE, PRODUCTIVITY, AND RESTORATION BY NONWORK ACTIVITIES

	%	# OF	PLEASURE[1]		PRODUCTIVITY[1]		RESTORATION[1]	
	Reporting	*Engagements*	M	SD	M	SD	M	SD
Computer	43/47	96	3.35	1.20	3.02	1.44	2.73	1.34
TV	35/47	75	3.53	1.02	1.88	1.34	2.83	1.26
Quiet leisure	34/47	81	4.04	1.28	3.32	1.40	3.41	1.31
Socializing	30/47	87	4.03	1.03	2.26	1.37	3.22	0.91
Exercise	24/47	38	3.79	1.02	3.92	1.17	3.32	1.42
Spiritual activities	15/47	28	4.14	11.01	3.75	1.48	4.32	0.91
Sports/recreation	8/47	10	4.50	1.28	2.80	1.81	4.60	0.52

Note. [1]Cell entries are mean scores coded on a 5-point scale from 1 "absent" to 5 "extremely high."

Discussion

Internal consistency of the PPR Profile was strong, suggesting that participants used the rating scale in a consistent, predictable way. Ratings used for pleasure, productivity, and restoration reflected the full range of function. These findings provide continued evidence of the internal structure of the PPR Profile. In addition, the differences in average pleasure, productivity, and restoration scores among individuals across the lifespan support the underlying assumptions that middle-aged adults often struggle with balancing work and expectations of others with time for self-care (Hakansson, Lissner, Bjorkelund, & Sonn, 2009; Jones, Burke, & Westman, 2006; Kerka, 2001). In addition, while there is not a statistically significant difference between average productivity scores between middle-aged and older adults, older adults in this study expressed on average higher levels of pleasure, productivity, and restoration than middle-aged adults. While our understanding of lifespan development might support higher pleasure and restoration scores among older adults, higher levels of productivity suggest the complexity of occupation and the need for further analysis that examines multiple variables at once and across a larger sample.

Review of the results in Tables 16-1 and 16-2 begins to support the assumption that activities can provide various levels of pleasure, productivity, and restoration at the same time, yet some activities may be seen as more pleasurable and/or restorative than others (e.g., sports and recreation compared to TV). These results appear to confirm ideas reported in the work-life balance literature, which suggests managing time is not sufficient for finding balance. Bird (2003) recommended finding achievement (productivity) and enjoyment (pleasure) in all areas of life to promote balance. McGee-Cooper, Trammell, and Lau (1992) suggested that adding joy (pleasure) and energy (restoration) into life was as important as managing time.

Although in the early stages of development, the initial results appear to support the PPR Profile's ability to provide a mechanism that allows participants to reflect on their daily experiences in a way that increases awareness without high participant burden reported. These results were similar to the findings reported earlier in Study 1. While caution must be taken, the ability to replicate these results may suggest that the design of the PPR Profile may lead to insights into how to address issues of burden that currently are identified with time-use methods measuring subjective experiences during daily activities (Kahneman et al., 2004).

The results of this study, however, cannot be generalized. The convenience sample of this study had the unique characteristics of being a highly educated group with the majority identifying their health as very good to excellent. Further development and analysis are required to continue to explore construct validity. Preliminary findings do, however, suggest that the PPR Profile may assist occupational scientists and occupational therapists with examining and measuring the objective and subjective experiences of daily life activities among young, middle-aged, and older adults.

CONTRIBUTIONS TO OCCUPATIONAL SCIENCE

Throughout the history of occupational science, there has been an emphasis on understanding the complexity of occupation (Yerxa, 1998; Yerxa et al., 1990). Methodologies and measures available to assist occupational scientists in the complexity of occupation, however, remain limited (Carlson & Clark, 1991). Because occupational science believes that occupational engagement is realized through the personal experience, the PPR Profile may provide an additional way to study this unique perspective. With continued development, the PPR Profile may offer a useful tool for occupational scientists to explicate the subjective experience of daily life, while potentially providing an objective measure that allows exploration of findings across larger groups of individuals, spans of time, or types of everyday occupations.

More specifically, the PPR Profile may be a means to (a) explore some of the constructs of occupational science (e.g., balance, occupational patterns) and (b) evaluate some of the underlying philosophical beliefs of occupational science. The PPR Profile is being designed to move beyond the identified impediments of examining health through measuring time spent in occupational categories. During the past few decades, occupational scientists and occupational therapists have suggested that examination of time spent in categories of self-care, work, and leisure may have limitations and be oversimplified (Hammell, 2009a; Jonsson, 2008; Pierce, 2001; Wilcock et al., 1998). The PPR Profile could become an alternative method to explore health and its relationship to occupational experiences of pleasure, productivity, and restoration, adding to the more recent developments of methodologies exploring occupational experience (Doble & Santha, 2008; Erlandsson & Eklund, 2006; Pentland & McColl, 2009; Persson & Jonsson, 2009).

By measuring the experiences of pleasure, productivity, and restoration, the PPR Profile may also provide a rich phenomenological perspective on how individuals organize their daily occupations to meet these three basic needs. As stated earlier, one of the underlying assumptions of occupational science is that humans have an innate need to engage in occupation (Clark et al., 1997; Pierce, 2003; Wood, 1998; Yerxa et al., 1990). In particular, fulfillment, pleasure, and rest have been articulated as innate needs met through engagement (Wilcock, 2006). The underlying foundation supporting the development of the PPR Profile conceptualizes occupation as the interwoven experiences of pleasure, productivity, and restoration within and across occupations.

Data from the PPR Profile may allow for examination of whether patterns of these three needs are unique or similar within specific groups of individuals (e.g., those living with stroke, mothers of toddlers, or individuals preparing to retire). In addition, examining how patterns of pleasure, productivity, and restoration change over time may be possible. Use of the PPR Profile over time could provide an additional means to understanding the lived experience following occupational changes, while allowing comparison between groups. One might explore the research question "How do individuals living with and without stroke experience pleasure or productivity over time?" Or "Do the same activities meet the same basic needs of pleasure, productivity, and restoration following illness or injury?"

Lastly, development of a reliable and valid tool that captures the subjective experiences of engagement in occupations across pleasure, productivity, and restoration may provide a means to study and understand a commonly ignored dimension of daily life and occupation, that of restoration (Greene, 2008; Howell & Pierce, 2000; Nurit & Michal, 2003). Past literature and recent research links life stress to acute and chronic illness (Christiansen, 2007; Hall & Buck, 1915; Winters & Bowers, 1957). A better understanding of the restorative dimension of occupation and the importance of individuals' successfully balancing pleasure, productivity, and restoration may help occupational scientists to produce basic knowledge of how occupations can be used to eliminate or cope with stress in order to renew individuals and enhance their performance, participation, and health.

IMPLICATIONS FOR OCCUPATIONAL THERAPY PRACTICE

The central focus of occupational therapy has always been to support people's engagement in occupations they need and want to do with the anticipated outcome of supporting their health and participation in life (American Occupational Therapy Association, 2008). I believe that the PPR Profile may have potential to assist occupational therapy practitioners and their clients throughout various aspects of the occupational therapy process. Discussion of the PPR Profile as an additional measure for use in practice is followed by my thoughts on how the PPR Profile may be used during intervention planning and implementation.

The PPR Profile may add to occupational therapy's repertoire of client-centered assessments because it is designed to allow individuals to reflect upon and record their subjective experiences of daily life. The richness of information gathered through the PPR Profile may allow the individual and therapist to collaboratively identify factors influencing their occupational experiences. These findings could guide individualized planning and implementation of interventions. While it is too early to say, perhaps the PPR Profile could be used to explore patterns of daily occupations among groups of individuals, thus providing an outcome measure that provides evidence supporting the use of occupation-based practice (Coster, 2006; Pollock, 1993).

The design and format of the PPR Profile not only facilitates reflection of what activities are performed, but also the associated experiences and contextual factors influencing those experiences, thus lending itself to being used as an occupational balance measure. Backman (2005) suggested that balance measures should be designed as client centered, allowing individuals to reflect and identify their own occupational concerns. Early findings in the first two studies reported on the use of the PPR Profile suggest that some individuals did gain awareness of occupational patterns. The use of the PPR Profile may help explicate the uniqueness and complexity of people's engagement in occupation. In addition, the results from the Well Elderly Study agree with Backman's perspective. These results demonstrated that interventions designed to increase awareness of one's occupations and their relationship to health enabled participants to create healthier occupations and routines (Clark et al., 1997, 2004). The PPR Profile may provide an additional way for individuals to recognize their occupational experiences.

Expansion of the use of the PPR Profile beyond assessment to assist with goal setting and individualizing occupational therapy services may also facilitate individuals taking on a more active role during occupational therapy and in daily life (Duggan, 2005). More importantly, the PPR Profile may elicit and offer additional information about the complexities of occupational engagement that might enhance the use of occupation in therapy and as an outcome of therapy. As an example, energy conservation is a common intervention strategy used with clients who may experience occupational challenges due to fatigue or pain (Pendleton & Schultz-Krohn, 2006; Radomski & Trombly Latham, 2008). Often, clients are educated about strategies for managing stress by planning, prioritizing, and pacing daily occupations (Pendleton & Schultz-Krohn, 2006). Using information gleaned from the PPR Profile, as well as facilitating discussions around its key concepts, may deepen clients' understanding of occupational engagement within daily contexts. For instance, discovering when, how, and which occupations actually restore the body and mind could be incorporated into daily life to support overall health. This could become a new way of incorporating the power of occupation into intervention and daily life.

LEARNING SUPPORTS

Exploring Your Own Experiences of Pleasure, Productivity, and Restoration

Purpose

- To increase awareness of experiences associated with daily occupations
- To increase awareness of the relationship between experiences of pleasure, productivity, and restoration and one's sense of well-being

Primary Concepts

- Pleasure, productivity, and restoration are innate needs met through engagement in daily occupations
- Personal experiences of occupation influence health and well-being
- Awareness and discovery of daily experiences can assist in balancing life and promoting health and well-being

Instructions

1. Choose a day to record your activities and related experiences. Use the column headings in Figure 16-1 to organize your recording. The definitions of pleasure, productivity, and restoration are listed on page 189.

2. During or immediately after recording your activities and experiences, jot down any thoughts or "a-ha's" you had.

3. On the following day, take time to review your activities, contextual factors (when, where, with whom), and related experiences. Use the following questions to guide your reflection:

    ○ What patterns if any do you notice related to your experiences of pleasure, productivity, and restoration?

    ○ What factors (what you did, where, when, and with whom) influenced your levels of pleasure, productivity, and restoration?

    ○ What is your perspective on the balance of your experiences?

    ○ What do you take away with you after recording and reflecting on your experiences?

    ○ In what ways might you use these thoughts to maintain or increase your satisfaction or well-being in life?

Discovering and Listening for Differences in Occupational Experiences

Purpose

- To appreciate the complexity and uniqueness of occupation

- To develop skills in listening to how innate needs are met through occupation

Primary Concepts

- Expressions and experiences of pleasure, productivity, and restoration are unique within and across individuals

Instructions

1. Select an occupation that you engage in often.

2. Reflect on the various experiences you have had engaging in this occupation. Consider your differing levels of pleasure, productivity, and restoration.

3. Identify what factors influenced or impacted your different experiences.

4. Talk to another person who engages in the same occupation.

5. Listen to how his or her experiences are similar or different.

6. Listen for how he or she shares or talk about his or her experiences. What is similar or different?

7. How will you ensure that you are able to discover one's personal experiences when you talk with him or her?

8. How will you ensure that you are not assuming that his or her experiences are the same as yours?

Exploring Restoration

Purpose

- To explore restoration and its interrelated connections to pleasure and productivity

Primary Concepts

- Pleasure, productivity, and restoration experiences are interrelated

Instructions

1. Brainstorm a list of all the words and phrases you connect with the concept of restoration defined as "being renewed by doing the activity."

2. Think about how your varying levels of restoration (absent to extremely high) impact your sense of pleasure.

3. Think about how your varying levels of restoration (absent to extremely high) impact your sense of productivity.

4. What is your perspective on the importance of restoration as a part of your daily occupations? Explain.

5. What is your perspective on the importance of restoration as it relates to your health and well-being? Explain.

6. Based on your perspectives of restoration, how would you integrate restoration into your occupational therapy services (assessment and intervention)? Explain.

7. Within a group, discuss your answers above.

8. In your group, discuss your thoughts related to the following quotes related to restoration, and identify how these ideas can be made more prominent in occupational therapy.

    ○ "It is in our daily lives that self-renewal is needed most. Renewal must be built into the ordinary ongoing rhythms of our lifestyles and work styles" (Hudson, 1999, p. 235).

    ○ While sleep is useful, it is not sufficient to restore one's capacity for daily living (Kaplan, 1995).

Exploring Characteristics of Assessments

Purpose

- To increase familiarity with assessments that measure occupation

- To critique assessments and their utility

Primary Concepts

- The design, format, and other characteristics of an assessment influence its purpose and use

Instructions

1. Select one of the three categories of assessments reviewed in the chapter (participation, client-centered, or balance measures).

2. Locate as many different assessments in this category as possible by examining the literature within and outside of occupational therapy.

3. Develop a chart that highlights key characteristics of the assessment. Include the following categories: the theoretical foundation, description or purpose, whom the assessment is designed to be used with, format, and clinical utility.

4. Identify how each assessment operationalizes occupation.

5. Discuss how you might integrate the use of these assessments into occupational therapy practice. Consider use in a variety of settings.

REFERENCES

American Educational Research Association. (1999). *Standards for educational and psychological testing.* Washington, DC: Author.

American Occupational Therapy Association. (2008). Occupational therapy practice framework: Domain and practice. *American Journal of Occupational Therapy, 62*(6), 625-683.

Atler, K. (2008). *Daily Experiences of Pleasure, Productivity and Restoration.* Unpublished assessment, Colorado State University, Fort Collins, CO.

Backman, C. (2005). Occupational balance: Measuring time use and satisfaction across occupational performance areas. In M. Law, W. Dunn, & C. Baum (Eds.), *Measuring occupational performance: Supporting best practice in occupational therapy* (pp. 287-298). Thorofare, NJ: SLACK Incorporated.

Benson, J., & Clark, F. (1982). A guide for instrument development and validation. *American Journal of Occupational Therapy, 36*(12), 789-800. doi:10.5014/ajot.36.12.789

Benson, J., & Schelly, B. (1997). Measurement theory: Application to occupational and physical therapy. In J. Deusen & D. Brunt (Eds.), *Assessment in occupational therapy and physical therapy* (pp. 3-24). Philadelphia, PA: W. B. Saunders.

Bird, J. (2003). Work-life balance defined: What it really means! Retrieved from http://www.worklifebalance.com/worklifebalancedefined.html

Carlson, M., & Clark, F. (1991). The search for useful methodologies in occupational science. *American Journal of Occupational Therapy, 45*(3), 235-241. doi:10.5014/ajot.45.3.235

Christiansen, C. (1996). Three perspectives on balance and occupation (A Wilma West lecture). In R. Zemke & F. Clark (Eds.), *Occupational science: The evolving discipline* (pp. 431-451). Philadelphia, PA: F. A. Davis.

Christiansen, C. (2007). Adolf Meyer revisited: Connections between lifestyles, resilience and illness. *Journal of Occupational Science, 14*(2), 63-76. doi:10.1080/14427591.2007.9686586

Christiansen, C., & Matuska, K. (2006). Lifestyle balance: A review of concepts and research. *Journal of Occupational Science, 13*(1), 49-61. doi:10.1080/14427591.2006.9686570

Clark, F., Azen, S., Zemke, R., Jackson, J., Carlson, M., Mandel, D., . . . Lipson, L. (1997). Occupational therapy for independent-living older adults: A randomized controlled trial. *Journal of the American Medical Association, 278*(16), 1321-1326. doi:10.1001/jama.1997.03550160041036

Clark, F., Jackson, J., & Carlson, M. (2004). Occupational science, occupational therapy and evidence-based practice: What the Well Elderly Study has taught us. In M. Molineux (Ed.), *Occupation for occupational therapists* (pp. 200-217). Malden, MA: Blackwell Publishers.

Coster, W. (2006). The road forward to better measures for practice and research. *OTJR: Occupation, Participation & Health, 26*(4), 131.

Creswell, J. (1998). *Quality inquiry and research design.* Thousand Oaks, CA: Sage Publications.

Csikszentmihalyi, M. (1990). *Flow: The psychology of optimal experience.* New York, NY: Harper & Row.

DeVellis, R. (2003). *Scale development: Theory and applications* (Vol. 26). Thousand Oaks, CA: Sage Publications.

Doble, S., & Santha, J. (2008). Occupational well-being: Rethinking occupational therapy outcomes. *Canadian Journal of Occupational Therapy, 75*(3), 184-190.

Duggan, R. (2005). Reflection as a means to foster client-centered practice. *Canadian Journal of Occupational Therapy, 72*(2), 103-112.

Eakman, A. (2007). *A reliability and validity study of the Meaningful Activity Participation assessment* (Doctoral dissertation). University of Southern California, Los Angeles, CA.

Eakman, A., Carlson, M., & Clark, F. (2010). Factor structure, reliability, and convergent validity of the Engagement in Meaningful Activities Survey for older adults. *OTJR: Occupation, Participation and Health, 30*(3), 111-121. doi:10.3928/15394492-20090518-01

Erlandsson, L., & Eklund, M. (2006). Levels of complexity in patterns of daily occupations: Relationship to women's well-being. *Journal of Occupational Science, 13*(1), 27-36. doi:10.1080/14427591.2006.9686568

Greene, J. (2008). Is mixed methods social inquiry a distinctive methodology? *Journal of Mixed Methods Research, 2*(1), 7-22.

Hakansson, C., Lissner, L., Bjorkelund, C., & Sonn, U. (2009). Engagement in patterns of daily occupations and perceived health among women of working age. *Scandinavian Journal of Occupational Therapy, 16*(2), 110-117. doi:10.1080/11038120802572494

Hall, H. (1910). Work-cure: A report of five years' experience at an institution devoted to the therapeutic application of manual work. *Journal of the American Medical Association, 54*(1), 12-15.

Hall, H., & Buck, M. (1915). *The work of our hands: A study of occupations for invalids.* New York, NY: Moffat, Yard & Co.

Hammell, K. (2004). Dimensions of meaning in the occupations of daily life. *Canadian Journal of Occupational Therapy, 71*(5), 296-305.

Hammell, K. (2009a). Sacred texts: A sceptical exploration of the assumptions underpinning theories of occupation. *Canadian Journal of Occupational Therapy, 76*(1), 6-13.

Hammell, K. (2009b). Self-care, productivity, and leisure, or dimensions of occupational experience? Rethinking occupational "categories." *Canadian Journal of Occupational Therapy, 76*(2), 107-114.

Harvey, A. (1999). Guidelines for time use data collection and analysis. In W. Pentland, A. Harvey, M. Lawton, & M. McColl (Eds.), *Time use research in the social sciences* (pp. 19-45). New York, NY: Kluwer Academic/Plenum.

Hemmingsson, H., & Jonsson, H. (2005). An occupational perspective on the concept of participation in the International Classification of Functioning, Disability and Health—some critical remarks. *The American Journal of Occupational Therapy, 59*(5), 569-576.

Howell, D., & Pierce, D. (2000). Exploring the forgotten restorative dimension of occupation: Quilting and quilt use. *Journal of Occupational Science, 7*(2), 68-72.

Hudson, F. (1999). *The adult years: Mastering the art of self-renewal* (rev. ed.). San Francisco, CA: Jossey-Bass.

Jones, F., Burke, R., & Westman, M. (Eds.). (2006). *Work-life balance: A psychological perspective.* New York, NY: Psychology Press.

Jonsson, H. (2008). A new direction in the conceptualization and categorization of occupation. *Journal of Occupational Science, 15*(1), 3-8.

Jonsson, H., & Persson, D. (2006). Towards an experiential model of occupational balance: An alternative perspective on flow theory analysis. *Journal of Occupational Science, 13*(1), 62-73.

Kahneman, D., Krueger, A., Schkade, D., Schwarz, N., & Stone, A. (2004). A survey method for characterizing daily life experience: The Day Reconstruction Method. *Science, 306*(5702), 1776-1780.

Kaplan, S. (1995). The restorative benefits of nature: Toward an integrative framework. *Journal of Environmental Psychology, 15*, 169-182.

Kerka, S. (2001). The balancing act of adult life. *Eric Digest, 229*.

Krefting, L. (1991). Rigor in qualitative research: The assessment of trustworthiness. *American Journal of Occupational Therapy, 45*(3), 214-222.

Law, M. (2002). Participation in the occupations of everyday life. *American Journal of Occupational Therapy, 56*(6), 640-649.

Law, M., Dunn, W., & Baum, C. (2005). Measuring participation. In M. Law, W. Dunn, & C. Baum (Eds.), *Measuring occupational performance: Supporting best practice in occupational therapy* (pp. 107-126). Thorofare, NJ: SLACK Incorporated.

McColl, M., & Pollock, N. (2001). Measuring occupational performance using client-centered perspective. In M. Law, C. Baum, & W. Dunn (Eds.), *Measuring occupational performance: Supporting best practice in occupational therapy* (pp. 66-76). Thorofare, NJ: SLACK Incorporated.

McGee-Cooper, A., Trammell, D., & Lau, B. (1992). *You don't have to go home from work exhausted: A program to bring joy, energy, and balance to your life.* New York, NY: Bantam Books.

Meijman, T., & Mulder, G. (1998). Psychological aspects of workload. In P. Drenth, H. Thierry, & C. D. Wolff (Eds.), *Work psychology* (pp. 5-33). East Sussex, UK: Psychology Press Ltd.

Meyer, A. (1922). The philosophy of occupation therapy. *Archives of Occupation Therapy, 1*, 1-10.

Miles, M., & Huberman, A. (1994). *Qualitative data analysis* (2nd ed.). Thousand Oaks, CA: Sage Publications.

Nurit, W., & Michal, A. (2003). Rest: A qualitative exploration of the phenomenon. *Occupational Therapy International, 10*(4), 227-238.

Pendleton, H., & Schultz-Krohn, W. (Eds.). (2006). *Pedretti's occupational therapy practice skills for physical dysfunction.* St. Louis, MO: Mosby.

Pentland, W., & McColl, M. (2009). Another perspective on life balance: Living in integrity with values. In K. Matuska & C. Christiansen (Eds.), *Life balance: Multidisciplinary theories and research* (pp. 165-179). Thorofare, NJ: SLACK Incorporated & AOTA Press.

Perenboom, R., & Chorus, A. (2003). Measuring participation according to the International Classification of Functioning, Disability and Health (ICF). *Disability and Rehabilitation, 25*(11-2), 577-587. doi:10.1080/0963828031000137081

Persson, D., Eklund, M., & Isacsson, A. (1999). The experience of everyday occupations and its relation to sense of coherence: A methodological study. *Journal of Occupational Science, 6*(1), 13-26.

Persson, D., & Jonsson, H. (2009). Importance of experiential challenges in a balanced life. In K. Matuska & C. Christiansen (Eds.), *Life balance: Multidisciplinary theories and research* (pp. 133-147). Thorofare, NJ: SLACK Incorporated & AOTA Press.

Pierce, D. (1997). The brain and occupational patterns: Productivity, pleasure, and rest. In C. Royeen (Ed.), *Neuroscience and occupation: Links to practice* (pp. 1-28). Bethesda, MD: American Occupational Therapy Association.

Pierce, D. (2001). Untangling occupation and activity. *American Journal of Occupational Therapy, 55*(2), 138-146.

Pierce, D. (2003). *Occupation by design: Building therapeutic power.* Philadelphia, PA: F. A. Davis Co.

Pollock, N. (1993). Client-centered assessment. *American Journal of Occupational Therapy, 47*(4), 298-301.

Portney, L., & Watkins, M. (2009). *Foundations of clinical research: Applications to practice* (3rd ed.). Upper Saddle River, NJ: Pearson Education.

Quiroga, V. (1995). *Occupational therapy: The first 30 years, 1900-1930.* Bethesda, MD: American Occupational Therapy Association.

Radomski, M., & Trombly Latham, C. (Eds.). (2008). *Occupational therapy for physical dysfunction* (6th ed.). Philadelphia, PA: Lippincott Williams & Wilkins.

Rochette, A., Korner-Bitensky, N., & Levasseur, M. (2006). "Optimal" participation: A reflective look. *Disability and Rehabilitation, 28*(19), 1231-1235. doi:10.1080/09638280600554827

Seligman, M., & Csikszentmihalyi, M. (2000). Positive psychology: An introduction. *American Psychologist, 55*(1), 5-14.

Slagle, E., & Robeson, H. (1941). *Syllabus for training of nurses in occupational therapy* (2nd ed.). Utica, NY: State Hospitals Press.

Sonnentag, S., & Fritz, C. (2007). The Recovery Experience Questionnaire: Development and validation of a measure for assessing recuperation and unwinding from work. *Journal of Occupational Health Psychology, 12*(3), 204-221. doi:10.1037/1076-8998.12.3.204

Ueda, S., & Okawa, Y. (2003). The subjective dimension of functioning and disability: What is it and what is it for? *Disability & Rehabilitation, 25*(11-12), 596-601.

van Hooff, M., Geurts, S., Beckers, D., & Kompier, M. (2011). Daily recovery from work: The role of activities, effort and pleasure. *Work & Stress, 25*(1), 55-74. doi:10.1080/02678373.2011.570941

Vaske, J. (2008). *Survey research and analysis: Applications in parks, recreation and human dimensions.* State College, PA: Venture Publishing Inc.

Wilcock, A. A. (1993). A theory of the human need for occupation. *Journal of Occupational Science: Australia, 1*, 17-24.

Wilcock, A. A. (2006). *An occupational perspective of health* (2nd ed.). Thorofare, NJ: SLACK Incorporated.

Wilcock, A., Arend, H., Darling, K., Scholz, J., Siddall, R., Snigg, C., & Stephens, J. (1998). An exploratory study of people's perceptions and experiences of wellbeing. *British Journal of Occupational Therapy, 61*(2), 75-82.

Willis, G. (2005). *Cognitive interviewing: A tool for improving questionnaire design.* Thousand Oaks, CA: Sage Publications.

Winters, E., & Bowers, A. (Eds.). (1957). *Psychobiology: A science of man.* Springfield, IL: Charles C. Thomas.

Wood, W. (1998). Biological requirements for occupation in primates: An exploratory study and theoretical analysis. *Journal of Occupational Science, 5*, 66-81.

Yerxa, E. (1998). Health and the human spirit for occupation. *American Journal of Occupational Therapy, 52*(6), 412-422.

Yerxa, E., Clark, F., Frank, G., Jackson, J., Parham, D., Pierce, D., . . . Zemke, R. (1990). An introduction to occupational science, a foundation for occupational therapy in the 21st century. *Occupational Therapy in Health Care, 6*(4), 1-17.

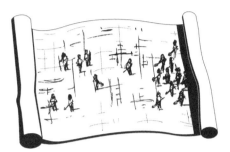

Development of the Self-Discovery Tapestry

Phyllis J. Meltzer, PhD, MSG, MS

The development of the Self-Discovery Tapestry (Figure 17-1), a life-review instrument, includes the study of how the instrument was developed within a social science discipline, how the research purposes of its development were achieved and interpreted, and how its utilization and recent developments contribute to occupational science and occupational therapy.

MY PERSONAL MOTIVATION FOR DEVELOPING THE TAPESTRY

The study of occupational science appealed to me because it appeared to synthesize several social science disciplines, some of which I had studied. I believed the degree in occupational science would allow me to combine my passion for the principles of adult learning and my knowledge of gerontology with the focus of occupational science on individuals' adaptive behaviors.

During my occupational science studies, I was struck by the book *Composing a Life*, by Mary Catherine Bateson (1989), in which she presented the idea that women improvise their lives. Bateson used many terms that were evocative of textiles: *weaving, patchwork,* and *threads.* Because I also work with textiles, I was inspired to weave a small tapestry of my life with woolen yarn. Colleagues suggested I adapt the tapestry idea to paper so that others might weave their lives with colored pens on a paper matrix form. To my amazement, the instrument seemed to evoke hitherto undisclosed insights, information, and connections for those who tried completing it. It became a very personal document for each person, especially those experiencing a transitional event.

I made the Self-Discovery Tapestry the basis for my dissertation research in order to ascertain if it was effective with mature women, like me, who were returning to education in order to change occupations. I was curious to discover how other women decided to return, how they adapted to their student occupations, and whether existing lifespan theories affirmed the changes these women were experiencing. Based on questions posed by individuals completing the matrix, as well as those suggested by lifespan theories, I added categories and refined the form. Because education is the longest strand in my own Self-Discovery Tapestry, the investigation seemed a natural progression in my own search for meaning. The year of administering the

Pierce, D. (Ed.).
Occupational Science for Occupational Therapy (pp. 201-210).
© 2014 SLACK Incorporated.

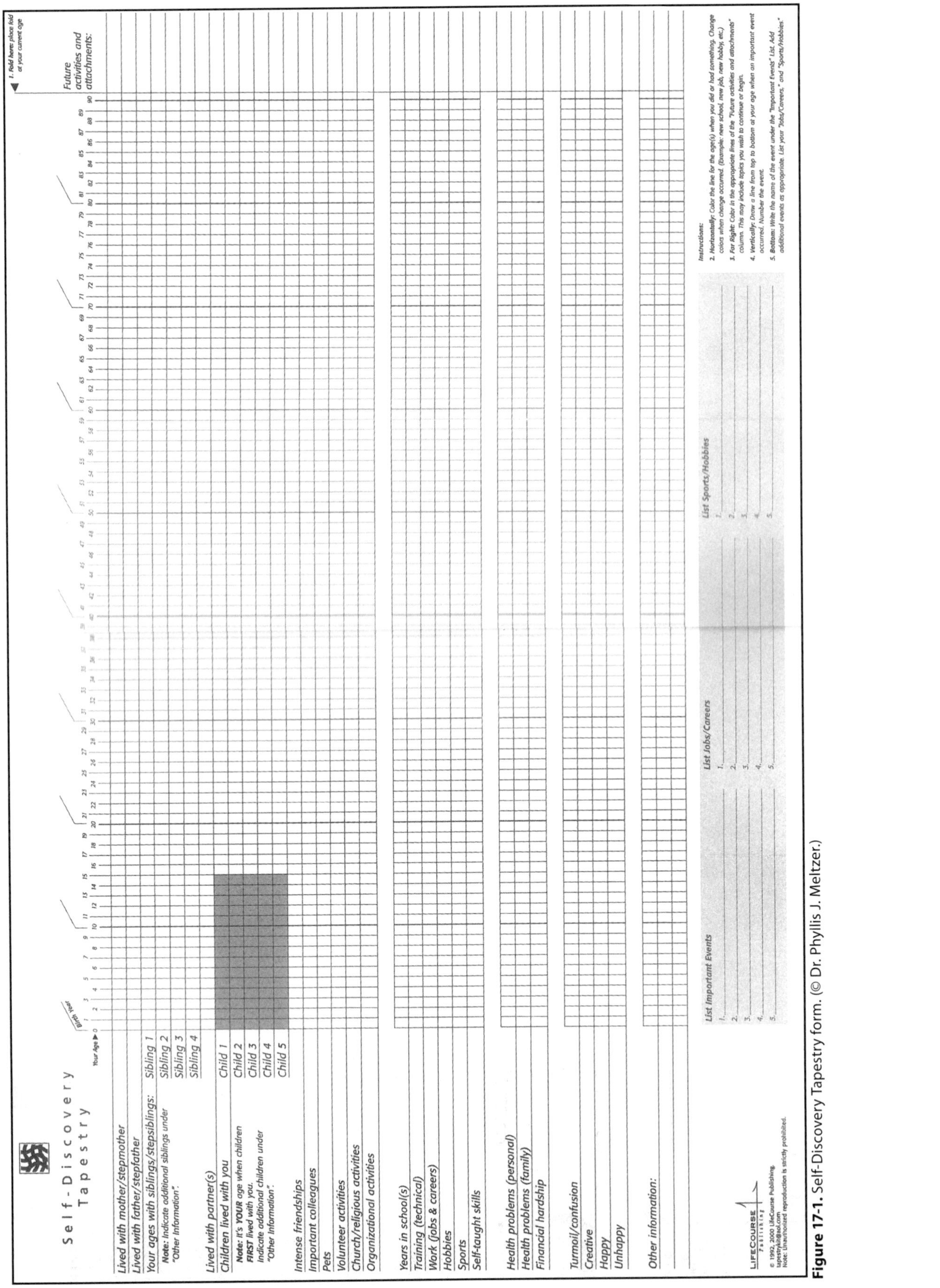

Figure 17-1. Self-Discovery Tapestry form. (© Dr. Phyllis J. Meltzer.)

Self-Discovery Tapestry to more than 100 men and women, and helping them analyze their Tapestries, while writing the dissertation according to its demanding academic forms, became one of the happiest and most fulfilling years of my life (Meltzer, 1997).

In the years since I published the Self-Discovery Tapestry (2000), it has found a place in the curricula of many universities and the private practices of therapists and has allowed thousands of people to "discover" their strengths and patterns of adaptation. The use of the Tapestry confirms many of the principles of occupational science as well as the theories used in gerontology and adult learning.

LITERATURE

Female Re-Entry Students

The need for the study became evident when preliminary research indicated that nearly one third of the enrollment of institutions of higher education in the United States were nontraditional students (those age 25 years and older) (U.S. Dept. of Education, 1987). More women are currently participating in the workforce, and all indications led to the conclusion that post-secondary education, either immediately following secondary education or throughout adulthood, provides financial as well as psychological benefits.

Female re-entry students have been studied from a variety of viewpoints. These women have chosen post-secondary education as their means of changing occupations (Glassner, 1994) or for job preparation. A growing number of popular and scholarly books indicate that many adults are viewing return to higher education as an acceptable means by which to change their occupations and perceived well-being, including economic stability or improvement. Occupational changes may be motivated by the need for a person to preserve his or her sense of productivity, self-esteem, and mental health by changing places of employment, marriage, or other toxic environments (Waskel, 1991). It should be noted that nearly all of the research on the effects of a college education has been conducted on traditional-age students who attend 4-year residential institutions. There is, at this time, "insufficient evidence to conclude that the factors that influence educational attainment are the same for [older nontraditional students] as there are for their traditional-age counterparts" (Pascarella & Terenzini, 1991, p. 414).

Gerontological Theories of Lifespan Development

Two lifespan development theories generally used in gerontology research were used to develop the Self-Discovery Tapestry: continuity theory and critical events theory. The concept of life review was also useful in developing the matrix. Life review may be defined as a somewhat "structured and comprehensive . . . sequential recounting from childhood to the present or an identification and systematic elaboration of developmental concerns. Certainly, more territory is covered in a life review and one gains an appreciation for the magnitude of one's life" (Haight & Webster, 1995, p. 277).

Continuity theory provides an explanation of the persistence of identity and essential authentic strands of occupations despite major life changes. Atchley describes continuity theory's central premise that adults "attempt to preserve and maintain existing internal and external structures" by applying "familiar strategies in familiar arenas of life" (Atchley, 1989, p. 184). Using the familiar can be a primary strategy for making occupational adaptations to changing conditions. Perseverance of occupational roles meshes with continuity theory as individuals attempt to maintain, for the most part, their roles as wives or partners, employees, and so forth. Even when assuming additional roles or occupations, people tend to maintain essential and familiar occupational behaviors as they continue to nurture their school-age children while attending educational institutions or working (Moorhead, 1969). Continuity theory provides for gradual change and "assumes evolution" (Atchley, 1989, p. 183). Occupying roles and taking on new ones over time—perhaps discarding others—has adaptive and improvisational aspects. The person is continuing his or her self as he or she evolves.

Events that interrupt the continuous evolution of the self are described as life events or critical events. "Life events usually include family, work, health, finances, and friendships" (Waskel, 1991, p. 76). Changes can cause stress as well as challenges for occupational adaptation. The degree of stress is an individual assessment and may be mitigated by its meaning for the individual and his or her social resources. Such occupational changes, if viewed in terms of critical events theory, almost certainly entail experiencing a personal crisis (Levinson et al., 1978; Osherson, 1980). Theorists describe a series of steps that the individual undergoes, yet the process also includes reflection back into personal history. In the beginning, the individual experiences a feeling of disorder and dissatisfaction with one's current life; a search into oneself is undertaken as identification of the source of the dissatisfaction is sought and separation is begun; feelings of loss, the abandonment of the formerly "wished-for self" is completed, and partial acceptance is gained; the grieving process for the self who was is experienced; and resolution for the pursuit of future directions in becoming the new self is gained after the crisis period, possibly after years of conflict, turmoil, and questioning (Osherson, 1980). Glassner (1994) uses more succinct terminology for the stages of transition: "cutting loose," "hanging out," and "moving on" (p. 185).

Levinson, among others, purports in his mid-life development theory (1978) that transitions in which individuals make commitment choices may occur, which then provide structure for their future years. Transitions can be a time of increasing individuation as people become more aware of themselves and those around them as well as the polarized discrepancies within themselves. Levinson's work, although using different vocabulary, reiterates the ideas of Trombly and Moorhead in the occupational therapy literature. Their work suggests that the recreation of the self is accomplished through the evolutionary, developmental process by which individuals come to conceptualize their interaction between their selves and their task-oriented environments by adopting and internalizing new occupational roles (Moorhead, 1969; Trombly, 1995).

Occupational Science Perspectives on Lifespan Development

Several principles from occupational science and occupational therapy were important in the development of the Self-Discovery Tapestry. Occupational science "accepts that people influence the state of their health through what they do" and that it is "the rigorous study of humans as occupational beings" (Wilcock, 2006, p. 262). Yerxa defined authenticity, stating, "In order to achieve authentic existence, man must have resolve to become his true self" (1967, p. 7). These definitions embrace the concept of occupational engagement as central to becoming one's authentic self.

Occupation and *occupational roles* are terms in common usage in the occupational science literature (Zemke & Clark, 1996). Occupational behavior includes the accumulation of skills and habits formed within occupational roles. The term *occupational career* refers to a "career of roles" (Black, 1976, p. 225) that individuals acquire over their lifetimes with varying strengths and weaknesses in each role. An individual's occupational career is a series of roles resulting from decisions that are influenced by personality, societal circumstances, gender, social class, and other variables, but are, nevertheless, subject to individual choices (Black, 1976). Atchley (1989) presents his similar concepts of continuity theory using a somewhat different vocabulary.

As individuals change careers through, for example, higher education, they demonstrate occupational adaptation. As individuals spiral through their occupational careers, they may experience similar occupations to which they have adapted, applying newly acquired skills and knowledge as needed. Schkade and Schultz (1992) posit that "occupation provides the means by which human beings adapt to changing needs and conditions, and the desire to participate in occupation is the intrinsic motivational force leading to adaptation, which is a normative process" (p. 829).

Occupational challenge is a concept derived from occupational therapy. It describes the individual's transitional state: the decision to pursue a new occupation due to the drive for self-mastery (Schkade & Schultz, 1992). Occupational challenges may occur within each person's life's activities at any time. Personal meaning is a motivator and also serves to organize behavior toward optimum functioning. People who change careers appear to have accepted the challenge of occupational adaptation, possibly as a result of gaining greater understanding of the meaning (or lack of meaning) of their current occupations and becoming willing to add additional occupations in their occupational careers.

Occupational persistence describes the habitual continuation of chosen or assumed occupations (e.g., mothering or accounting). This term, used by Carlson (1996), "refers to the phenomenon whereby an individual's participation in a given occupation is continued" (p. 144).

METHODS

The Tapestry was developed over several phases, as described by Benson and Clark (1982): Phase 1, purpose; Phase 2, literature review; and Phase 3, instrument evaluation.

Purpose of the Study

Although the matrix had been begun some years earlier while I was a student enrolled in gerontology classes, it required refinement to stand as a research tool. The Self-Discovery Tapestry was designed to assess the occupational behaviors of mid-life women in southern California who changed careers through higher education (my target group) to assist them in gaining insight into how they make occupational adaptations during transitions (domains), and to aid them as they assessed their occupational career patterns and transitions through this graphic life-review process (content area).

Pilot Studies

Evaluation of the instrument was completed through a series of pilot studies. The first was conducted with 23 students enrolled in a Certified Occupational Therapy Assistant's program. Each student responded to the written question "What have you discovered about yourself as a result of completing the Self-Discovery Tapestry?" Responses indicated most gained insights into patterns in their lives when they made transitions and said they enjoyed completing the instrument. When tallying the responses of critical events, I discovered as many students indicated the loss of a pet as the loss of a grandparent. I added "pets" as a topic within the interpersonal domain; this topic was supported by the literature (Sable, 1995).

A second pilot study was presented to a group of 25 individuals who regularly attend the post-polio support group in Los Angeles. Many were experiencing health problems related to late life changes affecting their post-polio conditions. Participants suggested adding a place on the matrix form where important events could be listed. This was added to the final design of the Tapestry form. Comments were generally favorable as individuals discovered continuing traits and values despite physical changes.

Several students in their early 20s at the University of Southern California, referring to the instrument's age lines (0 to 90 years), indicated they were happy to see they had a long time to grow and become successful.

A surprisingly negative response was expressed by a group of 10 elderly Black women who met regularly at a senior center in Central Los Angeles. All of the women, in their 70s and 80s, were born and raised in the South. None of the women completed the matrix: no one entered information beyond the second line (lived with father). When asked if they would like to complete them another day, each politely refused, "No, thank you, dear." This resistance to complete the matrix was puzzling. It raised hitherto unanticipated ideas regarding limitations of the form. Possible explanations may be that the researcher was a stranger to the group and of another race, or that, due to limited literacy, the women could not read the categories of the domains, could not see the words due to poor eyesight, or felt their privacy was being invaded. The reasons may have varied; no conclusions for their decisions to politely refuse to participate were reached.

Qualitative evaluation (face validation), suggested by Benson and Clark (1982), was conducted with four mental health staff members of a women's health organization. Each completed the Self-Discovery Tapestry and discussed their reactions to the instrument. Several suggestions were made regarding the design of the form, which two participants found confusing. They suggested making the written instructions more succinct. One psychologist suggested adding topics specific to the client-therapist dyad. This was regarded as too specific for the goals of the Tapestry.

Suggestions were evaluated and changes made. Instructions were made more succinct, and the size of the paper was increased to 11 x 17 inches for easier readability. Three shaded rectangles were added beneath the matrix in which participants were able to list the important (critical) events they indicated, careers or jobs they have held, and sports or hobbies in which they have participated. Due to the number of individuals who reported living with one parent or another following their parents' divorce, the category requesting information about the length of time lived with parents was changed into separate categories, asking length of time lived with each parent or stepparent. The topic of health concerns was enlarged to include family health problems. Additional horizontal areas were added in which individuals could indicate other important categories they felt had not been covered in the matrix.

Subject Domains of the Matrix

The domains in the matrix were amended and refined by the literature concerning re-entry women students (Edwards, 1993; Glassner, 1994) and occupational science (Clark, 1993; Clark et al., 1991; Schkade & Schultz, 1992), as well as guided by feedback proffered during pilot tests of the instrument. The domains are interpersonal relations, occupations, personal meaning, and self-evaluation. Each domain contains several topics in the horizontal plane that may be indicated as continuous elements (see Figure 17-1). For example, the first domain refers to interpersonal relationships. Interpersonal relationships may affect a person's ability to succeed in new occupations by offering or denying instrumental or emotional support for the endeavor. Prior experience in forming and maintaining interpersonal relations in a variety of social contexts may indicate that the participant has the skills to maintain relationships and values such relationships and should be able to continue to do so in new contexts and roles.

Matrix items in the occupational domain include years of formal education, employment and training, hobbies, sports, and self-taught skills. Educational and occupational pursuits, whether formal or informal, contribute to a person's ability to learn and to enhance her status in her private as well as public world. Following transitional events, she may be able to use and apply these experiences to other opportunities.

The third domain of the matrix, personal meaning, includes the topics dealing with chronic or prior personal health problems, family health problems, and financial hardships (both personal and familial).

The mood and productivity self-assessment domain, labeled self-evaluation, elicits personal review by the individual indicating periods of her life when she felt she was highly creative, happy, or unhappy. The topic of turmoil/confusion is included as a result of the literature in the area of mid-life transitions (Glassner, 1994). Resolution of this period of turmoil and confusion may be expressed on the matrix as an action that is termed an *important event* (Figure 17-2) or a mid-life transition (Levinson & Levinson, 1996) (e.g., the decision to re-enroll in college courses or deciding to leave a marriage or job). The participant may recall the intensity of the occupation of creativity as well as sustained emotional moods.

The final domain in the left-hand column is Other Information. Participants use these spaces to indicate some aspect of their lives they felt had not been included in another topic category, such as military service, living with a grandchild, or extended time spent traveling. This space has also been used to indicate the number of children or siblings who exceeded the allotted spaces within the body of the matrix.

Future Activities and Attachments heads a column on the right-hand side of the horizontal plane of the matrix.

The individual may indicate interest in beginning, continuing, or restarting a continuous element of his or her life by completing this column. Coloring aspects of this column corresponds with personal values such as interpersonal relations, continuing occupations or hopes for continued good health and creativity, and other factors. It is of vital interest to assess which future categories participants indicate they wish to continue or begin, in order to affirm the hypothesis that includes continuity theory as well as to determine the adaptability of the occupational transitions being pursued.

Instructions for completing the body of the matrix and writing personal information in the three shaded rectangles are included on the single-sheet of the Tapestry and in the Client Guide booklet. Instructions request the participant to indicate on the vertical plane her age(s) when important events occurred. Important events are those that are personally meaningful; for example, leaving home at age 18 may be regarded by one person as a usual part of maturing or as a wrenching action of separation by another. The term *important events* is used as a synonym for the theoretical term *critical events*. The category is used in order to gain information regarding substantiation of critical events theory. Occupations that appear to continue beyond critical events show evidence of being valued occupations. Adaptations may need to be made in order to continue, but it seems possible that occupational careers continue in an amended trajectory.

Important Events

- ❏ Met partner girlfriend/boyfriend
- ❏ Marriage
- ❏ Marital upheaval separation
- ❏ Divorce
- ❏ Birth of a child
- ❏ Death(s)
- ❏ School change(s)
- ❏ Start/finish college
- ❏ Religious event
- ❏ Illness/surgery
- ❏ Personal injury
- ❏ New Job
- ❏ Career change
- ❏ Financial loss
- ❏ Household move
- ❏ Immigration to U.S.
- ❏ Other _____

Figure 17-2. Important events widely indicated by group participants surveyed following completion of the Self-Discovery Tapestry. (© Dr. Phyllis J. Meltzer.)

A BRIEF OVERVIEW OF RESULTS FROM THE SELF-DISCOVERY TAPESTRY

The instrument assisted most informants in discovering patterns of adaptation as well as recalling meaningful events. The matrix was able to evoke affirmation of self-knowledge: several women said they had always known such things about themselves, such as their fortitude or resiliency. In several cases, the decision to re-enter or enter post-secondary education was the result of a critical event, such as a divorce or desertion, the death or breakdown of a parent, or in one case, the destruction of the family home by fire. Most of the participants exhibited adaptive behavior by requesting and receiving emotional or instrumental support from family members.

Occupational attenuation was the term I applied to the process in which the women students felt they were not performing their usual prior occupations as completely as they used to: less time was spent with the children, cleaning the house, working or volunteering outside the home, or spending time with friends. It was a striking and unexpected factor in the data analysis. The changes may demonstrate their enfolding multiple tasks, postponing, or delegating them. "I'll clean that room during winter break." Occupational attenuation may be the expression of the frustration they experienced in their roles of becoming successful students. "They're [school-age children] proud of me [for attending school], but they still want dinner on the table." Conflict is stated when the woman's academic goals are tempered by family needs, emotional conflicts, and occupational goals. Two participants were concerned about their children's anger at their student occupations. For the most part, however, mature students with children in the home maintained their mothering, housekeeping, and homemaker occupations, although in attenuated form. No woman questioned that the care of the children was her responsibility. Many of the participants reported a dual effect of their return to education. Not only did their children, for the most part, respect their efforts, but also the mothers developed new insights into their children's occupations as students. "I show him [her 12-year-old] test scores, and we kind of encourage each other and we say, 'that's good.'"

Theoretical bases for occupational changes were affirmed as participants related experiencing elements of both continuity and critical events in their Tapestry forms and transcribed personal histories. Most partici-pants also experienced periods of turmoil and confusion. Contemporary theorists strongly suggest that the lives of adults exhibit evidence, for the most part, of perpetua-tion of internal continuity that constitutes personality and behaviors as well as interpersonal support and resources (Atchley, 1989; Osherson, 1980). Tumultuous periods gen-erally surrounded a critical event, or even preceded the event, such as acknowledging the need to escape a bad mar-riage, or responding to a critical event, such as a disabling accident or losing one's job. It appeared that, for the most part, educational values, family connectedness, and inter-personal relationships, as well as unanimous feelings of personal stability, were supportive of internal and external continuity theory.

The Self-Discovery Tapestry meshed the theories used in the study of aging, adult learning, social psychology, and the principles put forth by the disciplines of occu-pational therapy and occupational science. It introduced students of occupational science to a greater range of the gerontology theoretical literature. Affirmation, rejection, or refined formulation of theories about occupational adaptation of mid-life re-entry students who were chang-ing occupations were derived from complete analysis of the data (Strauss & Corbin, 1990). These may add to the body of knowledge regarding occupational change and adaptation, continuity of selves, the effects of the percep-tion of critical events for mid-life re-entry women stu-dents, and patterns of transitional crisis resolution.

LATER DEVELOPMENT OF TAPESTRY MATERIALS

Following completion of my doctorate, I responded to requests for copies of the Tapestry for use in academic set-tings and with clients of occupational therapists. Application for copyright was made and awarded. The Tapestry form is printed on 11- x 17-inch card stock paper (see Figure 17-1). The Client Guide presents brief instructions and thought-ful introspective questions. A 21-page booklet, the Leader's Guide, provides a summary of the Tapestry's purpose, theo-retical background, components (domains), and suggested strategies for using the Tapestry. In addition, the Leader's Guide presents five case studies with proposed solutions. With the guidance of a skilled graphic designer, the three components were combined into a boxed kit with materials sufficient for 15 along with five colored pens. Workshops, presentations, and a colorful brochure were the main mar-keting tools.

Need led to the creation of additional forms. I pre-sented the Tapestry to a large class of honors freshmen at University of California—Los Angeles in October 2001; this was 2 weeks following the 9/11 tragedy in New York.

Not one student indicated that 9/11 was an important event for him or her. Their faculty and I were astounded although the students did speak later about their reactions in their small groups. In an attempt to understand their total lack of response to this event, I created the Self-Discovery Individual Summary, a one-page, two-sided form that asked the questions: (a) What elements or changes in your life have made your Tapestry "colorful"? (b) What patterns did you discover in your life review?/What adaptive skills did you employ when important change occurred? (c) Do you feel they were successful? (d) What ways, if any, did historical or political events impact your life? and (e) What thoughts about your future were changed or reinforced when you reviewed your Tapestry (Meltzer, 2001)?

The question in which I was most interested was, "What, if any, historical or political events impact your life?" The large majority of students felt that no political or historical event had impacted their lives. A number of instructors use the Individual Summary sheets along with the Self-Discovery Tapestry forms.

In response to requests by group leaders, I also created the Student Edition. The large envelope contains two copies each of the Tapestry forms. This package meets the needs of many instructors who assign students to use the Tapestry form as a research tool or as the basis for interviewing older adults after they have completed their own Tapestry.

Recently, the Self-Discovery Tapestry form, the Client Guide, and the Self-Discovery Individual Summary forms have been translated into Spanish. Antoine Bailliard and I, along with several advisors, completed the translations. We hope that many Spanish-speaking people will benefit by completing their life reviews using these forms of the Tapestry.

CONTRIBUTIONS TO OCCUPATIONAL SCIENCE

The Self-Discovery Tapestry can be viewed in com-parison with paper instruments developed within the practice of occupational therapy. Occupational therapists have devised several life history (review) instruments (Kielhofner, 1985, 1995; Matsutsuyu, 1969; Moorhead, 1969) with the goal of eliciting an individual's occupa-tional life story to assist in the choice of occupational goals and participation having the most therapeutic value for the patient. Life-review instruments have also been developed by professionals in other disciplines, such as personnel (Rounds, 1994; Super, 1984) and psychology (Schroots & ten Kate, 1989). It is, however, the first and, so far, the only instrument developed within the principles of occupational science.

IMPLICATIONS FOR PRACTICE

The Self-Discovery Tapestry is used in a variety of academic and practice settings. Many academics that teach occupational science or lifespan development present the exercise early in the term. Those conducting research projects on lifespan histories or adaptive strategies find the form valuable. Professionals who counsel individuals and individuals investigating family histories use the instrument.

Occupational therapy, occupational science, and gerontology students in post-secondary institutions in the United States and abroad probably use the Self-Discovery Tapestry most frequently. It is used as a classroom exercise in which students complete the Tapestry illustrating their own lives. The class as a group may share important (critical) transitional events and adaptive strategies and discuss possible events others may have experienced, although sensitive topics are always respected.

A form used as an overhead projection following the group's completion of the Tapestry during class lists 16 topics: a compilation gleaned from hundreds of completed Tapestries. Students are asked to indicate they have marked a particular topic as an "important event." The results are counted, usually by one of the students, and the totals announced. The topics listed are met partner, girl-friend/boyfriend, marriage, marital upheaval/separation, divorce, birth of a child, death, school change(s), start/finish college, illness/surgery, personal injury, new job, career change, financial loss, household move, immigration to the United States, other. An unusual personal topic may be recorded, usually a very personal event, such as getting on or off drugs, suffering a personal attack, or, more recently, losing a sweetheart to war.

Individual utilization varies, although completing the Tapestry is always an individual exercise. Adults who have been enrolled in workshops may use the completed Tapestry as a personal history document, referring to it periodically, updating their life's information, and seeing it as an affirmation of the meaningful aspects of their lives. One workshop I taught brought mothers and daughters together. Each completed her own Tapestry and then we, as a group, discussed differences and similarities. It was an afternoon of discovery!

Researchers in the United States, Australia, New Zealand, Scotland, United Kingdom, and elsewhere report successfully using the Tapestry and its component parts. It has been used by women parolees, drug addicts, and older women artists. Retirees enjoyed completing the Tapestry forms that they used as a guide to build their future occupations. The Self-Discovery Tapestry is a valuable tool when used to investigate and validate occupational science principles such as occupational adaptation, occupational careers, and occupational behaviors.

Although designed to be completed by the participants, the Self-Discovery Tapestry can be a valuable tool for therapists in private practice or those who meet individually to counsel clients or patients who have recently experienced dramatic transitions and who may be undergoing rehabilitation experiences. The Tapestry has recently been used by an occupational therapist in Colorado to help recently unemployed individuals assess their strengths and adaptive strategies.

The concept of creating a life-review instrument that imitated the creative process of weaving has been an occupational science journey incorporating, for me, a variety of continuous occupations with variations, finding meaning personally and helping others as they discover the means to explore their own lives. The use of the Tapestry by academic leaders, occupational therapists, and others offers rewards as they discover an instrument that allows them to teach lifespan development and occupational science principles as well as incorporate gerontology theories. The instrument continues to evolve when it is used as a counseling tool and as an aid for others to discover meaning in their lives.

LEARNING SUPPORTS

Analyze Narrative

Instructions

1. Analyze this narrative from an occupational therapist in rural New Zealand.

I completed the Tapestry kit personally to review my life difficulties and challenges. Plotting major difficult crisis through my life (such as childhood trauma, husband's brain tumor, daughter's year of undiagnosed seizures) gave me more understanding about myself. I took my completed Tapestry to some personal development sessions. Using a narrative approach, the counselor and I discussed my resilience and vulnerabilities during these times. I remembered activities I did to self-soothe/care for myself. I also noted the calm times in my life and what I was able to achieve during these periods. Our discussions enabled me to use the information at a much deeper level than when I was able to think through it by myself. (Diane Matsas, personal communication, November 16, 2009)

2. Which of the theories that underpin the Self-Discovery Tapestry are apparent in this narrative (continuity, critical events, or adaptation)? Justify your opinions.

Using Participant Responses to Make Future Occupational Choices

Purpose

Students will apply participants' life histories and values to their knowledge of counseling skills.

Primary Concepts

Combine all completed elements of the Self-Discovery Tapestry and apply to occupational therapy knowledge of personal counseling.

Instructions

1. Study the topics completed in the Future Activities and Attachments column and Jobs/Careers and Sports/Hobbies columns.

2. Prepare your notes for group case study.

Social and Political Environments

Primary Concepts

Apply knowledge of social and political environments in various settings.

Instructions

Jackson (1996) states that "occupations are carried out within a particular physical, social, political, and historical environment" (p. 342). Two weeks following the 9/11/2001 tragedy in New York, not one freshman student in a Southern California university noted the event on his or her completed Tapestry forms.

1. Students will review the description of the UCLA students' omission in the chapter text.

2. Discuss how the political event of 9/11 might have impacted your life.

3. How would you account for the students' omission of any reference to this event?

REFERENCES

Atchley, R. C. (1989). A continuity theory of normal aging. *The Gerontologist, 29*(2), 183-190. doi:10.1093/geront/29.2.183

Bateson, M. C. (1989). *Composing a life.* New York, NY: Penguin Books.

Benson J., & Clark, F. (1982). A guide for instrument development and validation. *American Journal of Occupational Therapy, 36*(12), 789-800. doi:10.5014/ajot.36.12.789

Black, M. M. (1976). The occupational career. *American Journal of Occupational Therapy, 30*(4), 225-228.

Carlson, M. (1996). The self-perpetuation of occupations. In R. Zemke & F. Clark (Eds.), *Occupational science: The evolving discipline* (pp. 143-157). Philadelphia, PA: F. A. Davis.

Clark, F. (1993). Occupational embedded in a real life: Interweaving occupational science and occupational therapy. *American Journal of Occupational Therapy, 47*(12), 1067-1078. doi:10.5014/ajot.47.12.1067

Clark, F. A., Parham, D., Carlson, M. E., Frank, G., Jackson, J., Pierce, D., . . . Zemke, R. (1991). Occupational science: Academic innovation in the service of occupational therapy's future. *American Journal of Occupational Therapy, 45*(4), 300-310. doi:10.5014/ajot.45.4.300

Edwards, R. (1993) *Mature women students: Separating or connecting family and education.* London, England: Taylor and Francis.

Glassner, B. (1994). *Career crash.* New York, NY: Simon & Schuster.

Haight, B. K., & Webster, J. D. (Eds.). (1995). *The art and science of reminiscing: Theory, research, methods, and applications.* Washington, DC: Taylor and Francis.

Jackson, J. (1996). Living a meaningful existence in old age. In R. Zemke & F. Clark (Eds.), *Occupational science: The evolving discipline* (pp. 339-361). Philadelphia, PA: F. A. Davis.

Kielhofner, G. (1985). *A model of human occupation: Theory and application.* Baltimore, MD: Williams and Wilkins.

Kielhofner, G. (1995). Appendix: Structured methods of data collected used with the model of human occupational. In G. Kielhofner (Ed.), *A model of human occupation: Theory and application* (2nd ed.). Baltimore, MD: Williams and Wilkins.

Levinson, D. J., Darrow, C. N., Klein, E. B., Levinson, M. H., & McKee B. (1978). *The seasons of a man's life.* New York, NY: Knopf.

Levinson, D. J., & Levinson, J. D. (1996). *The seasons of a woman's life.* New York, NY: Alfred A. Knopf.

Matsutsuyu, J. S. (1969). The interest check list. *American Journal of Occupational Therapy, 23*(4), 328.

Meltzer, P. J. (1997). *The Self Discovery Tapestry instrument used by mid-life women who are changing occupations through higher education* (Unpublished doctoral dissertation). University of Southern California, Los Angeles, CA.

Meltzer, P. J. (2000). *Self-Discovery Tapestry Kit.* Los Angeles, CA: Author.

Meltzer, P. J. (2001). *Self-Discovery Individual Summary.* Los Angeles, CA: Author.

Moorhead, L. (1969). The occupational history. *American Journal of Occupational Therapy, 23*(4), 329-334.

Osherson, S. D. (1980). *Holding on or letting go: Men and career change at midlife.* New York, NY: The Free Press.

Pascarella, E. T., & Terenzini, P. T. (1991). *How college affects students: Findings and insights from twenty years of research.* San Francisco, CA: Jossey-Bass Publishers.

Rounds, J. (1994). The Adult Career Concerns Inventory (ASSI). In J. T. Kapes, M. M. Mastie, & E. A. Whitfield (Eds.), *A counselor's guide to career assessment instruments* (pp. 242-247). Alexandria, VA: National Career Development Association.

Sable, P. (1995). Pets, attachment, and well-being across the life cycle. *Social Work, 40*(3), 334-431.

Schkade, J. K., & Schultz, S. (1992). Occupational adaptation: Toward a holistic approach for contemporary practice, Part 1. *American Journal of Occupational Therapy, 46*(9), 829-837. doi:10.5014/ajot.46.9.829

Schroots, J. J. F., & ten Kate, C. A. (1989). Metaphors, aging and the line interview method. *Current perspectives on aging of end of the life cycle* (Vol. 3). London, England: Jay Press.

Strauss, A., & Corbin, J. (1990). *Basics of qualitative research: Grounded theory procedures and techniques.* Newbury Park, CA: Sage Publications.

Super, D. E. (1984). The life career rainbow: Six life roles in schematic life space. In D. Brown & L. Brooks (Eds.), *Career choice and development.* San Francisco, CA: Jossey-Bass.

Trombly, C. A. (1995). Occupation: Purposefulness and meaningfulness as therapeutic mechanisms. *American Journal of Occupational Therapy, 49*(10), 960-972. doi:10.5014/ajot.49.10.960

U. S. Department of Education, Center for Education Statistics. (1987). *Survey of adult education: Current populations survey.* Washington, DC: Author.

Waskel, S. A. (1991). *Mid-life issues and the workplace of the 90s.* New York, NY: Quorum Books.

Wilcock, A. A. (2006). An occupational perspective of health (2nd ed.). Thorofare, NJ: SLACK Incorporated.

Yerxa, E. J. (1967). 1966 Eleanor Clarke Slagle lecture: Authentic occupational therapy. *American Journal of Occupational Therapy, 11*(1), 1-9.

Zemke, R., & Clark, F. (Eds.). (1996). *Occupational science: The evolving discipline.* Philadelphia: F. A. Davis.

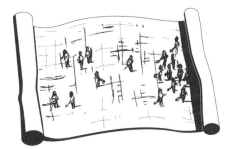

Researching Retirement
Studies That Lead to New Ways to Look at Freedom and the Categorization of Occupation

Hans Jonsson, OT(reg), PhD

The start of this long and continuing journey in research was a curious occupational therapist who had just left his clinical career to start a new one in education and research. I was working part-time as a research assistant at a geriatric research center in Stockholm, Sweden. In my clinical practice, I had felt an urgent need to base my practice in theories and models. The Model of Human Occupation was introduced in Sweden at that time (1985 to 1990). I was active in spreading the Model into clinical practice and education, and later in my own research. Flow theory was introduced in Sweden in 1989 by Dr. Elizabeth Yerxa as theory that was well-suited for occupational therapy practice. I wrote the first article about this theory in the Swedish occupational therapy journal (Jonsson, 1991). In her presentation in Stockholm, Dr. Yerxa said, "Occupational therapy represents an applied science in search of a unique science to apply" (Jonsson, 1993, p. 4). In my view, this statement was right on target for the state of the art in occupational therapy at that time. It pointed to the directions the field would take in the future. The public introduction of occupational science in 1990 (Yerxa, 1993; Yerxa et al., 1989) was a natural and much-needed continuation of knowledge development in occupational therapy.

I wanted to contribute to this research into occupation that was not necessarily connected to therapy or people with disabilities. Grounded in a geriatric research center where I worked with people at retirement age and older, the process of retirement was an obvious area in need of research. From an occupational perspective, retirement can be viewed as one of the largest changes in the life course. The major occupation of work, which has occupied a large proportion of waking time for 40 to 50 years, ends. Work time is replaced by unstructured time that looks more like vacation time. As the title goes of a Swedish book in which a woman reflects about her future retirement, *No Work To Go To . . . Whom Am I Now? . . . and What Should I Do? Have 20 Years of Vacation*? (Rollén, 2000). I was sure this transition would be interesting to research from the perspective of workers facing retirement in the near future: what strategies they had planned, how they viewed the change as newly retired, and how they saw it once they were more established in retirement.

This led to my PhD project, "Anticipating, Experiencing, and Valuing the Transition From Worker to Retiree: A Longitudinal Study of Retirement as an Occupational Transition" (Jonsson, 2000). It included five publishable

Pierce, D. (Ed.).
Occupational Science for Occupational Therapy (pp. 211-220).

TABLE 18-1

DEMOGRAPHIC CHARACTERISTICS OF PARTICIPANTS IN STUDIES 1 THROUGH 5

STUDY NO.	TOT.	MEN/ WOMEN		LIVING WITH PARTNER/ ALONE		BLUE COLLAR/WHITE COLLAR/MANAGEMENT (WHEN WORKING)			WORKING FULL-TIME/PART-TIME/ PENSION FULL-TIME		
		M	*W*	*Partner*	*Alone*	*BC*	*WC*	*M*	*W-FT*	*W-PT*	*P-FT*
Study 1	76	39	37	48	28	27	35	14	47	29	0
Study 2	32	16	16	19	13	11	15	6	14	18	0
Studies 3 + 5	29	15	14	18	11	8	15	6	2	8	19
Study 4	12	6	6	7	5	5	5	2	1	1	10

TABLE 18-2

PARTICIPANTS, AGE, DATA COLLECTION METHODS, AND METHODS OF ANALYSIS IN STUDIES 1 THROUGH 5

STUDY NO.	PARTIC.	AGE	DATA COLLECTION METHODS	METHODS OF DATA ANALYSIS
Study 1	76	63 to 64	Questionnaire	Descriptive statistics Chi-squared analysis
Study 2	32	63 to 64	Semistructured interview	Comparative analysis Narrative analysis
Study 3	29	65 to 66	Semistructured interview with individually tailored questions developed from Study 2	Comparative analysis Narrative analysis
Study 4	12	70 to 71	Semistructured interview with individually tailored questions developed from Studies 2 and 3	Comparative analysis Narrative analysis
Study 5	29	65 to 66	Same as in Study 3	Comparative analysis

studies. The longitudinal design in four of my studies meant that I followed about 30 Swedish men and women from when they still were working at the age of 63, over retirement as newly retired at the age of 66, and finally as more established retirees to the age of 70. Outside my dissertation, I later followed some participants until the age of 73.

The number of participants and some demographic characteristics are shown in Table 18-1. Data collection methods and methods of data analysis are shown in Table 18-2.

SUMMARY OF THE RESULTS OF THE FIVE STUDIES

Study 1

The aim of Study 1 was to explore and describe how work and retirement were viewed by a group of Swedish people about to retire (Jonsson & Andersson, 1999). At age 63, home

TABLE 18-3

POSITIVE AND NEGATIVE VALUES OF WORK AS EXPRESSED BY A GROUP OF PEOPLE AGED 63 YEARS

POSITIVE	NEGATIVE
Social contacts and fellowship	Undesired social contacts
Using one's knowledge and capacities	Uninteresting work and boring routines
Being a part of a larger whole	Structural changes of workplace and staff
Having something to do	Diversion of energy from preferred occupations
Being productive	Stress and the burden of responsibility
Having an external structure	Rigidity of external structure
Earning one's income	

and family was reported as the most important area in life for 50% of the participants. Work was most important for 39% of the participants and leisure/hobby for 11%. As many as 78% of participants had a positive attitude toward their own retirement. Only 4% reported a negative attitude. Fifty-four percent thought it would be easy to get used to being a retiree, while 17% thought it would be difficult. Neither gender nor type of work had any significant influence on attitude to retirement.

Present work was experienced in various ways. In terms of what characteristic of work was most important to participants, 40% reported financial reasons, 34% intrinsic motivators, 11% something to do, and 6% for social reasons.

About half of the participants (53%) were positive toward having some kind of paid work after retirement. For this factor, current type of work was of importance. Participants in management reported significantly more positive attitudes toward paid work after retirement than did participants with other types of work. Fifty-three percent of the participants also held positive attitudes toward volunteer work after retirement. In attitudes toward volunteer work, no significant differences for type of work were found.

Combining the responses related to paid and voluntary work, as many as 73% had a positive attitude toward some sort of work (paid or voluntary) after retirement. About three quarters of these participants reported needs besides financial as their most important reason for working after retirement.

Study 2

The aim of Study 2 was to explore and understand how participants about to retire experienced their current situation and anticipated their future retirement (Jonsson, Kielhofner, & Borell, 1997). Although most of the participants anticipated both positive and negative changes occurring upon retirement, it was possible to characterize the basic direction of the anticipated narrative slope for each participant's narrative. The three possible directions include a progressive slope, anticipating retirement as an improvement in life; a stable slope, anticipating no change in quality of life; and a regressive slope, anticipating retirement as a decrease in quality of life.

The different directions of the participants' narratives could be understood according to the experienced values of present work. Participants could experience several meanings of work both positive and negative (Table 18-3).

If present work was experienced overall as negative, leaving work was seen as something positive, and the narrative anticipating retirement had either a progressive or a stable direction. If present work was primarily perceived as positive, the narrative about retirement first led to reasoning about the possibility of replacing work values. This could be done either by finding similar values in other occupations of retirement life or with values in occupations that were seen as having at least the same importance. Participants with an overall positive interpretation of present work told narratives that had all three directions. Progressive narratives were told when the transition to retirement was seen as leaving something positive to do something even more positive in retirement. Narratives with a stable direction were told when participants anticipated a life in retirement about the same as when working. Regressive narratives were told when participants did not see the possibility of replacing work values with similar or new values in their future retirement life.

Study 3

Study 3 presents results from the second phase of the longitudinal studies of the retirement process (Jonsson, Josephsson, & Kielhofner, 2001b). The aim of this study was to explore and understand participants as new retirees. Their experiences of their current situation and the development of their retirement process were explored through analysis of the relationship between the present narrative and their earlier prospective narrative. The findings reveal that it was possible to characterize all but one of the participants' narratives about retirement in terms of its narrative slope (progressive, stable, or regressive). The narratives about the participants' actual experiences of retirement were interpreted in relation to each participant's former expectations of retirement.

For about one third of the participants, retirement turned out differently than they had expected. Some participants with regressive expectations of retirement actively avoided this outcome by continuing to work. Other participants' retirement went in unanticipated directions due to unexpected events and the unexpected consequences of the transition to retirement. The results of the study suggested that, while narratives do play a role in shaping the direction of a person's life, the narratives also interweave with, and change directions as a result of, ongoing life events and experiences.

Study 4

In the third and last of the longitudinal studies, the aim was to explore and understand the retirement process as an occupational transition over time for a group of participants, beginning with working and extending into life as established retirees (Jonsson, Josephsson, & Kielhofner, 2001a). The analysis resulted in themes that illustrate the complex relationship between life's stories and life's reality.

The transition to retirement was an interaction between the prospective narrative and the living world. Most of the participants found the transition to retirement more complex and unpredictable than they had imagined. This resulted in surprising experiences that caused either temporary periods of turbulence or a process of continuing difficulties in adaptation. Surprising experiences were found in different areas of the transition. First, some participants were surprised by the changing relationship between inner motivation and external demands. The absence of the external demands normally provided by work caused difficulty in feeling inner motivation. One participant said, "If you don't have anyone else who pulls the strings, you degenerate to be lazy." These participants experienced high-energy demands from always having to rely on their own choices in decisions of daily occupations. Second, the change of occupational rhythm caused surprising experiences related to lack of space in which

to perform in new occupations. One woman said, "When I'm going to do something today, it takes the whole day. Before, I had the time to do several things." Third, a change in occupational meaning took place when occupations were performed in the new circumstances created by retirement. "It is not the same any longer," said a man about going out to his summer cottage that before retirement was a place for relaxation after a hard working week. Fourth, a surprising change in social relationships was described where participants experienced that even extended social contacts with friends did not have the same valued type of socializing that they had experienced in the aspects of their work that had required discussion and problem solving together with other people.

The final theme in the analysis emerged out of a pattern that showed that the presence or absence of engaging occupations was closely related to a satisfying life in retirement. Engaging occupations were a set of activities that were done with great commitment and were narrated as a special type of occupation that stood out from other occupations. The analysis found six constituents in this type of occupation.

1. It was infused with positive meaning because it was experienced as especially enjoyable, interesting, and challenging.

2. It involved intense participation, meaning that the occupation was performed with a regularity that extended over time.

3. Engaging occupation consisted of a set of activities that were connected to each other and together formed this type of occupation.

4. An engaging occupation was performed for reasons beyond personal pleasure, and the commitment to the occupation was maintained whether the experience was good or bad.

5. An engaging occupation often involved an occupational community of people who shared a common commitment and worked together.

6. The engaging occupation was often summarized as "a sort of work" to describe the complexity of this type of occupation.

Study 5

The aim of Study 5 was to explore and describe how a group of people 65 to 66 years of age spent time in retirement, their experience of retirement, its influence on their occupational lives, and their plans and expectations for the future (Jonsson, Borell, & Sadlo, 2000). The findings showed that the participants developed new temporal structures as retirees. They described a preferable and less stressful rhythm, but with unexpected consequences. Their former plans of taking up new activities as retirees remained only plans because there was not enough time for them. Participants also described changed meanings for some well-known occupations, in part because this meaning had had a relationship to the whole occupational pattern that existed before retirement.

When work was no longer dominant in their lives, this was commonly experienced as new freedom and an opportunity to be a master of one's own time. The findings also revealed, however, that some retirees wished for more demands and more occupations, in order to regulate and structure their daily life. This finding was termed the *paradox of freedom*. That is, the appreciated and desired freedom was at the same time experienced as an emptiness that brought about an imbalance in the participants' occupational pattern. This did not mean that the participants wanted their former work back, but they experienced a need for some kind of regular commitment. This was often expressed as a need for a small job.

Finally, a pattern in most of the participants' future perspective was discovered in which maintaining stability was the participants' primary hope. The participants perceived that they had entered a period in life in which general capacities slowly decreased. With this in mind, the participants' hope of maintaining stability could be understood as an expression of a positive future perspective.

Summary

In the following paragraphs, I will discuss three of the most important results of these studies: the paradox of freedom (from Study 5 when participants where newly retired), the discovery of an occupation that stood out from others (from Study 4), and a potential experience-based categorization of occupation (from all studies).

The Paradox of Freedom

Of the participants who were full-time retired, some still looked upon part of their occupational life as being work: taking care of grandchildren, doing daily tasks at home, or taking care of the summer cottage (Jonsson et al., 2000). This was not a general pattern in the data, however, for the same task could be viewed either as work or leisure. One participant who had a summer cottage said, "I feel now that I have leisure all the time. I guess when one is a retiree this is the only time in life one really owns."

To own one's time meant that one was not forced to do anything and could decide for oneself. When the participants were working, work filled most of their daily schedule, and other types of occupations had to be pressed into the time that was left. When work was no longer present in daily life, this was described as "being the master of one's own time," a preferable change for most of the participants.

The freedom of being entirely master of one's own time was experienced in a paradoxical way. Some retirees wanted to have more demands of productive occupations to regulate and structure their daily lives. Participants experienced a lack of a valued part of life, described as paid work or volunteer work, although they did not want to go back to how life was before retirement. What several participants wanted was a regular commitment, described as the possibility to work 1 to 2.5 days per week, or a few hours a day:

> I would very, very, very much like to have a small job. Not like in the old company but some small job that I can manage. Like cutting the lawn or a hedge. Or go out with old people for a walk or shopping. (Jonsson, 2011)

Participants who did not describe this kind of need either had medical conditions that made them think that a higher level of productivity was not realistic or they were already highly involved in leisure activities/family obligations. These engagements were mostly regular commitments, such as being on the board of a leisure organization, were often described in terms similar to those used for work, and had work-like conditions.

Participants who described a lack of work in retirement had thoughts about possible ways to fill this lack, such as volunteer work or working as needed in their previous workplace. One of the strongest arguments for not realizing thoughts about paid work was that an "old-timer" should not take up work that younger people need, especially when unemployment figures were high. (Unemployment was rising during the period of the interviews and was commonly mentioned by the participants.) One woman expressed her view in this way:

> Why should I only walk around here and do nothing, I think. I ought to have real work. But on the other hand, I think, why should I work when there are so many people unemployed? (Jonsson, 2011)

Thoughts of being "tied down" also influenced decisions about whether or not to enter some kind of work. One woman said she had thoughts of doing some volunteer work but she also wanted freedom to be able to travel at short notice to visit her son and grandchildren.

The group of participants who still worked in some form valued this very positively. One man who worked 30% of full-time explained his view of being master of his own time, saying, "I have my time, it is my own. I can use it, and I don't want to use it as just free time. I want to use it actively, and it's a very nice feeling. Yes, that's freedom."

Another example is a woman who worked about half time. "I really have had an ideal situation during this time. Not to be just cut off, but to partly withdraw is really an advantage. Otherwise, it's just full-time work and the next day no work at all."

Asked to specify the reasons for working, participants expressed a need for more demands from the society or from outside of themselves, often expressed in statements like "having something organized to do" or "one is quite happy that one is needed, that's true." The chance to use the knowledge, skills, and experiences that people had acquired in working life was also valued. In addition, social contacts

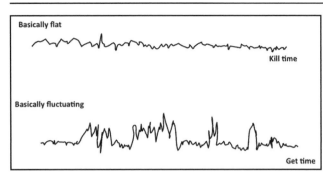

Figure 18-1. Differences in the structure and basic plot of narratives about retirement. (Reprinted with permission from Jonsson, H. [2008]. A new direction in the conceptualization and categorization of occupation. *Journal of Occupational Science, 15,* 3-8. doi:10.1080/14427591.2008.9686601)

in general and in connection with problem-solving situations at work were described.

The Discovery of an Occupation That Stood Out From the Others: Engaging Occupation

In Study 4, we could see a definite difference in pattern in narratives that were about a good and satisfying life as a retiree and those that were not. In fact, the narratives had different structures and different plots, as illustrated in Figure 18-1.

One type of narrative was basically flat in the structure, referring to how different occupations were narrated by the participant. It described a period (a day or a week) where one occupation came after another. The plot, kill time, described that the narrator tried to find things to do to make the time pass, as illustrated in the following quote from one participant telling about an ordinary day in retirement:

> And then I'll go and take a cup of coffee. So I'll walk around in town for a while. Then I'll take the metro home again. That will make this day pass. You can travel around a bit. You have to find something to make the time pass. (Jonsson, 2008)

This flat type of narrative contrasted with a fluctuating narrative that contained drama and engagement and where some occupations stood out from others. Time was not something to pass or kill. Rather, the desire was to get enough time for the occupations that stood out from others or, as this quote illustrates, to get to these occupations as quickly as possible: "It's Thursday almost every day. Thursday, then after only a few days, it's Thursday again."

Engaging Occupations

The occupations that stood out from others and that were narrated with intensity and engagement were called *engaging occupations*. From our analysis, we drew the following conclusions regarding engaging occupations (Jonsson, 2008).

- By looking at intensity and commitment in unfolding occupational narratives, it is possible to find different kinds of occupations that have different levels of importance for a person.
- Engaging occupation was present in many arenas of occupation, work, and leisure as well as in the family arena.
- Presence of engaging occupation was closely connected to a description of a good life as a retiree as well as a worker.

Engaging occupations had the following common characteristics: experienced as positive and highly meaningful; included intense participation, both in duration and regularity; consisted of a coherent set of activities; had evolved into a commitment or responsibility; involved a community of people who shared a common interest; gave an identity for the individual; and was often narrated as analogous to work.

The concept of engaging occupation relates to concepts like commitment (Manell, 1993), committed time (Ås, 1978), and serious leisure (Stebbins, 1997), the last used to describe a type of leisure distinguished from casual and relaxing leisure. These concepts are limited to the leisure arena and focus on the psychological identity provided by this kind of leisure. One concept from the literature that transcends the border between work and leisure is the concept of personal projects, developed out of constructs from personality psychology (Christiansen, Backman, & Nguyen, 1999; Christiansen, Little, & Backman, 1998; Little, 1998). Several of the characteristics of personal projects have parallels to the characteristics of engaging occupations. Personal projects could also be short-term engagements and might cover quite different kinds of goal-directed projects (e.g., improving a partner relationship). Some engaging occupations, which are an integrated part of an individual life, are also difficult to define within the concept of personal projects. Long-lasting engaging employment might, for example, be difficult to see as a personal project.

CONTRIBUTIONS TO OCCUPATIONAL SCIENCE

Toward an Experience-Based Categorization of Occupation

The concept of engaging occupation challenges the traditional way that occupational therapy and occupational science have viewed occupations. It puts emphasis on the experience of meaning and engagement rather than areas such as work, activities of daily living, or leisure. However, the area where occupation appears says very little about

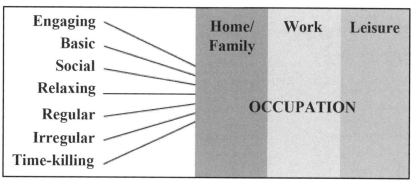

Figure 18-2. Seven experience-based categories of occupation transcending the arenas of home/family, work, and leisure. Based on *Occupational Narratives in the Transition to Retirement.* (Reprinted with permission from Jonsson, H. [2008]. A new direction in the conceptualization and categorization of occupation. *Journal of Occupational Science, 15,* 3-8. doi:10.1080/14427591.2008.9686601)

its quality and impact on the human being. Theoretical assumptions in the literature state close links between human occupation and health (e.g., Canadian Association of Occupational Therapists, 1997; Zemke & Clark, 1996). There is a need to further develop and deepen these statements regarding occupations. Not all occupations are of equal importance to a human being. The concept of engaging occupation offered a starting point for such development by identifying a special type of occupation with a specific positive influence and could be apparent in all arenas of human life. Beginning with the description of engaging occupations, we then turned back to the participants' data to search for further categories in their narrated occupational stories.

In this phase of the project, data were already collected for some participants at the age of 72 to 73 years. At that time, the retirement project had more than 90 interviews in different stages of the retirement process. To make an in-depth analysis possible, 10 interviews from 10 different participants were selected for analysis. Maximal variation was sought in regard to gender, marital status, type of employment, and employment status. The interviews were also representative for the time of the interviews (two at 63 years of age, three at 65/66 years of age, three at 70/71 years of age, and two at 72/73 years of age). The analysis used a constant comparative method (Bogdan & Bilken, 1992). In a process of open coding, the data were categorized into substantive codes and subsequently developed into theoretical codes that became the seven categories of occupation (Figure 18-2; Jonsson, 2008).

Engaging Occupations

As previously described, the first discovered category was that of engaging occupations, because they very much stood out within the narratives. Engaging occupations were present in all life arenas, such as paid employment, volunteer work, regularly taking care of your daughter's children, and going hiking in the mountains. The following participant had in retirement expanded his involvement in an engaging occupation: "I have my time, it is my own. I can use it, and I don't want to have it just as free time. I want to use it actively, and it's a very nice feeling. Yes, that's freedom."

Basic Occupations

Basic occupations were things one was obligated to do. Usually, these were part of a person's routine or habits for fulfilling basic needs, such as getting food, cleaning, and sleeping. Sometimes, it also could be a person's work, an occupation one had to do without putting more engagement in it than necessary. One participant said, "Then I get out of bed and take a shower, and then I tidy up a little, do some cleaning."

Social Occupations

Social occupations were those in which interactions with other people were the main purpose. Meeting friends, family, or co-workers were mentioned, as well as going to a meeting of a retiree organization to meet and socially interact with other people of the same age. A participant said, "I spend a lot of time with retired friends, too."

Relaxing Occupations

Relaxing occupations were those whose purpose was just relaxation. Reading the morning paper, doing crosswords, watching television, and taking an afternoon nap were all mentioned as relaxing occupations. One participant, who had a physically challenging occupation as his engaging occupation, relaxed with music. "We have some jazz meetings. But then you're not active in any way; it's more like relaxation."

Regular Occupations

Regular occupations were done once a month or even once a day, but without strong engagement. Daily walks were mentioned, as were visits to the church. "I take a walk every day, not to get stiff, so to say."

Irregular Occupations

Irregular occupations were those that were freely chosen and had positive meaning. They were done on an irregular basis across time. Going to a movie, the theater, or a vacation trip were narrated as irregular occupations. One participant said, "We go to the movies a lot, or maybe not a lot, we go to the movies."

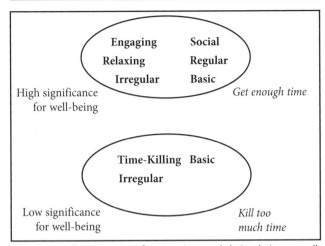

Figure 18-3. Two patterns of occupations and their relation to well-being. (Reprinted with permission from Jonsson, H. [2008]. A new direction in the conceptualization and categorization of occupation. *Journal of Occupational Science, 15*, 3-8. doi:10.1080/14427591.2008.9686601)

Time-Killing Occupations

Time-killing occupations lacked real engagement, and their purpose was to make the time pass. Fishing and shopping were mentioned as time-killing occupations: "But it is not real fishing, you are only standing there you know, and you can be there as much as anywhere else. It's a nice way of passing time." and "When we are out shopping, we go to different shopping centers a bit away from here. It's also a way of passing the time." Travels in the city, reading, taking walks, and listening to the radio were also mentioned as this type of occupation.

In summary, seven experience-based categories of occupation were detected in the second step of the analysis. They were not connected to a certain arena of occupation. Paid employment could have been an engaging occupation, a basic occupation, or a regular occupation. Reading the newspaper was reported as part of an engaging occupation, a relaxing occupation, or a time-killing occupation. Going to church could be an irregular occupation as well as a part of an engaging occupation. The form of the occupation was of minor importance. What was important was how it was experienced and the general pattern of which it was a part.

Two Distinct Patterns of Occupations

Looking back to the two types of narratives (see Figure 18-1) that led to the discovery of engaging occupations, it became obvious that they represented two distinct patterns of occupations that had only some occupations in common. The two patterns and their occupations are illustrated in Figure 18-3 (Jonsson, 2008).

One pattern has a number of categories where an engaging occupation is central to the narrative. Relaxing occupation was often narrated in relation to the importance of not

being involved and active in your engaging occupations all the time. Few, if any, time-killing occupations existed in these narratives, because the theme in the narrative is to get enough time for their engaging occupation. This pattern of categories was connected to the experience of well-being in work as well as in retirement.

The second pattern had fewer categories. Basic occupations created a base for the narrative and provided a daily structure to life. Inside that structure, the participants were occupied with passing time through occupation. As one participant said, "You got to find something to make the time pass." In this pattern, different time-killing occupations were an important part of their narrative. Some irregular occupations were also part of the narrative. They were seen as randomly occurring, but quite meaningful, occupations. This pattern was not connected to the experience of well-being in work nor in retirement.

Future Directions

A critical view of the way we look at and categorize occupation from the results of these retirement studies has started an ongoing discussion in our field (see for example Hammell, 2009a, 2009b). This type of discussion is necessary to theory development and to the establishment of the discipline within academia. In an intensive and unending dialogue, occupational science can develop into a strong and well-respected science, adding an occupational perspective on health and development for human beings.

IMPLICATIONS FOR OCCUPATIONAL THERAPY

Engaging Occupation as a Concept in the Public Arena

So far, knowledge development in the retirement project has focused on interdisciplinary development regarding retirement, occupation and well-being, and development of an experience-based categorization of occupation. This new knowledge also has potential at a public and societal level to enhance quality of life in individuals facing retirement. The research project received broad interest in the Swedish media, with articles in the largest morning paper, television interviews, and radio programs (i.e., Dagens Nyheter, 1998; Sveriges Radio, 2006). The research also resulted in an invitation to lecture before a committee of the Swedish parliament that was outlining policy for the elderly of Sweden in the 21st century. In the final report of the committee, concepts like the paradox of freedom and engaging occupations have been incorporated in the policy-making texts (Senior 2005, 2002). National retiree organizations have also showed interest in the results, and a popular science article has been used in courses for people facing retirement (PRO-Pensionären, 1999).

This research about retirement, especially the concept of engaging occupations, has also served as a source of inspiration for occupational therapists internationally. A government-funded, action-oriented project called "Do It Now," which promoted participation in engaging occupations, was conducted by Dr. Alison Wicks at the Australasian Occupational Science Centre at the University of Wollongong in Shoalhaven, Australia. The aim of the project was to help seniors to plan participation in engaging occupations (Wicks, 2006a, 2006b). The project involved 171 residents, aged 55 and older, in 20 programs. Its aim was to raise their awareness about the importance of planning what they are going to do in retirement and then staying involved in community activities during their retirement. In a summary of the outcome of the project, the report stated the following:

> Do It Now has achieved outcomes at all levels. Some participants have reported making lifestyle changes to increase their engaging occupations during retirement. Conference presentations have raised awareness of an occupational perspective of health and its relevance to the aging population for local planning officers and agencies, as well as national policy makers. (Wicks, 2006b, p. 1)

Both of these examples show how an occupational perspective can contribute relevant knowledge and new perspectives. Within the role of retiree, there is potential for engaging in different occupations that goes beyond personal leisure and contributes to society (e.g., in volunteer work). Occupational therapy can help to spread this knowledge and support engagement in occupation for the well-being of both individuals and society.

Research development in an academic discipline is a never-ending story where small pieces of knowledge add to the whole body of knowledge. This research about the transition to retirement demonstrates how an occupational perspective can bring added relevance. It also shows the international character of knowledge. In one part of the world (Sweden), knowledge was developed that inspires researchers on the opposite part of the globe (Australia) to apply this in preventive work in the community. This produced inspiring examples of new areas where occupational therapists can work in a way that expands our view of the profession.

the categorization in this chapter of seven experience-based categories of occupation:

- Engaging occupations
- Basic occupations
- Social occupations
- Relaxing occupations
- Regular occupations
- Irregular occupations
- Time-killing occupations

2. The group puts this together and then discusses similarities and differences found between individuals in the group.

3. Pick one or two individual patterns in the group that has engaging occupation—and imagine that their engaging occupation/s is no longer possible to perform (due to one of the following reasons: unemployment, economic problems, disability, functional problems, illness).

4. Discuss the impact of this change on quality of life and well-being. Discuss also possible adaptations and alternatives that could develop engaging occupations.

What Happens in an Occupational Transition Like Retirement?

Interview a person who has been a retiree for 2 years or more. Ask about his or her experiences of the transition and if something has surprised him or her in this transition. What engaged him or her in his or her working life? What engages him or her now? Is there a change in the person's experience of participation/involvement in society/community/family? Reflect on and discuss the results of your interview from the results of the retirement study.

Qualities of Daily Life in an Institution

Interview a person in a nursing home or in another institution about an ordinary day in this institution and if the days in the week differ from each other. Go through the descriptions in his or her interviews from the experience-based categorization—which categories can you find and which not?

LEARNING SUPPORTS

Qualities in What We Do That Impact on Life Quality and Well-Being

1. In a group of four to six students, each individual goes through his or her occupations over a single day using

REFERENCES

Ås, D. (1978). Studies of time-use: Problems and prospects. *Acta Sociologica, 2,* 125-141. doi:10.1177/000169937802100203

Bogdan, R. C., & Bilken, S. K. (1992). *Qualitative research for education—An introduction to theory and methods* (2nd ed.). Needham Heights, MA: Allyn and Bacon.

Canadian Association of Occupational Therapists. (1997). *Enabling occupation: An occupational therapy perspective.* Toronto, Ontario, Canada: Author.

Christiansen, C. H., Backman, C., & Nguyen, A. (1999). Occupations and well-being: A study of personal projects. *American Journal of Occupational Therapy, 53,* 91-100. doi:10.5014/ajot.53.1.91

Christiansen, C. H., Little, B. R., & Backman, C. (1998). Personal projects: A useful approach to the study of occupation. *American Journal of Occupational Therapy, 52,* 439-446. doi:10.5014/ajot.52.6.439

Dagens Nyheter (1998, November 14). *Skönt att styra sitt eget liv Nybliven pensionär. Viktigt att ha en uppgift i livet visar forskning (Nice to rule your own life as new retiree. Research shows it is important to have a task in life).* Interviewer: Hans Jonsson.

Hammell, K. W. (2009a). Sacred texts: A skeptical exploration of the assumptions underpinning theories of occupation. *Canadian Journal of Occupational Therapy, 76,* 6-13.

Hammell, K. W. (2009b). Self-care, productivity, and leisure, or dimensions of occupational experience? Rethinking occupational "categories." *Canadian Journal of Occupational Therapy, 76,* 107-114.

Jonsson, H. (1991). Flow Theory—en viktig byggsten i arbetsterapeutisk teoribildning. Arbetsterapeuten nr 5.

Jonsson, H. (1993). The retirement process in an occupational perspective: A review of literature and theories. *Physical and Occupational Therapy in Geriatrics, 11*(4), 15-35.

Jonsson, H. (2000). *Anticipating, experiencing and valuing the transition from worker to retiree: A longitudinal study of retirement as an occupational transition* (Doctoral dissertation). Karolinska Institutet, Solna, Sweden. Retrieved from http://diss.kib.ki.se/2000/91-628-4076-2/

Jonsson, H. (2008). A new direction in the conceptualization and categorization of occupation. *Journal of Occupational Science, 15*(1), 3-8. doi:10.1080/14427591.2008.9686601

Jonsson, H. (2011). The first steps into the third age: The retirement process from a Swedish perspective. *Occupational Therapy International, 18,* 32-38. doi:10.1002/oti.311

Jonsson, H., & Andersson, L. (1999). Attitudes to work and retirement: Generalization or diversity? *Scandinavian Journal of Occupational Therapy, 6*(1), 29-35. doi:10.1080/110381299443825

Jonsson, H., Borell, L., & Sadlo, G. (2000). Retirement: An occupational transition with consequences on temporality, rhythm and balance. *Journal of Occupational Science, 7,* 5-13. doi:10.1080/14427591.2000.9686462

Jonsson, H., & Josephsson, S. (2005). Occupation and meaning. In C. H. Christansen, C. M. Baum, & J. Bass-Haugen (Eds.), *Occupational therapy: Participation, participation and well-being* (3rd ed.). Thorofare, NJ: SLACK Incorporated.

Jonsson, H., Josephsson, S., & Kielhofner, G. (2001a). Evolving narratives in the course of retirement. *American Journal of Occupational Therapy, 54,* 463-476. doi:10.5014/ajot.54.5.463

Jonsson, H., Josephsson, S., & Kielhofner, G. (2001b). Narratives and experience in an occupational transition: A longitudinal study of the retirement process. *American Journal of Occupational Therapy, 55,* 424-432. doi:10.5014/ajot.55.4.424

Jonsson, H., Kielhofner, G., & Borell, L. (1997). Anticipating retirement: The formation of narratives concerning an occupational transition. *American Journal of Occupational Therapy, 51*(1), 49-56. doi:10.5014/ajot.51.1.49

Little, B. R. (1998). Personal projects pursuit: Dimensions and dynamics of personal meaning. In P. T. P. Wong & P. S. Fry (Eds.), *The human quest for meaning: A handbook of psychological research and clinical applications.* Mahwah, NJ: Lawrence Erlbaum Associates.

Manell, R. C. (1993). High-investment activities and life satisfaction among older adults. In J. R. Kelly (Ed.), *Activity and aging: Staying involved in later life.* Newbury Park, CA: Sage Publications.

PRO-Pensionären. (1999). *Priset för friheten är att inte längre vara behövd. (The National Retiree Association—The Retiree Journal. The price for freedom is to no longer be needed).* No. 7.

Rollén, B. (2000). *Inget jobb att gå till...Vem är jag nu då ... och vad ska jag göra? Ha semester i 20 år? (No work to go to ... Whom am I now? and What should I do? Have 20 years of vacation?).* Stockholm, Sweden: Cebastos AB.

Senior 2005 (2002). *Riv åldertrappan: Livslopp I förändring.* SOU 2002:29. *(Tear down the stairs of aging: Life courses in change).* Stockholm, Sweden: Nordstedts tryckeri.

Stebbins, R. A. (1997). Serious leisure and well-being. In J. T. Haworth (Ed.), *Work, leisure and well-being* (pp. 117-130). New York, NY: Routledge.

Sveriges Radio (2006, December 19). I ntervju i programmet Tendens. (National Radio Broadcast. Interview).

Wicks, A. (2006a). *Do it now: A project promoting participation in engaging occupations.* Presented at the meeting of the 39th National Conference of the Australian Association of Gerontology. Australian Association of Gerontology, Sydney, Australia.

Wicks, A. (2006b). *Do it now: A project promoting participation in engaging occupations.* Retrieved from http://shoalhaven.uow.edu.au/aosc/publications/do_it_now.pdf

Yerxa, E. J. (1993). Occupational science: A new source of power for participants in occupational therapy. *Journal of Occupational Science, 1,* 3-10. doi:10.1080/14427591.1993.9686373

Yerxa, E. J., Clark, F., Frank, G., Jackson, J., Parham, D., Pierce, D., . . . Zemke, R. (1989). An introduction to occupational science, a foundation for occupational therapy in the 21st century. *Occupational Therapy in Health Care, 6*(4), 1-17. doi:10.1080/J003v06n04_04

Zemke, R., & Clark, F. (Eds.). (1996). *Occupational science: The evolving discipline.* Philadelphia, PA: F. A. Davis.

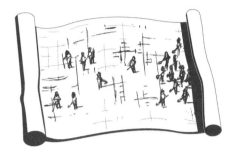

Understanding the Development of Occupational Potential Over Time Through the Analysis of Life Stories

Alison Wicks, PhD, MHSc(OT), BAppSc(OT)

Effective occupational therapy practice requires an understanding of ourselves and our clients from an occupational perspective as well as knowledge about different occupations and what influences people's occupational choices and patterns. Occupational science contributes to occupational therapists' requisite understanding and knowledge by investigating relevant concepts, constructs, and contextual factors that shape people's engagement in occupation. This chapter describes my qualitative doctoral study that explored the construct of occupational potential and how it develops over time. *Occupational potential*, which in simple terms refers to a person's capacity to do, was a relatively new construct in occupational science at the time of my study yet one that has always been fundamental to occupational therapy. The aim of the study was to research the development and realization of occupational potential from the perspectives of six older Australian women. The study adopted a life history approach using life stories to obtain a comprehensive view of the occupational experiences of the women. Life stories are the stories that people tell about what they have done throughout their lives. As such, life stories are valuable

resources for occupational scientists who seek to generate knowledge about occupation. The women's life stories were the study data that were analyzed and interpreted to comprehend the construct of occupational potential and the influences that facilitated and constrained the women's occupational experiences at different stages of their lives. Findings from the study provide significant insight about people as occupational humans that occupational therapists can apply in practice.

LITERATURE REVIEW

A review of the occupational science and occupational therapy literature undertaken when the study began found only Wilcock's (1998) description of occupational potential. Wilcock referred to occupational potential, an essential component of her theory of the human need for occupation (Wilcock, 1993), as "future capability, to engage in occupation towards needs, goals and dreams for health, material requirement, happiness and well-being"

Pierce, D. (Ed.).
Occupational Science for Occupational Therapy (pp. 221-231).

(1998, p. 257). However, the review did identify references to the realization of potential through engagement in occupations (Fidler & Fidler, 1978; Townsend, 1997), as well as references to the relationship between doing and the attainment of personhood (Bateson, 1990) and doing and identity formation (Christiansen, 1999, 2000). A review of the generic literature on human needs, capacities, and potential was subsequently undertaken to fully investigate the construct of occupational potential and gain an appreciation of its role in the occupational development of humans.

There were ample references in the psychology literature on theories about human needs and what influences human behavior (Bandura, 1986; Cannon, 1939; Erikson, 1965; Maslow, 1954; Pavlov, 1927; Piaget, 1950). Theories of intrinsic motivation, such as the theory of flow (Csikszentmihalyi, 1990) and the theory of the drive for competence (White, 1971), provided relevant background material. Literature on human cognitive and intellectual capacities (Coleman, Butcher, & Carson, 1980; Gardner, 1983), individual differences in regard to capacities (Ornstein & Sobel, 1988), and the human need to exercise capacities (Maslow, 1968) also served as a useful resource. The writings of the humanists (Allport, 1955; Maslow, 1968; Perls, Hefferline, & Goodman, 1951; Rogers, 1961) provided insight into human potential and were useful in highlighting the humanist assumptions underpinning occupational therapy (Meyer, 1922) as well as occupational science (Yerxa, 1998). An educational perspective on human potential (Gardner, 1993; LeVine & White, 1986; Scheffler, 1985) was particularly useful when considering influences on the realization of potential.

Given that the study participants were Australian women, classic feminist texts (Curthoys, 1988; de Beauvoir, 1988; Friedan, 1963) and Australian feminist writings (Connell, 2002; Lake, 1999; McDowell & Pringle, 1992) were reviewed for the study. Such woman-centered literature challenged biological assumptions about women's nature and identified gender role socialization and sexual discrimination as keys to understanding gender inequalities (Connell, 2002; Germov, 1998). Consequently, such literature raised my awareness of the importance of acknowledging and explaining the social, economic, and political constraints on the women's occupational participation and their subsequent influence on the development of the women's occupational potential. Interestingly, in the occupational science literature, only Primeau's (2000) work on housework discussed the interaction between gender ideologies and occupation.

In summary, the literature review process highlighted a lack of research and literature on occupational potential and on women's occupational development. The review subsequently shaped the two main questions that guided the study, and these questions determined the appropriate methodology for the study.

METHODS

Purpose of the Study

The principal question that guided this study was "What is occupational potential, and how does it develop over time?" A specific question that focused on the older women's perceptions of their occupational life course was "How was the development of the women's occupational potential facilitated and constrained over time?" Because the study questions were largely about the women's experiences, a qualitative approach, focusing on the way the women interpreted their experiences and their worlds (Holloway, 1997), was deemed the most appropriate means of addressing the questions.

Philosophical Foundations of and Approaches to the Study

The qualitative research paradigm is underpinned by the philosophy that people's experiences are real (a subjectivist ontology) and that through sharing experiences we are able to know this reality (a relativist epistemology) (DePoy & Gitlin, 1998). In this study, the reality was each woman's personal perceptions of her occupational experiences over time. It was the interaction between the researcher and the participants during in-depth individual interviews that enabled their realities to be known, interpreted, and understood. In qualitative research, the researcher's subjectivity is as significant as that of the participant's and, according to Hasselkus (1997), should be "acknowledged and celebrated" (p. 82) because it is the starting point of the research, enabling, rather than limiting, the research process. In this study, my pre-understandings were shaped by my own experiences as an Australian woman and linked to the assumptions and beliefs of my profession, occupational therapy.

The two research approaches to my study were aligned philosophically. First, a narrative approach, which uses narratives—the stories people tell about the things they do—shaped the structure of the study. Developed from an exploration of the form and content of narratives (Bruner, 1986; Ricoeur, 1985), the narrative approach uses the sequential nature of narratives and the cohesive role of narrative plots to reflect on experiences that people recall (Grbich, 1999). Narratives, the basic medium through which humans speak and think, are ubiquitous, universal. As such, narratives are uniquely suited for comprehending human lives in culture and in time (Freeman, 1997) and particularly suitable for understanding people's occupational experiences (Clark, Carlson, & Polkinghorne, 1997; Polkinghorne, 1988). My study adopted a life history approach, a specific narrative approach that uses life stories to reconstruct and interpret whole lives in order to obtain a continuous-time and comprehensive view of people (Frank, 1996). A life story is "the story a person chooses to tell about a life he or she has lived, told as completely and honestly as possible, what is remembered of it and what the teller wants others to know of it" (Atkinson, 1998, p. 8).

The second distinct approach that guided my study was a hermeneutic orientation to phenomenology. Based on the philosophical works of Heidegger (1962) and Gadamer (1975), hermeneutic phenomenology is both descriptive and interpretive in that it endeavors to illuminate and understand human phenomena. Profoundly reflective, hermeneutic phenomenology involves uncovering the essence of a phenomenon by gathering stories from those living it and then interpreting those stories (van Manen, 1997). The data of hermeneutic studies are personal experiences. Van Manen (1997) maintained that the aim of a hermeneutic phenomenological approach is to borrow other people's experiences in order to learn from them and develop a richer, deeper comprehension of a human phenomenon. In my study, the women's stories of their occupational experiences over time were interpreted as a means of learning more about the concept of occupational potential.

Two theoretical perspectives were used to make sense of the study data. Given that occupational science set the boundaries of this study, the primary theoretical perspective was an occupational one, viewing people as occupational humans who need to do meaningful and purposeful things (Wilcock, 1993, 1998). However, because the study participants were women, a feminist perspective was also adopted to critically reflect on how power and social structures influenced aspects of their everyday lives (Townsend, 1998).

Study Sequence

Following approval of the study by the Charles Sturt University Ethics Committee in September 2000, the study was conducted from 2001 to 2003. The setting for the study was the Shoalhaven, a rural local government area located on the south coast of New South Wales, Australia.

The study began with recruitment of participants by means of newspaper advertisements, personal invitations, and word of mouth. The criteria for participation were being female, aged over 65 years, and currently living in the Shoalhaven. Thirty-four women volunteered to participate in the study on the basis of informed consent.

Following recruitment, there were three phases to the study, each with a specific purpose. Phase 1 was a pilot study consisting of a focus group with six women randomly selected from the recruitment pool and life story interviews with one woman purposively selected from the pool. The aim of the pilot was to evaluate the proposed research methods and to collect some preliminary data for trial analysis.

Phase 2 involved two focus groups, one with nine randomly selected volunteers and the other with seven. The initial aim of the focus groups was to identify significant themes embedded in the occupational experiences that the women shared with each other. These themes were later explored in depth during the life story interviews. The second aim of the focus groups was to explore those social, historical, political, and economic events that had influenced the women's occupational life courses. Societal expectations around women's education and employment options and the call to action to support the World War II effort emerged as powerful influences that had, respectively, constrained and enhanced their occupational choices. These influences provided the context against which the life stories were interpreted.

The third phase consisted of life story interviews with six women purposively selected from participants in the three focus groups ($n = 22$) on the basis of their differences in educational background, marital status, and breadth of life experience. All six women, whose pseudonyms were Sylvia, Maureen, Fran, Doris, Mary, and Alice, had already demonstrated in the focus groups their ability to reminisce and reflect. The aim of the interviews was to collect life story data for narrative analysis. The individual interview sessions were conducted face to face, in a relaxed manner, with each woman choosing a setting in which she felt comfortable. In total, there were 21 individual interview sessions, 16 for data collection and discussion and 5 for data clarification. The number of data collection and discussion sessions with each woman ranged from three to four. These sessions were concluded when it was mutually agreed that there was enough data (Dickie, 2003). Only the data collection component, which ranged from 70 to 110 minutes, was taped recorded and therefore available for transcription and subsequent narrative analysis. However, field notes relating to the discussion component, which ranged from 60 to 100 minutes, were always made, forming an important part of my reflexive journal. The field notes helped inform the analysis and interpretation phases of the study. In the data clarification sessions, the women had an opportunity to check their stories, modifying or expanding them as they wished.

Analysis

The manner in which life story data were analyzed and interpreted evolved over a lengthy period into a custom-made process. The process was developed in response to interaction with the life stories and informed by hermeneutic phenomenology and narrative theory. Polkinghorne's (1995) narrative analysis was especially influential because it emphasizes the wholeness of the narratives, retaining the integrity and uniqueness of each story rather than dissecting it into elements. A goal of the analysis was to celebrate and honor each life story by focusing on its individual quality.

Becoming steeped in the world of the participants was an important part of the analysis process. The intention of total saturation in the women's stories was to pick up nuances that would enable interpretation, or making sense of, important occupational aspects of their lives. Illuminating the themes woven through their stories was another part, one that I found was analogous to shifting and sifting sand. Shifting sand can be a lengthy procedure, and at times it can feel that you are not making progress. Thematic analysis, like sifting sand, requires fine mesh and a keen eye to find just the grain of insight that you are seeking.

Interpretation was a key part of the analysis, beginning during the data collection phase and continuing through the writing phase. In essence, the interpretation involved analyzing the data by deciphering how the women themselves explained the phenomenon of occupational potential to answer the research question. My interpretation of the data was influenced by my life world (Heidegger, 1962) and by the study's theoretical framework and approaches. It was also shaped by the occupational and feminist lenses I wore while reading and rereading the stories to understand the influences on the women's occupational potential.

Though the actual processes involved in the analysis are important, it is useful for new or intending researchers to appreciate the personal experience of doing qualitative studies. For me, at times, the analysis was tortuous, circuitous, and messy, just as described by Dickie (2003). In fact, I have described some of my personal experiences during analysis as "being fog bound" (Wicks, 2004, p. 16), being unable to understand anything, and feeling that I had completely lost all sense of direction. At times during the analysis I was unable to move my thinking forward, backward, or sideways. In fact, there were times when I felt cognitively paralyzed. Such an experience created feelings of incompetency as a researcher and increased self-doubt about my ability to complete the journey. "Losing sight of the forest" (Wicks, 2004, pp. 16-17), or concentrating too much on minor, irrelevant details and going off on unnecessary tangents, rather than keeping a focus on the big picture, was another personal experience during analysis. At times, I needed my supervisor to remind me to readjust my focus and get back on track. But the emotional energy involved in analysis of life history research is not the only challenge for researchers. As with most qualitative research, large amounts of time need to be invested in the gathering and then interpreting of life stories. This type of research is not for those who prefer a preplanned research journey with a predetermined time schedule.

RESULTS

The synthesis of the findings from the analysis and interpretation of the life stories illuminated some general features of occupational potential, thus addressing the study's principal question. Additional understandings, gathered when a feminist perspective was applied to the data, highlighted the gendered nature of occupational potential and addressed the secondary question.

Features of Occupational Potential

The main understanding gained from the study was that occupational potential is a highly complex construct. Because "occupation is a complex multidimensional phenomenon" (Yerxa, 1989, p. 6), it is not surprising that occupational potential was revealed in my study as a multidimensional and dynamic human phenomenon that encompasses a person's needs and capacities, which reflect and are influenced by characteristics of the person and the environment. Some core features of occupational potential were also elucidated.

The first feature that emerged was that occupational potential evolves over time. Rather than being predetermined by specific personal attributes, occupational potential was revealed as a fluid phenomenon, developing as capacities were exercised at different stages of the women's lives. Doris's story effectively illuminates how people undergo occupational reinventions in the process of realizing their occupational potential. Her story shows that people do not necessarily stay transfixed once they become who they want to be. For example, Doris loved school and enjoyed being a student. With the financial and moral support from her uncle, she was enabled to stay on at high school to become a senior student. Then, she wanted to become a student at teachers' college. On completion of her tertiary studies, she became a teacher. After several years working in the field, she undertook further studies at university, part-time, to become more highly qualified. At the time of the study, Doris was an older woman, using her teaching skills at a local museum.

The second core feature that emerged from the analysis was the relationship between the realization of occupational potential and the women's patterns of occupational participation. The life stories revealed how patterns and diversity of participation facilitated the development of occupational potential. For example, Mary and Sylvia, the two women who traveled overseas as young adults, were exposed to a rich variety of social, cultural, and political experiences that undoubtedly broadened their views of who they were and subsequently shaped their ideas as to who they wanted to become. The women who had comparatively limited occupational experiences in the childhood and adolescent stages of their lives, such as Maureen and Fran, had somewhat narrower occupational aspirations.

The third feature is that each person's occupational potential is unique, as a result of the diverse interactions between personal capacities and characteristics and environmental influences. The noticeable differential in the occupational potential of Fran and Doris effectively exemplifies how this uniqueness is created. Although both female, and both born into working-class families during a similar period in Australia's social and economic history, their subsequent occupational life courses varied significantly, as did their reflections of their occupational potential over time. It was evident from their stories that the interaction between each woman's personal characteristics, and her family and social supports, influenced the way she managed the occupational opportunities as they were presented to her. The infinite variety of possible outcomes resulting from interactions between the individual and the environment makes the difference. That the development of each person's occupational potential is unique adds to the complex nature of the concept.

Influences on the Development of Occupational Potential

Adopting a feminist perspective for analysis of the women's stories revealed that different environmental influences, at different stages of their lives, shaped the women's occupational potential. Furthermore, the study findings revealed that such influences were either enhancing or constraining. Within the environment, there were micro, meso, and macro influences (Bronfenbrenner, 1979).

The microlevel of the environment includes the family unit and the person's network of close friends. Within the family, a person engages in personally meaningful occupations and develops significant interpersonal relationships with family members. Such engagement reflects family values, to a greater or lesser extent, and reinforces the development of personal belief systems. In turn, the personal belief system influences the development of occupational interests of the family member. The availability of role models and various means of support from within the family and friendship network also play major functions in developing occupational potential. Doris's life story exemplifies this particular point. Although she chose not to be a practicing Jehovah's Witness, as was her mother, Doris has internalized some of the Jehovah's Witness values, particularly those values relating to the productive use of time.

The mesolevel incorporates larger groups and institutions, such as school and the workplace. At this level, it is apparent that a person may or may not have the opportunity to engage in activities that enable the development of skills, abilities, and general occupational competence. The third level of the environment that influences the development of occupational potential is the macroenvironment, or the broader society, within which the micro- and mesoenvironments are embedded. The study revealed how Australian economic and social policies as well as historical events influenced the development of the women's occupational potential. During their early adult years, the legislative constraints that deprived the women of certain career options and the relative freedom in relation to social occupations bestowed on them during World War II are two such examples.

Various personal influences also significantly shaped the realization of the women's occupational potential. These personal influences could be categorized as personal needs, goals, and values; personal capacities; and occupational persona, "that dimension of self ... which is predisposed to as well as driven towards, engagement in certain types of occupations" (Whiteford & Wicks, 2000, p. 48). The different travel experiences recounted by Maureen and Mary effectively illustrate how their occupational personae, shaped by very different biological and sociocultural factors, influenced the development of their occupational potential. In the interviews, Maureen presented as conservative and pragmatic, and her story revealed that she was occupationally constrained, to some extent, by limited finances, family responsibilities, a fear of flying, and a susceptibility to seasickness. Consequently, at the age of 72, Maureen had only traveled interstate, by car or train, on a few occasions and had still not fulfilled her long-held dream of traveling to Perth. On the other hand, Mary, as a young, single woman, traveled by ship to the United Kingdom, where she lived on the estate of wealthy and privileged family friends. Mary then returned home, traveling overland in a double-decker bus from England to Karachi, and reveling in the adventures, occupational challenges, and romance along the way. Needless to say, the occupational experiences that each woman recounted in her life story were quite different, due to each woman's unique occupational persona. Occupational persona influences a person's patterns of occupational participation, which can affect the realization of capacities and subsequently influence the development of occupational potential.

Being a woman was certainly illuminated by this study as having a significant influence on the development of occupational potential throughout the women's lives. The study showed that the occupations associated with being a woman, and the options for occupational participation available to women were, to some extent, biologically and socially determined. Moreover, there was an interaction between these determinants and the women's personal values, interests, and aspirations. The interaction of biological and social determinants is illustrated most clearly by the following example. Childbearing is one of the two biologically determined occupations for women, the other being breastfeeding (Alston, 1995). As the stories revealed, five of the women in this study became mothers, and one chose to abort a pregnancy. Although their decisions about motherhood were probably based on their personal needs and interests, and likely made in conjunction with their partners, there were also significant social expectations of women during the post–World War II period, when the women in this study were having their families. Australian women were encouraged to populate the country and, as a result, there was a high birth rate in the period of 1945 to 1961, and so the children of the women in this study are all members of the postwar baby boom cohort. There was also a social expectation at this time that children would be born to married couples, which possibly explains Mary's personal decision to have an abortion. Though the women in this study had some choice about becoming mothers, some other significant factors that deprived the women of opportunities for participating in self-chosen occupations, due to the politics of gender, emerged from their stories.

Gendered power relationships, which were embedded within the prevailing Australian patriarchal ideology, became apparent as important influences on the development of the women's occupational potential. In addition, the explicit and tacit social expectations about women's occupations as well as the gender-based division of occupations reduced the occupational opportunities and choices of the women, thereby influencing their occupational experiences. In the study, it was Fran who was the most dependent on her husband. After she was married, she did not undertake any paid employment and was totally reliant on her husband for money. On reflection, Fran realized how much she would have loved to work and earn money in her own right, to meet some of her personal occupational needs. Alice also never undertook paid employment outside the home. However, as was usual for farmers' wives, she was allocated the task of managing the accounts for the family farm business. In some respects, this task enabled her to regain some power, because she was able to keep informed of the financial status of the business. Sylvia, who recounted how she had witnessed the debilitating effects of patriarchy on her mother, vowed that she would always work, at least part-time, because she realized that money was, in many respects, power. Though each woman adapted to the patriarchal society in her own way, it nevertheless affected the development of her occupational potential. Each woman had to create ways of acquiring income or compensating for lack of income so that she was able to do the things she needed and wanted to do.

A particularly interesting finding of the study was that the women developed unique occupational strategies in response to the gender-specific influences on the realization of their occupational potential. These strategies, coined as "women's ways of doing" (Wicks, 2006), were instrumental in developing and realizing their occupational potential as they were designed to enable them to cope with and adapt to interruptions to their participation and overcome some of the occupational deprivations and tensions they experienced. The primary purpose of all of the strategies was to create opportunities for meaningful participation. Although each woman developed strategies in response to her own situation, there were

some common features. The strategies were developed and refined over time. There was a relationship between the quantity and quality of strategies and the woman's level of participation, and strategies were sometimes used subconsciously (Wicks & Whiteford, 2005). For example, Maureen's strategy of entering a convent so that she could become a teacher is an example of creating occupational opportunities. Sylvia's strategy for learning about political thought and world events, despite being prohibited from pursuing school and tertiary education, is an excellent example of refinement of occupational strategies over time. As a young girl, Sylvia used to sit very still, not saying a word, so she could stay up and listen to the discussions among her father's intellectual friends. Later, as an adult, she worked for 4 years as a secretary for an academic at the Australian National University, attending evening classes in political science and international relations as a nonexaminable student. Today, Sylvia continues her self-education in political affairs by being an active member of a political party.

Summary of Results

The in-depth analysis, from an occupational perspective, of the life stories of the six older women in this study enhanced understanding of the construct of occupational potential. The study revealed that rather than following a predetermined course, the developmental course of a person's occupational potential is largely unpredictable, due to a host of environmental and personal influences that affect its trajectory. Occupational potential and its realization over time emerges from the dynamic interaction between the environment and the individual, and the specific features of each that are brought to this interaction are what render it unique.

When the life stories were also analyzed from a feminist perspective, the effect of gender on the development of occupational potential emerged as significant. The study revealed that being a woman shapes the development of occupational potential at each stage of the life course as biological and social determinants of gender interact. Yet, despite constraints on the development of their occupational potential, women use occupational strategies that are gradually refined over time, in order to create opportunities for meaningful occupational participation. In this way, they can continue to reinvent themselves occupationally and realize their potential. When considered collectively, these findings formed the basis of a new description of occupational potential. It is proposed that occupational potential be described as a person's capacity to do what is required and within available opportunities in order to become who he or she has the potential to be.

CONTRIBUTION TO OCCUPATIONAL SCIENCE

This study has contributed to occupational science in several ways. First and foremost, the study has increased understanding of occupational potential, a significant construct in the theory of the human as an occupational being, by revealing its complexity. Second, this study, like most research, has generated more questions than answers, and the findings presented in this chapter possibly represent just the tip of the iceberg in relation to occupational potential, the gendered nature of occupational potential, and the influences that affect the development and realization of women's occupational potential. Topics for further research on occupational potential by occupational scientists include whether and how gender influences men's occupational potential, occupational experiences of other groups within Australian society, and cross-cultural studies of occupational potential. Such research will help to clarify the general features of occupational potential identified in this study and identify whether there are additional features of occupational potential that are specific to particular groups in society.

A third contribution is the raising of awareness of some significant issues when researching occupation. For example, in relation to feminist research, this study, which had women as subjects rather than objects of research, supports Smith's (1990) proposal for research from the standpoint of women, incorporating women's interests and perspectives. In addition, the focus on the "dailiness" (Aptheker, 1989, p. 39) of the everyday lives of ordinary Australian women (as opposed to the lives of high-achieving women who are usually the subjects of biographies) has proven to be particularly valuable in this instance, because such typical women represent the majority of women and their life experiences. In addition, for occupational scientists, this study has highlighted the value of adopting a continuous-time approach to ensure a comprehensive understanding of the occupational natures of humans. Moreover, the value of life stories for gathering a person's occupational experiences and the effectiveness of life stories for understanding aspects of the occupational human have been further demonstrated. The life stories used in this study provided subjective accounts of the women's occupational experiences throughout their lives. Individually, each life story revealed rich information about a life lived. When considered as a group, they provided an appreciation of the broad sociocultural, political, economic, and historical issues that shape the occupational life course. Upon reflection, the use of life stories as the data for this study satisfied the majority of criteria for occupational science research: they preserved the integrity of the women; acknowledged the women's experiences as credible; viewed the women as interacting with the environment; included the past,

present, and future; and enabled study of their occupational behaviors over the lifespan (Yerxa et al., 1990).

IMPLICATIONS FOR PRACTICE

This study's findings can be transformed into useful knowledge and skills for incorporation into practice. However, because the findings of this interpretive study are tentative and remain grounded in the stories of the six women, it is not possible, or appropriate, to identify specific implications in relation to occupational potential for occupational therapy. Yet, despite this limitation, there are some broad, rather than specific, implications and recommendations for practice arising from my study.

Occupational Therapists Need to Be Politically Aware and Socially Responsive

In view of the findings about the social and political influences on the development of occupational potential, the recommendation that occupational therapists become politically aware and socially responsive (Pollard, Sakellariou, & Kronenberg, 2009) and the World Federation of Occupational Therapists' (2006) position statement on human rights are supported by my study. By adopting a broad view of the individual, a view that recognizes that individuals are embedded and embodied (Fay, 1987) within their societies and that the social organization is the locus through which individuals find expression (Mumford, 1967), occupational therapists can effectively enable individuals to realize their occupational potential. My study has particularly highlighted the need for occupational therapists to be aware of the influence of gender constructions on occupational participation (Primeau, 2000) and to acknowledge the influence of being a woman on the development and realization of occupational potential.

Some ways in which occupational therapists can become politically and socially active include moving beyond traditional roles of occupational therapists and becoming part of health promotion, public health, and community development teams. Within such teams occupational therapists will have opportunities to develop working relationships with politicians, social planners, research bodies, and the media. The development of these relationships will broaden the dissemination of understanding and ideas about occupation, health (Wilcock & Whiteford, 2003), and gender. If more occupational therapists become entrenched within the public health domain and local and state government organizations, they can use available opportunities to focus debate on the underlying factors that prevent people from realizing their occupational potential, such as having limited occupational choices and lacking opportunities for occupational satisfaction, balance, and meaning. Advocating for more community-based occupation-focused programs, such as the Men's Shed program (Ballinger, Talbot, & Verrinder, 2009) for older retired men who often risk social isolation once they leave work, would be one way of enabling people to do the things they need and want to do.

Occupational Therapy Practice Should Be Contextually Relevant

Given that a significant influence of the environment on the development and realization of a person's occupational potential has emerged from this study, it is essential that the sociocultural, historical, economic, and political contexts within which people live, work, and recreate are considered in practice (Wilcock & Whiteford, 2003). Accordingly, it is recommended that occupational therapists undertake community practice; that is, practice that acknowledges Hillery's view that community involves "moral commitment, social cohesion and continuity in time" (Fazio, 2001, p. 4) and is undertaken within the community (i.e., within the locale). This recommendation is consistent with the current trend in health care, which, in many countries, involves a shift away from an institutional to a community focus (World Health Organization, 2009).

Occupational Therapy Practice Should Be Client Centered and Conducted Within an Enablement Framework

In view of the influence of personal factors on the development of occupational potential, the study has reinforced the importance of occupational therapy practice being client centered. Client-centered practice involves respecting clients' values, belief systems, and choices; giving clients ultimate responsibility for decisions about daily occupations and occupational therapy services; facilitating client participation in all aspects of occupational therapy services; fostering collaborative and partnership relationships; and enabling clients to solve occupational issues (Law, Baum, & Baptiste, 2002; Townsend, 1999).

In this recommendation, the term *client* refers to an individual, a group, or a community. Client-centered, enabling occupational therapy practice strives for clients to become their authentic selves (Palmer, 2000) and realize their occupational potential.

CONCLUSION

My study used life stories of older women to explore the construct of occupational potential, now described as a person's capacity to do what is required and within available opportunities, in order to become who he or she has the potential to be. It has reinforced the fundamental objective of occupational therapy practice. Based on this study, it would appear consistent with occupational therapy philosophy and assumptions that occupational therapists should focus on enabling people to develop and realize their occupational potential. That is, the goal of occupational therapy practice should be to enable people, regardless of their backgrounds and the physical, cognitive, and emotional challenges that may constrain them, to become whom they have the capacity and opportunity to become. Maintaining such a focus will enable occupational therapy to realize its potential as one of the great ideas of the 21st century, by enabling people in all walks of life, across the globe, to achieve health and well-being through occupation (Yerxa, 1991).

LEARNING SUPPORTS

Building Insight Into Everyday Occupations

Purpose

To develop an awareness of gender-based occupations in everyday life.

Primary Concepts

Observation, gender-based occupations, dailiness (everyday occupations), and subjectivity.

Instructions

1. Go to the local shopping mall with a fellow student or colleague and find a comfortable place to sit for 1 hour and observe what people do.

2. Independent of each other, record on paper the various occupations you observe, making notes about what people are doing, the different roles and responsibilities undertaken by various people, and gendered occupations (who is doing what).

3. Think about the dailiness of what you observe, from the perspective of an occupational therapist enabling clients to do what they need and want to do every day. Consider possible barriers or difficulties for people with physical impairments.

4. Think about some recommendations you could provide the management of the shopping mall to ensure equity of access for all customers.

5. At the end of the hour when you compare your notes and discuss your thoughts, consider the reasons for the similarities and differences of your observations and ideas.

Building Insight Into the Practical Issues of Interviewing

Purpose

To appreciate the equipment, skills, and time required for recording and transcribing an interview.

Primary Concepts

Qualitative research, narratives, interviews, and storytelling.

Instructions

1. Read this journal article: Wicks, A., & Whiteford, G. (2006). Conceptual and practical issues in qualitative research: Reflections on a life history study. *Scandinavian Journal of Occupational Therapy, 13*(2), 94-100. doi: 10.1080/11038120600654676

2. Ask a friend, fellow student, or family member for permission to be interviewed by you for 15 minutes.

3. Propose several topics for the interview and invite the interviewee to select one (e.g., my last holiday, my work, my hobbies).

4. Make arrangements for the interview on a day and at a time that is mutually convenient and at a place that is appropriate.

5. Prepare your equipment for the interview and think about some questions you will ask and how you will ask them.

6. Record the interview and then transcribe it verbatim (word for word).

7. Reflect on the experience by asking yourself questions such as: Was I an effective interviewer? Did the interview go as I expected—if not, why not? What would I do differently next time? What does the transcript tell me about the way people tell stories?

Building Insight Into the Personal Strategies You Have Developed to Do What You Want to Do

Purpose

To gain an appreciation of your personal occupational strategies.

Primary Concepts

Occupational strategies, "ways of doing," opportunities, barriers, enablers, and understanding yourself as an occupational human.

Instructions

1. Think of a situation in the past when you were unable to do something you needed and wanted to do. Perhaps you had an impairment (e.g., you sustained a fracture to your arm prior to the school swimming carnival); maybe your parents had instructed you not to do something (e.g., you could not stay at a party after midnight); or possibly there was legislation or a policy that restricted you doing something (e.g., you were below the legal age for purchasing an alcoholic drink).

2. Reflect on your feelings at the time.

3. Did you satisfy your occupational need at that time? If so, how did you do that? What strategy did you develop? Have you continued using that strategy? What did you learn about yourself in that situation?

4. Consider some clients who have been restricted from doing something they need and want to do. Based on your personal experiences, how do you think they would be feeling? What is your role as an occupational therapist to enable them to meet their needs?

REFERENCES

Allport, G. (1955). *Becoming: Basic considerations for a psychology of personality.* New Haven, CT: Yale University Press.

Alston, M. (1995). Women on the land: The hidden heart of rural Australia. Kensington, New South Wales, Australia: University of New South Wales Press.

Aptheker, B. (1989). *Tapestries of life: Women's work, women's consciousness and the meaning of daily experience.* Amherst, MA: University of Massachusetts Press.

Atkinson, R. (1998). *The life story interview.* Thousand Oaks, CA: Sage Publications.

Ballinger, M., Talbot, L., & Verrinder, G. (2009). More than a place to do woodwork: A case study of a community-based Men's Shed. *Journal of Men's Health, 6*(1), 20-27. doi:10.1016/j.jomh.2008.09.006

Bandura, A. (1986). The explanatory and predictive scope of self-efficacy theory. *Journal of Social and Clinical Psychology, 4*(3), 359-373.

Bateson, M. (1990). *Composing a life.* Middlesex, England: Penguin Books.

Bronfenbrenner, U. (1979). *The ecology of human development. Experiments by nature and design.* London, England: Harvard University Press.

Bruner, J. (1986). *Actual minds, possible worlds.* Cambridge, MA: Harvard University Press.

Cannon, W. (1939). *The wisdom of the body.* London, England: Routledge & Kegan Paul.

Christiansen, C. (1999). Defining lives: Occupation as identity: An essay on competence, coherence, and the creation of meaning. *American Journal of Occupational Therapy, 53*(6), 547-558. doi:10.5014/ajot.53.6.547

Christiansen, C. (2000). Identity, personal projects and happiness: Self construction in everyday action. *Journal of Occupational Science, 7*(3), 98-107. doi:10.1080/14427591.2000.9686472

Clark, F., Carlson, M., & Polkinghorne, D. (1997). The legitimacy of life history and narrative approaches in the study of occupation. *American Journal of Occupational Therapy, 51*(4), 313-317. doi:10.5014/ajot.51.4.313

Coleman, J., Butcher, J., & Carson, R. (1980). *Abnormal psychology and modern life* (6th ed.). Glenview, IL: Scott, Foresman & Co.

Connell, R. (2002). *Gender.* Malden, MA: Polity/Blackwell.

Csikszentmihalyi, M. (1990). *Flow: The psychology of optimal experience.* New York, NY: Harper & Row.

Curthoys, A. (1988). *For and against feminism.* Sydney, Australia: Allen & Unwin.

de Beauvoir, S. (1988). *The second sex* (H. Parshley, Trans.). London England: Picador.

DePoy, E., & Gitlin, L. (1998). Philosophical foundations. In *Introduction to research: Understanding and applying multiple strategies* (2nd ed., pp. 25-37). St. Louis, MO: Mosby.

Dickie, V. (2003). Data analysis in qualitative research: A plea for sharing the magic and effort. *American Journal of Occupational Therapy, 5,* 49-56. doi:10.5014/ajot.57.1.49

Erikson, E. (1965). *Childhood and society.* Harmondsworth, England: Penguin.

Fay, B. (1987). *Critical social science: Liberation and its limits.* Cambridge, England: Polity Press.

Fazio, L. (2001). *Developing occupation-centered programs for the community.* Upper Saddle River, NJ: Prentice-Hall.

Fidler, G., & Fidler, J. (1978). Doing and becoming: Purposeful action and self actualisation. *American Journal of Occupational Therapy, 32,* 305-310.

Frank, G. (1996). Life histories in occupational therapy clinical practice. *American Journal of Occupational Therapy, 50*(4), 251-264. doi:10.5014/ajot.50.4.251

Freeman, M. (1997). Why narrative? Hermeneutic, historical understanding and the significance of stories. *Journal of Narrative and Life History, 7*(1-4), 169-176.

Friedan, B. (1963). *The feminine mystique.* London, England: Victor Gollancz.

Gadamer, H. (1975). *Truth and method* (G. Barden & J. Cumming, Trans.). New York, NY: Seabury Press.

Gardner, H. (1983). *Frames of mind. The theory of multiple intelligences.* New York, NY: Basic Books.

Gardner, H. (1993). *Frames of mind. The theory of multiple intelligences* (10th ed). New York, NY: Basic Books.

Germov, J. (1998). *Second opinion: An introduction to health sociology.* Melbourne, Australia: Oxford University Press.

Grbich, C. (1999). Qualitative research design. In V. Minichiello, G. Sullivan, K. Greenwood, & R. Axford (Eds.), *Handbook for research methods in health sciences* (pp. 124-145). Sydney, Australia: Addison Wesley Longman.

Hasselkus, B. (1997). In the eye of the beholder: The researcher in qualitative research. *Occupational Therapy Journal of Research, 17*(2), 81-83.

Heidegger, M. (1962). *Being and time* (J. Macquarrie & E. Robinson. Trans.). London, England: SCM Press.

Holloway, I. (1997). *Basic concepts for qualitative research.* Oxford, United Kingdom: Blackwell Science.

Lake, M. (1999). *Getting equal—The history of Australian feminism.* St. Leonards, Australia: Allen & Unwin.

Law, M., Baum, C., & Baptiste, S. (2002). *Occupation-based practice. Fostering performance and participation.* Thorofare, NJ: SLACK Incorporated.

LeVine, R., & White, M. (1986). *Human conditions.* New York, NY: Routledge & Kegan Paul.

Maslow, A. (1954). *Motivation and personality* (1st ed.). New York, NY: Harper.

Maslow, A. (1968). *Toward a psychology of being* (2nd ed.). New York, NY: D. Van Nostrand.

McDowell, L., & Pringle, R. (1992). *Defining women: Social institutions and gender divisions.* Cambridge, England: Polity Press.

Meyer, A. (1922). The philosophy of occupation therapy. *Archives of Occupational Therapy, 1,* 1-10. (Reprinted from *American Journal of Occupational Therapy* [1997], *31*[10], 639-642.)

Mumford, L. (1967). *The myth of the machine.* London, England: Secker & Warburg.

Ornstein, R., & Sobel, D. (1988). *The healing brain: A radical new approach to health care.* London, England: Macmillan.

Palmer, P. (2000). *Let your life speak: Listening for the voice of vocation.* San Francisco, CA: Jossey-Bass.

Pavlov, I. (1927). *Conditioned reflexes: An investigation of the physiological activity of the cerebral cortex* (G. Anrep. Trans.). London, England: Oxford University Press.

Perls, F., Hefferline, R., & Goodman, P. (1951). *Gestalt therapy: Excitement and growth in the human personality.* New York, NY: Penguin Books.

Piaget, J. (1950). *The psychology of intelligence* (M. Piercy & D. Berlyne, Trans.). London, England: Routledge & Paul.

Polkinghorne, D. (1988). *Narrative knowing and the human sciences.* Albany, NY: State University of New York Press.

Polkinghorne, D. (1995). Narrative configuration in qualitative analysis. *Qualitative Studies in Education, 8*(1), 5-23.

Pollard, N., Sakellariou, D., & Kronenberg, F. (2009). *A political practice of occupational therapy.* London, England: Elsevier.

Primeau, L. (2000). Household work: When gender ideologies and practices interact. *Journal of Occupational Science, 7*(3), 118-127. doi:10.1080/14427591.2000.9686474

Ricoeur, P. (1985). *Time and narrative* (Vol. 2, K. McLaughlin & D. Pellauer, Trans.). Chicago, IL: Chicago University Press.

Rogers, C. (1961). *On becoming a person.* Boston, MA: Houghton Mifflin.

Scheffler, I. (1985). *Of human potential: An essay in the philosophy of education.* Boston, MA: Routledge & Kegan Paul.

Smith, D. (1990). *Texts, facts and femininity: Exploring the relations of ruling.* London, England: Routledge.

Townsend, E. (1997). Occupation: Potential for personal and social transformation. *Journal of Occupational Science, 4*(1), 18-26. doi:10.1080/14427591.1997.9686417

Townsend, E. (1998). *Good intentions overruled.* Toronto, Ontario, Canada: University of Toronto Press.

Townsend, E. (1999). Enabling occupation in the 21st century: Making good intentions a reality. *Australian Occupational Therapy Journal, 46,* 147-159. doi:10.1046/j.1440-1630.1999.00198.x

van Manen, M. (1997). *Researching lived experience: Human science for an action sensitive pedagogy* (2nd ed.). London, Ontario, Canada: Althouse Press.

White, R. (1971). The urge toward competence. *American Journal of Occupational Therapy, 25,* 271-274.

Whiteford, G., & Wicks, A. (2000). Occupation: Persona, environment, engagement and outcomes. An analytical review of the *Journal of Occupational Science* Profiles. Part 2. *Journal of Occupational Science, 7*(2), 48-57. doi:10.1080/14427591.2000.9686465

Wicks, A. (2004). Reflecting on the interpretive practice of a doctoral student conducting qualitative research. In G. Whiteford (Ed.), *Qualitative research as interpretive practice* (pp. 10-20). Bathurst, New South Wales, Australia: Centre for Research Into Professional Practice, Learning and Education.

Wicks, A. (2006). Older women's ways of doing: An occupational perspective of health. *Ageing International, 31*(4), 263-275.

Wicks, A., & Whiteford, G. (2005). Gender, occupation and participation. In G. Whiteford & V. Wright-St Clair (Eds.), *Occupation and practice in context* (pp. 197-212). Sydney, Australia: Churchill Livingstone.

Wicks, A., & Whiteford, G. (2006). Conceptual and practical issues in qualitative research: Reflections on a life history study. *Scandinavian Journal of Occupational Therapy, 13*(2), 94-100. doi: 10.1080/11038120600654676

Wilcock, A. (1993). A theory of the human need for occupation. *Journal of Occupational Science, 1,* 17-24. doi:10.1080/14427591.1993.9686375

Wilcock, A. (1998). *An occupational perspective of health.* Thorofare, NJ: SLACK Incorporated.

Wilcock, A., & Whiteford, G. (2003). Occupation, health promotion and the social environment. In L. Letts, P. Rigby, & D. Stewart (Eds.), *Using environments to enable occupational performance* (pp. 55-70). Thorofare, NJ: SLACK Incorporated.

World Federation of Occupational Therapists. (2006). *World Federation of Occupational Therapists position statement on human rights.* Retrieved from http://www.wfot.org/office_files/Human%20 Rights%20Position%20Statement%20Final%20NLH%281%29.pdf

World Health Organization. (2009). *Community based rehabilitation.* Retrieved from http://www.who.int/disabilities/cbr/en/

Yerxa, E. (1989). An introduction to occupational science. A foundation for occupational therapy in the 21st century. *Occupational Therapy in Health Care, 6*(4), 1-17. doi:10.1080/J003v06n04_04

Yerxa, E. (1991). Seeking a relevant, ethical and realistic way of knowing for occupational therapy. *American Journal of Occupational Therapy, 45*(3), 199-204. doi:10.5014/ajot.45.3.199

Yerxa, E. (1998). Health and the human spirit for occupation. *American Journal of Occupational Therapy, 52*(6), 412-418. doi:10.5014/ ajot.52.6.412

Yerxa, E. J., Clark, F., Frank, G., Jackson, J., Parham, D., Pierce, D., . . . Zemke, R. (1990). An introduction to occupational science, a foundation for occupational therapy in the 21st century. *Occupational Therapy in Health Care, 6,* 1-18. doi:10.1080/J003v06n04_04

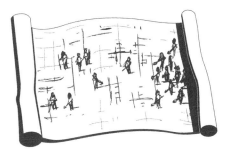

20

The Exploration of Quality of Life Through Q Methodology

Susan Corr, DipCOT, MPhil, PhD and Alexandra Palombi, BSc OT (hons), MSC OT

This chapter will illustrate how researching the concept of quality of life from an occupational perspective can generate predictive knowledge to support occupational therapy. Hocking (2000) suggested that it is valid to conduct research that demonstrates the influence of occupation on other phenomena such as health. This Q methodology study was undertaken to investigate the perceptions of healthy individuals over 50 years of age of their quality of life.

LITERATURE

Defining Quality of Life

There are many definitions of *quality of life* (Kind, 2003). Bowling and Normand (1998) considered it to be a broad concept, greater than just health status and one that takes social well-being into account. Bogousslavsky, Hommel, and Bassetti (1998) suggested that there are many different issues to take into account when considering what constitutes quality of life. These include orientation, physical independence, mobility, occupation of time, social integration, and economic self-sufficiency (Bogousslavsky et al., 1998). Traditionally, health-related quality of life has been described as feelings one had as a response to change in health (Guyatt et al., 1997) and not on aspects such as finances or the quality of the environment. The distinction between quality of life and health-related quality of life, however, is not clear. One aspect may influence the other, making it difficult to separate all of the contributing viewpoints to quality of life. Health-related quality of life is now considered the extent to which an individual person maintains physical, emotional, and intellectual function, as well as the ability to perform in valued activities within the workplace, family, and community (Naughton & Shumaker, 2003).

Quality of Life Dimensions

Cella and Nowinski (2002) described the dimensions of quality of life as including physical, functional, social, and emotional well-being but not external contributors, such as the environment and work influences. Harvey (1993) argued that quality of life is in fact closely connected with how an individual carries out his or her daily routine and the relationship between his or her environment, choices, and

Pierce, D. (Ed.).
Occupational Science for Occupational Therapy (pp. 233-245).
© 2014 SLACK Incorporated.

behavior. However, Brownson and Marjorie (2001) acknowledged that health and disability can affect how individuals carry out their daily routines, how they function in their environment, their choices, and their behaviors.

Felce (1997) suggested three key aspects to quality of life: objective life conditions, subjective feelings of well-being, and personal values and aspiration. Both he and Hammell (2004a) emphasized the importance of the subjective viewpoint when defining quality of life.

Choice, Control, and Quality of Life

The Canadian Association of Occupational Therapists (1997) also noted that quality of life relates to people having choice and control in their lives. Meaningful occupations may not only influence the quality and meaning of living but also survival itself (Hammell, 2004a).

Many researchers have identified the importance of control (the exercise of choice) to the experience of a life worth living with a serious illness or impairment (Abresch, Seyden, & Wineinger, 1998; Conneeley, 2003; Hammell, 2004b; Laliberte Rudman, Valiant, Cook, & Polatajko, 1997; Plahuta et al., 2002; Vrkljan & Miller Polgar, 2001). Yerxa et al. (1989, p. 5) stated that "to engage in occupations is to *take control*." Research has found that people whose lives have been disrupted by illness or injury such as AIDS and spinal cord injury often made conscious decisions to take control of their lives (Carpenter, 1994; Gloersen et al., 1993; Hammell, 1998; Reynolds, 2003; Vrkljan & Miller Polgar, 2001). A key manner in which they did this was through reengagement in occupations they found personally meaningful. It has been suggested that people gain a sense of control by choosing, shaping, and managing their daily occupations (Clark & Jackson, 1989; Hammell, 2004a). The strong emphasis placed on self-determination by people whose lives have been disrupted by illness or impairment, as well as their perceived need to be in control of their own lives, supports a client-centered approach to occupational therapy (Hammell, 2004a). Central to the experience of quality of life is the ability and opportunity to enact choices and assert control over one's occupations and one's aspirations.

Occupational Therapy Literature and Quality of Life

The occupational therapy literature defines many concepts that surround overall well-being and may be equated to quality of life. Laliberte Rudman et al. (1997) found in a qualitative study that physical, social, and mental activity is reported to contribute to the well-being and quality of life of older adults. The participants of the study described activities as essential to continue one's existence and to promote one's sense of well-being. Jackson, Carlson, Mandel, Zemke, and Clark (1998; also see Chapter 25) found in their

study of well elders that engaging in meaningful occupation was essential to well-being in older adults. Four contributing qualities of occupation were highlighted: (a) the need to control one's participation in the activity, (b) participation in new occupations, (c) changing the environment to increase accessibility to an occupation, and (d) maintaining a social connectedness through the occupation. These reflect some of the issues that have been also explored in a qualitative study of quality of life of elderly Chinese persons (Lau & McKenna, 2002). In particular, the "locus of control" (Lau & McKenna, 2002, p. 210) is reported to be an important issue that contributes to the quality of life of elderly Chinese persons. The importance of an individual having control may be attributed to its relationship with motivation.

Christiansen (1994) proposed that having control of one's situation or having free choice contributes to an individual's intrinsic needs and thus increases motivation. Although motivation as a concept is not the purpose of this chapter, it has strong links with occupation and contributes to the domains that make up quality of life (Christiansen, 1994; Felce, 1997). Motivation has also been seen to link directly with the value one may place on an activity that is meaningful to oneself. Naughton and Shumaker (2003) stressed the importance of understanding health-related quality of life as the value an individual places on activities, rather than on how well that person performs these activities.

Occupation and Quality of Life

Occupations enrich lives. Being able to do something that is meaningful enhances daily existence. But this is a very individualized experience. Rollerblading may bring excitement to an uneventful day for one person, whereas being able to sit and talk to a loved one may be pleasurable to another person. The phrase *quality of life* encompasses this concept. However, quality of life can mean different things to different people. For some, quality of life is being involved in outdoor sports, for others this phrase means reading to one's children, and to still others, quality of life may mean simply being alive and able to interact in some meaningful way with others. It is critical that the individual be able to define his or her significant occupations (Hinojosa, Kramer, Royeen, & Luebben, 2003).

Yuan (2001) highlighted the belief that quality of life appears to be directly related to a person's capability or "the ability or the potential to do or to be something" (p. 128). This is consistent with Wilcock's (1993) description of occupations as the mechanism by which individuals express their value and worth to society through achievement.

The Quality of Life Research Unit at the University of Toronto identified quality of life as the degree to which a person enjoys life's possibilities in three major domains: being, belonging, and becoming. The being domain is inclusive of personal identity and personal physical, psychological, and spiritual viewpoints. The belonging domain includes personal fit within the physical, social, and community environment. The becoming domain includes engagement in purposeful activities to meet personal needs and goals, including those of a practical, leisure, and growth nature.

Do Rozario (1992) identified five principal themes to illustrate peoples' perceptions and experiences related to coping viewpoints that facilitate health and well-being. These are the power of hope, the need for personal control, the contribution of positive external support, the need for meaningful activity and creative participation in life, and the healing effect of spiritual experiences.

Congruent with the self-focused and individualistic values of Western culture, occupational therapy theory has traditionally privileged goal-oriented, purposeful occupations that have economic and social benefits. However, the evidence base supporting the effectiveness of this approach is inconclusive at best. Research supports the importance of engagement in purposeful occupations when these are personally meaningful and valuable to the individual (Gloersen et al., 1993; Hammell, 2004b; Vrkljan & Miller Polgar, 2001). However, despite an alleged commitment to meaningful occupations, occupational therapists have only rarely explored the meaning of occupational engagement (Vrkljan & Miller Polgar, 2001) or whether engagement in purposeful occupations is sufficient to imbue life with meaning (Hammell, 2004b).

Rationale for This Research

The above research challenged our understanding of quality of life from an occupational perspective. An initial study was conducted to establish the perceptions of quality of life of individuals with neurological conditions (Corr & Palombi, 2009). The findings suggested three viewpoints of quality of life relating to independence, choice, and control; maintaining dignity, values, and aspirations; and actively contributing to society. Though it was thought that these findings helped occupational therapists understand this client group and their needs, it also raised the question as to what views individuals without a neurological condition held on quality of life.

METHODS

There is a consensus in the literature that quality of life is a complex human phenomenon that is difficult to measure and may not always be measured when using standardized quality of life questionnaires. It is therefore desirable to approach this concept with a form of research that can illuminate its subjective nature (Vestling, Ramel, & Iwarsson, 2005). According to Iso-Aloha (1980), the most important

aspect of quality of life is perceptions. It is the individual's own perceptions that underlie his or her personal definition of the quality of life.

Q methodology is an approach that draws on both qualitative and quantitative paradigms of research (Corr, 2006). British physicist-psychologist William Stephenson invented Q methodology in 1935 (Brown, 1996). Since then, Q methodology has received much attention in the sociology and political science literature (Brown, 1996). It was designed by Stephenson to provide a basis for a science of subjectivity. It is a method of measuring subjective views in a mathematical and rigorous fashion, thereby combining the strengths of qualitative and quantitative research (Brown, 1996). The value of Q methodology for identifying opinion clusters for a studied population (Cross, 2005; Valenta & Wigger, 1997; Watts & Stenner, 2012) suggested it as being appropriate for exploring perceptions of quality of life by healthy adults.

It was intended to explore the concept of quality of life in a qualitative way, in order to allow space for subjectivity and not influence the results and to provide the researchers with a clear reflection on the needs of the client group.

The first step in Q methodology is the development of a sort pack of statements relevant to the topic being studied (Corr, 2006). A list of statements, or statement pack, is generated from the literature using everyday language. Then, the participants sort these statements via a ranking process, or Q-sort, to express their point of view. After administration of the Q-sort, interpretation of the data uses statistical analysis to complete a viewpoint analysis (Corr, 2001). The findings are viewpoints that present the combined perspectives of the participants. Q methodology is a useful tool for occupational therapists to use for exploring attitudes to illness, health (Cross, 2005), and occupations (Corr, 2006).

Developing the Q-Sort

The Q-sort for this study was developed using current quality of life literature in order to ensure a broad spectrum of opinions (McKeown & Thomas, 1998). Key articles that defined, explored, and described issues, concepts, and dimensions of quality of life in older people or in persons with a neurological population were explored. Ninety-seven statements relating to quality of life were extrapolated from the key articles. These were then grouped into categories such as health, contributing to society, and self-realization.

In order to have equal representation in the statement pack of all categories and to maintain the spectrum of opinions (McKeown & Thomas, 1998), the 17 categories were merged into 7. These were health; independence, choice, control; emotional well-being; family, friends, and intimacy; finance and civic well-being; being productive; and beauty.

Categories with only one statement were considered equally important to the others and were represented in the statement pack. A thorough literature review is essential to

── TABLE 20-1 ──

EXAMPLES OF STATEMENTS

1. Quality of life means good physical and mental health.
2. Quality of life is being able to eat, wash, and dress independently.
3. Quality of life is being happy with oneself and having good self-esteem.
4. Quality of life is freedom to seek personal fulfillment and pursue one's desires.
5. Quality of life is actively contributing to society.
6. Quality of life is having your friends and family close to you.
7. Quality of life is when one has intimacy and is sexually active.
8. Quality of life is having financial security.
9. Quality of life is being physically pleasing.
10. Quality of life is feeling safe and feeling that I am not at risk (e.g., of falling or being mugged).

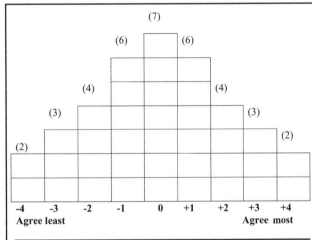

The numbers in brackets refer to the number of statements to be placed in each column.

Figure 20-1. Thirty-seven statement grid.

address content validity of the Q-sort (Valenta & Wigger, 1997). Face validity is addressed by leaving the statements in everyday readable language that is appropriate for the participants in the study (Valenta & Wigger, 1997).

Next, duplicate statements were eliminated. Statements that were similar were combined or eliminated. Statements that were ambiguous or difficult to understand were simplified. Although further minor changes were made, the statements were not further reduced in this phase beyond 41 statements in English. Corr, Phillips, and Capdevila (2003) found that, for participants who had had a stroke, sorting 47 statements became tiring and reduced concentration.

Because the participants in this study were individuals from a community center in Italy, the statements were then translated and checked for clarity by four Italian individuals. As a result, the statement pack was further reduced to 37 statements. Certain concepts were eliminated because they become redundant with translation. The statements were then back-translated into English to ensure that the translation was accurate. Table 20-1 contains examples of statements in the final pack.

Administering the Q-Sort

Once the final Q-sort was developed, a grid with the −4 to +4 spectrum was created (Figure 20-1). The grid enabled participants to place statements in the position they wanted along a least agree to most agree continuum.

Participants

A convenience sample was recruited from all individuals who participated in various activities in a community center in Italy. Individuals volunteering for the study gave their name to a secretary who set up an appointment. All individuals over the age of 50 years were included unless they had reading, cognitive, or speech problems that might have affected their understanding or execution of the Q-sort task.

All potential participants were given an information sheet and consent form to read by the secretary of the community center. Further verbal explanation was given as necessary. Participants could withdraw at any stage of the research. The study was approved by the School of Health Ethics Committee at the University of Northampton, United Kingdom.

A total of 22 participants were recruited for the study. Ten (45.5%) were male. Their ages ranged from 53 to 83 years old. The mean age was 68 years ($SD = 8.4$).

Seventeen (78%) of the participants were pensioners and 8 (22%) were still employed. All participants lived at home with their families and were independent in their daily activities as well as driving or using public transport to move around in the community.

Data Collection

The participants carried out the sorting process seated at a table in the community center. A large grid was drawn on a piece of cardboard and then cut out. The participants used this to sort out their statements, which were on individual cards. One statement was typed on each card. They were first asked to divide their cards into three piles—first pile "most agree" cards, second pile "least agree" cards, and third pile all the statements in between. This was in order to facilitate the sorting process of numerous statements on the grid. The "most agree" pile would be prioritized on the positive right end of the large grid. The "least agree" pile would be sorted out on the negative left end of the grid and the "middle pile" in the middle of the grid. Only one statement could be placed in one square of the grid. The participants could not place two statements in one square of the grid. They were urged to prioritize each statement. When completed, the participants were able to see all of their statements placed on the grid and had the opportunity to make any final changes.

Each sorting session lasted approximately 1 hour and the participants were invited to make further comments. Once completed, the researcher recorded all of the statement numbers and comments made by the participants on a smaller representation of the grid on a piece of paper.

Research Process Challenges

There were a number of challenges to overcome. First, the translation of the statements from English to Italian required carefully checking to ensure that there was no loss of meaning in translation. There was also a requirement to ensure that the statements were culturally relevant to an Italian population. The nationality mix of the research team and bilingual skills of some research team members ensured that this was not a problem.

A second challenge was locating a healthy population of the right age range who did not have a neurological condition. A community center was determined to be the best location because it was well attended by older people directly from the community, was easily accessible by the research team, and had sufficient space to undertake the data collection.

Explaining the purpose of the study to the participants was also a challenge. They were aware that the research team consisted of people in health care professions but it was necessary to conduct an initial interview with each participant to explain that the study was not about health services but about their perceptions of their quality of life. It was felt that these interviews ensured that the participants understood the research and their involvement in it to their satisfaction.

Statistical Analysis

The completed Q-sorts were analyzed using PQMethod, a data input computer package specific for Q-sort analysis. The viewpoint extraction method used was principal component analysis with varimax rotation (McKeown & Thomas, 1998) and automatic flagging. Statistical analysis typically follows three stages in Q methodology: correlation, viewpoint analysis, and computation of viewpoint scores (McKeown & Thomas, 1998).

In this study, the correlation between sorts identified which individual sorts (participants) correlated significantly with each other in their opinion of what quality of life means to them, using a standard error ($SE = 1/\sqrt{N}$) of 0.40. The correlation process identifies like groups of opinions, which are called *viewpoints* (Brown, 1996). Each viewpoint has an eigenvalue that indicates the significance of the viewpoint. This is calculated by squaring the viewpoint loadings (i.e., how much each sort, or participant, loads onto a viewpoint and therefore represents the proportion of variance; McKeown & Thomas, 1998). An eigenvalue needs to be greater than the numerical value of 1 for a viewpoint to be considered significant.

There are several techniques that can inform decision making in regard to how many viewpoints to retain (Bryant, Green, & Hewison, 2006). One recommendation is to select viewpoints with eigenvalues above the numerical value of 1. Mrtek, Tafesse, and Wigger (1996) recommend using the Q-sorts of individuals with a viewpoint loading of 0.6 or greater ($p < .001$). Eight viewpoints were identified with having a significant value (eigenvalue > 1). However, four of these were determined only by one or two Q-sorts or participant viewpoints. Therefore, it was decided that the four significant viewpoints or opinions with more than two Q-sorts or participant viewpoints would be extracted for this study. Each viewpoint or opinion is represented as a Q-sort grid (see Figure 20-1). This facilitates comparison between the four viewpoints (McKeown & Thomas, 1998).

RESULTS

Four viewpoints, or opinions on quality of life, were identified in the study. They were as follows:

- Viewpoint 1: Socially busy
- Viewpoint 2: Looking and feeling good
- Viewpoint 3: Accepting and feeling hopeful
- Viewpoint 4: Being independent

	-4	-3	-2	-1	0	+1	+2	+3	+4
(6)					35.Quality of life is feeling safe and feeling that I am not at risk (ex fall or being mugged)				
(4)				5.Quality of life is when one has a good appetite and is able to sleep well	22.Quality of life means having personal dignity	26.Quality of life is freedom to seek personal fulfilment and pursue one's desires			
				25.Quality of life is being able to work and earn money and feel productive	19.Quality of life is the degree which one has a positive appraisal and feelings about their lives as a whole	28.Quality of life is having your friends and family close to you			
(3)			37.Quality of life is being young	20.Quality of life depends on the mood ones in that day	18.Quality of life depends on one's values, hopes and aspirations	12.Quality of life is having control over one's life and being able to make ones own decisions.	21.Quality of life is having spiritual wellbeing		
(2)		2.Quality of life means the absence of pain	32.Quality of life is having a good home and neighbourhood.	9.Quality of life is being able to eat, wash and dress independently	17.Quality of life is when your expectations of a good life is fulfilled	11.Quality of life means to be able to rely on oneself and lead an active lifestyle	23.Quality of life is when one is able to accept themselves for who they are and accept their situation	29.Quality of life is being able to form relationships with other people	
	36.Quality of life is being physically pleasing	33. Quality of life is having material wellbeing	31.Quality of life is having financial security	8.Quality of Life is being able to move freely and exercise	16.Quality of life is to be able to habituate to changes in ones life (good and bad)	3.Quality of life means physical and psychological and emotional wellbeing	15.Quality of life is being able to cope with changes in one's life	24.Quality of life is being able to pass time meaningfully	34.Quality of life is having civic wellbeing
	4.Quality of life is not being disabled	30.Quality of life is when one has intimacy and is sexually active	6.Quality of life means living longer and feeling better	7.Quality of life is maintaining reasonable physical, emotional and intellectual functioning	14.Quality of life is having a sense of self worth and feel that life is worth living	1.Quality of life means good physical and mental health	10.Quality of life is not being a burden to family members	13.Quality of life is being happy with oneself and having a good self esteem	27.Quality of life is actively contributing to society

Figure 20-2. Viewpoint 1: Socially Busy.

Figure 20-2 presents Viewpoint 1 in full detail, showing all of the statements along the continuum of least agreed (–4) to most agree (+4). All four viewpoints were represented using this format, in order to facilitate analysis and interpretation of the viewpoints.

Viewpoint 1: Socially Busy

This viewpoint suggested that quality of life meant having good social relationships and being able to pass time meaningfully (see Figure 20-2). By positioning statement 34 in the +4 (most agree) position, it could be considered that having the right to vote, being safe in their community, and having social access were important to participants. This viewpoint had a strong social trend. Placing statement 13 and statement 24 in the +3 position gave it a personal value that one needed to accept one's self and pass personal time meaningfully. This suggested that being actively part of, and having an impact on, the community was vital, but having choice and freedom to pursue time as one wished was also essential for a good quality of life. Valuing material well-being and being sexually active did not relate to quality of life in this viewpoint. In addition, having pain and being disabled were not considered to have an impact on quality of life.

Viewpoint 2: Looking and Feeling Good

In this viewpoint, spiritual well-being and having personal dignity were considered important to quality of life (Table 20-2). There was strong agreement that quality of life depended on being independent and being physically pleasing. Being able to form relationships was also considered important. This suggested that the physical state was valued in order to be accepted socially and to maintain dignity. Similar to Viewpoint 1, this viewpoint suggests that material well-being and not being disabled did not contribute strongly to quality of life. This is contradictory to the value placed on being physically pleasing. In addition, spiritual well-being is not considered important as well as one's perception of one's health.

Viewpoint 3: Accepting and Feeling Hopeful

This viewpoint has a somewhat contradictory perspective in regard to the placement of certain statements (Table 20-3). Although good physical, mental, emotional, and psychological well-being was valued by the placement of statements 1 and 3, this viewpoint also valued the ability to accept one as is. The strong agreement of statement 8, however, emphasized the importance of being physically well. There was also a strong value placed on having expectations fulfilled and therefore demonstrating the importance of hope that all will go well. So, on one hand there was a hope that all will go well, and on the other hand it was recognized that if it did not, one needs to accept the situation. Similar to Viewpoints 1 and 2, material well-being and being young or physically pleasing were not considered important for quality of life.

TABLE 20-2

VIEWPOINT 2: LOOKING AND FEELING GOOD

MOST LIKE/ UNLIKE	NO.	STATEMENT
+4	7	Quality of life is maintaining reasonable physical, emotional, and intellectual functioning.
+4	9	Quality of life is being able to eat, wash, and dress independently.
+3	22	Quality of life means having personal dignity.
+3	29	Quality of life is being able to form relationships with other people.
+3	36	Quality of life is being physically pleasing.
-3	4	Quality of life is not being disabled.
-3	5	Quality of life is when one has a good appetite and is able to sleep well.
-3	21	Quality of life is having spiritual well-being.
-4	19	Quality of life is the degree to which one has a positive appraisal and feelings about one's life as a whole.
-4	33	Quality of life is having material well-being.

TABLE 20-3

VIEWPOINT 3: ACCEPTING AND FEELING HOPEFUL

MOST LIKE/ UNLIKE	NO.	STATEMENT
+4	1	Quality of life means good physical and mental health.
+4	23	Quality of life is when one is able to accept oneself for who one is and accept one's situation.
+3	3	Quality of life means physical and psychological and emotional well-being.
+3	8	Quality of life is being able to move freely and exercise.
+3	17	Quality of life is when your expectations of a good life are fulfilled.
-3	25	Quality of life is being able to work and earn money and feel productive.
-3	30	Quality of life is when one has intimacy and is sexually active.
-3	33	Quality of life is having material well-being.
-4	36	Quality of life is being physically pleasing.
-4	37	Quality of life is being young.

Viewpoint 4: Being Independent

Having no pain and being in control of one's activities of daily living were considered important in this viewpoint, as illustrated by the placement of statements 2 and 9 (Table 20-4). This suggested that having dominance over the physical world is important in order to have self-worth, which was valued in order to have a good quality of life (see placement of statement 14). Interestingly, no value was given to maintaining physical, mental, and psychological health. Being young and having intimacy was also not considered for a good quality of life in this viewpoint.

⌐ TABLE 20-4 ⌐

VIEWPOINT 4: BEING INDEPENDENT

MOST LIKE/ UNLIKE	NO.	STATEMENT
+4	1	Quality of life means good physical and mental health.
+4	4	Quality of life is not being disabled.
+3	2	Quality of life means the absence of pain.
+3	9	Quality of life is being able to eat, wash, and dress independently.
+3	14	Quality of life is having a sense of self-worth and feeling that life is worth living.
-3	3	Quality of life means physical and psychological and emotional well-being.
-3	5	Quality of life is when one has a good appetite and is able to sleep well.
-3	37	Quality of life is being young.
-4	30	Quality of life is when one has intimacy and is sexually active.
-4	7	Quality of life is maintaining reasonable physical, emotional, and intellectual functioning.

CONTRIBUTION TO OCCUPATIONAL SCIENCE

This study offers to occupational science an enhanced understanding of quality of life as it is expressed through occupation. As such, it supports the value of the science across disciplines concerned with the study of quality of life, as well as contributing to the development of a central concept for the young science.

The literature suggests that there are many different definitions of quality of life (Kind, 2003), and the findings of this study support that. The four viewpoints that emerge represent different viewpoints from the perspectives of the individuals studied. It is interesting to note that all four viewpoints have both concrete and abstract elements in the expression of what is necessary for a good quality of life. Although all statements in the Q-sort were given equal potential, each viewpoint that emerged was on two levels and consistent with the way we proposed defining quality of life.

These results suggest that certain abstract values are needed for a good quality of life. For example, there needs to be certain "doing" elements. In Viewpoint 1, forming relationships and passing time meaningfully lead to self-acceptance, which is necessary for a good quality of life. In Viewpoint 2, independence and being physically pleasing lead to maintaining dignity. In Viewpoint 3, being in good physical, mental, and psychological health helps fulfill one's aspirations and provides hope. In Viewpoint 4, independence and physical well-being lead to self-worth, which is important for a good quality of life.

The statements defining Viewpoint 1: Socially Busy suggest that this group values social access, contributing to society, and control beyond their personal sphere into their community. This viewpoint suggests that it is not enough to achieve basic capabilities and control daily routines. It is also important to maintain roles in society. Wilcock (1993) noted that, through doing, individuals can express their value and worth to society. This is consistent with Jackson et al.'s (1998) view that an important quality of an occupation is that it allows social connectedness. It also reflects that the element of control is an important issue for good quality of life, not just in daily routines but also in long-term commitments involving the wider community (Lau & McKenna, 2002). Reynolds (2003) considered the importance of a competent, able self involves both self-perception and the perceptions of others. Reciprocal relationships that encourage perceptions of value and competence, connecting, and belonging are also important (Hammell, 2004a; Laliberte Rudman et al., 1997; Reynolds, 2003).

Viewpoint 4: Being Independent implies that this group of participants value independence and being in control of their daily routines. This supports other literature that suggests that having choice and control over life is essential to quality of life. This is also consistent with Harvey's (1993) theory that quality of life is closely related to daily routine. This is supported by the occupational therapy literature. The need to control one's participation in occupation and to increase accessibility to an occupation is important for a good quality of life (Jackson et al., 1998). In addition, Christiansen (1994) suggested that having free choice contributes to meeting an individual's intrinsic needs.

Do Rozario (1992) acknowledged that personal control and meaningful activity are coping viewpoints that facilitate health and well-being. This is also consistent with the Canadian Association of Occupational Therapists (1997), who stated that freedom of choice and control over one's life are closely related to quality of life.

The concepts of Viewpoint 3: Accepting and Feeling Hopeful resonate with Felce's (1997) definition of quality of life. Viewpoint 3 implies that faith, respect, resilience, and hope are important. These reflect two of do Rozario's (1992) principles, the power of hope and the healing ability of spiritual experience. It recognizes that individuals aspire to new things. Believing in the potential to do or be something is consistent with Yuan's (2001) description of a good quality of life.

The issue of self-worth in Viewpoint 4: Being Independent reflects how people gain a sense of control when choosing, shaping, and carrying out their daily occupations (Clark & Jackson, 1989). Qualitative research among people with physical impairments has identified five dimensions of experiencing and expressing meaning through doing. These include the need/opportunity to keep busy, have something to wake up for, explore new opportunities, envision future time engaged in valued activities, and contribute to others (Hammell, 1998, 2004a). These themes were characterized by the participants' implied need for a sense of purpose and fulfillment. The ability to be able to execute daily occupations enabled individuals to increase their feelings of competence and fostered feelings of self-worth (Hammell, 2004a).

The four viewpoints emerging from this study illustrate how certain concepts that define quality of life are important to healthy Italian individuals. Qualitative research has shown that when people lose their ability to do those occupations that are important to them, this erases their perceptions of themselves as capable and competent, such that they describe feeling useless and valueless (Hammell, 1998; Reynolds, 2003). Conversely, researchers have observed a connection between engagement in personally valued occupations and perceptions of being competent, capable, and valuable (Hammell, 1998; Vrkljan & Miller Polgar, 2001). In the presence of an illness or disability there may be a shift in priorities and therefore further studies need to be carried out with people with different illnesses or disabilities to establish their perceptions. It cannot be assumed that everyone agrees that enabling choice, control, social connectedness, hope, and aspiration are important for a good quality of life and therefore further studies including establishing the viewpoints of service providers are necessary.

IMPLICATIONS FOR PRACTICE

Occupational therapy is defined as "the profession concerned with promoting health and well-being through occupation" (World Federation of Occupational Therapists, 2010, p. 1). Occupational therapists are equipped with a broad spectrum of skills that allow them to work with those who experience barriers to participation (World Federation of Occupational Therapists, 2010). Occupational therapy "enables people to do the day-to-day activities that are important to them despite impairments, activity limitations, or participation restrictions or despite risks for these problems" (Moyers, 1999, p. 252). The occupational therapist is therefore responsible for treating the individual who has an increase in dependency due to disease, in order to maximize his or her participation in daily activities.

The findings of this Q methodology study suggest that occupational therapists need to be able to determine which aspects of occupation, as well as which occupations, are valued by their clients, in order to implement an intervention that will enhance quality of life. It supports arguments by Hammell (2004a) that forms of practice that are preoccupied with self-care, productivity, and leisure activities may be inadequate to address clients' needs for meaning. Instead, occupational therapy is most relevant and useful when it addresses meaning, values, and purpose as these are experienced and expressed by clients through their chosen occupations. As Hammell stated, "Engagement in personally meaningful occupations contributes, not solely to perceptions of competence, capability and value, but also to the quality of life itself" (2004a, p. 303).

This Q methodology study can be a framework from which occupational therapists can work to determine specific occupational characteristics that are appropriate for every client. Establishing which viewpoint a client holds would assist the therapist to understand what concepts are important in order for that client to have a good quality of life. This could then provide guidance in the implementation of the intervention.

LEARNING SUPPORTS

Q Methodology

This simplifies the Q methodology process for beginners and uses the previous study as an example.

Introduction

- Developed in 1935 by British physicist-psychologist William Stephenson.

- Described as the science of subjectivity.

- Measures subjective views in a mathematical and rigorous fashion.

- Uses factor analysis (correlations)—individuals measure subjective opinions and those are then intercorrelated.

TABLE 20-5

LITERATURE SEARCHING SOURCES AND TERMS

LITERATURE SEARCH	SEARCH TERMS	BOOLEAN TERMS
• Ingentaconnect	• Quality of life	• Use "AND", "OR" to narrow search
• AMED	• Older people	
• CINAHL	• Elderly	
• Medline	• Neurological conditions	
• Ovid	• Definition or defining	
• Swetswise	• Perceptions	
• Medscape	• Measuring	
• Cochrane library		
• Journal Web sites (e.g., *American Journal of Occupational Therapy*)		

- A combination of quantitative and qualitative measures of research.

- This allows the researcher to explore everyday common language, concepts, and attitudes that are difficult to measure.

- Allows for analysis of one statement in relation to other statements and not only the level of agreement as found in other forms of research.

- The pack of statements is generated from the literature and then the participants will use these statements to perform the Q-sort.

Process of Q Methodology Using "Quality of Life" Example

1. Literature search process used for development of qualify of life statement pack. Can also conduct focus groups to develop statements (Table 20-5).

2. Development of statements for Q-sort (Table 20-6).

3. Examples of statements from quality of life study:
   - 2—"Quality of life means the absence of pain."
   - 10—"A good quality of life means able to wash, dress, and eat independently."
   - 14—"A good quality of life is having a sense of self-worth."
   - 28—"A good quality of life is having your friends and family close to you."

4. Data analysis: Can be done using free software from the World Wide Web called PQMethod (http://schmolck.userweb.mwn.de/qmethod/downpqwin.htm)

- PQMethod generates factors for discussion.

- Factors are common patterns that arise from the grids entered into the package.

- The factors with the strongest weighting are accepted (usually two to four).

- These will be represented as new grids.

- The data will then be analyzed qualitatively; that is, a consensus of perceptions of this population group are explored.

5. Viewpoints (emerged factors) are qualitatively interpreted and discussed (see Watts & Stenner, 2012).

Connecting Results of the "Quality of Life" Study of Healthy Older Adults With the Characteristics of Occupation

This illustrates how Q methodology results can be applied to and inform practice.

1. Search for literature related to occupational therapy.
   - According to Jackson et al. (1998), there are four qualities to engaging in occupation. These can be linked to quality of life and are as follows:
     - Choice: Control of participation
     - Opportunity: Participation in new occupations
     - Access: Environmental changes to increase one's accessibility to occupations
     - Contact: Social connectedness through occupations

TABLE 20-6

STEPS FOR DEVELOPING Q-SORT PACK

STEPS	QUALITY OF LIFE STUDY STEPS
1. Identify key literature, conduct focus groups	1. 12 key articles located
2. Generate potential statements	2. 97 statements generated
3. Identify themes and categories	3. Themes and categories identified
4. Eliminate duplicates and ambiguities (final pack usually 40 to 80 statements)	4. Duplicates and ambiguities eliminated
5. Pilot statements	5. Translated and piloted
6. Provide each statement with a unique number	6. Final 37 statements numbered
7. Create grid with two statements, then three statements in outer extremes	7. Grid created (see Figure 20-1)

TABLE 20-7

QUALITY OF LIFE STUDY FINDINGS MAPPED

VIEWPOINTS (FACTORS)		OCCUPATION CHARACTERISTICS
Viewpoint 1	• Contribute to society	Social access
	• Having social relationships	Contact
	• Pass time meaningfully	
	• Satisfied with oneself	
Viewpoint 2	• Being independent and physically well	Contact
	• Physical intimacy and physically pleasing	
	• Maintaining dignity	
Viewpoint 3	• Physical and mental well-being	Opportunity
	• Accept different situations	Choice
	• Choice	
	• Make decisions and realize one's expectations	
Viewpoint 4	• Physical well-being	Contact
	• Absence of pain	
	• Independence	
	• Being useful	

2. Link to results of study: Table 20-7 illustrates how the findings of the quality of life study have been mapped against Jackson et al.'s (1998) characteristics of occupation.

3. Reflection: Once a therapist understands what is valuable to his or her client, he or she can cater his or her intervention to that individual. Once a Q methodology study has been made and the various opinions have

emerged, the therapist can develop a questionnaire using the significant statements to understand where a person lies and which viewpoint represents him or her. If the therapist knows that his or her client is represented by Viewpoint (Factor) 1, he or she can choose occupations that give that person social access and contact. There are other occupational characteristics not described here (e.g., having a successful outcome). However, this characteristic for individuals represented by Viewpoint 1 is important because they need to be satisfied with themselves, so the therapist needs to take this into consideration. It is not just the case of choosing an activity that may interest the client but also that has a characteristic that satisfies his or her needs that renders it an occupation. Eating is an activity of daily living that can be completed as such or it can be done in a social context, which adds the characteristics of social contact. If the client then cooks for guests, it adds the characteristic of social contribution.

The better the therapist knows his or her client group, the better he or she can organize his or her service to satisfy needs. Knowing the occupational characteristics can help overcome possible resource difficulties if the therapist does not have a variety of occupations to offer his or her client when looking at individual interests. It is important that the occupation chosen for the client has the characteristics necessary to have an impact on the well-being of the client and on his or her quality of life.

REFERENCES

Abresch, R. T., Seyden, N., & Wineinger, M. (1998). Quality of life. Issues for persons with neuromuscular diseases. *Physical Medicine and Rehabilitation Clinics of North America, 9,* 233-248.

Bogousslavsky, J., Hommel, M., & Bassetti, C. (1998). Stroke. In M. Swash (Ed.), *Outcomes in neurological and neurosurgical disorders* (pp. 61-93). Cambridge, England: Cambridge University Press.

Bowling, A., & Normand, C. (1998). Definition and measurement of outcome. In M. Swash (Ed.), *Outcomes in neurological and neurosurgical disorders* (pp. 14-34). Cambridge, England: Cambridge University Press.

Brown, S. (1996). Q methodology and qualitative research. *Qualitative Health Research, 6*(4), 561-567. doi:10.1177/104973239600600408

Brownson, C. A., & Marjorie, E. S. (2001). Occupational therapy in the promotion of health and the prevention of disease and disability statement. *American Journal of Occupational Therapy, 55,* 656-660. doi:10.5014/ajot.55.6.656

Bryant, L., Green, J., & Hewison, J. (2006). Understandings of Down's syndrome: A Q methodological investigation. *Social Science & Medicine, 63,* 1188-1200. doi:10.1016/j.socscimed.2006.03.004

Canadian Association of Occupational Therapists. (1997). *Enabling occupation. An occupational therapy perspective.* Ottawa, Ontario, Canada: Author.

Carpenter, C. (1994). The experience of spinal cord injury: The individual's perspective—Implications for rehabilitation practice. *Physical Therapy, 74,* 614-629.

Cella, D., & Nowinski, C. J. (2002). Measuring quality of life in chronic illness: The functional assessment of chronic illness therapy measurement system. *Archives of Physical Medicine and Rehabilitation, 83*(12, Suppl.), s10-s17. doi:10.1053/apmr.2002.36959

Christiansen, C. (1994). Classification and study in occupation a review and discussion of taxonomies. *Journal of Occupational Science: Australia, 1*(3), 3-21. doi:10.1080/14427591.1994.9686382

Clark, F. A., & Jackson, J. (1989). The application of the occupational science negative heuristic in the treatment of persons with human immunodeficiency infection. *Occupational Therapy in Health Care, 6,* 69-91.

Conneeley, A. L. (2003). Quality of life and traumatic brain injury: A one-year longitudinal qualitative study. *British Journal of Occupational Therapy, 66*(10), 440-446.

Corr, S. (2001). An introduction to Q methodology, a research technique. *British Journal of Occupational Therapy, 64*(6), 293-297.

Corr, S. (2006). Exploring perceptions about services using Q methodology. In G. Kielhofner (Ed.), *Research in occupational therapy: Methods of inquiry for enhancing practice* (pp. 389-400). Philadelphia, PA: F.A. Davis.

Corr, S., & Palombi, A. (2009, October). *Establishing the perceptions of quality of life of individuals with neurological conditions using Q-methodology.* Paper presented at the Society of the Study of Occupation Annual Meeting, New Haven, CT.

Corr, S., Phillips, C., & Capdevila, R. (2003). Using Q methodology to evaluate a day service for younger adult stroke survivors. *Operant Subjectivity, 27*(1), 1-23.

Cross, R. (2005). Exploring attitudes: The case for Q methodology. *Health Education Research, 20*(2), 206-213.

do Rozario, L. (1992). Subjective well-being and health promotion factors: Views from people with disabilities and chronic illness. *Health Promotion Journal of Australia, 2*(1), 28-33.

Felce, D. (1997). Defining and applying the concept of quality of life. *Journal of Intellectual Disability Research, 41,* 126-135. doi:10.1111/j.1365-2788.1997.tb00689.x

Gloersen, B., Kendall, J., Gray, P., McConnell, S., Turner, J., & Lewkowicz, J. (1993). The phenomena of doing well in people with AIDS. *Western Journal of Nursing Research, 15,* 44-58. doi:10.1177/019394599301500104

Guyatt, G. H., Naylor, D., Juniper, E., Heyland, D. K., Jaeschke, R., & Cook, D. J. (1997). How to use articles about health-related quality of life measurements. *Journal of the American Medical Association, 277,* 1232-1237. doi:10.1001/jama.1997.03540390062037

Hammell, K. W. (1998). Client centred occupational therapy: Collaborative planning, accountable intervention. In M. Law (Ed.), *Client centred occupational therapy* (pp. 123-144). Thorofare, NJ: SLACK Incorporated.

Hammell, K. W. (2004a). Dimensions of meaning in the occupations of daily life. *Canadian Journal of Occupational Therapy, 71*(5), 296-305.

Hammell, K. W. (2004b). Using qualitative evidence to inform theories of occupation. In K. W. Hammell & C. Carpenter (Eds), *Qualitative research in evidence based rehabilitation* (pp. 14-26). Edinburgh, Scotland: Churchill Livingstone.

Harvey, A. (1993). Quality of life and the use of time theory and management. *Journal of Occupational Science, 1*(2), 27-30. doi:10.1080/14427591.1993.9686381

Hinojosa, J., Kramer, P., Royeen, C. B., & Luebben, A. J. (2003). Core concept of occupation. In P. Kramer, J. Hinojosa, & C. Royeen (Eds.), *Perspectives in human occupation: Participation in life* (pp. 1-17). Philadelphia, PA: Lippincott Williams & Wilkins.

Hocking, C. (2000). Occupational science: A stock take of accumulated insights. *Journal of Occupational Science, 7*(2), 58-67. doi:10.1080/14427591.2000.9686466

Iso-Ahola, S. (1980). *The social psychology of leisure and recreation.* Dubuque, IA: W.C. Brown.

Jackson, J., Carlson, M., Mandel, D., Zemke, R., & Clark, F. (1998). Occupation in lifestyle redesign: The Well Elderly Study Occupational Therapy Program. *American Journal of Occupational Therapy, 52*(3). doi:10.5014/ajot.52.5.326

Kind, P. (2003). Using standardised measures of health-related quality of life: Critical issues for users and developers. *Quality of Life Research, 12*, 519-521.

Laliberte Rudman, D. L., Valiant Cook, J., & Polatajko, H. (1997). Understanding the potential of occupation: A qualitative exploration of seniors' perspectives on activity. *American Journal of Occupational Therapy, 51*(8), 640-650. doi:10.5014/ajot.51.8.640

Lau, A., & McKenna, K. (2002). Perception of quality of life by Chinese elderly persons with stroke. *Disability and Rehabilitation, 24*, 203-218. doi:10.1080/09638280110072922

McKeown, B., & Thomas, D. (1998). *Q methodology (Quantitative applications in the social sciences).* London, England: Sage Publications.

Moyers, A. (1999). The guide to occupational therapy practice [Special issue]. *American Journal of Occupational Therapy, 53*(3), 251-255. doi:10.5014/ajot.53.3.247

Mrtek, R., Tafesse, E., & Wigger, U. (1996). Q-methodology and subjective research. *Journal of Social and Administrative Pharmacy, 13*(2), 54-64.

Naughton, M. J., & Shumaker, S., A. (2003). The case for domains of function in quality of life assessment. *Quality of Life Research, 12*, 73-80.

Plahuta, J. M., McCulloch, B. J., Kasarshis, E. J., Ross, M.A., Walter, R. A., & McDonald, E. R. (2002). Amyotrophic lateral sclerosis and hopelessness: Psychosocial factors. *Social Science and Medicine, 55*, 2131-2140. doi:10.1016/S0277-9536(01)00356-2

Quality of Life Research Unit, University of Toronto. (n.d.). Retrieved from http://www.utoronto.ca/qol/qol_model.htm

Reynolds, F. (2003). Exploring the meanings of artistic occupation for women living with chronic illness: A comparison of template and interpretive phenomenological approaches to analysis. *British Journal of Occupational Therapy, 66*(12), 551-557.

Valenta, A. L., & Wigger, U. (1997). Q-methodology: Definition and application in health care informatics. *Journal of the American Medical Informatics Association, 4*, 501-510.

Vestling, M., Ramel, E., & Iwarsson, S. (2005). Quality of life after stroke: Well-being, life satisfaction, and subjective aspects of work. *Scandinavian Journal of Occupational Therapy, 12*, 89-95.

Vrkljan, B., & Miller Polgar, J. (2001). Meaning of occupational engagement in life-threatening illness: A qualitative pilot project. *Canadian Journal of Occupational Therapy, 68*, 237-346.

Watts, S., & Stenner, P. (2012). *Doing Q methodological research: Theory, method and interpretation.* London, England; Sage Publications.

Wilcock, A. (1993). A theory of the human need for occupation. *Journal of Occupational Science, 1*(2), 17-24. doi:10.1080/14427591.1993.9686375

World Federation of Occupational Therapy. (2010). Statement on occupational therapy. Retrieved from http://www.wfot.org.au/

Yerxa, E. J., Clark, F., Frank, G., Jackson, J., Parham, D., Pierce, D., & Zemke, R. (1989). Occupational science: The foundations for new models of practice. *Occupational Therapy in Health Care, 6*, 1-17.

Yuan, L. (2001). Quality of life case studies for university teaching in sustainable development. *International Journal of Sustainability in Higher Education, 2*, 127-138. doi:10.1108/14676370110388345

IV

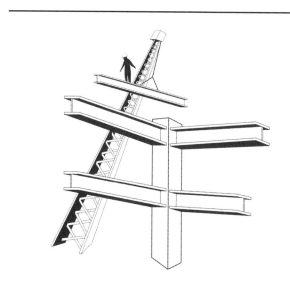

Level 4 Research

*How Does Occupational Science
Enhance Occupational Therapy Through
Research on Occupation in Practice?*

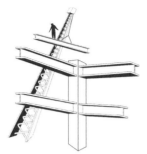

Occupation in Practice

Doris Pierce, PhD, OTR/L, FAOTA

PRESCRIPTIVE RESEARCH: THE LEVEL HISTORICALLY FAMILIAR TO OCCUPATIONAL THERAPY

Research on how occupation is implemented in practice has always been the research type of greatest interest to occupational therapy. The profession has developed with little descriptive, relational, or predictive knowledge regarding occupation. Knowledge needs at lower levels have been met only by borrowed knowledge and therapist intuition, which has provided a rather rickety foundation for practice. For many years, the best approaches in the field have been interdisciplinary systems models, cobbled together from various extradisciplinary theories that did not include research on occupation. Because the profession has continued to develop despite these deficiencies, it has not been obvious how much stronger and more effective occupational therapy could be if it did have a knowledge base that was more responsive to the needs of practitioners. Elizabeth Yerxa (1995) argued that

autonomous and valued professions must bring to the table a knowledge base that is not provided by any other profession. It was her vision that launched occupational science, in order to create that unique professional knowledge base for occupational therapy.

PRECURSORS TO OCCUPATIONAL SCIENCE RESEARCH AT LEVEL 4

Because occupational therapy has always been interested in research on the use of occupation in practice, occupational therapy and occupational science have their closest research match at Level 4. Two key lines of occupational therapy research especially set the stage for the emergence of occupational science.

Occupational Behavior Research

Occupational science emerged from a particular approach to occupational therapy: occupational behavior.

Pierce, D. (Ed.).
Occupational Science for Occupational Therapy (pp. 249-253).
© 2014 SLACK Incorporated.

Combining interdisciplinary theories of the 1960s with the field's interests in occupation, Mary Reilly and her students at the University of Southern California studied and researched occupation in practice at a holistic level and across the lifespan. The theory of occupational behavior was best expressed in Dr. Reilly's (1974) book, *Play as Exploratory Learning*, which described the progression from childhood play to adult competence in work. Mary Reilly was a voracious scholar of the theories and meta-theories of her time, keeping her graduate students researching within these frameworks. Her interest in systems theory, complexity, and a Kuhnian (1962) perspective on science can be seen in the work of her students on the model of human occupation (Kielhofner, Burke, & Igi, 1980). Her interest in the developmental unfolding of occupation was expressed in the work of her students on the occupation of play (Florey, 1971, 1981; Knox, 1974; Robinson, 1977; Takata, 1974).

Under the influence of Reilly and her students, it was nearly impossible to discuss occupational therapy theory during the 1980s without reference to paradigm shifts, systems models, or developmental progressions in occupation. The occupational behavior treatment approach used whole occupations as they were viewed and valued by the persons enacting them, with the goal of advancing the occupational development of that person. Mary Reilly's ultimate impact was to insist that the profession recognize and respond to the therapeutic potential of a holistic use of the core concept of occupation, rather than only addressing the components of occupation (Reilly, 1961). By doing so, she paved the way for occupational science.

Purposeful Activity Research

In this historical period, the profession was deeply engaged with the important question of the relative effectiveness of a holistic, occupation-based approach versus a more biomedical, component-focused approach. Of course, at that time, it was not referred to in that way. Rather, the question concerned the relative effectiveness of "rote" versus "purposeful" activity (American Occupational Therapy Association, 1983). That is, the profession was embroiled in a heartfelt ideological struggle over the role of occupation itself in occupational therapy services. Biomedical approaches that produced their therapeutic effects through changes to muscles and joints as a result of repetitive motions appealed to occupational therapists. They fit well within medical culture, had a sound theoretical base in anatomy and kinesiology, and required expert technical knowledge from the therapist. The occupational approach, on the other hand, had an underdeveloped knowledge base that was not easily supplemented from other disciplines, required occupational therapists to explain their unique approach across disciplinary boundaries within medical settings, and seemed less scientific.

Looking back from the vantage point of an established science of occupation, the importance of this early research into the relative effectiveness of rote versus purposeful activity is clear. Beginning in the 1980s, a series of researchers set out to examine this question by comparing therapeutic outcomes between groups who did the same movements with and without a perceived purpose (Chisholm, Dohli, & Schreiber, 2004). Of course, the "purpose" clients experienced in these studies was not defined with the theoretical and methodological depth and rigor of today's Level 4 occupational science research. Instead, purpose was the difference between jumping with or without a rope (Bloch, Smith, & Nelson, 1989; Kircher, 1984), pedaling or pedaling to operate a drill press (Steinbeck, 1986), simple shoulder movement versus wall stenciling (Mullins, Nelson, & Smith, 1987), pretending to kick something versus kicking a balloon (DeKuiper, Nelson, & White, 1993), pinch and grip movements versus using a computer game (King, 1993), and shoulder flexion versus playing basketball (Zimmerer-Branum & Nelson, 1995).

This line of research, which clearly demonstrated the greater effectiveness of purposeful activity in comparison to rote activity, was ongoing for many years. The most frequent researcher in this area was David Nelson, working in research partnerships with a series of master's students. Eventually, the research began to change from the early "added purpose" studies to studies of real engagements in valued activity in comparison to doing rote activity. This controversy over purposeful versus rote activity generated a research effort that provided the earliest evidence in regard to occupation-based practice. It was within this atmosphere of questioning and calling for research on occupation in practice that occupational science was born. Occupational science still retains strong research commitments to the effectiveness of occupation-based practice.

THE DEVELOPMENT OF OCCUPATIONAL SCIENCE RESEARCH ON PRACTICE

Expanding Occupational Science to Level 4 Prescriptive Research

Initially, occupational science was envisioned as a Level 1, descriptive science (Clark et al., 1991). The thinking was, if we provided research that described occupation well, therapists would use that understanding to inform and strengthen their practices. And in part this is still true. It did not take long, however, for occupational scientists to realize that they needed not just to describe occupation in people's lives but also to examine occupation as it was used in practice and to assist in translating descriptive occupational science into occupation-based practice (Pierce, 2001). So, soon after the initiation of the science, occupational scientists, who are almost all occupational therapists, began to do Level 4, prescriptive research on occupation in practice.

Compared to occupational science at its start 25 years ago, Level 4, prescriptive occupational science has increased dramatically, especially in the United States. The movement of the science into studies of occupation within interventions was led by Florence Clark (1993) in her Slagle Lecture on narrative in intervention as well as in collaboration with other researchers of the Well Elderly Study (Clark et al., 1997; see Chapter 25). In 1998, the profession responded to the emergence of occupational science with a special issue of the *American Journal of Occupational Therapy* on occupation-based practice, guest edited by Wendy Wood (1998) and including key articles on occupation-centered assessment (Coster, 1998) and occupation as the ends and means of practice (Gray, 1998).

Clinical Reasoning and Outcomes Research

At this fourth level of research, occupational science has been especially productive in two areas: therapists' reasoning and therapy outcomes. Occupational science studies of how therapists reason about occupation in practice translate smoothly into supports to practice (Burke, 2001; Estes & Pierce, 2012; Jackson, 1998; Price, 2008; Price & Miner, 2007, 2009; Price & Stephenson, 2009; Ward, Mitchell, & Price, 2007). Chapters 23 and 24 are exemplars of research into therapist reasoning concerning occupation-based practice. Examples of innovative occupation-based practice include the Los Angeles Street Kids Program, a gang prevention initiative by occupational therapists (Snyder, Clark, Masunaka-Noriega, & Young, 1998), and Hoppes and Segal's (2010) use of occupation in accommodating the death of a family member. Braveman and Page's (2012) blending in their new book, *Work,* of a theoretical focus on the occupation of work with a review of work interventions, is an interesting demonstration of the profession's present gradual migration toward a more holistic, occupation-based approach to practice.

It is a classic statement that occupational therapy uses occupation as both the ends and the means of practice (Gray, 1998). Occupational therapy's recent "outcomes panic" (Lieberman & Scheer, 2002, p. 345) has especially accelerated research to produce evidence of the effectiveness of occupation in practice in response to tightening health care budgets. Some of the most well-known research on the outcomes of occupation-based practice is the research of the Lifestyle Redesign Group at the University of Southern California, which is described in detail in Chapter 25.

Recently, Law and McColl (2010) provided a comprehensive review of studies of the effectiveness of occupational therapy with adults and older adults. They described interventions as they are focused on the person (training, skills development, or education), the occupation (task adaptation, occupational development), or the environment (modification, supports, information). Intervention outcomes are examined for participation, self-care, work, leisure, environmental change, cognitive-neurological function, and physical, sociocultural, and psychosocial determinants of occupation. This focused review of occupational therapy outcomes research for one age group offers general insights into how occupation is considered in such studies: the degree to which occupation is reduced to a protocol or depersonalized and the degree to which evidence of effectiveness is or is not measured as changed occupational capacities of individuals. It is interesting to consider how, over 30 years, occupational therapy's research interest in the comparative effectiveness of rote versus purposeful activities has evolved into a rich diversity of sophisticated studies that are, at heart, still exploring the usefulness of occupational therapy's core concept, occupation.

QUESTIONS FOR OCCUPATIONAL SCIENCE AT LEVEL 4

Within occupational science, Level 4 research emerged last but not least. Prescriptive occupational science is the type of research most familiar to, and most valued by, the profession. Many important Level 4 prescriptive research questions call for attention in occupational science. The potential for occupational science to strengthen and coevolve with occupational therapy has no limit at the predictive level.

How Does Occupation Operate in Practice?

We are only beginning to understand occupation-based practice, the reasoning that drives it, its key factors and effectiveness, and its differential use across ages, populations, and settings. A further consideration might be what activities are most used as interventions and how this varies with setting and population. Such a survey of practice would be highly useful to therapists. Bringing an occupational science perspective to these questions can only benefit occupational therapy.

How Does the Use of Occupation Differ Across Practice Settings?

How does practice in settings natural to the client, as opposed to more artificial clinical settings, impact the effectiveness of applications of occupation? Where are our best examples of programs that use the natural contexts of occupation to provide highly effective services within industry, schools, homes, and communities? How can we study and learn from their successes?

How Do We Impact Occupational Injustice?

Occupational science has made great progress in describing injustice in relation to occupation. Now, at Level 4, our challenge is to study and develop approaches to address, reduce, and ameliorate occupational injustices. It is highly likely that this research will highlight the need for occupational science to begin policy work as a population-level approach to occupational injustice.

Section Chapters Illustrating Level 4, Prescriptive Occupational Science Research

This section of *Occupational Science for Occupational Therapy* features some of occupational science's most exciting Level 4 work. Together, these chapters provide a summary view of the potential of research into occupation in practice. The emergence of disciplinary instruments to measure change in the occupations of persons receiving occupational therapy is illustrated in Catana Brown and Melisa Rempfer's chapter on the Test of Grocery Shopping Skills, an elegant assessment that uses the performance of an everyday occupation to examine occupational capabilities of persons within the natural context of a familiar neighborhood grocery (Chapter 22). Pollie Price, the leading theorist on occupation in practice, provides a chapter describing the specific occupation-based strategies therapists use during intervention (Chapter 23). Joanne Estes and I offer a study of how therapists negotiate between children's worlds and medical culture in their experience of providing pediatric occupation-based practice (Chapter 24). Members of the Lifestyle Redesign Team of the University of Southern California—Florence Clark, Jeanne Jackson, and Elizabeth Pyatak—describe their perspectives on the sequential development of occupation-based approaches that have been examined at the level of randomized clinical trials (Chapter 25). Michele Berro and Lisa Deshaies, two occupational therapists from Rancho Los Amigos National Rehabilitation Center, describe how the entire occupational therapy department of this leading service setting revised its approach to practice to be more occupation based (Chapter 26). Donna Colaianni and Ingrid Provident provide insights into what is often considered to be the most challenging practice within which to use an occupation-based approach: hand therapy (Chapter 27). The Youth

Research Group at Eastern Kentucky University, which includes Elaine Fehringer, Amy Marshall, Karen Summers, and myself, describes our ongoing efforts to develop occupational therapy services to adolescents (Chapter 28). Together, this grouping of chapters will revolutionize your understanding of what it means to use occupation as the key therapeutic approach of the profession of occupational therapy, your appreciation of its power, and the bright future that lies ahead of the profession as it comes into a more fully developed and effective occupational science knowledge base.

References

American Occupational Therapy Association. (1983). Purposeful activities. *American Journal of Occupational Therapy, 37*, 805-806. doi:10.5014/ajot.37.12.805

Bloch, M., Smith, D., & Nelson, D. (1989). Heart rate, activity, duration and affect in added-purpose versus single-purpose jumping activities. *American Journal of Occupational Therapy, 43*, 25-30. doi:10.5014/ajot.43.1.25

Braveman, B., & Page, J. (2012). *Work: Promoting participation and productivity through occupational therapy.* Philadelphia, PA: F.A. Davis.

Burke, J. P. (2001). How therapists' conceptual perspectives influence early intervention evaluations. *Scandinavian Journal of Occupational Therapy, 8*, 49-61. doi:10.1080/11038120121303

Chisholm, D., Dohli, C., & Schrieber, J. (2004). *Occupational therapy intervention resource manual: A guide for occupation-based practice.* Clifton Park, NY: Thomson Delmar Learning.

Clark, F. A. (1993). Occupation embedded in a real life: Interweaving occupational science and occupational therapy. *American Journal of Occupational Therapy, 47*, 1067-1078. doi:10.5014/ajot.47.12.1067

Clark, F. A., Azen, S. P., Zemke, R., Jackson, J., Carlson, M., Hay, J., . . . Lipson, L. (1997). Occupational therapy for independent-living older adults: A randomized controlled trial. *Journal of the American Medical Association, 278*(16), 1321-1326. doi:10.1001/jama.1997.03550160041036

Clark, F. A., Parham, D., Carlson, M. E., Frank, G., Jackson, J., Pierce, D., . . ., Zemke, R. (1991). Occupational science: Academic innovation in the service of occupational therapy's future. *American Journal of Occupational Therapy, 45*, 300-310. doi:10.5014/ajot.45.4.300

Coster, W. (1998). Occupation-centered assessment of children. *American Journal of Occupational Therapy, 52*(5), 337-344. doi:10.5014/ajot.52.5.337

DeKuiper, W., Nelson, D., & White, B. (1993). Materials-based occupation versus imagery-based occupation versus rote exercise: A replication and extension. *Occupational Therapy Journal of Research, 13*, 183-197.

Estes, J., & Pierce, D. (2012). Pediatric therapists' perceptions of occupation-based practice. *Scandinavian Journal of Occupational Therapy, 19*, 17-25. doi:10.3109/11038128.2010.547598

Florey, L. (1971). An approach to play and play development. *American Journal of Occupational Therapy, 25*, 275-280.

Florey, L. (1981). Studies of play: Implications for growth, development, and for clinical practice. *American Journal of Occupational Therapy, 35*, 519-524. doi:10.5014/ajot.35.8.519

Gray, J. M. (1998). Putting occupation into practice: Occupation as ends, occupation as means. *American Journal of Occupational Therapy, 52*(5), 354-364. doi:10.5014/ajot.52.5.354

Hoppes, S., & Segal, R. (2010). Reconstructing meaning through occupation after the death of a family member: Accommodation, assimilation, and continuing bonds. *American Journal of Occupational Therapy, 64,* 133-141. doi:10.5014/ajot.64.1.133

Jackson, J. (1998). The value of occupation as the core of treatment: Sandy's experience. *American Journal of Occupational Therapy, 52*(6), 466-473. doi:10.5014/ajot.52.6.466

Kielhofner, G., Burke, J. P., & Igi, C. H. (1980). A model of human occupation, part IV. Assessment and intervention. *American Journal of Occupational Therapy, 32*(12), 777-788.

King, T. (1993). Hand strengthening with a computer for purposeful activity. *American Journal of Occupational Therapy, 47,* 635-637. doi:10.5014/ajot.47.7.635

Kircher, M. (1984). Motivation as a factor of perceived exertion in purposeful versus non-purposeful activity. *American Journal of Occupational Therapy, 38,* 165-170. doi:10.5014/ajot.38.3.165

Knox, S. (1974). A play scale. In M. Reilly (Ed.), *Play as exploratory learning* (pp. 247-266). Beverly Hills, CA: Sage Publications.

Kuhn, T. (1962). *The structure of scientific revolutions.* Chicago, IL: University of Chicago Press.

Law, M., & McColl, M. (2010). *Interventions, effects, and outcomes in occupational therapy: Adults and older adults.* Thorofare, NJ: SLACK Incorporated.

Lieberman, D., & Scheer, J. (2002). AOTA's evidence-based literature review project: An overview. *American Journal of Occupational Therapy, 56,* 344-349. doi:10.5014/ajot.56.3.344

Mullins, C., Nelson, D., & Smith, D. (1987). Exercise through dual-purpose activity in the institutionalized elderly. *Physical and Occupational Therapy in Geriatrics, 5,* 29-39. doi:10.1300/J148v05n03_04

Pierce, D. (2001). Occupation by design: Dimensions, creativity, and therapeutic power. *American Journal of Occupational Therapy, 55,* 249-259.

Price, P. (2008). Therapeutic relationship. In E. B. Crepeau, E. Cohn, & B. B. Schell (Eds.), *Willard and Spackman's occupational therapy* (11th ed., pp. 328-342). Philadelphia, PA: Lippincott Williams & Wilkins.

Price, P., & Miner, S. (2007). Occupation emerges in the process of therapy. *American Journal of Occupational Therapy, 61,* 441-450. doi:10.5014/ajot.61.4.441

Price, P., & Miner, S. (2009). Mother becoming: Learning to read Mikala's signs. *Scandinavian Journal of Occupational Therapy, 16*(2), 68-77. doi:10.1080/11038120802409739

Price, P., & Stephenson, S. M. (2009). Learning to promote occupational development through co-occupation. *Journal of Occupational Science, 16*(3), 180-186. doi:10.1080/14427591.2009.9686660

Reilly, M. (1961). The Eleanor Clarke Slagle Lecture. Occupational therapy can be one of the great ideas of 20th century medicine. *American Journal of Occupational Therapy, 16,* 1-9.

Reilly, M. (1974). *Play as exploratory learning.* Beverly Hills, CA: Sage Publications.

Robinson, A. (1977). Play, the arena for acquisition of rules of competent behavior. *American Journal of Occupational Therapy, 31,* 248-253.

Snyder, C., Clark, F., Masunaka-Noriega, M., & Young, B. (1998). Los Angeles street kids: New occupations for life program. *Journal of Occupational Science, 5*(3), 133-139. doi:10.1080/14427591.1998.9686441

Steinbeck, T. M. (1986). Purposeful activity and performance. *American Journal of Occupational Therapy, 40,* 529-534. doi:10.5014/ajot.40.8.529

Takata, N. (1974). Play as prescription. In M. Reilly (Ed.), *Play as exploratory learning* (pp. 209-246). Beverly Hills, CA: Sage Publications.

Ward, K., Mitchell, J., & Price, P. (2007). Occupation-based practice and its relationship to social and occupational participation in adults with spinal cord injury. *OTJR: Occupation, Participation & Health, 27*(4), 149-156.

Wood, W. (1998). Nationally speaking: Is it jump time for occupational therapy. *American Journal of Occupational Therapy, 52*(6), 403-411. doi:10.5014/ajot.52.6.403

Yerxa, E. (1995). Nationally speaking: Who is the keeper of occupational therapy's practice and knowledge? *American Journal of Occupational Therapy, 49,* 295-299. doi:10.5014/ajot.49.4.295

Zimmerer-Branum, S., & Nelson, D. (1995). Occupationally embedded exercise versus rote exercise: A choice between occupational forms in elderly nursing home residents. *American Journal of Occupational Therapy, 49,* 397-402. doi:10.5014/ajot.49.5.397

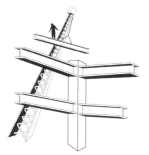

The Test of Grocery Shopping Skills
Assessing Occupation in a Natural Environment

Catana Brown, PhD, OTR/L, FAOTA and Melisa Rempfer, PhD

Grocery shopping is a common occupation, yet its familiarity belies its complexity. Like many of the activities that make up our everyday lives, most people could not tell you how they acquired the ability to grocery shop. In all likelihood it was not a formal process but one that came about through observation, practice, and trial-and-error learning. With some reflection, however, it becomes obvious that the process of grocery shopping is highly complex. The size of the physical space; the sheer number of products, people, and aisles to negotiate; and the marketing strategies used to influence decisions come together to create a challenging situation. There is individual variability in where individuals shop, why, and who they are shopping for, as well as the actual process of looking and choosing items, yet most people figure out strategies for creating a grocery shopping experience that works for them. Without these strategies, grocery shopping would be too overwhelming for most people to manage. For example, upon entering a new store, how do you know where to find a head of lettuce? How do you go about choosing the brand, flavor, and size of yogurt you want? How do you minimize the necessity to return to an aisle of the store you have already perused? These are just a few of the questions that were considered when the

developers of the Test of Grocery Shopping Skills (TOGSS; Brown, Rempfer, & Hamera, 2009) became interested in creating a measure to assess this complicated occupation.

This chapter reviews the TOGSS by (a) introducing issues related to the assessment of occupational performance, (b) discussing the process and evidence related to developing the TOGSS and investigating its reliability and validity, (c) identifying the contribution of the TOGSS to occupation science, and (d) presenting clinical implications of the TOGSS. The TOGSS was initially developed to assess the occupation of grocery shopping in people with serious mental illness. Therefore, much of the information in this chapter will be presented in relation to the literature and evidence associated with serious mental illness.

Background on Measuring Occupations in People With Serious Mental Illness

In the last decade, there has been a great deal of interest in the functional outcomes associated with serious mental illness (e.g., Heinrichs, Ammari, Miles, & McDermind Vaz, 2010; McKibbin, Brekke, Sires, Jeste, & Patterson, 2004). The multidisciplinary literature typically utilizes the term

Pierce, D. (Ed.).
Occupational Science for Occupational Therapy (pp. 255-263).
© 2014 SLACK Incorporated.

function or *functional outcomes* to describe what occupational therapists refer to as *occupation* or *occupational performance*. There are differences in the constructs, but for the purposes of this chapter grocery shopping can be considered both a function and an occupation. This section of the chapter will utilize both terms depending on the context and the literature on which the discussion is based.

Advancements in drug treatments have brought improved management of psychiatric symptoms; however, it is clear that residual difficulties in cognitive and psychosocial functioning impact occupational performance for many individuals with serious mental illness. With this emerging recognition of occupation as a key outcome variable, there is increased scrutiny of existing measures of community functioning and independent activities of daily living (Dickerson, Ringel, & Parente, 1997; McKibbin et al., 2004; Miles, Heinrichs, & Ammari, 2011; Wallace, 1986). Researchers and clinicians are exploring various methods of assessing occupational performance. Recent authors have examined the available assessment strategies associated with functional outcomes and have divided them into the following: self- or informant reports, simulated performance measures, and real-world performance measures (e.g., McKibbin et al., 2004; Patterson, Goldman, McKibbin, Hughs, & Jeste, 2001). Briefly, the status of these approaches to assessment of people with serious mental illness will be examined.

Self- and informant report (asking people whether they perform a particular occupation and sometimes asking about the quality of the performance) is a common method for measuring functioning in a variety of domains. Self-report is widely used to assess quality of life and social functioning because it is an efficient method to obtain the desired information (e.g., Becker, Diamond, & Sainfort, 1993; Lehman, Possidente, & Hawker, 1986; Lehman, Postrado, & Rachuba, 1993). However, self-report measures can be unreliable due to problems with insight and cognitive impairment (Dickerson et al., 1997; McKibbin et al., 2004; Patterson, Goldman, et al., 2001) and consequently their validity has been questioned (Atkinson, Zibin, & Chuang, 1997; Rohland & Langbehn, 1997). Other measures of functioning are designed to be completed by informants such as case managers, clinicians, or family members and some also have self-report versions (Birchwood, Smith, Cochrane, Wetton, & Copestake 1990; Glazer, Aaronson, Prusoff, & Williams, 1980; O'Malia, McFarland, Barker, & Barron, 2002; Schooler, Hogarty, & Weissman, 1979; Wallace, Liberman, Tauber, & Wallace, 2000). Ratings by informants are limited by the amount of knowledge the rater has about the individual and the demands created by the physical and social environment where the person lives. For example, a case manager may be fairly involved with an individual in relation to his or her money management but have little opportunity to observe or learn about that individual's ability to socialize with others, prepare a meal, or utilize public transportation. Furthermore, Brekke (1992); Rogers, Holm, Goldstein, McCue, and Nussbaum (1994); and Dickerson, Parente, and Ringel (2000) have found only modest convergent validity between different functional measures. This means that when self- and informant ratings are collected together, they tend to reveal different results, suggesting that the ratings are not interchangeable. It is generally unknown whether self-report or informant report is more accurate.

The limitations of self- and informant ratings have led to interest in more objective measures that directly assess occupational performance in simulated as well as "real-world" settings (McKibbin et al., 2004; Patterson, Goldman, et al., 2001; Rempfer, Hamera, Brown, & Cromwell, 2003). Measures of direct assessment range from basic activities of daily living, which may be more applicable to an inpatient population or people with serious physical disabilities (Thompson, 1992), to assessment of independent living skills (Patterson, Moscona, McKibbin, Davidson, & Jeste, 2001) in individuals living in the community. Despite the advantages of these performance-based measures, currently there are few measures available for people with serious mental illness. McKibbin and colleagues (2004) identified only eight measures of direct assessment of functional abilities that have been used with people who have schizophrenia. Further, a major methodological limitation of these simulated or role-play assessments is the question of whether the simulation reflects real-world performance. One recent study in persons with schizophrenia (Heinrichs et al., 2010) found that in terms of predicting real-world functioning, a simulated performance measure (the UCSD Performance Based Skill Assessment; Patterson, Goldman, et al., 2001) did not provide any additional information over traditional measures of cognition.

In summary, the review indicates that there are several prominent limitations in the existing functional assessment literature. Due to ease of administration, there tends to be an overreliance on self-report and informant ratings and little direct observation of behavior using performance-based assessments. Even among direct measures of functioning, most are simulated and/or role-play measures that are conducted in clinical or research settings. These simulated assessments are incapable of capturing the authenticity and complexity of real-world environments. This may be particularly important when it comes to assessing those occupations that (a) require a great deal of interaction with the environment and (b) take place in an environment that is multifaceted and therefore difficult to recreate. For example, it would be extremely challenging to simulate the environment necessary to assess the occupation of using public transportation. Asking an individual to read a bus schedule or identify stops does not incorporate all of the negotiations necessary for getting on the correct bus and getting off at the desired location. On the other hand, it is fairly easy to simulate the complete process of finding a phone number and placing a phone call. Grocery shopping is more like using public transportation than it is like placing a phone call. Grocery shopping requires multiple interactions with a large environment full of a wide variety of things to sort through and people that may or may not require some sort of dealings. When it came to developing a measure of grocery shopping, it was important to consider the relevance of the environment. Consequently, the TOGSS was designed to provide an ecologically focused approach to measuring occupational performance in the real world.

Overview of the Test of Grocery Shopping Skills

This chapter explores the development and application of a performance assessment, the TOGSS (Brown et al., 2009), which focuses on the person's ability to carry out the occupation of grocery shopping. The TOGSS was initially developed as a performance assessment for individuals with serious mental illness but is relevant for other conditions in which cognition interferes with occupational performance. Grocery shopping was targeted as a relevant area of assessment for people with serious mental illness because (a) it is important for successful community living, (b) it requires a variety of cognitive abilities that tend to be compromised in people with serious mental illness (e.g., attention, memory, executive function), and (c) the activity is made more challenging due to the complexity of the physical environment (other performance-based assessments for people with serious mental illness have tended to focus on the social environment). The cognitive requirements of grocery shopping (e.g., selectively attending to the relevant cues in the environment, remembering what is on your list including what you have already located and what still needs to be found, and making choices based on preferences and price, among many options) entails highly complex thinking. Consequently, when assessing grocery shopping, the occupational therapist can determine the individual's ability to carry out this occupation and simultaneously through observation make clinical inferences about the cognitive abilities that are affecting performance.

The TOGSS administration involves shopping for 10 grocery items from a list in an actual grocery store. Three separate subscales include accuracy, time, and redundancy. Accuracy includes the ability to select the correct item, at the correct size, and at the lowest price. Total accuracy scores can range from 0 to 30. Time indicates the elapsed time from when the individual enters the store until he or she enters the checkout line, and redundancy is the number of times the individual enters an aisle/section of the store. Time and redundancy may be considered together as measures of grocery shopping efficiency. There are two forms (or grocery lists) for the TOGSS so that the measure can be used as a pre-/post-test without concern that the individual will learn the list and location of items from the first administration.

When selecting the grocery store for test administration, it is important to determine the purpose of the assessment. In clinical situations, it may make the most sense to select a store that is familiar to the participant, so that the occupational therapist can better assess performance in that individual's real-life shopping setting. For research purposes, the TOGSS is typically administered in an unfamiliar store so that all participants start out with an equal level of knowledge about the context in which the assessment takes place. Once the store is selected, the therapist must develop a store map to use for the scoring of the redundancy subscale, which involves marking the spot each time the individual enters a new aisle or section. Specific instructions are provided in the TOGSS manual for scoring redundancy, time, and accuracy (Brown et al., 2009). The occupational therapist scoring the TOGSS follows the participant while shopping in order to score the measure as well as to make clinical observations. The occupational therapist does not provide cues or answer questions that might provide additional information; however, the individual who is doing the shopping may ask others in the store for help.

STUDIES OF THE TEST OF GROCERY SHOPPING SKILLS

The first study of the TOGSS was published more than a decade ago (Hamera & Brown, 2000), and the work on the measure started a few years before the publication. Today we are still conducting studies with the TOGSS. Clearly, this is a lengthy process and really there is no end to the investigation that can be done. This section of the chapter will describe a series of studies focusing on (a) instrument development, (b) instrument validation, and (c) use of the TOGSS as a clinical measure.

Instrument Development Studies

The first step was creating the measure. It was essential to us that the initial process of instrument development focused on creating a measure that was relevant to people with serious mental illness and authentic in terms of replicating the process of grocery shopping in an actual store (Hamera & Brown, 2000). First, 10 individuals with schizophrenia were interviewed about grocery shopping to identify where they typically shop, how they get to the grocery store, what foods they choose, and what issues they consider when making those food choices. In addition, one of the researchers (CB) accompanied three individuals with schizophrenia while they conducted their regular grocery shopping. During this observation period, the researcher asked questions about what the person was thinking when making a selection and what he or she found difficult about the experience. We then took this information to determine the aspects of grocery shopping that made it most challenging for individuals with serious mental illness. As a result, the TOGSS focuses on measuring the finding of desired items in the store and choosing the lowest price for the desired item. In addition, the TOGSS includes measures of efficiency because many individuals found the grocery store overwhelming and difficult to navigate.

An initial aim of TOGSS development was to create two comparable shopping lists so that different lists could be used at pre- and post-test. This was important because if the same list was used, learning might occur during the pretest. This turned out to be an arduous process. Initially a list of 27 grocery products was generating using the following criteria: (a) items commonly used by persons with serious mental illness, (b) items offering a number of choices (in terms of flavors, ingredients, sizes, etc.) to make finding a specific item fairly difficult, and (c) variety in the items such that they would be distributed throughout the different sections of the store.

Twenty individuals with schizophrenia participated in a study in which they located all 27 items in an unfamiliar grocery store (Hamera & Brown, 2000). An item analysis was conducted on the list to find items we wanted to keep and comparable items that could be paired across the two lists. The final lists were created by (a) selecting items with a difficulty index between 20% and 65%, (b) finding equivalent pairs of items in terms of item difficulty, and (c) dividing 10 pairs of items into Form 1 and Form 2 so that each list had items distributed throughout the store.

Subsequently, the two alternate forms of the TOGSS were compared in an initial reliability study (Hamera & Brown, 2000). Both forms were administered to 26 individuals with schizophrenia or schizoaffective disorder. The order in which the forms were administered was counterbalanced and the administration occurred on two separate days. In terms of reliability, this study simultaneously examined the equivalence of the two forms as well as test–retest reliability. Consequently, it would be expected that the reliability coefficient would be lower than if either aspect of reliability (equivalence or test/retest) was examined separately. The resulting correlations were statistically significant, ranging from 0.64 to 0.83. Interrater reliability was examined in the same study. Using highly trained research assistants, the interrater reliability for scoring the TOGSS was extremely high, with correlations of 0.99 for Form 1 and perfection correlations of 1.00 for Form 2. At this point we felt fairly comfortable with the comparability of the two forms, their test–retest reliability, and the interrater reliability. At this point we moved onto validity studies.

Instrument Validation Studies

Much of the validity work on the TOGSS was guided by the work of Samuel Messick (1995a). Instead of considering different aspects of validity such as content validity, criterion-related validity, and so on, Messick suggested that validity may be viewed as a unitary concept and all validity is construct validity. This approach emphasizes that validation is an ongoing process—a test is never a perfectly valid test but your belief in a test's validity is based on the degree to which accumulated evidence supports the intended use of a particular test. In other words, does the test actually measure what it is purported to assess?

Some of the previously described test development research provides some of the most important validity information for the TOGSS. According to Messick (1995b), a major threat to test validity involves construct underrepresentation. For a test to be representative, great care must be taken in selecting items that best characterize the performance domain. Consequently, the process of developing the TOGSS as described previously was crucial for developing a measure that would accurately represent the construct of grocery shopping.

Another aspect of validity involves examining the ability of a measure to discriminate different individuals in an expected direction. To this end, we conducted a study that compared TOGSS performance in individuals with serious mental illness to individuals without mental illness (Hamera, Brown, Rempfer, & Davis, 2002). The study included a sample of 26 persons with schizophrenia, 19 persons with a nonschizophrenia psychiatric diagnosis, and 19 persons with no psychiatric diagnosis who were recruited from a local community agency and were matched in terms of socioeconomic status. Two groups were expected to perform similarly (the two groups with psychiatric diagnoses) but differently from those without psychiatric diagnoses. The results indicated that persons without a psychiatric diagnosis took less time and were more efficient in terms of not returning to aisles or going to unnecessary sections of the store as they completed the TOGSS than individuals with schizophrenia or other psychiatric diagnoses. There was no difference between the groups on accuracy of finding items, although this finding is difficult to interpret due to confounded age differences between groups. Further research comparing TOGSS performance across different samples is ongoing. Currently we are involved in a study examining TOGSS performance in individuals with traumatic brain injury.

Additional validity evidence for the TOGSS has come from studies that compare performance on the TOGSS to cognitive performance. It is well known that cognition in serious mental illness is related to occupational performance across multiple domains (social functioning, activities of daily living, etc.; Heinrichs et al., 2010). Thus, one important dimension of validity evidence for the TOGSS concerns its relationship with domains of cognition that are known to impact occupational performance in this population. In a study of 73 community-dwelling individuals with schizophrenia or schizoaffective disorder (Rempfer et al., 2003), participants completed the TOGSS as well as a cognitive evaluation that assessed verbal memory, processing speed, sustained attention, and executive functioning. Accuracy was related to processing speed, sustained attention, and verbal memory. Efficiency was also associated with verbal memory and was related to several measures of executive functioning. Providing additional support for the validity of the TOGSS, these results also provide evidence that the accuracy and efficiency subscales of the TOGSS require somewhat different cognitive abilities.

The study by Rempfer and colleagues (2003) suggested that the TOGSS may have particular relevance as a measure of the cognitive abilities known as *executive functioning*. As a follow up, Zayat, Rempfer, Gajewski, and Brown (2011) examined the validity of the TOGSS as a measure of executive function. In this study, 80 participants with schizophrenia or schizoaffective disorder completed the TOGSS and a battery of cognitive tests that assess the executive functions of planning, problem solving, task persistence, and working memory for individuals with schizophrenia. Canonical correlation was used to examine the relationship between the two variable sets (TOGSS variables and executive function variables). Once again this study supported the concept that accuracy and efficiency provide unique information. The canonical correlation revealed that one set of cognitive variables was associated more with accuracy and the other set was associated most with efficiency. More specifically, simple correlations and the canonical analyses identified a significant effect on shopping *accuracy* from the working memory variables and a significant effect on shopping *efficiency* from the problem-solving and planning variables. This is important information for occupational therapy practice. Most measures focus on accuracy—in other words, can a person perform a particular task? Though accuracy is important, efficiency should also be considered and for some people may be the aspect of performance that is most problematic.

Future publications that examine the TOGSS as a specific (as compared to a global) assessment with ecological validity that provides distinct measures of accuracy and efficiency are underway (Rempfer & Brown, 2012). This study examines the relationship of the TOGSS to self- and informant-reported measures of community functioning. Briefly, this work suggests that (a) the TOGSS is more similar to other specific measures of grocery shopping than it is to more global measures of community functioning and (b) the accuracy subscale of the TOGSS (but not the efficiency subscale) is related to other measures of community functioning.

In summary, several validity studies were conducted that provide support for the TOGSS as a real-world measure of

a specific area of occupational performance. The TOGSS distinguishes performance among people with and without mental illness, it is associated with cognitive performance, and it provides distinct measures of accuracy and efficiency.

Studies of the Test of Grocery Shopping Skills as a Clinical Outcome Measure

There are specific features of the TOGSS that make it useful as a clinical outcome measure. First, it is among only a few published, validated measures that assess performance in the real world, an outcome of increasing importance in treatment and rehabilitative settings. Further, a unique feature of the TOGSS is the availability of two alternate forms of the shopping list, which allow for comparison of pre- and post-treatment performance. In initial work, the TOGSS was utilized as a clinical measure to assess skill improvements following a nine-session grocery shopping skills training program (Rempfer, Brown, & Hamera, 2011), as described next.

A primary aim of this study was to examine cognitive predictors of skill improvements following skills training. In particular, we examined the role of learning potential, which has been found in previous research to be a predictor of rehabilitation readiness (Fiszdon et al., 2006) and treatment outcome (Watzke, Brieger, Kuss, Schoettke, & Wiedl, 2008; Wiedl, 1999) in people with schizophrenia. In comparison to traditional, static cognitive assessment, learning potential is based on dynamic assessment and evaluates performance improvement following training. As a dynamic approach to understanding cognition, learning potential may be particularly relevant to more complex aspects of occupational performance (Rempfer et al., 2011), such as the real-world cognitive, social, and environmental demands associated with performance on the TOGSS. This study was intended to extend the existing learning potential and rehabilitation outcome literature by examining skill acquisition in terms of skill performance in a natural setting, as measured by the TOGSS.

Study participants included 25 persons between the ages of 18 and 25 who were diagnosed with serious mental illness. Psychiatric diagnoses were confirmed with the *Structured Clinical Interview for DSM-IV* (First, Spitzer, Gibbon, & Williams, 2002) and included bipolar disorder ($n = 8$), unipolar (major) depression ($n = 8$), and schizophrenia or schizoaffective disorder ($n = 9$).

Participants in this study participated in a nine-session grocery shopping skills training intervention in small groups. Each session included didactic instruction, as well as in vivo skill practice at local grocery stores. The training was modeled after existing social and independent living skills programs (e.g., Wallace, Liberman, MacKain, Blackwell, & Eckman, 1992) and focused on teaching the subskills necessary for effective grocery shopping (e.g., finding items within a store and choosing items based on desired features of size, flavor, price, etc.). Grocery shopping skill was assessed pre- and post-intervention with the TOGSS. The two equivalent TOGSS shopping lists were counterbalanced across participants for pre- and post-testing. The outcome variable of interest was TOGSS skill acquisition, as measured by the change in TOGSS accuracy scores from pre- to post-testing.

Participants also completed cognitive assessment with the Wisconsin Card Sorting Test (WCST; Kongs, Thompson, Iverson, & Heaton, 2000) to assess static performance and learning potential. Consistent with learning potential assessment, the WCST was administered in a test–train–test format to generate both static and learning potential indices (e.g., Wiedl, 1999). Briefly, the WCST requires participants to match a deck of cards to one of four key cards and evaluates problem solving and abstraction. In the present study, three consecutive administrations of the test were given. The first deck was administered in a traditional format and therefore yielded the static, or standard, measure of performance (Trial 1). The second deck (Trial 2) was administered with enhanced training and feedback (Wiedl, 1999); in other words, the participants were taught how to determine the category and match the cards. Finally, a third deck (Trial 3) was administered in a standard format post-training. This dynamic method of assessment is intended to go beyond the initial static measurement to determine whether the individual can benefit from training. Studies of dynamic assessment with the WCST and people with schizophrenia have consistently identified three groups:

1. High performers or individuals who do well initially and consistently throughout all three administrations

2. Learners or individuals who start out poorly but benefit from instruction

3. Nonlearners or individuals who start out poorly and do not improve their performance with instruction

The results of this study indicate that although this skills training intervention did not prove effective at improving overall group performance on the TOGSS, individual gains in TOGSS performance were predicted by the measure of learning potential. Learners as assessed by the WCST were able to derive more benefit from the grocery shopping intervention than were nonlearners. This study adds to the growing learning potential literature by examining outcome in terms of real-world skill performance on the TOGSS. As this study highlights, performance in dynamic, real-world environments places specific demands on functioning (Rempfer et al., 2003) and may be best captured by dynamic, rather than standard, approaches to assessment.

CONTRIBUTION TO OCCUPATIONAL SCIENCE

In her model of occupation by design, Pierce (2001) described three components of occupation that contribute to therapeutic power: appeal, accuracy, and intactness. *Appeal* is the desirability of the occupation, and *accuracy* is the consistency or match that the occupation has with the individual's therapeutic goals. However, it is the construct of *intactness* in which the TOGSS probably makes the greatest contribution to occupational science. Intactness is defined as "the degree to which a therapeutic occupation occurs in the usual spatial, temporal and sociocultural conditions in which it would usually occur for that client if it were not being used as an intervention" (Pierce, 2001, p. 254). However, instead of intervention, in this case the issue is related to the contextual relevance of the assessment process. Like with intervention, there is power associated with the naturalness of the environment in which assessment takes place.

There are several measures of occupation or instrumental activities of daily living (IADL) like grocery shopping that are performance based; however, the majority of these measures simulate the occupation in a clinical environment. For example, the Kohlman Evaluation of Living Skills ([KELS] Thompson, 1992) combines interview items with simulated performance. The KELS is practical to administer in a clinical setting, because it requires limited equipment and can be administered in 30 to 45 minutes. Seventeen living skills are addressed in the areas of self-care, safety and health, money management, transportation and telephone, and work and leisure. The measure was designed so that the results can be used by occupational therapists to make recommendations regarding the client's living situation.

However, Brown, Moore, Hemman, and Yunek (1996) found that simulated items on the KELS were not necessarily predictive of performance of the same tasks in the natural environment. In this study, two of the KELS tasks were administered: making a purchase in the store and using the bus. The participants were then asked to perform the same tasks in the natural environment. This involved purchasing a bar of soap in an actual store and taking the bus to a place the person had never been before. The results of the purchasing task were fairly consistent in both administrations, although 2 individuals who were independent on the KELS required assistance in the real store. On the other hand, 6 of the 16 participants identified as independent on the KELS were unsuccessful in utilizing public transportation independently. Although the KELS and similar measures provide useful information, the simulation of the setting and the occupation being measured may not be close enough to real life to provide a truly accurate measure of specific areas of occupational performance. On the other hand, and as described previously, the TOGSS was associated with the real-life occupation of grocery shopping when individuals were observed during an actual grocery shopping experience. The natural environment provides a level of authenticity that is difficult to replicate in simulated experiences.

IMPLICATIONS FOR PRACTICE

There are two primary purposes for using the TOGSS in practice: (a) assessing grocery shopping skills to develop an intervention plan and (b) evaluating the efficacy of an intervention targeting grocery shopping.

Using the Test of Grocery Shopping Skills in Intervention Planning

Most obviously, the TOGSS serves as a measure of grocery shopping ability, particularly for people with cognitive impairments that might interfere with occupational performance. The use of a specific assessment that was developed with information from individuals with serious mental illness lends itself to better construct representation. In other words, the TOGSS was developed with the intention of measuring those aspects of grocery shopping that best reflect real-world performance and that address the most significant areas of concern for the population. One of the unique features of the TOGSS is the inclusion of outcome measures of accuracy and efficiency. Few measures consider efficiency, yet in some cases this can be the aspect of performance that is most troublesome. Occupational therapists can use the TOGSS to determine an individual's abilities related to accurately and efficiently performing the occupation of grocery shopping.

Scoring of the measure provides just one piece of information for clinical reasoning. Because the therapist observes the individual during the performance of the TOGSS, the observational data provide additional information that can be particularly useful in determining the specifics about what is interfering with successful performance. As mentioned previously, TOGSS outcomes are associated with cognition, and there is support for the use of the TOGSS as a measure of executive function. When observing performance during the administration of the TOGSS, the therapist may identify underlying cognitive impairments that interfere with grocery shopping. For example, the occupational therapist may consider the following:

- Attention—Is the individual able to screen out distractions and selectively attend to relevant information such as naturally occurring cues (e.g., overhead signs, salient label information)?
- Working memory—Is the individual able to remember which items on the list have been located and which items he or she is still looking for?

- Planning—Does the individual appear to have a systematic method for finding the items or does he or she randomly wander the store to find the items on the list (this is often reflected by behaviors such as searching for each item in the order it appears on the list instead of where it is found in the store, returning to aisles that the person has already shopped, going down every aisle even when no item on the list is on that aisle)?
- Decision making—Observations regarding selecting the correct flavors, size, etc. Is the individual able to identify the relevant information needed to make a decision? Even with the necessary information the individual may be reluctant or slow to make decisions.
- Problem solving—Determining the lowest priced item among many choices requires identification and comparisons with like items; there is also problem solving involved in making educated guesses about where an item might be located.

There are other observable behaviors that can provide information regarding barriers to successful grocery shopping performance. Some individuals may have limited frustration tolerance or perseverance and give up before completing the task. Others may be reluctant to ask for help even when that would be the most efficient method of locating a difficult-to-find item. Once the occupational therapist identifies aspects of grocery shopping that are difficult and/or the barriers that are interfering with the performance, the occupational therapist can develop an intervention plan with those targets in mind.

Using the Test of Grocery Shopping Skills to Evaluate the Efficacy of an Intervention

The alternate forms of the TOGSS enhance its usefulness as an efficacy measure. In this context, the TOGSS can be used either to assess the progress of an individual who has received a grocery shopping intervention or it may be used as a program evaluation to determine the efficacy of a particular approach to grocery shopping training. As an outcome measure, the pre- and post-test scores can be compared to determine whether an improvement occurs and, if so, in what areas. The occupational therapist can then determine what aspects of the intervention are effective and where the intervention needs to be modified.

CONCLUSION

The appeal for occupation-based practice has focused on the intervention piece of the occupational therapy process. However, to increase the authenticity of practice, it is important for occupational therapists to have measures that assess particular occupations in their natural environments. The TOGSS may serve as one example upon which others might draw as the profession moves toward practices where occupation is a central value.

Learning Supports

Considering the Influence of Context

Select a grocery store item that you have never shopped for before and one that you are not sure where it would be located. First, locate that item in the grocery store where you typically shop. Then, look for that same item in a store that is unfamiliar to you. Consider the following questions:

1. What strategies did you use to find the item in each setting? How effective were your strategies? Were the strategies you used the same or different in each of the settings?

2. What cognitive processes were most challenged in each of the situations?

3. What aspects of the environment supported your performance? What aspects of the environment presented challenges to your performance?

Instrument Development

Identify a particular IADL and begin to think about how you would go about developing an ecologically valid performance measure of that particular occupation.

Complete the following:

1. What is the IADL of concern?

2. Who is the target population?

3. Who would you interview and/or observe to collect information about the scope, performance variables, and specific setting for this IADL? Specifically, how would you go about collecting this information?

4. How would you conceptualize accuracy for this IADL?

5. How would you conceptualize efficiency for this IADL?

6. Are there other aspects of performance you would be interested in measuring?

7. Possibly create a score sheet that illustrates your measurement of accuracy and efficiency.

8. Describe studies you would design to gather data related to the reliability of the measure.

9. Describe studies you would design to gather data related to the validity of the measure.

References

Atkinson, M., Zibin, S., & Chuang, H. (1997). Characterizing quality of life among patients with chronic mental illness: A critical examination of the self-report methodology. *American Journal of Psychiatry, 154*, 99-105.

Becker, M., Diamond, R., & Sainfort, F. (1993) A new patient focused index for measuring quality of life in persons with severe and persistent mental illness. *Quality of Life Research, 2*, 239-251.

Birchwood, M., Smith, J., Cochrane, R., Wetton, S., & Copestake, S. (1990). The Social Functioning Scale: The development and validation of a new scale of social adjustment for use in family intervention programs with schizophrenic patients. *British Journal of Psychiatry, 157*, 853-859. doi:10.1192/bjp.157.6.853

Brekke, J. S. (1992). An examination of the relationships among three outcome scales in schizophrenia. *Journal of Nervous & Mental Disease, 180*(3), 162-167. doi:10.1097/00005053-199203000-00003

Brown, C., Moore, W. P., Hemman, D., & Yunek, A. (1996). Influence of instrumental activities of daily living assessment method on judgments of independent. *American Journal of Occupational Therapy, 50*, 202-206. doi:10.5014/ajot.50.3.202

Brown, C., Rempfer, M., & Hamera, E. (2009). *Test of Grocery Shopping Skills manual*. Bethesda, MD: AOTA Press.

Dickerson, F. B., Parente, F., & Ringel, N. (2000). The relationship among three measures of social functioning in outpatients with schizophrenia. *Journal of Clinical Psychology, 56*(12), 1509-1519. doi:10.1002/1097-4679(200012)

Dickerson, F. B., Ringel, N. B., & Parente, F. (1997). Ratings of social functioning in outpatients with schizophrenia: Patient self-report versus caregiver assessment. *Evaluation and Program Planning, 20*, 415-420. doi:10.1016/S01497189(97)00020-7

First, M. B., Spitzer, R. L., Gibbon, M., & Williams, J. W. (2002). *Structured clinical interview for DSM-IV Axis I disorders (SCID I/P)* (Research ver., patient ed.). New York, NY: Biometrics Research, New York State Psychiatric Institute.

Fiszdon, J. M., McClough, J. F., Silverstein, S. M., Bell, M. D., Jaramillo, J. R., & Smith, T. E. (2006). Learning potential as a predictor of readiness for psychosocial rehabilitation in schizophrenia. *Psychiatry Research, 143*, 159-166. doi:10.1016/j.psychres.2005.09.012

Glazer, W. M., Aaronson, H. S., Prusoff, B. A., & Williams, D. H. (1980). Assessment of social adjustment in chronic ambulatory schizophrenics. *Journal of Nervous and Mental Disease, 168*, 493-497.

Hamera, E., & Brown C. (2000). Developing context-based performance measures: Grocery shopping skills in individuals with schizophrenia. *American Journal of Occupational Therapy, 54*, 20-25. doi:10.5014/ajot.54.1.20

Hamera, E., Brown, C., Rempfer, M., & Davis, N. C. (2002). Test of grocery shopping skills: Discrimination of people with and without mental illness. *Psychiatric Rehabilitation Skills, 6*, 296-311. doi:10.1080/10973430208408440

Heinrichs, R. W., Ammari, N., Miles, A. A., & McDermind Vaz, S. (2010). Cognitive performance and functional competence as predictors of community independence in schizophrenia. *Schizophrenia Bulletin, 36*, 381-387. doi:10.1093/schbul/sbn095

Kongs, S. K., Thompson, L. L., Iverson, G. L., & Heaton, R. K. (2000). *Wisconsin Card Sorting Test—64 card version*. Odessa, FL: Psychological Assessment Resources.

Lehman, A. F., Possidente, S., & Hawker, F. (1986). The quality of life of chronic patients in a state hospital and in community residences. *Hospital and Community Psychiatry, 37*, 901-907.

Lehman, A. F., Postrado, L. T., & Rachuba, L. T. (1993). Convergent validation of quality of life assessments for persons with severe mental illnesses. *Quality of Life Research, 2*, 327-333. doi:10.1007/BF00449427

McKibbin, C. L., Brekke, J. S., Sires, D., Jeste, D. V., & Patterson, T. L. (2004). Direct assessment of functional abilities: Relevance to persons with schizophrenia. *Schizophrenia Research, 72*, 53-67. doi:10.1016/j.schres.2004.09.011

Messick, S. (1995a). Standards of validity and the validity of standards in performance assessment. *Educational Measurement: Issues and Practice, 14*(4), 5-8. doi:10.1111/j.1745-3992.1995.tb00881.x

Messick, S. (1995b). Validity of psychological assessment: Validation of inferences from persons' responses and performances as scientific inquiry into score meaning. *American Psychologist, 50*, 741-749.

Miles, A. A., Heinrichs, R. W., & Ammari, N. (2011). "Real world" functioning in schizophrenia patients and healthy adults: Assessing validity of the Multidimensional Scale of Independent Functioning. *Psychiatry Research, 186*, 123-137.

O'Malia, L., McFarland, B. H., Barker, S., & Barron, N. M. (2002). A level of functioning self-report measure for consumers with severe illness. *Psychiatric Services, 53*(3), 326-331. doi:10.1176/appi.ps.53.3.326

Patterson, T. L., Goldman, S., McKibbin, C. L., Hughs, T., & Jeste, D. V. (2001). UCSD Performance-Based Skills Assessment: Development of a new measure of everyday functioning for severely mentally ill adults. *Schizophrenia Bulletin, 27*(2), 235-245.

Patterson, T. L., Moscona, S., McKibbin, C. L., Davidson, K., & Jeste, D. V. (2001). Social skills performance assessment among older patients with schizophrenia. *Schizophrenia Research, 48*, 351-360. doi:10.1016/S09209964(00)00109-2

Pierce, D. (2001). Occupation by design: Dimensions, therapeutic power and creative process. *America Journal of Occupational Therapy, 55*, 249-259. doi:10.5014/ajot.55.3.249

Rempfer, M., & Brown, C. (2012). *The Test of Grocery Shopping Skills: A specific real world assessment of accuracy and efficiency.* Manuscript in preparation.

Rempfer, M. V., Brown, C. E., & Hamera, E. K. (2011). Learning potential as a predictor of skill acquisition in people with serious mental illness. *Psychiatry Research, 185*, 293-295.

Rempfer, M. V., Hamera, E. K., Brown, C. E., & Cromwell, R. L. (2003). The relations between cognition and the independent living skill of shopping in people with schizophrenia. *Psychiatry Research, 117*, 103-112. doi:10.1016/S01651781(02)00318-9

Rogers, J. C., Holm, M. D, Goldstein, G., McCue, M., & Nussbaum, P. D. (1994). Stability and change in functional assessment of patients with gerophyschiatric disorders. *American Journal of Occupational Therapy, 48*(10), 914-918. doi:10.5014/ajot.48.10.914

Rohland, B. M., & Langbehn, D. R. (1997). Self-reported life satisfaction. *American Journal of Psychiatry, 154*, 1478-1479.

Schooler, N., Hogarty, G. E., & Weissman, M. M. (1979). Social Adjustment Scale II (SAS-II). In J. E. Sorenson (Eds.), *Resource materials for community mental health program evaluators* (DHEW No. 79-328). Washington, DC: Superintendent of Documents.

Thompson, L. K. (1992). *Kohlman Evaluation of Living Skills* (3rd ed.). Bethesda, MD: AOTA Press.

Wallace, C. J. (1986). Functional assessment in rehabilitation. *Schizophrenia Bulletin, 12*, 604-630.

Wallace, C. J., Liberman, R. J., MacKain, S. J., Blackwell, G., & Eckman, T. A. (1992). Effectiveness and replicability of modules for teaching social and instrumental skills to the severely mentally ill. *American Journal of Psychiatry, 149*, 654-658.

Wallace, C. J., Liberman, R. P., Tauber, R., & Wallace, J. (2000). The Independent Living Skills Survey: A comprehensive measure of the community functioning of severely and persistently mentally ill individuals. *Schizophrenia Bulletin, 26*(3), 631-658.

Watzke, S., Brieger, P., Kuss, O., Schoettke, H., & Wiedl, K. (2008). A longitudinal study of learning potential and rehabilitation outcomes in schizophrenia. *Psychiatric Services, 59*, 248-255. doi:10.1176/appi.ps.59.3.248

Wiedl, K. H. (1999). Cognitive modifiability as a measure of readiness for rehabilitation. *Psychiatric Services, 50*, 1411-1413.

Zayat, E., Rempfer, M., Gajewski, B., & Brown, C. E. (2011). Patterns of association between performance in a natural environment and measures of executive function in people with schizophrenia. *Psychiatry Research, 187*, 1-5.

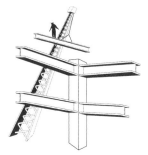

How Occupation Emerges in the Practices of Occupational Therapists
Therapeutic Strategies That Address Occupation

Pollie Price, PhD, OTR/L

In this chapter, I will describe the steps that I have undertaken to create a research program over the past 14 years. The series of four studies and their findings reported in this chapter emerged from my dissertation research (Price, 2003) examining the therapeutic processes of two therapists, each working with two service recipients. Although the four studies vary in participant selection criteria and practice setting, they employed similar methods to examine a single research question: How does occupation, as a central idea in occupational therapy, emerge in the practices of occupational therapists as they work with clients in the therapy process?

LITERATURE

From the inception of the discipline of occupational science, the intent of its founders was to nurture occupational therapy by generating knowledge that would enhance and substantiate practice (Clark et al., 1991, 1993; Yerxa, 1991). With its unique focus on the study of humans as occupational beings and the relationship of engagement in occupation to health and well-being, the developing science prom-

ised to legitimize occupational therapy. It would do this by giving therapists a language, a more explicit understanding of the power of human occupation to influence health and well-being, and more relevant therapeutic approaches leading to more potent outcomes in people's lives. All of these intents of the science have the potential to sharpen occupational therapy's professional identity. Occupational science was birthed to explore and manifest the philosophical roots of the occupational therapy profession (Molke, Laliberte Rudman, & Polatajko, 2004). In turn, occupational therapy can support global occupational science research by providing examples of its application embedded in the local social and cultural contexts in which therapy is practiced (Blanche & Henry-Kohler, 2000).

Wilcock (2005) criticized occupational therapy for getting distracted by evidence-based practice, standardized assessments, activities of daily living, and equipment selection. These distractions cause therapists to lose the true focus of the profession on helping people "transcend difficulties and reach toward potential" (Wilcock, 2005, p. 10). She asserted that the profession has not embraced the ethic of having occupation as the basis of practice. She argued that occupational science could help occupational therapy

Pierce, D. (Ed.).
Occupational Science for Occupational Therapy (pp. 265-280).
© 2014 SLACK Incorporated.

by providing rigorous research that would demonstrate client-driven outcomes regarding the influence of occupation on health. In order to impact public understanding of the relationship between occupation and health, occupational therapists have to understand this relationship so that they can articulate it, what Pierce (2001) called "walk[ing] the walk" (p. 250). The ability to understand and articulate this relationship would enhance public appreciation of occupational therapy philosophy and practice.

Clark (2006) argued that occupational scientists should conduct outcome studies that support occupational therapy policy and practice and provide real value to key stakeholders, including the public, people receiving services, policy makers, and insurers. She further stated, "Continuing to demonstrate the efficacy of practice through science, we hope occupational therapists will become known as highly professional life designers" (Clark, 2006, p. 177). Clark and colleagues (1997) published their landmark study "Occupational Therapy for Independent-Living Older Adults: A Randomized Controlled Trial" in the *Journal of the American Medical Association*, the largest study to date of the effectiveness of occupational therapy (see Chapter 25). The lifestyle redesign model has been disseminated in occupational therapy journals and has been replicated by several scholars. The scholarship of practice or practice-scholar model (Crist, Muñoz, Hansen, Benson, & Provident, 2005; Kielhofner, 2005; Taylor, Fisher, & Kielhofner, 2005) is being used to conduct research on successful practices that emphasize occupation-based approaches and outcomes, thus contributing to an emerging body of evidence-based research about those practices.

Although there is an emerging body of theoretical research about occupation and its applications in practice, few studies have been conducted in which the researcher has observed therapists and their clients as they work through the therapeutic process to examine aspects of occupation-based practice and how occupation, as the central idea of occupational therapy, emerges in the therapy process. Prior to my dissertation study, I had conducted a pilot study with seven doctoral students and faculty affiliated with the University of Southern California Department of Occupational Science. The study involved a series of interview questions. I found that the interviews yielded more theoretical perspectives than actual stories of how they were integrating occupational science concepts in their practices. This is likely because very few were actually practicing at the time of the interviews or had practiced since immersion in the occupational science program. This caused me to want to conduct observations as well as interviews with practitioners who were actually practicing. The aim of the series of studies described in this chapter was to explicate the approaches, processes, and features that make practices occupation based. Drawing upon the occupational science and occupational therapy literature, for the purposes of this research, I defined occupation as:

> The constellation of activities and their related roles in which an individual wants and needs to do in daily life and across time. Occupations are particular in form as they are engaged in in the individual's natural contexts, including home, school, extended family and community, work, and therapy situations (Clark, Wood, & Larson, 1998).

> Occupations have personal and cultural meaning, are related to identity creation, health and life satisfaction, and connect individuals through shared interests. Occupations have aspects of learning, problem solving, and skill acquisition and maintenance, all of which are called upon in circumstances that require adaptation. (Price, 2003, p. 15)

Synthesizing the literature that attempts to define occupation-based practice, and examining my own experiences and assumptions, I anticipated that therapists practicing from an occupation-based perspective would attempt to create therapeutic experiences through activities and contextual conditions that would be meaningful and relevant to the person's occupational life and priorities (Mattingly, 1998). I also expected that therapists would use activities that were occupations of the service recipient as therapeutic interventions and that they would also use:

> Activities and procedures that were not necessarily the clients' occupations, but that would be linked narratively, symbolically and experientially in words and/or actions to what the individual cares about working toward. I expected that outcomes would relate to an individual's competence for doing relevant occupations in natural contexts with others, and confidence, which I suggest is related to adaptiveness, to engage in their social worlds after therapy has ended. (Price, 2003, pp. 15-16)

A Research Program on Occupation in Practice

Study 1: The Dissertation

Methods

This series of studies and their findings emerged from my dissertation research (Price, 2003). As previously stated, though the research question was the same and the methods were similar across all of the studies, the methods, therapist selection criteria, and practice settings did evolve with each study. I will discuss the rationale for these decisions as I move through the succession of studies (Table 23-1).

Selection of Participants

For the dissertation, I solicited nominations from occupational therapy faculty, doctoral students, and clinicians to identify two occupational therapists considered to be particularly concerned with occupation in their practices. Understanding the uniqueness of each therapy process, given my own experiences as a therapist, I wanted to see how

TABLE 23-1

CHART OF PARTICIPANTS FOR ALL STUDIES

THERAPIST	SETTING	CLIENT(S)
Erin	Tertiary neonatal intensive care (15+ years' experience)	Rachel: born 23.5 weeks' gestation; Mira: first-time mother, educated professional Mikala: full-term newborn twin, respiratory condition; Carmen: experienced mother of 4, insurance professional
Nancy	Private practice "after school club" (15+ years' experience)	Hannah: 3.5 years old, labeled "just different"; Susan: new mom, art professional Andrew: 4 years old, developmentally delayed; Roxanna: new mom, ESL teacher, Spanish descent
Dani	Hospital-based outpatient rehabilitation (11+ years' experience)	Rosa: 30 years old, South American descent, college student, 5 years post-C6 SCI, mom and cousins Kevin: 27-year-old body builder, 3 years post-C6 SCI; aide and best friend Tim, brother Jim
Brian	Community-based outpatient rehabilitation (12+ years' experience)	Peter: mid-50s, Scandinavian descent, elite athlete, 1 year post–incomplete cervical SCI Sam: late 30s, glass worker, moderate TBI
Fran	Acute cardiac ICU (8 years' experience)	Joe: early 50s, artificial heart transplant, not working, husband and father; partner Mika
Kenneth	Inpatient rehabilitation (8 years' experience)	Sandra: 80, mother, grandmother, wife, cervical tumor, tetraplegia; husband Tom retired
Lisa	Inpatient rehabilitation (5 years' experience)	Jared: 19, Hispanic, paraplegia, gang member; mom Lena
Rikki	Inpatient rehabilitation (8 years' experience)	Janet: White, 40s, mother, grandmother
Katie	Hippotherapy— community based (5 years' experience)	Danny: 3 years old, multiple developmental issues; mom Terri, wife and mother of two Hank: 35, brainstem TBI; wife Cindy
Annie	Sensory integration clinic— free-standing hospital (12 years' experience)	Jeremy: 7, autism; mom Sherise, wife and mother of three Heather: 8, sensory-motor deficits; mom Danielle
Jennifer	Inpatient rehabilitation, SCI (5 years' experience)	Emily: 43, anoxic TBI, bilateral CVA; involved brother, father Reina: 53, left CVA

Note. ESL=English as a second language, SCI=spinal cord injury, TBI=traumatic brain injury, ICU=intensive care unit, CVA=cerebrovascular accident.

each therapist and client would work together to address the client's occupational life. I expected that the forms of occupation and the approaches, processes, and features of the therapy process would have similarities and differences across therapists and practice settings, which is why I wanted to observe the therapists with two different clients. I expected that understanding those similarities and differences would contribute to a more complex and applicable understanding of occupation-based practice. I screened the therapists by asking them to characterize their practices, to identify the kinds of outcomes with which they were concerned, and to describe a successful and not-so-successful case. In the dissertation study, I examined the therapeutic processes of the two therapists as they each worked with two clients over the course of service. Both of the therapists worked with infants and young children; therefore, the mothers were also involved as research participants. Erin (pseudonym of her choice) worked in a tertiary neonatal intensive care unit (NICU) with the most fragile babies and their parents, and Nancy (pseudonym of my choice) worked with young children up to late adolescence who had problems with friendship in a private practice modeled as an "after-school club." Both therapists talked about therapy processes that promoted adaptation and participation in occupations and social or family life. Each therapist selected for participation the two children and their set of two parents who most adequately represented her best practices.

Data Collection

This ethnographic study required deep immersion into a particular area of practice. Following the methods that Mattingly and Fleming (1994) used in their seminal study to examine the clinical reasoning of occupational therapists, I conducted both interviews and in-depth observations of the therapists and the mothers over the course of the therapy process. This approach was used to understand not only what a therapist says about his or her practice but also what he or she does and how (Hoshmand & Polkinghorne, 1992; Mattingly, 1998; van Maanen, 1983). I also collected anecdotal data from casual hallway conversations between the therapist and other professionals, team meetings, parent education sessions, and a reunion for the NICU babies and families. Following institutional review board approval, and prior to beginning data collection, I conducted the screening interview previously described and "hung out" with the therapists for varying lengths of time prior to starting data collection with a specific parent and child. I used this approach to help the therapists be more comfortable with my presence so that their behaviors and interactions would, in theory, return to normal. I intended to start data collection as close to the beginning of the therapy process as possible, in order to see how the therapy process evolved and became more individualized and relevant for the child and/or family. Initial questions with the therapists included "What kind of outcome do you envision for this person? Have you worked with similar persons in the past?" I conducted interviews with the therapist before and after each session to ask, "What do you have planned for the session today? Has anything happened to cause you to change your vision of the outcome? How do you feel the session went?" I observed a minimum of three sessions and, in some cases, completed seven or more observations between a therapist and a client. I also interviewed the parent, and the child when possible, near the beginning of the service and at the end of service, asking, "What are your hopes and dreams? How did you come to seek occupational therapy? What do you hope to achieve in occupational therapy?" and at the end of service, "Has occupational therapy made a difference in your child's day-to-day life?" (Table 23-2).

The interviews were audiotaped and transcribed verbatim into texts for analysis. I audiorecorded and took in-depth field notes of the observed sessions. The observations were transcribed verbatim and integrated into the interview texts for analysis. Although I had initially planned to enroll 10 participants, because of the expansive depth of the data collected, I decided to complete the study with the two therapists.

Data Analysis

I have used several approaches to data analysis, including narrative analysis (Polkinghorne, 1995; Reissman, 1993), narrative microanalysis (Mattingly, 1998), narrative smoothing (Polkinghorne, 1995), and constant comparative method (Boeije, 2002). However, the primary method has been narrative microanalysis (Mattingly, 1998). This method involves analyzing data following each data collection session and examining the entire transcript line by line to look for the narrative theme that holds together a particular "therapy story" or therapeutic process. The constant comparative method is useful when looking across cases to compare and contrast approaches, processes, and features within the therapeutic process (Boeije, 2002), which we have come to call *therapeutic strategies* or *microprocesses* (Price, 2003; Price & Miner, 2007).

Results

The key findings of the dissertation study were that the therapists used a variety of activities and contexts to promote the children's occupational development, including occupations, and purposeful activities. The use of context was circumscribed for Erin; the NICU was the infant's context. Nancy used both the natural context and the social context of the after-school club in her office suite. Although co-occupations (occupations that cannot be done without another person; Humphry & Thigben-Beck, 1997; Pierce, 2003; Zemke & Clark, 2006) were often used in the NICU, such as feeding, playing, and bathing, in the after-school club, occupation, as a more abstract idea, often existed in a narrative form about who the child was becoming. Improving participation in generic preschool activities in play with peers promoted belonging and becoming a particular kind of friend in natural contexts of home and school. For example, Nancy used pretend play with Hannah to expand her play repertoire and her ability to engage in the preschool setting with other little girls, although Hannah did not like pretend play (Price & Miner, 2007).

Analysis also revealed that the therapeutic relationship and strategies were an important part of occupation-based practice (Price & Miner, 2007). Numerous therapeutic strategies already found in the literature were confirmed (Kielhofner, 2002; Mattingly & Fleming, 1994) and new ones were identified. We concluded that therapists use complex reasoning to create a therapy process that included activity forms and strategies to move a process toward occupational outcomes. The second key finding is that occupation is both a discreet doing and a process of becoming and fosters adaptiveness (Fidler & Fidler, 1978; Price & Miner, 2007).

┌── TABLE 23-2 ──────────

INTERVIEW QUESTIONS

QUESTIONS FOR THERAPISTS

Screening Questions

- Describe a successful case you have had in practice.
- What would you consider a successful outcome?
- How would you characterize your practice?
- What kinds of outcomes do you address?
- Describe a case that was not so successful.

Initial Interview

- Tell me about this individual. How do you envision his or her outcome?
- Have you worked with similar persons?
- Before each subsequent observation:
  - What have you planned for today?
  - What do you hope to achieve?
  - Has anything happened that has influenced your plans or vision of the outcome?

After the Session

- How did the session go today?
- What worked and what did not go as hoped?
- How do you see the therapy evolving?
- What do you think about the next session?

QUESTIONS FOR CLIENTS AND/OR THEIR PROXIES

- What do you hope to gain from occupational therapy?
- What are your hopes and dreams for your family member?
- Periodically throughout the therapy process:
  - How was therapy today?
  - Is therapy going the way you hoped?
  - Is therapy affecting your daily life?
  - What do you hope to accomplish in therapy?

Within 1 Year of Termination of Therapy Services

- How satisfied are you with your daily life?
- What is your definition of a good life and where do you think your life falls on this continuum?
- How important is it for you to be able to participate in meaningful activities? Does this influence your perceived quality of life?
- Do you make your own decisions and does this influence your quality of life?
- What social activities do you participate in and what responsibilities do you have?
- How do you contribute and what is your role in the group?
- What aspects of your therapy were most useful in helping you resume your life?
- What are looking forward to?

The third key finding was that both of these therapists saw the parents, in all cases mothers, as needing support, modeling, and instruction so that they could promote their child's development and advocate for their needs with confidence and competence (Price, 2003; Price & Miner, 2009a, 2009b; Price & Miner Stephenson, 2009). As the mothers observed and learned effective approaches, they were able to replicate them at home and in the community and advocate for their children at school.

Therapeutic Strategies

I have selected a few of the therapeutic strategies that were identified in the dissertation study to discuss and illustrate in this section; more will be discussed in subsequent sections. Each of these microprocesses held narrative meaning about movement toward or away from the occupational outcome goal—a concept that I will illustrate in this chapter using excerpts from observations and interviews in which they emerged.

Scaffolding

In this observation, Carmen, mother of newborn Mikala, and Erin, an occupational therapist, are in the NICU. Erin is teaching Carmen to help Mikala learn to coordinate drinking from a bottle and breathing while watching her oxygen level. Later, Carmen summarized her interactions with Erin in this way:

> She'd kind of give me tips if I'd hold her too far back. You know, she told me, "Kind of hold her up straight, listen for how she breathes," and I started catching on. So, you know, she'd be like my standby. So, now, I feel comfortable um, being able to feed her on … my own. She did good. So, she helped me out a lot … there's certain techniques that she showed me, or things to look for, and made me feel comfortable in coming in at night and doing the feeding on my own. (Price & Miner, 2009b, p. 72)

We extended the theory developed by Wood, Bruner, and Ross (1976) in which teachers used a scaffolding process to teach a task to young children. Using the three phases of scaffolding (Wood et al., 1976), Erin first demonstrated to Carmen the techniques and strategies to feed Mikala while making sure she was breathing, and in subsequent sessions, Carmen would feed Mikala with Erin as a "backup." In the final sessions, Carmen was feeding Mikala successfully on her own at night, and Erin acted as a validator, confirming that Carmen was the expert in feeding Mikala and even teaching the nurses at night. What made this case occupational was the narrative context within which this highly technical training took place. Carmen felt that Mikala was fragile and that she was doing something wrong; Erin countered that Mikala was "lucky to have such an experienced mother." Through scaffolding, Erin helped Carmen to develop the competence and confidence to parent Mikala and to visualize her running and playing alongside her siblings.

Promoting Generalization / modeling

Roxanna was a keen observer of the after-school club Andrew attended with his occupational therapist, Nancy. Over time, Roxanna began recreating similar social opportunities and activities in their home and with the children of neighbors and friends. She frequently arranged play dates to provide social opportunities for Andrew and created a "mini-preschool" at home with several activity choices.

> We can do anything in the world he wants to. … Before, it was really like … pulling teeth. … We make mud puddles … we bake, he likes Legos. … There's 12 centers: pictures, table toys, sand … and we did that for home, so he has to choose what he wants to do … so that's helping. (Price & Miner Stephenson, 2009, p. 183)

As a result, Roxanna began to experience a different relationship with Andrew and began seeing him interact more with other children at home and at preschool.

> He's done really well in school. Really well. He loves school. He loves his friends. He really just has bonds and ties. And he's just talking a lot more with the kids, and he stands his ground. … If somebody takes his chair or if somebody stands in front of him, he'll just really speak his mind. And that, to me, is everything. You know, "I wanted that" and "This is for me" … and to follow the rules, and "I'm number three" and [stand in line]. So that gives me a lot of [encouragement]. If he's sad, if he argues, that would be fine too. I need him to be really strong, he has to really use his words, so … he's growing, he's definitely growing. Before, he used to be very much the shadow, the follower. Completely. Now, he's bringing ideas and the kids pick up on that so then they in turn treat him differently. … And he's getting into trouble, too, in school in front of the teachers, and that's always good, you know, when the teacher yells, "Andrew and Joey, you guys aren't" whatever. In that whole social scheme of preschoolers, that's pretty cool to get in trouble in front of everybody. (Price & Miner Stephenson, 2009, p. 184)

Nancy had the perspective that parents are the experts on their own children, and she did not directly coach parents in how to be with their children. However, she did provide modeling for parents, and by watching Nancy, Roxanna learned how to interact with Andrew in a different way. This is when the relationship between Andrew and Roxanna changed, in turn supporting Roxanna to create similar conditions that helped Andrew to generalize his new social skills and increase his participation in home, school, and community life (Price & Miner Stephenson, 2009).

Occupational Storytelling and Storymaking

Another narrative micronegotiation is storytelling and storymaking. Mattingly (1991) introduced the concept of storytelling and storymaking, and Clark (1993) extended the concept to occupational storytelling/storymaking. This is a process through which the therapist and client cocreate a vision or story of a meaningful future despite the presence of disability. In this illustration from the data, which occurs in the NICU, Erin is teaching Mira how to touch her baby, Rachel, born at 22½ weeks gestation, even though at this point, she is too fragile to hold. Through a narrative process, she is helping Mira to come to appreciate that Rachel is more than "a bundle of nerves" (mom's words) but that she is a little person who is becoming. Erin believes that an infant's development is promoted the best through the occupations and co-occupations of the family, especially those of the mother. Here, therapist and mother are talking, standing on either side of the isolet.

> Erin: I think she's saying she wants you to keep your hands just like that, and don't do anything else. … I think she's always liked your hand on her head like that, kind of supporting her like that. I think it helps her settle back down and stay asleep.

> Mira: Well, she's starting to act like a baby. … I'm getting this feeling, like she's a baby, you know? The crying and the, you know, your ups and downs.

> Erin: The awake times.

> Mira: She was like really, really tiny, you didn't see much of … a personality.

> Erin: How would you describe her personality?

> Mira: Oh, that she has a mind of her own!

> Erin: That's right … you were saying … she had inherited it from your side of the family.

> Mira: Oh yes! From me. Definitely from me. Definitely feisty! (Price, 2003, pp. 272-273)

In Erin's practice, the parents are as much the client as are the infants. It is important to note here that the baby cannot live outside of the NICU. Therefore, this highly biomedical context is her home, and Erin naturalizes it as much as she can by creating opportunities for Mira and Rachel to engage in co-occupations such as feeding, bathing, and rocking routines at times when Rachel is more "robust." This is storymaking through the actions and interactions of therapy (Mattingly, 1998) about who Rachel is becoming and who they are becoming as a mother–child pair.

Changing Conditions

Nancy began seeing Hannah when she was 2½ years old. Hannah could not be around anyone except her mother without crying and being terrified; this included her father. Hannah was evaluated for autism but was labeled "just different." When Nancy started seeing Hannah, she attempted to see her at Hannah's local park, but Hannah was frightened by the other children. Nancy saw Hannah in the "little kid's room" (Price, 2003) with her mother present. When Hannah would become upset, Nancy would help her to relax by breathing. Nancy also found little routines that Hannah liked, like blowing bubbles, to start each session. As Hannah began to trust Nancy, Nancy changed the therapeutic conditions by either adding a peer or having Hannah participate in activities that stretched her play repertoire, such as making pretend food with play dough. When I

first started observing their sessions, Nancy had Hannah playing with a young child who was actually less capable than Hannah, someone she could actually support and encourage. Over the next few months, Nancy moved her into a bigger group of more diverse children. Over several observations, including an observation of Hannah at her new preschool, Hannah did begin to play reciprocally with other children, but I never saw her verbally communicate. However, when she was alone with Nancy, she was quite verbal and animated. Changing conditions and grading challenges were just two of numerous strategies I observed Nancy using with Hannah to move her toward her goal of going to school.

The dissertation study added complexity to the understanding of occupation-based practice that is present in the literature. Some scholars have argued for using the natural context (Fidler, 2000; Hocking, 2001; Humphry & Wakeford, 2006), and others have empirically shown that using a variety of contexts and activities promoted occupational outcomes (Gray, 1998; Jackson, 1998; Lawlor, 2003). This series of studies supports Pierce's (2003) notion of intactness and her challenge to therapists to think critically about the choice of context and activity to create the most powerful change. These data support the use of complex reasoning to do just that. This analysis also demonstrates the power of the therapy relationship and the dynamic use of therapy strategies and activities to move the process in a symbolic way toward occupational goals. Each of the strategies discussed in this section emerge in most of the therapy dyads in the subsequent studies.

Study 2: How Occupation Emerges in Practice Across Settings

Methods

After completing my doctoral degree and taking a faculty position in another state, I chose to replicate the study with new participants. I decided to broaden the study to include 10 occupation-based occupational therapists and 20 clients (2 clients per therapist) from a diversity of settings, age ranges, and conditions. This decision was based on my expectation that forms of occupation and the approaches, processes, and features of practices in these diverse conditions would yield common aspects of occupation-based practice as well as important differences shaped by factors such as setting, reimbursement, or medical versus social versus educational orientation. For this study, I added quantitative measures to the methods: the Health-Related Quality of Life Measure (short form) (Sherbourne & Ware, 2011) and the Satisfaction with Life Scale (Diener, Emmons, Larsen, & Griffin, 1985). I also included a follow-up interview with the client and/or family at 1 year postdischarge, unless the client was continuing with other occupational therapy services. This study ultimately included only three therapists who worked in adult rehabilitation settings: one in a community-based setting, one in a hospital-based outpatient program, and one in an inpatient acute rehabilitation center. Reasons for stopping at three participants will be further explained later. Data were collected with six clients, three of whom had spinal cord injuries, one who sustained a traumatic brain injury, one who sustained an anoxic brain injury, and one who sustained a cerebral vascular accident.

Results

Key findings of this second study confirmed the dissertation findings, uncovered new therapeutic strategies, and added complexity to some identified therapeutic strategies. The findings also revealed that occupation-based practice was more constrained in inpatient biomedical rehabilitation settings than in community and outpatient settings. However, the therapists used a variety of activities and contexts, including occupational activities and natural contexts, in the community to move the clients toward occupational outcome goals. Another important finding was seeing how the therapy processes started out either client directed or therapist directed and then moved toward a therapeutic partnership.

Doing With–Doing Together

Doing with–doing together seems to be an important aspect of occupation-based practice, because it emerged in several of the therapy processes with the participants. This process seems to have both a practical problem-solving feature as well as a social feature and is closely related to the next theme of being a social partner.

An example of this therapeutic strategy comes from an observation of Kevin, his therapist Dani, Kevin's caregiver, and Kevin's brother as they went out to eat at an outdoor mall. Dani and Kevin used wheelchairs and took the city train to meet the others at the mall. By also using a wheelchair, Dani could experience the trip as Kevin did and was able to facilitate problem solving as situations arose. Another intended objective of this outing was to expose Kevin to a different form of transportation. The following dialogue took place:

Kevin: Look at me. I'm trying this now. I don't like it, but I'm doing it.

Dani: Kevin's out of his comfort zone.

Kevin: That's right, totally out of my comfort zone. (Price, 2010)

Several researchers have looked at the importance of learning how to transition from one's "former body" to the "new body." Guidetti, Asaba, and Tham (2009) found that their participants with stroke and spinal cord injury experience a "sense of alienation—a disconnection between the self and the new body—and also a disconnection in the interaction between the body and the world in different kinds of activities" (p. 329). In order to facilitate a reconnection, the authors asserted that individuals need to try their new bodies in an activity because this gives them a sense of their potential development and possible future.

Doing With–Being a Social Partner

Doing with–doing together has a social quality; however, therapists develop relationships with their clients that seem more like friendships; we came to call this feature *being a social partner*. Peter talked a lot about his relationship with his occupational therapist, Brian. Having been a ski instructor for several years, Peter knew the value of the relationship to the process of teaching and learning.

Brian was able to give me his undivided attention, moments when I came in and when I was troubled, he would give me that two minutes of voicing what was really important to me, and then he would sort of push me. I view that time with fondness; that guy helped me do this. … It was a great time, and I got stronger, and I was able to use my hands more. (Price, 2008a)

Peloquin (1995) described therapists as covenanters, when they take up the journey with the client, staying with the client and encouraging him or her until he or she can journey on his or her own. Gahnström-Strandqvist, Tham, Josephsson, and Borell (2000) called this *emotional competence* and suggested that this is not just the "art of practice" but that it is an essential skill required of occupational therapists.

Narrative Micronegotiating

As was true of Peter and Brian, at the beginning of his therapy process with Dani, Kevin wanted to focus mainly on gaining strength and was not interested in working on occupations. Peter had been an elite athlete and Kevin had been a body builder. Both valued exercise as an occupation and as part of their identities. Additionally, Peter, who had an incomplete cervical injury, felt that as he gained strength and coordination, his function would return. Conversely, both felt that accepting modifications would mean giving up on potential. Over the course of service, both therapists continually talked to their clients about how the exercise therapy would help them to achieve an occupational goal and would negotiate with them to try different occupations. Over the next few months, Kevin began to participate in functional tasks in various contexts in order to gain strength and ability. Here we see a micronegotiation about what they were up to in therapy.

Dani: Talk to me about what's working. Instead of me telling you. What activities do you need to be able, what are you thinking of an activity that you want your triceps for?

Kevin: Everything … pushing, grabbing, reaching, extending my arm, even trying to transfer. … I never knew that triceps were so important … if I can learn … what exercise I can do to try to strengthen that.

Dani: Do you want to know my opinion? How does it get stronger?

Kevin: Through function.

Dani: [You are] totally reaching … grabbing things.

Kevin: Looking like a stud. … If you don't look good doing it, don't do it. That's my motto.

Dani: Fashion not function … you are talking to the wrong girl … function not fashion. Speaking of research. Functional movement … and repetition improves your movement.

Kevin: Function and repetition improves movement. (Price, 2010)

Getting Commitment

An aspect of micronegotiating is getting commitment. Dani felt that Kevin could do more for himself. As he began to try more tasks, she pushed him to commit to practicing things they were working on in therapy at home. In the following excerpt, she is attempting to get his commitment to practice bed transfers at home.

Dani: That's the next step Kevin … doing this stuff more at home.

Kevin: Yeah, I gotta work in the bed. I just gotta find time for it.

Dani: So when, could you get it in in the morning?

Kevin: I don't know, I've got to think about it.

Dani: I mean, okay, so let's talk. How badly do you want to be able to do this on your own?

Kevin: I'd love to. I just got to, uh, figure out some time.

Dani: Kevin, we gotta get you practicing this at home. … We're going to figure out how many we could do in 15 minutes. … 15 minutes a day.

Kevin: I don't have 3 minutes.

Dani: Could you get up 15 minutes earlier? Could you go to sleep 15 minutes later?

Kevin: Yeah, it doesn't bother me.

Dani: You would double your progress if you did it at home … like teamwork. Like we do it here, you go home and do your part there.

Kevin: Oh I understand it. It's not without homework. … I won't get anywhere just practicing it once. (Price, 2010)

Several months into therapy, Kevin had this to say:

The more patterns and routine I'm doing here the more I take it home and it's almost like homework and then it becomes fluid, routines. So I wake up in the morning and the first thing I want to do is get in the kitchen and see what I can do. You know, brush my teeth independently. That

was something I wasn't even doing. And ah, I even got that down in time. There are so many things that are so minute but when you put them all together you get a bigger picture and it becomes very routine at home. And all the sudden you, you know even, I don't even notice that I was doing things more regularly, almost like an able-bodied person like I was before I got hurt because it just becomes second nature. So, um, I'm definitely taking it home and it's working out better. (Price, 2010)

Jennifer was a therapist who worked in an inpatient rehabilitation unit. She discussed how challenging it is to work in a large medical center and sustain an occupation-based approach, saying, "I struggle with doing the best occupational therapy for the patient and fitting into a medical model in a large hospital. I feel like I am in constant conflict" (Price, 2010). However, therapeutic activities with both clients included occupational activities such as putting on makeup and doing hair, going shopping for a dress for a child's graduation, and cooking fajitas. Jennifer continued:

Emily was really excited to go out to lunch. We can't go out to lunch every day. But wow, if we could have … she would have been more engaged and excited because that was her interest and that's what she likes to do. And just the restriction of "You have to feel good because right now is when I have you scheduled." (Price, 2010)

In contrast, Dani stated,

[In an outpatient setting] you're not limited by, "I've got a week's stay. I've got to get them home" … and I think as I've changed to outpatient, I've really seen the opportunity to be able to look more at the long term. (Price, 2010)

Although Brian saw Peter in a community-based program, except for conducting a driving evaluation with him, Brian was only able to engage Peter occupationally in a narrative form, giving him ideas for cooking and other home modifications, strategies for getting paperwork completed, and return-to-work strategies. However, Brian worked with his other client, Sam, at his home, conducted a driving evaluation, and helped him to transition back to work. One research question that arose from this study is this: Is using natural settings that are not the client's (e.g., not his neighborhood grocery store) as impactful in promoting adaptiveness as using the client's natural settings (e.g., his own bank)?

This analysis demonstrates how potent therapy processes are inherently client centered, complex, and dynamic in their structure. Rosa started off very passive in her therapy with Dani. As she became more occupationally competent, however, she became more of a partner in determining which occupations they would address and where she and Dani would work. Both Peter and Kevin directed their therapy in the beginning. The previous data demonstrated how Dani and Kevin became a "we union" (Guidetti, Asaba, & Tham, 2009) in determining which occupations they would work on. This was also true of setting. Dani asked Kevin early on whether they could work in his home on his occupations activities, but he declined.

Over the year, as Kevin gained more trust in Dani and as she convinced him that working on activities would help him gain strength, they took the train to the mall, worked in his home on transfers, visited the grocery store, completed meal prep in the rehab kitchen, and completed a driving evaluation. Therapists must be client centered if they are to sustain good therapy relationships with clients. This often resulted in the therapists using exercise and purposeful activities that were more meaningful. However, as we see in the previous scenarios, through narrative micronegotiations, the therapy process became a partnership that moved the therapy toward mutually desired occupational outcomes.

Study 3: How Occupation Emerges in Practices of Those Who Use Single Modalities

Methods

As is true of much of faculty research, this research program has been supported by occupational therapy graduate students who complete a research project as part of degree requirements. Students have participated in each of the three studies, including this one, assisting in collecting and analyzing one or two cases each. I have often asked the graduate research advisees whether they were interested in sampling from a particular setting or condition.

Selection of Participants

For this study, one of the students was interested in studying a therapist she knew of who worked in a horse arena using hippotherapy as the therapeutic modality, an area of practice that I probably would not have considered as occupation based. Two other groups of students were interested in studying the practice of a therapist who uses a sensory integration approach in a hospital-based outpatient clinic who had been recommended to me for the study.

Data Collection

For these four cases, we explored whether and when purposeful activity yielded occupational outcomes and, if they did, under what conditions. Purposeful activities are defined as goal-directed activities used in therapy in order to promote performance of occupation (American Occupational Therapy Association, 2008). With the exception of shoe tying and tooth brushing, which may or may not have had meaning to the child, most of the therapy activities observed in these settings could be considered purposeful or preparatory. Although the therapists regularly linked the therapy procedures to the child's occupational life, such as when Annie said to Flo, "So all of those things, you remember we said, are part of your job as being a kid… as being a second grader."

Results

One of the most significant findings in this study was that the therapists expected that improvements in sensory integration and sensory motor function in the clinic or arena would promote improvements in occupational performance and social participation at home and school. The therapists counted on the mothers to promote generalization by providing similar opportunities at home and encouraging teachers and others in the child's natural context to use therapy strategies. Flo's mother stated,

> I was very pleased with the suggestions and the ideas and the forethought that she had put into it as far as making some practical suggestions as far as how you can attack this and that… and I think the biggest challenge… is taking what she gave you and then incorporating it into life which is crazy and hectic. (Price, 2011)

The social aspect of doing with, as discussed under Study 2, was also prominent in this study. Perhaps because these participants were children, the doing with had the narrative qualities of promoting the child's becoming. The narratives were often gendered, with the therapists using words like *cowboy*, *train conductor*, or *gymnast*. We came to call this doing with–being a play partner.

Annie is an occupational therapist who practices in a free-standing hospital clinic and reports practicing from a sensory integration perspective. Jeremy has a diagnosis of autism and has sensory, sensory motor, and social issues. In the following excerpt, Annie and Jeremy are working in the gym on a bolster swing suspended from the ceiling. Mom is sitting to the side.

Annie: Oh my word! Where are you? On a boat, a train, or an airplane?

Jeremy: A train.

Annie: A train. OK, so you're the train driver? Where are you going to today, train driver?

Jeremy: Mm … the other side of the world.

Annie: Oh … the other side of the world? Oh my gosh, it's going to take us forever!

Jeremy: Whoa! [One foot begins to fall off of swing.]

Annie: I better get you a train seat. … Whoa! [J falls off of the swing. A brings a square foam seat for J to sit on] Get back on the train! Hurry before it drives away, quick! [J begins to get back on swing with help from A.]

Jeremy: When will it drive?

Annie: Say it again?

Mom: When will it drive? [interpreting]

Annie: Not until the driver's in place. [J gets on top of the square on top of swing with some assistance from A] Phew! It's very important to have the driver or else it's a runaway train, my goodness!

Jeremy: What is a runaway train?

Annie: A train that is out of control, and we want you to be in control. OK, you put your hands on here. [A shows J where to place his hands on the ropes of the swing. A adjusts the seat.] Sit right in the middle. And it looks like your body is kind of … off on the side. OK, here we go train driver. [J pulls and pushes the ropes to make the swing go back and forth.]

Jeremy: Woo woo.

Annie: Woo woo. [Makes train whistle motion with arm.] Pull your whistle. [A and J make whistle sound together.]

Jeremy: Woo woo.

Annie: Full steam ahead. (Woo woo) There you go, J, you got it better that time. (Woo woo) …

Annie: Now stay on. No falling off the train until we pull into the station. (Woo woo) What number station are we going to?

Jeremy: 10. (Price, 2011)

Following the session, Annie talked about Jeremy:

And with Jeremy … just as a part of his diagnosis, they … are fine with isolation, they're fine with kind of going off into their own thing. … So that's an interesting point with someone like him … that's when I know we're socially doing the right thing therapeutically, because we're actually connected. Like we're doing it together … both going to the train station. We're together. He easily can kind of go on his own thing and he's fine with that. … And he doesn't necessarily ask for help or need help, that's why I offer that all the time, you know. "Let me know if you need some help" to bring him back to, oh, there's somebody over here. [Laughs.] Playing with you. (Price, 2011)

Guidetti et al. (2009), Lawlor (2003), and Price and Miner (2007) have highlighted the importance of the social relationship between therapist and client. The participants with spinal cord injury in Guidetti et al. (2009) often referred to their relationship with their therapists as a "we union." The three themes, *doing with–doing together, being a social partner*, and *being a play partner* all share a social feature; however, they have subtle aspects that are unique. Doing with–doing together has a feature of problem solving, whereas being a social partner is more about conveying "you are worth being with." Being a play partner is inserting oneself as a peer in the process of playing.

In three of the four cases, the mothers helped to scaffold the skills the child was learning in therapy to home and school and reported to the therapists that the child was improving in occupational performance and social relationships at home and in school. Flo's mother stated,

I've seen huge improvements in her eye–hand coordination … and I think that helps a lot socially on the playground. … She wouldn't be playing with friends because they would be playing with balls or something so she would just sit out and watch and I think she participated more. (Price, 2011)

Flo agreed, "Yeah, like I started playing four square this year and I [used to not be able to] at all, so I wouldn't go play" (Price, 2011).

Despite these apparent occupational and social outcomes, we were still left with a question: Could the outcomes be more potent if the therapists had added a social component through peer play, or followed a hippotherapy session with homework, or had seen the child in his or her home or school environment, even just once? Katie reflected on this limitation of a single modality:

I've seen this at other places, but ideally, from a therapeutic standpoint, it would be ideal to have our own little gym next to the rink … immediately see some functional outcomes. [Like] "Let's sit down and try to do some of your homework" and see how he does. … That's the whole point, right? To see how "the how" is transferring from here to there, right? (Price, 2011)

The assumption of generalization of occupational therapy to occupational life is an area that we feel needs more research. Another question that needs further research is the assertion that purposeful activities become occupations as meaning is created (Price, 2003; Price & Miner, 2007). An example arose in the case of Hannah: Nancy used pretend play with Hannah even though she didn't like it. Her ability to participate in it, however, had symbolic meaning that she would be able to play with other little girls once she went to preschool. Therefore, a purposeful activity acquired meaning and became occupation.

Study 4: Consideration of Occupation in the Practices of Specialists

Methods

By the time I reached Study 4, I decided to again broaden the participant criteria to include therapists who were considered specialists with a certain condition (e.g., spinal cord injury, cardiac rehabilitation) but may or may not be thought of as occupation based in their practice. The intent of this decision was to begin to more specifically identify aspects of occupation-based practice and to identify approaches, processes, and features that might not be included in such a definition. This study included four therapists: one who worked on an acute surgical unit with persons who had heart transplants and three who worked in two different inpatient rehabilitation units. The clients included a man who had an artificial heart transplant and two women and one young man with paraplegic spinal cord injuries.

Results: Missed Opportunities

We found in these four cases that, although generally the therapists had developed rapport and the clients seemed to trust them, the therapy was much more prescriptive, therapist directed, and functionally oriented. That is, we did not see collaborative goal setting or intervention planning between the therapist and the client. Safety, efficiency, and a mild degree of problem solving with respect to functional mobility and self-care performance were observed. Almost no narrative storytelling and storymaking were observed, with many missed opportunities to address the person's desired occupations, anticipated future, and identity; who they hoped to become; or how they might belong in their social worlds. Two of the therapists blamed their clients for not pushing themselves hard enough to meet independence goals, but neither really explored the psychosocial aspects of why the clients were reluctant to fully engage. In these cases, getting commitment through micronegotiating, a therapeutic strategy discussed in Study 2, was missing.

Rikki's client, Janet, had several broken ribs and associated pain, and she was often tearful and fearful about her spinal cord injury and whether she would walk again. Although it might have occurred in other sessions that were not observed, Rikki did not seem to feel that addressing Janet's fears or hopes for the future was part of her skilled service. Neither did she seem to collaborate with the social worker on these issues. Rikki also missed opportunities to address Janet's occupations of grooming and hygiene. Janet loved to look beautiful, and these kinds of activities might have been incorporated to address Rikki's biomechanical goals as well as give her a sense of connection to the person she was and could continue to be. During the exit interview, Rikki stated, "Janet definitely had some obstacles in her way that impeded her progress. … She didn't meet all of my goals that I set for her originally." In contrast, Kevin had this to say about the "we union" (Guidetti et al., 2009) he had with Dani, "With what [the outpatient clinic] can do and what they offer, how we worked together, I think we did very well. We really did, I think we did a good job."

The following excerpt illustrates a missed opportunity to use narrative approaches to promote identity and to create a hopeful future. Fran worked on an inpatient cardiac unit that specialized in heart transplants. Her client, Joe, had undergone a heart transplant and she was seeing him to advance his self-care skills, teach him to manage the heart battery, and promote energy conservation. This conversation transpired during one of the observed sessions.

Joe: Yeah, I'm on regular food.

Fran: How does that feel?

Joe: Oh it's good. It's just … they ain't got nothing up there that they got that I want.

Fran: [Laughs.] What do you want?

Joe: I want the all meat … something that I can cook, you know.

Wife: [Laughs.]

Fran: Not bad. Are you a good cook?

Joe: Oh yeah. I think I am, anyway.

Fran: Well you like it. What do you like to cook?

Joe: Everything.

Fran: Oh, come on. Give me an example.

Joe: Oh my favorite's, like, uh, brown beans and fried taters and cornbread, you know. But I don't make it much 'cause she don't like it, you know. And I don't like her to come up to me when I do, you know. And, of course, my trick to my brown beans is I cook 'em for about 24 hours.

Fran: Do ya?

Joe: And I put them in a pot with, uh, with your ham hock and cut up like a whole onion.

Fran: Uh huh.

Joe: Oh man. And I put a little, uh, uh, salt in, a little garlic and, uh, oh what's that other stuff that … cumin. Put a little cumin in it and let them cook for about 24 hours. I used to put them on like at six or probably six the day before and then I could eat them at about five or six the next day.

Fran: Wow, that's great. Can I move this?

Joe: Okay.

Fran: Oh! That's good. Do you remember what we were going to do today?

Joe: No not yet.

Fran: Okay. What I'd like to do is have you get dressed and then go to the sink and brush your teeth. Well, we'll play it by ear on how you're feeling. But the first step is getting dressed. (Price, 2008a)

We saw this as a missed opportunity to acknowledge that Joe had been on the brink of death, quite debilitated and waiting for a heart transplant, not knowing whether he would live or die. Now he has a new heart and a new chance at life. This might have been an opportunity to discuss what he was most looking forward to upon returning home and perhaps incorporate some of his occupations, such as cooking, into therapy, if not physically doing then through narrative storytelling (Clark, 1993; Mattingly, 1991).

Two of the clients transitioned to skilled nursing, and the outcome of the gentleman with the heart transplant is unknown because he returned home to another state.

Again, we are left with a question: Do narrative approaches, client-centered collaborative goal setting and intervention planning, and occupation as means lead to more potent occupational outcomes?

Kenneth, an inpatient rehabilitation therapist reflected:

It just seems like everything's so superficial that you're just, that all we're concerned about is moving to the next step. You know we forget these people are even people ... you are now at this diagnosis and you have this many days and so here's my checklist. You know, it's like all on barriers and impairment and ... we've got to get away from that. I mean so addressing her needs as a person, not just her physical means. And that's where, you know, it would be fun to be her outpatient therapist and say, you know, I don't care if you can get to the toilet or not you know. ... What do you need you know? ... Because your whole life's been turned on its head, where do we need to go to make you smile again, you know? (Price, 2008a)

These data illustrate the tensions and challenges to practice from an occupation-based perspective that exist in traditional biomedical settings. Several scholars have asserted that stronger occupation-based practice occurs when therapy is done in the person's natural setting (Fidler, 2000; Hocking, 2001; Humphry & Wakeford, 2006; Pierce, 2001) and when using his or her typical occupations as means (Gray, 1998; Kielhofner, 2002; Pierce, 2003). Pierce cautioned that traditional clinical settings are the most challenging to occupation-based practice, asserting that therapists have a moral and ethical imperative to ask, "If we could go anywhere, when, where, and with whom would this intervention work best for this client?" (p. 224).

A radical response to this question would be to advocate that occupational therapists should pull out of working in institutional settings and focus on community-based services through which therapy can better facilitate occupational and role functioning in their natural contexts. This assertion raises many questions. Does occupational therapy, when provided in an occupation-based, client-centered way, contribute to potent outcomes in traditional biomedical settings? If we pull away from medically based settings and medical reimbursement, will reimbursement move with the client into the community? Will the profession be able to thrive in community-based settings through grants and/or other social services funding? If occupational therapy does remain, as it most certainly will, in traditional clinical settings, consideration of the most effective setting for occupation-based practice can, at the least, provide therapists with valuable insights into the interventions they provide. Exploring the contrast between the client's usual occupational settings and the clinical setting will spur thinking about how to mediate the artificiality of the setting in order to support effectiveness of occupation-based practice.

CONTRIBUTIONS TO OCCUPATIONAL SCIENCE

This research program addressed the original intent of occupational science in the United States to produce knowledge that would substantiate occupational therapy practice (Clark et al., 1991, 1993; Yerxa, 1991). It also answers the call to conduct studies focused on outcomes that provide real value to clients, insurers, policy makers, and the public (Clark, 2006; Wilcock, 2005). This program of research contributes to occupational science by providing tangible examples of the ways in which occupation was addressed and facilitated by occupational therapists in a variety of practice settings through the therapy process in real time. These findings contribute to the development of theory of occupation-based occupational therapy practice.

Although this is only one line of research on occupation-based practice, it is unusual in its methods. Observations and interviews were conducted over the course of 18 therapy processes, which enabled a close and deep examination of the concept of occupation and its presence or absence in those processes across diverse settings, therapists, and clients. Building on the work of Clark (1993), Kielhofner (1995), and Mattingly and Fleming (1994), this research has yielded numerous therapeutic strategies (also called *microprocesses*) that therapists use to move the therapy process toward occupational outcomes. The therapeutic relationship is a central aspect of understanding a client's occupational life, identity, fears, and desires for the future. Client-centeredness is a key aspect of a collaborative therapeutic partnership through which therapist and client determine the occupational outcome goals and the therapeutic activities and contexts. Showing *how* therapists addressed clients' occupational lives and produced occupational outcomes contributes to the evolving theory of occupation-based practice, conducting research that demonstrates the effectiveness of occupational therapy (Clark, 2006).

IMPLICATIONS FOR OCCUPATIONAL THERAPY

Occupation-based practice is a term that is laden with mystery and assumptions, embraced by some occupational therapists and considered a threat by others. Recently, a fairly new graduate told me, "It's hard to be occupation based in a large, medical rehabilitation center. When I came out of school, I had bought into all of that." These study results suggest that being occupation based is not an either–or dichotomy. Rather, this research suggests that there is a continuum of approaches, processes, and features that would be considered occupation based. The study provides an opening, an opportunity, and an invitation for occupational therapists to reflect on their practices, to acknowledge when they are being occupation based, and to consider ways in which they could strengthen their occupation-based practices. In this time of limited health care resources, occupational therapists must not shrink away from their training in order to look like other professionals and emulate the medical model. Rather, it is time for them to step into the light and articulate and demonstrate that what they have to offer is unique and provides real value to the people they serve. It is time to, as Wilcock (2005) urged, "help people transcend difficulties and reach toward potential" (p. 10). Davis (2010) recently wrote, "Our time has come—our time is now—for us to lead in the realm of occupation-based practice" (p. 17).

This study demonstrates the complexity of occupation-based practice. It illustrates that occupation-based practice is not simply using an individual's typical occupations as a therapeutic modality in the individual's natural context. Rather, therapists use complex reasoning to design therapeutic conditions that will promote occupational outcomes and adaptiveness in their clients. This change is not only physical and functional. It is a change in who the client wishes to be and become in the world. It is social and emotional and requires adaptation and recreation of identity; it is finding a new way to be in the world while still being connected to who one was in the past. The findings show the many microprocesses that therapists used to propel the therapy process forward toward mutually identified occupational outcomes. The therapy process facilitated confidence and competence to move out into the world as a social actor who, despite disability, has a lot to offer to the world. These processes include, but are not limited to, scaffolding, promoting generalization, occupational storytelling and storymaking, doing with–doing together, doing with–being a social partner, doing with–being a play partner, narrative micronegotiating, and getting commitment. The fourth study revealed what an occupation-based practice is not: prescriptive, therapist directed, lacking in understanding of the client's life and desires, focused on "the next step" instead of the occupations and roles of future life, and promoting function rather than adaptiveness.

The founders of occupational science in the United States intended the science to support occupational therapy practice by giving the profession a stronger understanding and a language to describe occupation. It is important, however, that this information be pragmatic, accessible, and useful to practitioners who are providing services to clients every day. This series of studies also offers therapists glimpses of real scenarios that demonstrate ways in which therapists practice from an occupation-based perspective. The findings show how therapists address clients' occupational lives through a complex therapy process that looks to the future and values and honors clients' adaptations.

LEARNING SUPPORTS

Research Methods to Study Occupational Therapy Practice

Purpose

The purpose of this learning activity is to understand more deeply the value of the methods used in this study and how to implement them in a limited replication of the study.

Primary Concepts

- What makes a practice occupation-based
- Missed opportunities to address an individual's occupational life
- Occupational versus functional outcomes
- Therapeutic strategies
- Therapeutic partnership
- Collaboration

Instructions

1. Identify a therapist who is willing to let you observe three therapy sessions with a client as part of a class assignment. This therapist could be self-identified or identified as occupation based or not.

2. Ensure that the therapist has gotten permission from the client for you to observe three sessions, audiotape them, and take notes without identifying the client.

3. Schedule the sessions, either one at a time as you go or all at once, making a note of which scheduling approach the therapist chose.

4. Use Table 23-2 to complete the initial and exit interviews, the interviews before and after the sessions, and interviews with the client.

5. Attend the sessions; take notes just on what you see happening in the session between therapist, client, and any others; and audiotape the sessions. Do not interpret what you are seeing at this point—write down how hard or easy it is to not judge.

6. Using the concepts to be examined outlined above, listen to the audiotapes and review your observation notes. Mark or make note of therapy actions or interactions that seem to reflect the above concepts.

7. Write a five- to seven-page reflection paper on the occupation-based nature of this three-session process.

Literature Review

Purpose

The purpose of this literature review is for you to examine any new theoretical or data-based literature in occupational science or occupational therapy about occupation-based occupational therapy.

Primary Concepts

- The use of occupational science by occupational therapists to study practice
- Occupational science research that supports occupation-based practice

Instructions

1. Generate a list of search words to help you search the databases. You can ask your instructor for suggestions.

2. Search the literature using your key words. Start with these databases: OT Search (American Occupational Therapy Foundation) and CINAHL. Limit your search to the past 10 years.

3. If your search yields a large volume of abstracts, you may limit your search by selecting an area of your interest (e.g., refugees, women with multiple sclerosis, returning vets, persons with persistent mental illness, etc.).

4. Read the abstracts and select five that you feel are the most relevant to understanding occupation-based practice and how it is implemented in practice (theoretical or data based).

5. Summarize the articles using a critical appraisal task model or another model that your instructor suggests.

6. Write a five-page synthesis of your literature review, using a format from a journal publication, your research text, or another guideline that your instructor suggests.

Theoretically Abstract Research

Purpose

The purpose of this activity is to compare and contrast this research method with the methods in learning activity.

Primary Concepts

- What makes a practice occupation-based
- Missed opportunities to address an individual's occupational life
- Occupational versus functional outcomes
- Therapeutic strategies
- Therapeutic partnership
- Collaboration

Instructions

1. Identify two or three practicing occupational therapists who may or may not be identified as practicing from an occupation-based perspective.

2. Contact the therapists and ask for permission to audiotape and interview to get their perspectives on occupation-based practice.

3. Generate a list of interview questions that are different from those in Table 23-2 (e.g., Please define occupation. Please define occupation-based practice. What are your views about occupation-based practice in your setting? Would you consider yourself as practicing from an occupation-based perspective?).

4. Listen to the audiotapes and any notes you might have taken. Mark or make note of any parts of the narrative that reflect the primary concepts to be examined.

5. Write a five- to seven-page paper that summarizes the therapists' theoretical views and any examples they gave. Compare and contrast these methods with the methods in the first Learning Activity and their utility for understanding how to implement occupation-based practice.

REFERENCES

American Occupational Therapy Association. (2008). Occupational therapy practice framework: Domain and process (2nd ed.). *American Journal of Occupational Therapy, 62*, 625-683. doi:10.5014/ajot.62.6.625

Blanche, E., & Henry-Kohler, E. (2000). Philosophy, science, and ideology: A proposed relationship for occupational science and occupational therapy. *OT International, 7*(2), 99-110. doi:10.1002/oti.110

Boeije, H. (2002). A purposeful approach to the constant comparative method in the analysis of qualitative interviews. *Quality and Quantity, 36*, 391-409. doi:10.1023/A:1020909529486

Clark, F. (1993). Occupation embedded in a real life: Interweaving occupational science and occupational therapy. 1993 Eleanor Clark Slagle Lecture. *American Journal of Occupational Therapy, 47*, 1067-1078. doi:10.5014/ajot.47.12.1067

Clark, F. (2006). One person's thoughts on the future of occupational science. *Journal of Occupational Science, 13*(3), 167-179. doi:10.1080/14427591.2006.9726513

Clark, F., Azen, S. P., Zemke, R., Jackson, J. M., Carlson, M. E., Hay, J., . . . Lipson, L. (1997). Occupational therapy for independent-living older adults: A randomized controlled trial. *Journal of the American Medical Association, 278*(16), 1321-1326.

Clark, F., Parham, D., Carlson, M. E., Frank, G., Jackson, J., Pierce, D. E., . . . Zemke, R. (1991). Occupational science: Academic innovation in service of occupational therapy's future. *American Journal of Occupational Therapy, 45*, 303-310. doi:10.5014/ajot.45.4.300

Clark, F., Wood, W., & Larson, E. A. (1998). Occupational science: Occupational therapy's legacy for the 21st century. In M. E. Neidstadt & E. B. Crepeau (Eds.), *Willard and Spackman's occupational therapy* (9th ed.). Philadelphia, PA: J. B. Lippincott.

Clark, F., Zemke, R., Frank, G., Parham, D., Neville-Jan, A., Hedricks, C., . . . Abreu, B. (1993). Dangers inherent in the partition of occupational therapy and occupational science. *American Journal of Occupational Therapy, 47*(2), 184-186. doi:10.5014/ajot.47.2.184

Crist, P., Muñoz, J. P., Hansen, A., Benson, J., & Provident, I. (2005). The practice-scholar program: An academic–practice partnership to promote the scholarship of "best practices." *Occupational Therapy in Health Care, 19*(1-2), 71-93. doi:10.1300/J003v19n01_06

Davis, J. (2010). Our time is now. *OT Practice, 15*, 14-17.

Diener, E., Emmons, R. A., Larsen, R. J., & Griffin, S. (1985). The Satisfaction With Life Scale. *Journal of Personality Assessment, 49*, 71-75.

Fidler, G. S. (2000). Beyond the therapy model: Building our future. *American Journal of Occupational Therapy, 54*, 99-101. doi:10.5014/ajot.54.1.99

Fidler, G. S., & Fidler, J. W. (1978). Doing and becoming: Purposeful action and self-actualization. *American Journal of Occupational Therapy, 32*, 305-310.

Gahnström-Strandqvist, K., Tham, K., Josephsson, S., & Borell, L. (2000). Actions of competence in occupational therapy practice: A phenomenological study of practice in narrative form. *Scandinavian Journal of Occupational Therapy, 7*(1), 15-25. doi:10.1080/110381200443580

Gray, J. M. (1998). Putting occupation into practice: Occupation as ends, occupation as means. *American Journal of Occupational Therapy, 52*(5), 354-364. doi:10.5014/ajot.52.5.354

Guidetti, S., Asaba, E., & Tham, K. (2009). Meaning of context in recapturing self-care after stroke or spinal cord injury. *American Journal of Occupational Therapy, 63*(3), 323-332. doi:10.5014/ajot.63.3.323

Hocking, C. (2001). Implementing occupation-based assessment. *American Journal of Occupational Therapy, 55*, 463-469. doi:10.5014/ajot.55.4.463

Hoshmand, L. T., & Polkinghorne, D. (1992). Redefining the science–practice relationship and professional training. *American Psychologist, 47*, 55-66. doi:10.1037/0003-066X.47.1.55

Humphry, R., & Thigben-Beck, B. (1997). Caregiver role: Ideas about feeding infants and toddlers. *Occupational Therapy Journal of Research, 17*, 237-264.

Humphry, R., & Wakeford, L. (2006). An occupation-centered discussion of development and implications for practice. *American Journal of Occupational Therapy, 60*(3), 258-267. doi:10.5014/ajot.60.3.258

Jackson, J. (1998). The value of occupation as the core of treatment: Sandy's experience. *American Journal of Occupational Therapy, 52*, 466-473. doi:10.5014/ajot.52.6.466

Kielhofner, G. (1995). A scholarship of practice: Creating discourse between theory, research, and practice. *Occupational Therapy in Health Care, 19*, 7-16.

Kielhofner, G. (2002). *A model of human occupation: Theory and application* (3rd ed.). Baltimore, MD: Lippincott Williams & Wilkins.

Kielhofner, G. (2005). A scholarship of practice: Creating discourse between theory, research and practice. *Occupational Therapy in Health Care, 19*(1-2), 7-16. doi:10.1300/J003v19n01

Lawlor, M. C. (2003). The significance of being occupied: The social construction of childhood occupations. *American Journal of Occupational Therapy, 57*(4), 424-434. doi:10.5014/ajot.57.4.424

Mattingly, C. (1991). The narrative nature of clinical reasoning. *American Journal of Occupational Therapy, 45*(11), 998-1005. doi:10.5014/ajot.45.11.998

Mattingly, C. (1998). *Healing dramas and clinical plots: The narrative structure of experience.* Cambridge, England: Cambridge University Press.

Mattingly, C., & Fleming, M. H. (1994). *Clinical reasoning: Forms of inquiry in a therapeutic practice.* Philadelphia, PA: F.A. Davis.

Molke, D. K., Laliberte Rudman, D., & Polatajko, H. J. (2004). The promise of occupational science: A developmental assessment of an emerging academic discipline. *Canadian Journal of Occupational Therapy, 71*(5), 269-280.

Peloquin, S. M. (1995). The fullness of empathy: Reflections and illustrations. *American Journal of Occupational Therapy, 49*(1), 24-31. doi:10.5014/ajot.49.1.24

Pierce, D. (2001). Occupation by design: Dimensions, therapeutic power, and creative process. *American Journal of Occupational Therapy, 55*, 249-259. doi:10.5014/ajot.55.3.249

Pierce, D. (2003). *Occupation by design: Building therapeutic power.* Philadelphia, PA: F. A. Davis.

Polkinghorne, D. (1995). Narrative configuration in qualitative analysis. *International Journal of Qualitative Studies in Education, 8*, 5-23. doi:10.1080/0951839950080103

Price, P. (2003). *Occupation-centered practice: Providing opportunities for becoming and belonging* (Doctoral dissertation). Retrieved from Dissertation Abstracts International. (UMI No. 3133327)

Price, P. (2008a). [Consideration of occupation in the practices of specialists]. Unpublished raw data.

Price, P. (2008b). Therapeutic relationship. In E. B. Crepeau, E. Cohn, & B.A.B. Schell (Eds.), *Willard and Spackman's occupational therapy* (11th ed., pp. 328-342). Philadelphia, PA: J. B. Lippincott.

Price, P. (2010). [How occupation emerges in practice across settings]. Unpublished raw data.

Price, P. (2011). [How occupation emerges in practices of those who use single modalities]. Unpublished raw data.

Price, P., & Miner, S. (2007). Occupation emerges in the process of therapy. *American Journal of Occupational Therapy, 61*, 441-450. doi:10.5014/ajot.61.4.441

Price, P., & Miner, S. (2009a). Extraordinarily ordinary moments of co-occupation in a neonatal intensive care unit. *OTJR: Occupation, Participation and Health, 29*(2), 72-78. doi:10.3928/15394492-20090301-04

Price, P., & Miner, S. (2009b). Mother becoming: Learning to read Mikala's signs. *Scandinavian Journal of Occupational Therapy, 16*(2), 68-77. doi:10.1080/11038120802409739

Price, P., & Miner Stephenson, S. (2009). Learning to promote occupational development through co-occupation. *Journal of Occupational Science, 16*(3), 180-186. doi:10.1080/14427591.2009.9686660

Reissman, C. K. (1993). *Narrative analysis.* Newbury Park, CA: Sage Publications.

Sherbourne, C. D., & Ware, J. E. (2011, September). SF-36 Health Survey and SF-36v2 Health Survey (SF-36/SF-36v2). Retrieved from http://www.proqolid.org/instruments/sf_36_r_health_survey_and_sf_36v2_health_survey_sf_36_r_sf_36v2

Taylor, R. R., Fisher, G., & Kielhofner, G. (2005). Synthesizing research, education, and practice according to the scholarship of practice model: Two faculty examples. *Occupational Therapy in Health Care, 19*(1-2), 107-122. doi:10.1300/J003v19n01_08

van Maanen, J. (1983). A fact of fiction in organizational ethnography. In J. van Maanen (Ed.), *Qualitative methodology* (pp. 37-53). Beverly Hills, CA: Sage Publications.

Wilcock, A. A. (2005). Occupational science: Bridging occupation and health. *Canadian Journal of Occupational Therapy, 72*(1), 5-12.

Wood, D., Bruner, J., & Ross, G. (1976). The role of tutoring on problem-solving. *Journal of Child Psychology and Psychiatry, 17*, 89-100. doi:10.1111/j.1469-7610.1976.tb00381.x

Yerxa, E. J. (1991). Seeking a relevant, ethical, and realistic way of knowing for occupational therapy. *American Journal of Occupational Therapy, 45*, 199-204. doi:10.5014/ajot.45.3.199

Zemke, R., & Clark, F. (2006). *Occupational science: The evolving discipline.* Philadelphia, PA: F. A. Davis.

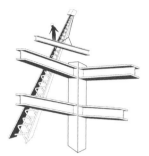

24

Pediatric Therapists' Perceptions of the Dynamics of Occupation-Based Practice

Joanne Phillips Estes, MS, OTR/L and Doris Pierce, PhD, OTR/L, FAOTA

The premise that engagement in occupation supports health and well-being is foundational to occupational therapy (Meyer, 1922/1975). A paradigm shift occurred in the 1940s whereby the profession deviated from this holistic, occupation-based approach and became aligned with a more powerful biomedical model of practice (Jackson, 1998). It was not long after this paradigm shift that professional leaders called for a return to the profession's roots, a call that continues in current literature (Baum, 2000; Pierce, 2003). Though the desire for a return to the centrality of occupation in practice remains strong, a competing pull toward practice aligned with the more culturally dominant medical model has created a tension in the profession (Burke, 2001). Change from biomedical, impairment-driven practice to occupation-based practice has been slow to take hold (Baum, 2000), especially in medical settings (Chisholm, Dolhi, & Schrieber, 2000).

According to Schell (2003), shifts in clinical reasoning would be required to enhance occupation-based practice. Clinical reasoning is defined as a "process used by therapists to plan, direct, perform, and reflect on client care" (Schell, 2003, p. CE-1). It is the mental process used by occupational therapists to make practice decisions in order to provide the best interventions possible. Several modes of clinical reasoning have been identified (Mattingly & Fleming, 1994) and include thought processes associated with both occupation-based practice and medical model practice.

Although increasing in recent years, literature is sparse regarding the dynamics of occupation-based practice and the experiences of therapists in its implementation. Furthermore, there is no research addressing the influence of clinical reasoning on occupation-based practice. This seemed to us a central question for occupational therapy. Thus, our aim in this study was to explore therapists' perceptions of supports and barriers to occupation-based practice in a pediatric medical center.

Literature

Occupation-Based Practice Defined

Although several explanations of aspects of occupation-based practice have been published, a clear and comprehensive definition is lacking (Price & Miner, 2007). At its

Pierce, D. (Ed.).
Occupational Science for Occupational Therapy (pp. 281-290).
© 2014 SLACK Incorporated.

most basic level, occupation-based practice can be defined as "using occupation as the framework for intervention" (Goldstein-Lohman, Kratz, & Pierce, 2003, p. 242). Goldstein-Lohman et al. (2003) went on to note that two conditions for using occupation in practice were that the occupation must be viewed from the client's perspective and that careful attention must be paid to the context of occupations. Gray (1998) referred to occupation-based practice as the application of occupation as a means or as an end of therapy. In other words, occupation can serve as either the intervention modality or as the intervention goal. Though not explicitly defining occupation-based practice, the American Occupational Therapy Association's (AOTA) *Occupational Therapy Practice Framework: Domain and Process, 2nd ed.* (2008), states that occupational therapists help clients perform and this performance leads to participation in valued occupations.

Occupation-Based Practice Research

In 1997, a seminal study documenting the effectiveness of an occupation-based intervention was published in the *Journal of the American Medical Association* (Clark et al., 1997). This randomized controlled trial studied the effectiveness of a 9-month wellness program with three groups of elderly: an occupation-based occupational therapy group, a social group, and a nonintervention group. "Significant benefits for the occupational therapy preventive treatment group were found across various health, function, and quality-of-life domains" (Clark et al., 1997, p. 1321). The authors concluded that an occupation-based intervention was effective in mitigating health risks in older adults.

Goldstein-Lohman et al. (2003) studied two therapists' implementations of occupation-based services in an independent- and assisted-living center for the elderly. The analysis produced five themes: distinguishing among four practice approaches; the therapists' multiple moral contracts; the tension that exists when using both occupation-based and component-focused approaches; working with occupational identity; and using context as intervention. These findings describe the complex dynamics of doing occupation-based practice.

More recently, Wilding and Whiteford (2007) facilitated a participatory action research study about doing occupation-based practice at an acute medical facility in Australia. They concluded that therapists in this setting experienced challenges to engaging in occupation-based practice due to a conflict between philosophical underpinnings of occupation and the more dominant biomedical paradigm. However, the participants in this study were able to make changes toward a more occupation-based practice through collective reflection and a supportive practice community.

Using a single case study approach, Price and Miner (2007) observed one therapist's interventions with a single child and completed in-depth interviews regarding

intervention strategies. The results contributed to the understanding that it is "the interaction of the therapeutic relationship, therapeutic process, and forms of intervention that makes a practice occupation-based" (p. 448). That is, central aspects of occupation-based practice include the therapeutic relationship and creating meanings as part of the therapeutic process (Price & Miner, 2007).

Other recent research about pediatric occupation-based practice focuses on co-occupations between parents and infants/toddlers. Two case studies describe occupation-based practice in a neonatal intensive care unit, a traditionally strong biomedical setting. The therapist in each of these case studies included the infant's mother as a client and focused on the co-occupation of learning to nurture her infant and manage the infant's medical needs as a member of her family (P. Price & Miner, 2009) and the co-occupation of parenting and becoming a family (M. P. Price & Miner, 2009). Another case study described a process of occupational development for a toddler through participation in co-occupations with his mother (Price & Miner Stephenson, 2009).

Clinical Reasoning

Interest in clinical reasoning was stimulated by Rogers' 1983 Slagle Lecture and was further developed by Mattingly and Fleming's (1994) well-known study, funded by the AOTA and American Occupational Therapy Foundation (Leicht & Dickerson, 2001). Mattingly and Fleming (1994) concluded that clinical reasoning involves multiple types of thinking, each level employed for a different purpose, including procedural, conditional, and interactive reasoning.

Procedural reasoning occurs when a therapist decides which treatment activities or intervention procedures he or she could employ to mitigate functional deficits resulting from a patient's disease or condition (Fleming, 1991). This type of reasoning is more impersonal and sequential in nature and can be based on the diagnosis or may reflect the culture of the institution (Schell & Schell, 2008). Interactive reasoning, on the other hand, involves the therapist's knowing of the patient's occupational nature, in order to better align interventions with client concerns, preferences, and interests (Fleming, 1991). Narrative reasoning is similar to interactive reasoning in that the focus is on the client and the impact of his or her condition on occupational performance (Schell & Schell, 2008). Conditional reasoning is used to construct an image of the possible treatment outcome, or "revised condition" (Fleming, 1991, p. 1012).

Pragmatic reasoning is a fourth form of clinical reasoning first identified by Schell and Cervero (1993) and features factors related to context. Contextual factors include issues related to patients as well as those related to the occupational therapist, on both personal and practice levels. Pragmatic reasoning is "used to fit therapy possibilities into the current realities of service delivery" (Schell & Schell, 2008, p. 7), such as available equipment and other resources, reimbursement, time pressures, or departmental culture (Unsworth, 2004).

METHODS

Design

The purpose of the study was to describe therapists' perceptions of supports and barriers to occupation-based practice in a pediatric medical center. The design was qualitative, in the tradition of grounded theory (Bryant & Charmaz, 2007; Strauss & Corbin, 1998). A qualitative approach was used because theories were not readily available to explain the phenomenon and initial description was needed (Creswell, 1998). The intent of grounded theory is to generate a substantive theory that describes aspects of practice at a level of descriptive detail that will be useful to practitioners.

Participants

A purposive sample (Patton, 2002; *N* = 22; 18 females, 4 males) of occupational therapists was recruited from a Midwestern pediatric medical center. Participants' mean experiences as occupational therapists was 9.4 years and mean duration of employment at this facility was 5.3 years. Therapists' caseloads consisted of infants, children, and adolescents with the typical spectrum of conditions seen in pediatric occupational therapy practice. Patients were seen as inpatients and outpatients at the main hospital and at four suburban satellite facilities.

Data Collection and Analysis

Prior to data collection and at the request of the department director, the first author provided an in-service presentation to the occupational therapy staff. The presentation consisted of an overview of occupation-based practice and related concepts, including a definition (Gray, 1998); assessments; the power of occupation (Pierce, 2003); and change theory (Langley, Nolan, Nolan, Norman, & Provost, 1996; Wheatley, 2001). The presentation concluded with an invitation to therapists to participate in the study at a later date.

Ethical approvals from participating institutional review boards were obtained and data collection commenced 15 months following the in-service presentation. Each therapist participated in an individual, semistructured interview lasting an average of 30 to 45 minutes. A schedule of interview questions was used, but therapists were encouraged to diverge into any areas on which they wished to make additional comments. Interviews

were transcribed verbatim, producing 268 double-spaced pages of transcription. Analysis was a collaborative process between the first and second authors, using grounded theory techniques (Figure 24-1).

RESULTS

We discovered six overarching and related themes that describe how this group of pediatric occupational therapists viewed occupation-based practice. These themes are that occupation-based practice expresses professional identity, is rewarding, is more effective, requires certain supports, could be difficult in the clinic, and requires "creativity to adapt."

Expression of Professional Identity Through Occupation-Based Practice

Occupation Is Key to Professional Identity

Intrinsic perceptions of what it means to be an occupational therapist drove the degree to which therapists used an occupation-based practice approach. Nine of the 22 participants indicated that occupation-based practice formed the core of their identity as occupational therapists: "That's what an occupational therapist does. If you're not using occupation then what are you doing? And what's the difference between what you do and what another ... professional is doing?"

Influence of Education on Intervention Approach

Six therapists described the degree to which their educational programs influenced them to practice with a focus on occupation. Academic and fieldwork portions of their professional histories were mentioned as strong influential factors in how they practiced. Some mentioned that their strong training in biomechanical practice prevented them from using an occupation-based approach. Other participants' professional education supported the doing of occupation-based practice. One participant said, "I went to [school name]. It was very occupation-centered. ... It was 'don't be the therapist that sits there and stacks cones.'"

Occupation-Based Practice Is More Rewarding

According to the therapists' interviewed, occupation-based practice was more personally satisfying to them because it is more fun and also more rewarding. One therapist indicated that it was for this reason that she chose a career in occupational therapy. Customizing interventions, being creative, changing and adapting for each child, and

Figure 24-1. Data analysis process.

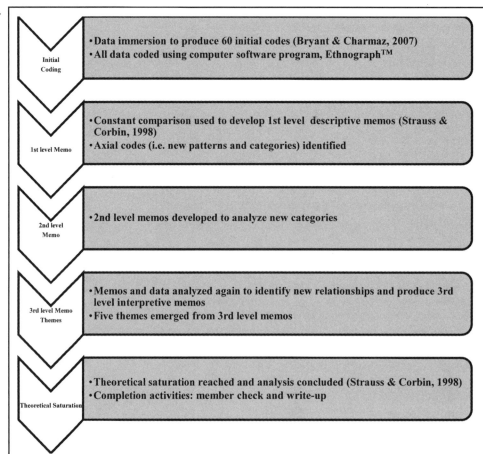

playing with the children made her work as an occupational therapist more interesting.

> I think to really make it occupation-based [in a way] that is meaningful for the child, you really need to think about each child and what the needs are with that child; what's going to motivate that child; what's going to be fun for that child; what's going to be fun for that parent; what's going to be fun for you as a therapist. (Estes & Pierce, 2012)

Six participants also noted that it was rewarding, and therefore motivating, for them to see children progress into engagement in everyday, age-typical activities. It was personally rewarding for therapists to see that the child and parents were happy or excited about progress made in therapy.

> When I … do treatment that's meaningful to them, to the child and to the parent, … it's much more rewarding. They are happier and … more motivated and that to me is more rewarding. And I think that we get better results and I am sure if you try to force them to do things that they don't want to do, we wouldn't [get such good results]. (Estes & Pierce, 2012)

Using an Occupation-Based Approach Is More Effective

Occupation-based practice was considered by many of the therapists in the study to be a better intervention:

12 of the 22 participants specifically stated that it produced more successful outcomes. They attributed the effectiveness of occupation-based practice to its customization, family centeredness, support of client motivation, and stronger generalization.

Because It Is Highly Customized, Occupation-Based Practice Is More Effective

Ten therapists felt that individualization, or customized design, of interventions for each child is a key component of occupation-based practice. To customize treatments, therapists match the child with occupations specifically selected for his or her needs. What works for one child might not work for another. Four participants referred to the ways in which they allowed the child to guide what activities are used in interventions. Six acknowledged the importance of setting aside their own plans for treatment or enfolding those plans into the desired activities of the child in order to maximize results.

> I think OTs have to be creative. … I mean, I think over half of my caseload are kids with sensory processing disorders and I just don't think any of them would be progressing as well if I used the same exact same thing with each one of them. … I really have to be creative. (Estes & Pierce, 2012)

Because Children and Families Value and Understand Occupations, Occupation-Based Practice Is More Family Centered

According to the interviewees, individualization of treatment occurs through a collaborative process between therapists, children, and families. This process is a defining feature of client-centered and family-centered care. The children's and families' goals for therapy usually referred to specific occupations in which they would like the child to be more successful, rather than as improvements in biomechanical, cognitive, or emotional components. Eight participants observed that parents more easily observed progress when they saw improved performance in valued tasks and were able to communicate this progress more easily when they could describe it in terms of everyday activities.

> A lot of times the parent's goal is an occupation and that is what you want to be accomplishing. So why not just work on the occupation and break it down even into its small [steps] … and have them do … what they are wanting to do? (Estes & Pierce, 2012)

Because Children Value and Understand Occupations, Occupation-Based Practice Is More Motivating

Fourteen therapists described how children appear more invested and participate better because customized treatment revolves around occupations that are important to them. As noted by six of the interviewees, the children were more engaged when therapeutic activities were of interest to them, rather than just imposed by the therapist. Some stated that there was no power struggle when occupations were well designed to match the unique occupational nature of each child.

> I think that patients' participation level is better with occupation-based practice. … Between doing therapeutic activities or therapeutic exercise and then switching to an occupation-based activity, I've seen improvements in [range of motion] just because it's more goal oriented than say, you know, "Raise your arms over your head." I've noticed it just because they are not as aware of what they are doing, they are aware of the activity that they are focused on. I feel like it produces better results, greater participation with the patient. (Estes & Pierce, 2012)

Because Families Value and Understand Occupations, Occupation-Based Practice Generalizes Better to Daily Life

According to the therapists interviewed, not only are children more motivated to participate in occupation-based interventions, but so are their families. This multiplies the impact of therapy. Home program implementation was also better when interventions consisted of child/family-centered, valued occupations. Three therapists described the greater ease with which families were able to engage children in home programs tailored to their occupational interests. Four participants also observed that an occupation-based approach made families more successful in implementing the home program. Two participants observed that there was not good follow-through at home if the program consisted of occupations deemed important by the therapist but not by the parents.

> Because I think that motivation is also very key in any child that we are treating, not only the child but the family. If they are not motivated to let the kid do something by themselves, they are not going to practice at home and then working on it once a week is not really going to be effective. Research shows occupation-based practice is more effective. (Estes & Pierce, 2012)

Good Occupation-Based Practice Requires Certain Supports

Participants described three factors that need to be present in order to effectively implement occupation-based practice: good family involvement, mind-shifting to occupation as ends, and creativity to adapt.

Good Family Involvement

Lack of good family involvement actually presents a barrier to high-quality occupation-based practice. Five participants described how difficult it could be to communicate with families about treatment and home programs. It may be difficult for parents to implement the home program due to competing demands for their time. In addition, some parents were not able to attend therapy sessions, requiring the therapist to explain the home program to whoever brought the child to clinic.

Mind-Shifting to Occupation as Ends

Twelve of the therapists reported that, although they used a component-focused approach, they perceived their work as still addressing the occupational needs of the child. This has been described as "occupation as ends" by Gray (1998) and others. For example, strengthening intrinsic hand muscles in preparation for handwriting was a component-focused intervention that was viewed as direct preparation for occupational functioning.

> In my mindset, I use it all the time because I have to know a reason for why I am going to tie it in, in the end, for me. For me, when I am doing an exercise program or if I am doing strengthening and that sort of thing, it's always with the end goal of this is what I am going to be doing it for. (Estes & Pierce, 2012)

The Clinic Can Make Occupation-Based Practice Difficult

Occupation-Based Practice Takes More Time, and Time Is in Short Supply

For the therapists of this study, the biggest barrier to occupation-based practice was time. Twenty of the 22 interviewees stated that occupation-based practice takes longer than component-focused approaches. Interventions must be planned, prepared, implemented, and cleaned up, and time for this is not built into the schedule. This contributed to the perception that it may be more efficient to do less occupation-based interventions.

> I think it goes back to the time. ... You know we have patients back to back. ... We are starting at nine and we are ending at nine fifty-eight and you know, we have got two minutes sometimes to get to the next. (Estes & Pierce, 2012)

The Artificiality of the Clinical Environment Makes Occupation-Based Practice Difficult

Eighteen of the 23 therapists believed that the "artificiality" of the clinic limited occupation-based interventions. Twelve specifically discussed their perceptions that observing the authentic behavior of the child was especially difficult, because the clinic shaped the child's behavior in such a different way than did home or community settings. In a similar vein, enacting a natural occupation or functional behavior in the clinic was also seen as challenging. In the clinic, the problem of concern to the family may not have even been observable, preventing the effective targeting of a solution.

> Even some of my sensory kids, I have parents that come in, they are talking about specific issues that they are seeing at home and I don't see them here because this environment is so different and we are a lot more enclosed and structured. ... We really don't [have a way] to really see what the child is like in their home environment. (Estes & Pierce, 2012)

The clinic environment itself has characteristics that do not support occupation-based practice. Ironically, one participant pointed out that it was a problem that the clinic is designed to elicit the child's most successful performance, in marked contrast to the child's real performance at home or in school.

> Because in a clinic you kind of have it set up a certain way and you can a lot of times prevent certain distractions and things that the kids have at home. So I think it's really important that the parents work with the child and try to use some of the techniques that we educate them on. But a clinic is a clinic. Which then I guess goes back to a little bit of a barrier because it's, you know, a structured setting. (Estes & Pierce, 2012)

Many of the therapists expressed the desire to observe the child in the natural context of school, home, and community. They believed that parental reports of a child's behavior in a natural context did not provide them with the same degree of detailed and relevant information that direct observation does. Participants also felt that they would be able to design more effective interventions if they could see the child in his or her daily life contexts and more accurately identify factors limiting successful performance.

> So I think that it would be interesting too to spend ... a day with some of our clients in their world, like really in their world, and seeing all the little things. They come to

us in the clinic saying, "Oh, they can't get dressed," but you could come up with, if you watched them in their home, maybe five or six other little things that you can give real simple suggestions and that might make them feel much more successful. (Estes & Pierce, 2012)

Lack of Space and Objects Impacts the Quality of Occupation-Based Practice

Spatial issues impacted the implementation of occupation-based practice for 17 of the participants. They described challenges in accessing designated spaces due to crowding (and its influence on patients' behavior) and lack of storage. Participants also voiced a need for additional types of spaces, especially at satellite units. Specific spaces designed for advanced activities of daily living treatment (e.g., cooking, bathing) was desired. Activities had to be simulated, as was noted by four participants. Two participants observed that the treatment space was primarily designed for younger children's play activities, which created a barrier to occupation-based practice with adolescents.

> I would say environment is the biggest barrier. ... If the child is driven to a certain activity during a treatment session, if it's not available, if that space is not available or that equipment is not available due to space, then we are not necessarily going to do that activity that was top on the child's priority list. (Estes & Pierce, 2012)

Although interviewees agreed that toys, equipment, and supplies were plentiful at this facility, there were also problems in terms of object availability. Three therapists found that toys available for use in treatment were usually not appropriate for older children, could be in poor repair, or were often unsuitable for children with greater degrees of impairment. Finally, for those working in patient rooms, access to toys, equipment, and supplies was necessarily difficult.

Occupation-Based Practice Can Be Impeded by the Traditional Medical Culture

Three participants commented that the gatekeeper role of physicians controls access to clients. This could be problematic, due to physicians' lack of knowledge of occupational therapy services, their lack of understanding of the evidence supporting an occupation-based approach, or their writing of referrals that overspecified strictly biomechanical interventions.

Six participants indicated that reimbursement from third-party payers influenced the types of goals they wrote and the interventions they implemented. Two participants noted that limited numbers of reimbursable visits prevented them from targeting desired occupations. Some participants perceived insurance companies as preferring documentation through quantified measures of progress, which they found to be more difficult to provide in regard to a child's occupations than it would be in terms of biomechanical components. Similarly, some found it difficult to write occupation-based goals that they thought would be acceptable to insurance companies because noted improvements might not be reported in quantifiable units of functional performance. Here, one participant who worked with adolescents with emotional and behavioral disorders gives an example.

> [This child] will get mad at me when [I give] a redirection or correction. [He] walked all the way down here [to my office], stood at the door, and turned around and stuck his tongue out at me. … From my standpoint, that was a huge improvement. He didn't go and hit his mom. He did give me the bird, but he knew enough to hide it, and he came back. He got the anger out in an appropriate way. … That's a huge improvement. It's very important to mom. And how do I write a goal for that? (Estes & Pierce, 2012)

Creativity to Adapt

One participant termed her efforts to increase the degree to which she provided occupation-based interventions within the constraints of the clinic as *creativity to adapt*. Other therapists also described the need to create innovative solutions and interventions and to move beyond the opportunities that existed within the clinic environment. They generally expressed that the department's culture supported their creativity in service of an occupation-based approach; 12 stated that they were free to be as creative as they wished. For example, 5 therapists reported taking children to outdoor spaces not formally designated for treatment. Although being outdoors had disadvantages (e.g., weather, safety issues such as geese or cars in parking lot), the advantages of being able to use certain activities (e.g., wheelchair mobility over curbs, playing basketball) was perceived as outweighing the disadvantages.

Treating children confined to their rooms was a situation in which creativity was essential. The environment was adapted as much as was possible. For example, mats were brought in to provide opportunities for floor play. (For infection control, floor play is not allowed, but the mats are sterile.)

> Especially in the ICU, I get made fun of. My kids want to play, they are stuck supine, and they have a halo. … I make tape balls out of wash cloths and tape and we draw on them and we become friends and we can talk about emotions on them, and so I get made fun of for my tape balls, but I think it's an ingenuity thing. (Estes & Pierce, 2012)

CONTRIBUTION TO OCCUPATIONAL SCIENCE

The findings from this study affirm the existence of an additional, more dynamic, and reciprocal relationship between occupational science and occupational therapy.

Occupation is a defining feature of both occupational therapy and occupational science (Molineux, 2010). Occupational science has made occupation the focus of research, and it is up to occupational therapists to apply this knowledge and make occupation the focus of occupational therapy practice (Whiteford, Townsend, & Hocking, 2000). Occupational science and occupational therapy operate under a system of shared values that include the centrality of occupations in health and well-being, the belief that humans actively shape their lives, and a focus on everyday living and on the individual (Clark et al., 1991). Occupational science was initiated to justify and enhance practice (Clark et al., 1991). The influence of occupational science and acceptance of its focus on the centrality of occupation in human functioning is readily apparent in the practice patterns of these participants. Consistent with occupational science, most of these therapists think in occupational terms and view their patients as occupational beings. Their embracing of an occupational perspective on practice affirms occupational science's tenets and research.

Pierce (2003) asserted that in order for the knowledge produced by occupational science to be applied as occupation-based practice, three bridges must be built: a generative discourse regarding occupation-based practice, occupation-based educational programs, and demonstration programs on occupation-based practice. The findings from this study contribute to this generative discourse and can support the further development of educational and demonstration programs that are focused on an occupation-based approach.

IMPLICATIONS FOR PRACTICE

Clinical Reasoning and Occupation-Based Practice

It is apparent from the voices of these therapists that several modes of clinical reasoning are inherently used in occupation-based practice. Specifically, these include procedural, interactive, conditional, and pragmatic reasoning modes. Procedural reasoning, as it was applied in practicing from an occupation base, was more evident in therapists who described mind-shifting to occupation as ends. That is, procedural reasoning was used when therapists thought about the patient's physical condition and component-focused intervention, in terms of how these impacted his or her function (Mattingly & Fleming, 1994). Though therapeutic processes overtly addressed component deficits, the desired end result was improvement in occupational performance.

One important aspect of occupation-based practice was the application of interactive reasoning processes. Interactive reasoning was used to get to know the occupational nature

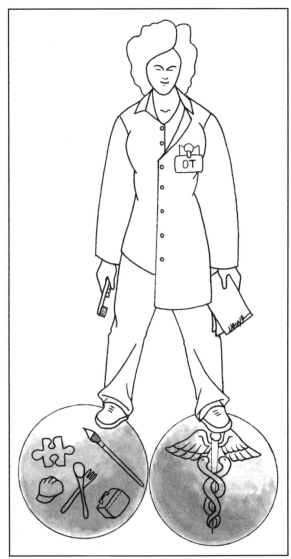

Figure 24-2. Standing in two worlds.

interventions. One therapist even imagined spending a day in the patient's world in order to better understand his or her needs and to provide more effective intervention.

Therapists' descriptions of the realities and limitations of doing occupation-based practice in a medical center clinic are pragmatic reasoning processes. Pragmatic reasoning addresses the impact of factors external to the therapist–patient relationship (Schell & Schell, 2008). Pragmatic issues challenging occupation-based practice in this study included physical space, limited resources (i.e., time, space, objects), and the traditional medical culture.

Standing in Two Worlds

Beyond clinical reasoning, these findings also serve as affirmation for therapists who are experiencing the same rewards and challenges of occupation-based practice. Participants in this study experienced the tensions of standing between two worlds in wanting to practice the ideal (i.e., occupation-based practice) within the realities of a clinic-based, medical model practice (Figure 24-2). The self-reinforcing supports of occupation-based practice promote the desire to practice in accordance with this holistic model despite the impediments inherent in clinic practice.

Enhancing Occupation-Based Practice

Finally, this study's findings can be especially useful in guiding improvements to occupation-based practice. Therapists can use these results as a springboard for shared problem solving, in order to influence institutional policies and procedures and promote changes that would strengthen the occupation base of their practice. Creative changes in space design, object choice, and practice management strategies could support occupation-based interventions. A forum for sharing daily experiences of the rewards, perceived effectiveness, child and family centeredness, and creativity of occupation-based practice could improve support to therapists who aspire to excellent occupation-based practice.

and everyday experiences of the client so that intervention could be more individually tailored to meet his or her needs (Mattingly & Fleming, 1994). As noted previously, customizing interventions made therapists' work more enjoyable. Because customized intervention was more meaningful to patients and families, it also served to motivate better participation in therapy, thus producing more successful outcomes. Getting to know the patient and collaborating with him or her along with his or her family was the essence of client-centered and family-centered intervention.

Conditional reasoning was used when therapists considered their patients' needs as they existed within a real-life context (Mattingly & Fleming, 1994). Therapists in this study identified understanding their patients' natural contexts as a factor important to the therapeutic process. That is, they observed that the artificiality of the clinic environment impeded more authentic, and hence more effective,

Learning Supports

Ethical Reflections on Occupation-Based Practice

Purpose

Provide an opportunity for critical reflection on how occupation-based practice is ethical practice.

Primary Concepts

Ethical reasoning.

Instructions

1. Form small groups of three or four students.

2. On an individual basis, each student will brainstorm for 5 to 10 minutes a defense of occupation-based practice as ethical practice and include references to the AOTA's ethics documents to support his or her argument.

3. After everyone has completed brainstorming, discuss what each person has written.

4. As a group, compile a list of the top three reasons why occupation-based practice is ethical practice and include supportive references.

Occupation-Based Practice Versus Medical Model Practice

Purpose

Provide an opportunity to critically examine the benefits of occupation-based practice.

Primary Concepts

Theoretical concepts about the doing of occupation-based practice.

Instructions

1. Read the following case study:

You are beginning a third Level II fieldwork rotation at a pediatric hospital. Your supervisor, Joan, has approximately 25 years of experience and strongly believes in a medical model approach to treatment. You observe her treating Tommy, an 8-year-old child with developmental motor coordination disorder. Treatment activities consist of skipping along a line, stacking cones, and stringing beads. Tommy looks bored, constantly asks why he is doing these activities, and complains about having to come to therapy. Joan then asks you to develop a treatment plan for Tommy. Your treatment plan consists of doing occupations that Tommy and his mother have said he enjoys. Joan reads your treatment plan and then asks you to redo it, stating, "This isn't therapy."

2. Reflect on the following questions:

   ○ What is your initial (internal) response to Joan's directive?

   ○ What strategy will you use to respond to Joan (e.g., cite literature, describe your observations, others)?

   ○ Compose a list of five arguments to defend your position.

What Research Will You Do Next?

Purpose

Understand the experience of designing research and promote occupation-based practice research.

Primary Concepts

Research methods.

Instructions

1. Form small groups of three to four students.

2. As a group, develop an answer to each of the following questions, being sure that you discuss a rationale for each.

   ○ What is the purpose of the study and why have you chosen this purpose?

   ○ What is your research question?

   ○ What type of design (i.e., qualitative or quantitative) will you use?

   ○ Describe who your participants will be.

   ○ What data will you collect?

How Will You Practice?

Purpose

To reflect upon how this chapter has influenced your thinking about best practice in occupational therapy.

Primary Concepts

Occupation-based practice theory.

Instructions

Reflect in writing upon the findings of this study. Describe how they will influence your practice as an occupational therapist. What will you make sure you do when treating patients? What will you make sure you do not do? What are characteristics of the ideal treatment setting?

References

American Occupational Therapy Association. (2008). Occupational therapy practice framework: Domain and process (2nd ed.). *American Journal of Occupational Therapy, 62*, 625-683.

Baum, C. (2000, January 3). Occupation-based practice: Reinventing ourselves for the new millennium. *OT Practice*, pp. 12-15.

Bryant, A., & Charmaz, C. (2007). *The Sage handbook of grounded theory.* Thousand Oaks, CA: Sage Publications.

Burke, J. (2001). How therapists' conceptual perspectives influence early intervention evaluations. *Scandinavian Journal of Occupational Therapy, 8*, 49-61.

Chisholm, D., Dolhi, C., & Schrieber, J. (2000, January 3). Creating occupation-based practice in a medical model clinical practice setting. *OT Practice, 5*, CE-1-CE-8.

Clark, F., Azen, S. P., Zemke, R., Jackson, J., Carlson, M., Mandel, D., . . . Lipson, L. (1997). Occupational therapy for independent-living older adults: A randomized controlled trial. *Journal of the American Medical Association, 278*(16), 1321-1326.

Clark, F. A., Parham, D., Carlson, M. E., Frank, G., Jackson, J., Pierce, D., . . . Zemke, R. (1991). Occupational science: Academic innovation in the service of occupational therapy's future. *American Journal of Occupational Therapy, 45*(4), 300-309.

Creswell, J. (1998). *Qualitative inquiry and research design: Choosing among five traditions.* Thousand Oaks, CA: Sage Publications.

Estes, J., & Pierce, D. E. (2012). Pediatric therapists' perspectives on occupation-based practice. *Scandinavian Journal of Occupational Therapy, 19,* 17-25.

Fleming, M. (1991). The therapist with the three-track mind. *American Journal of Occupational Therapy, 45*(11), 1007-1014.

Goldstein-Lohman, H., Kratz, A., & Pierce, D. (2003). A study of occupation-based practice. In D. Pierce (Ed.) *Occupation by design: Building therapeutic power* (pp. 239-261). Philadelphia, PA: F.A. Davis.

Gray, J. (1998). Putting occupation into practice: Occupation as ends, occupation as means. *American Journal of Occupational Therapy, 52*(5), 354-364.

Jackson, J. (1998). The value of occupation as the core of treatment: Sandy's experience. *American Journal of Occupational Therapy, 52,* 466-473.

Langley, G., Nolan, K., Nolan, T., Norman, C., & Provost, L. (1996). *The improvement guide: A practical approach to enhancing organizational performance.* San Francisco, CA: Jossey-Bass.

Leicht, S., & Dickerson, A. (2001). Clinical reasoning, looking back. *American Journal of Occupational Therapy, 14*(3/4), 105-130.

Mattingly, C., & Fleming, M. (1994). *Clinical reasoning: Forms of inquiry in a therapeutic practice.* Philadelphia, PA: F. A. Davis.

Meyer, A. (1922/1975). The philosophy of occupational therapy. *American Journal of Occupational Therapy, 31*(10), 639-642.

Molineux, M. (2010). Occupational science and occupational therapy: Occupation at center stage. In C. Christiansen & E. Townsend (Eds.), *Introduction to occupation: The art and science of living* (2nd ed., pp. 359-383). Upper Saddle River, NJ: Pearson.

Patton, M. (2002). *Qualitative research and evaluation methods* (3rd ed.). Thousand Oaks, CA: Sage Publications.

Pierce, D. (2003). How can the occupation base of occupational therapy be strengthened? *Australian Occupational Therapy Journal, 50,* 1-2.

Price, M. P., & Miner, S. (2009). Mother becoming: Learning to read Mikala's signs. *Scandinavian Journal of Occupational Therapy, 16,* 68-77.

Price, P., & Miner, S. (2007). Occupation emerges in the process of therapy. *American Journal of Occupational Therapy, 61,* 441-450.

Price, P., & Miner, S. (2009). Extraordinarily ordinary moments of co-occupation in a neonatal intensive care unit. *OTJR: Occupation, Participation, and Health, 29*(2), 72-78.

Price, P., & Miner Stephenson, S. (2009). Learning to promote occupational development through co-occupation. *Journal of Occupational Science, 16*(3), 180-186.

Rogers, J. C. (1983). Eleanor Clarke Slagle Lectureship—1983. Clinical reasoning: The ethics, science and art. *American Journal of Occupational Therapy, 37*(9), 601-616.

Schell, B. (2003, October 6). Clinical reasoning and occupation-based practice. *OT Practice, 8,* CE-1-CE-8.

Schell, B., & Cervero, R. (1993). Clinical reasoning in occupational therapy: An integrative review. *American Journal of Occupational Therapy, 47,* 605-610.

Schell, B., & Schell, J. (2008). *Clinical and professional reasoning in occupational therapy.* Philadelphia, PA: Lippincott Williams & Wilkins.

Strauss, A., & Corbin, J. (1998). *Basics of qualitative research: Techniques and procedures for developing grounded theory* (2nd ed.). Thousand Oaks, CA: Sage Publications.

Unsworth, C. (2004). Clinical reasoning: How do pragmatic reasoning, worldview, and client centeredness fit? *British Journal of Occupational Therapy, 67*(1), 10-19.

Wheatley, M. (2001). *Leadership and the new science: Discovering order in a chaotic world.* San Francisco, CA: Berrett-Koehler Publishers.

Whiteford, G., Townsend, E., & Hocking, C. (2000). Reflections on a renaissance of occupation. *Canadian Journal of Occupational Therapy, 67*(1), 61-69.

Wilding, C., & Whiteford, G. (2007). Occupation and occupational therapy: Knowledge paradigms and everyday practice. *Australian Occupational Therapy Journal, 54,* 185-193.

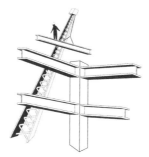

25

Developing an Integrated Occupational Science Research Program
The USC Well Elderly and Pressure Ulcer Prevention Studies

Florence A. Clark, PhD, OTR/L, FAOTA; Jeanne Jackson, PhD, OTR, FAOTA; and
Elizabeth A. Pyatak, PhD, OTR/L

The discipline of occupational science has, since its inception, navigated the borderlands between the social and biological sciences and between the academic discipline and the profession of occupational therapy (Clark & Lawlor, 2008). Entering such uncharted territories naturally involves diverging opinions on how best to traverse them. This chapter will trace four controversies that arose regarding the development of occupational science and the nature of its relationship to occupational therapy. In doing so, it will simultaneously illustrate the approach the authors and the investigative teams with which they have been associated have taken in resolving these concerns through the process of building an integrated research program. We will also proffer a translational research blueprint that evolved organically in the course of building our research programs, which incorporates both basic and applied components as well as qualitative and quantitative methodologies. This blueprint contin-

ues to guide our research efforts today. Its eight steps were followed as we successfully grew our extramurally funded National Institutes of Health (NIH) research program aimed at translating basic science with a focus on occupation and everyday living into cost-effective occupational therapy intervention approaches. These research programs demonstrate how occupational science is a "science of everyday living" that can enable the building of theoretical knowledge as well as its translation into evidence-based therapeutic applications. In our presentation of these studies we illustrate how our engagement in this research required us to effectively manage these tensions. We did not have the luxury of approaching them as merely abstract issues; rather, these were real-world tensions that were ultimately resolved or rendered irrelevant through our development of occupational science-informed research programs.

Pierce, D. (Ed.).
Occupational Science for Occupational Therapy (pp. 291-309).
© 2014 SLACK Incorporated.

Literature

The Four Polemics: Debates on Approaches to Occupational Science Research

Technically, the first occupational science PhD programs were established by the 1990s in the United States at the University of Southern California (USC) and in Australia at the University of South Australia (Wilcock, 1991; Yerxa et al., 1989). However, it was the debates surrounding its development that were being ignited primarily in the American occupational therapy community that influenced the directions our research would take. At USC, occupational science had been described at its onset as a basic science focused on the organization and transmission of basic knowledge on occupation but as also supporting and maintaining a close relationship with the profession of occupational therapy (Clark et al., 1991; Yerxa et al., 1989). Questions soon arose in the United States regarding the relationship between the discipline of occupational science and the profession of occupational therapy and the appropriate roles and contributions of the discipline and profession in relation to one another. Specifically, tensions flared up regarding the following concerns: (a) whether the science should undertake basic or applied research, (b) the types of methodologies that were appropriate to adopt for its research, (c) the relative advantages of focusing on well populations or people who have illnesses and/or disabilities, and (d) the question of how occupational science research could satisfy practitioners' growing need for evidence to support the practice of occupational therapy.

The Basic Versus Applied Science Controversy

The question of whether occupational science should undertake basic or applied research sharply divided scholars, particularly because it had implications for resource allocation. Central to this debate was the issue of whether occupational science should exist as a wholly separate entity from occupational therapy, unconcerned and indeed barred from considering the clinical implications of its research, or should maintain a relationship through which occupational science would develop not only foundational theoretical knowledge on occupation but insights that would inform therapeutic processes and techniques. One school of thought led by Mosey (1992, 1993) argued that occupational science and occupational therapy should be completely partitioned from one another. In this view, the discipline of occupational science would exclusively provide basic research and theory building without regard for the therapeutic applicability of its research findings. In contrast, the profession of occupational therapy would

solely focus on conducting applied research directly related to clinical practice and on drawing from the social and biological sciences (including but not limited to the nascent science of occupation) for its knowledge base. Beyond this, it argued for a total separation of resources (both financial and personnel), theoretical approaches, and research methodologies. The rationale to justify this division was that the discipline and profession had different aims and responsibilities and should pursue their work independently, precluding the dual risks of occupational science developing an "unhealthy dependence" (Mosey, 1992, p. 852) on occupational therapy and of its research pursuits being ill-conceived or unfocused as a result of combining both basic and applied scientific inquiry. Consistent with this view, Mosey opined that the two research approaches were dichotomous and could not be incorporated within a single study without detracting from its scientific rigor.

This perspective was countered by scholars at USC, who argued that a complete partitioning of occupational science from occupational therapy would be harmful to both the discipline and the profession (Carlson & Dunlea, 1995; Clark et al., 1993). They viewed Mosey's proposed division of labor as a false dichotomy unnecessarily restricting occupational scientists from conducting research with potential practical application in therapeutic contexts. If the work of conducting basic and applied research was strictly allocated to the discipline and profession, respectively, there was a danger of producing theory of limited or no relevance to practice and of practice stagnating because of a paucity of new theoretical frameworks to guide it. These authors made the case that the spectrum of basic versus applied research is continuous rather than dichotomous and that studies could contain components of both, thus conserving resources and enhancing scholarly productivity without compromising the results or implications of either.

Scholars at USC also argued that, although the research of other disciplines in the social and biological sciences did produce insights useful to occupational therapy, there existed no integrated corpus of knowledge on occupation. They asserted that a science of occupation, with the study of humans as occupational beings as its core area of concern, would yield more coherent and directly applicable information for occupational therapy, strengthening the profession's identity and stimulating innovations in its practice (Parham, 1998). In fact, by 1996, proponents of this school of thought were describing occupational science as interlinked with occupational therapy, focusing on occupation in all contexts including therapeutic contexts, and as encompassing basic and applied research (Zemke & Clark, 1996).

Appropriate Methodologies

The second debate that arose with the founding of occupational science was concerned with the methodologies that were appropriate for its research. It should be noted that this debate predates advances in research methodology that allow for more sophisticated management of complex variables and the current emphasis on translational science, which renders the methodological debate somewhat obsolete. The scientific climate at the time was one of reductionism, which heavily favored positivistic or quantitative approaches. However, naturalistic or qualitative approaches including narrative, life history, ethnography, and phenomenological analysis were gaining recognition as valid and relevant means of obtaining information on the meaning and interpretation of human experience, subject matter that cannot be easily reduced to quantifiable variables. The appropriateness of using quantitative methods to answer questions within the humanistic field of occupational science, which seeks to understand the whole person in interaction with the environment within the stream of time rather than the health or pathology of individual body systems, was questioned, most notably by Yerxa (1991). Yerxa (1991) recommended that researchers studying occupation employ qualitative methods, which have the capacity to deal with this complexity, rather than quantitative approaches, which typically reduce occupation to decontextualized variables, potentially resulting in a distorted or inaccurate view of the subject of study. Further, she argued that qualitative approaches were more congruent with our ethical commitment, stemming from our roots in occupational therapy, to individuals living with chronic disease or disability, whose perspectives were typically undervalued or silenced entirely under positivistic paradigms.

Duchek and Thessing (1996) challenged this view, questioning whether qualitative methods (specifically singling out narrative and life history approaches) were adequate in meeting the research objectives of occupational therapy and whether sufficient funding existed to support research employing qualitative methods. They argued that qualitative studies are deficient in meeting the totality of occupational therapy's research needs because they lack the power to predict and control variables and thereby test the outcomes of interventions. Duchek and Thessing (1996) further asserted that those in positions of power within funding agencies value positivist approaches and view naturalistic inquiry as suspect. In order to advance the status of occupational science as an academic discipline, they maintained that we should conform to the expectations of the traditional scientific community and engage in quantitative research to gain extramural funding and the respect it engenders.

This view was disputed by Clark, Carlson, and Polkinghorne (1997), who provided evidence of the growing interest of extramural granting agencies in funding qualitative research. For example, Boundary Crossings, a longitudinal ethnographic study examining cross-cultural health care encounters headed by Mary Lawlor and Cheryl Mattingly, had just been awarded a $688,894 grant from the

Maternal and Child Health Bureau (MCH). This research program would go on to attract a total of $5,481,459 in federal funding through the MCH and the NIH. They further noted that, as a multidisciplinary science pursuing diverse research questions, occupational science should draw from multiple methodologies congruent with the aims of the studies being conducted, including both qualitative and quantitative approaches where appropriate. This perspective, foregrounding the research question as the key factor in determining which methods to utilize, is consistent with the conclusions previously reached by Carlson and Clark (1991) and Ottenbacher (1992) with regard to the methodology debate.

Populations and Evidence of Practice Efficacy

The remaining two polemics surrounding the development of occupational science were closely intertwined: namely, the concern with whether its research should focus on people living with chronic disease or disability versus the well population and the issue of whether occupational science could meet occupational therapy practitioners' growing need for evidence to support the efficacy of their practice. The political issue at hand within these debates was the extent to which occupational science should address the immediate need of occupational therapy practitioners for evidence supporting their intervention approaches versus attending to the broader task of developing a generic theory on occupation that contributes to the universe of knowledge. The first approach would maximize the discipline's ability to respond to pressing concerns and policy issues relevant to the profession. The second, by accruing scientific capital, could fortify the profession's future by securing its foothold in academia where, at the time, basic research tended to be appropriated greater value than applied research. Finally, if occupational science broadened its focus to include the general public as well as individuals with chronic diseases or disability, it was clear that its relevance would extend to new stakeholders. However, inherent in taking this course was the danger that occupational science would ultimately neglect to adequately address significant concerns of the populations the profession had traditionally served.

Shades of these debates were present in the tensions surrounding whether occupational science should pursue basic or applied research, notably in the concern that occupational science would poach scarce resources needed by occupational therapy to conduct applied research on its interventions (Mosey, 1992). However, these debates are distinct from one another in that the basic versus applied research debate questioned the relationship between occupational science and occupational therapy, whereas this debate centered on whether the very existence of occupational science as an academic discipline was justified, versus a science of occupational therapy that would serve as the disciplinary foundation of the practice profession. Kielhofner (2002a) took up this issue in his keynote address to the World Federation of Occupational Therapists, arguing that devoting resources to developing the discipline of occupational science is unwise because the generation of knowledge about occupation is unlikely to translate into improved occupational therapy practice, at a time in which society is demanding such improvements and evidence of the efficacy of occupational therapy. Asserting that "the growth of such knowledge in the field has not led to an identifiable renaissance in occupation-based practice" (Kielhofner, 2005, p. 237), he proposed the alternative model of a scholarship of practice in which knowledge emerges from occupational therapy practice (Kielhofner, 2002b). In this approach, academics, practitioners, and consumers work together in a participatory model of research, with the idea that knowledge generated from within a specific practice context would be more readily translated than improvements to occupational therapy practice more generally.

We do not dispute the potential of the scholarship of practice approach in generating new and important insights for occupational therapy practice. However, the research programs we describe in this chapter provide solid evidence to make explicit an "identifiable renaissance in occupation-based practice" (Kielhofner, 2005, p. 237). First, through these studies we will demonstrate that occupational science is not diverting resources from occupational therapy research and practice. Second, our studies illustrate that the underlying assumption that knowledge about the nature of human occupation cannot readily translate into the application of occupation as a therapeutic modality is patently untrue. The founders of occupational science have repeatedly asserted that their intent was not to develop a "pure" science wholly divorced from and unconcerned with issues related to occupational therapy practice (Clark & Lawlor, 2008; Yerxa et al., 1989; Zemke & Clark, 1996); in fact, we consider the concept of a scholarship of practice to be a solid type of occupational science with much clinical utility.

Moreover, when we take the broader range of occupational science work into account beyond our own studies, we would argue that the threats with which Kielhofner was concerned have not been borne out in the years hence. First, an analysis of the first decade of occupational science research determined that its three primary research directions were the following:

1. Identifying the nature of occupation

2. Investigating how occupations are experienced and enacted

3. Determining the relationship of occupation to health, quality of life, and other outcome variables (Hocking, 2000)

Second, studies such as the USC Well Elderly Studies outlined in this chapter have demonstrated the utility of research inclusive of both disabled and well populations. Finally, the very existence of this edited book as a whole, aimed at providing occupational therapy students and professionals with occupational science research addressing contemporary practice concerns, is evidence that occupational science continues to honor its initial commitment to generate knowledge relevant to occupational therapy.

As our research program grew, these four polemics permeated the zeitgeist to varying degrees depending on the decade. Although it would be disingenuous to claim that we had set out with a preconceived plan to explicitly redress these tensions, over the course of the past two decades, albeit inadvertently, we found ways to resolve them. Instead of choosing between basic and applied research, we conducted hybrids—with elements of both. Rather than selecting qualitative or quantitative methods, our studies blended them, which ultimately created coherence and efficiencies that optimized the science. Although we conducted a large-scale randomized controlled trial on a public health population without disability, we are currently focusing our research on adults with spinal cord injury, a group for which occupational therapists have traditionally been service providers. In addition, our studies have demonstrated how basic science on occupation can be explicitly used to create innovative, theoretically driven, occupational therapy interventions. Finally, to meet the most pressing concerns of therapists today, we have completed outcome and cost-effectiveness studies pertaining to these interventions.

In the end, within the context of our research programs, we have been able to work through the polemics that had emerged. In the new process, a new occupational therapy intervention, which we call Lifestyle Redesign, was manualized (Figure 25-1). Through discussions with our colleagues in light of our respective research programs, a fresh conceptualization of occupational science as "the science of everyday living" began to be embraced. This conceptualization dispossesses a strict separation of occupational science from occupational therapy. It views the discipline as focused on deepening our understanding of the everyday lives of people, furnishing basic knowledge to guide the development of innovative treatment approaches, and providing solid evidence of the efficacy, effectiveness, and cost effectiveness of innovative occupational therapy interventions.

SEQUENCE OF STUDIES

The Seeds of Lifestyle Redesign: The Penny Richardson Study

In 1992, the first author of this chapter was named the Eleanor Clarke Slagle Lecturer for the American Occupational Therapy Association. Preparation for the lectureship, which would take place in 1993, required a

1988	First submission of proposal to University of Southern California Graduate School for a PhD Program in Occupational Science
1989	Second submission of proposal to University of Southern California Graduate School for a PhD Program in Occupational Science approved; Commencement of PhD Program
1990	Florence Clark attends workshop at Key West sponsored by AHCPR to train allied health researchers in developing federal research grants
1992-1993	Penny Richardson study undertaken in preparation for Florence Clark's Eleanor Clarke Slagle lecture
1993	Journal of Occupational Science launched at the University of South Australia; becomes a joint publication of the University of South Australia, the Auckland University of Technology, and USC
1993	Formation of Well Elderly Research Team
1994-1998	First USC Well Elderly Study: *"The Effectiveness of Two Occupational Therapy Treatments for the Elderly"* (NIH #R01 AG11810)
2000-2004	Pressure Ulcer Prevention Study: *"Daily Living Context and Pressure Sores in Consumers with Spinal Cord Injury"* (DOE/NIDRR #H133G000062)
2004-2010	Second USC Well Elderly Study: Health Mediating Effects of the Well Elderly Program (NIH # 5R01AG021108-04)
2008-2013	Lifestyle Redesign® for Pressure Ulcer Prevention in SCI Study (LR-PUPS) (NIH # 5R01HD057152-02)

Figure 25-1. Key events in the Lifestyle Redesign research programs.

year of research. She now refers to this research as the Penny Richardson Study, an in-depth case study of a stroke survivor. The first of her research programs she formally designated as occupational science, it also led to her conceptualization of occupational therapy as a life design process. Inadvertently, however, it also gave rise to preliminary stands with respect to the four polemics previously discussed, which were becoming more contentious in the occupational therapy professional community at the time. Publications on the basic versus applied debate were appearing in the *American Journal of Occupational Therapy* (Clark et al., 1993; Mosey, 1992, 1993), following forums at professional meetings at which clashing perspectives had been presented. Similarly, two key papers addressing

appropriate research methodologies for occupational science appeared in the literature (Ottenbacher, 1992; Yerxa, 1991). In undertaking the Penny Richardson Study, the first author hoped to resolve these tensions.

Further, the study was designed to be responsive to another emerging strand in occupational therapy practice that was gaining popularity—interest in narrative. A now classic paper had just been published in the *American Journal of Occupational Therapy* by Cheryl Mattingly (1991), based on her doctoral dissertation work in which she studied the clinical reasoning of occupational therapists. Her in-depth qualitative analysis revealed the complex ways in which occupational therapists employed narrative in clinical encounters to move patients into future lives they hoped to gain. The first author of this chapter admired and was influenced by this work but was unsure how it could be explicitly related to occupational science. She hoped that the Penny Richardson Study would foreground how occupation per se played out in recovery narratives. If, in fact, it was central, narrative would be better situated within the conceptual boundaries of occupational science. At the time, narrative theory was gaining momentum across several social sciences and the first author aimed to clarify how an occupational science approach to narrative would be distinctive.

To tackle these concerns head on, the first author set out to describe the ways in which the childhood occupations of Penny Richardson were influential in character development, stroke recovery, and the subsequent reclaiming of self after catastrophic disability. More specifically, the study was aimed at illustrating (a) the usefulness of narrative inquiry focused on occupation as a research method for occupational science; (b) the centrality of one's childhood occupational experiences for securing future possibilities; (c) the unique contribution that occupational science could make when focused on disability concerns; and, most important, (d) the importance of occupational science for furthering occupational therapy.

The study methodology entailed conducting nine interviews totaling 20 hours as well as employing participant observation while taking several excursions into the community. All interviews were recorded, transcribed, and analyzed over a 9-month period. With respect to the original aims, the findings illustrated that a research approach called *narrative analysis*, through which life histories are constructed based on qualitative data, could be particularly useful for providing complex understandings of the ways in which experience in childhood occupations could be recycled to positively influence recovery from stroke. They also demonstrated that when focused on disability concerns, occupational science provided a unique lens through which to understand rehabilitation processes, community reintegration, and the production of therapeutic outcomes. Finally, they showed that even at the most basic level of simply creating a more in-depth understanding of patients and their everyday living experiences, occupational science had the potential to enrich occupational therapy.

However, the resulting publications based on this study (Clark, 1993; Clark, Ennevor, & Richardson, 1996) revealed that the findings had unanticipated implications beyond the four previously listed aims. An unforeseen and stunning finding was that this in-depth case study spawned a new intervention approach focused on the intersection of life design, occupation, reflection, and experience. What became clear as the study progressed and the data were analyzed was that engagement in the interview process became, in and of itself, therapeutic, a springboard for the ways in which the participant would go on to redesign her life using occupations as the building blocks. As Penny Richardson described this process, the interviews became opportunities to put her concerns into words, reflect on them, and transmute them into intentions. Typically, this process resulted in emerging plans for the things she would subsequently do to accelerate her recovery and to be better able to deal with the situations that threatened her emotional and physical well-being. The plans incorporated carefully thought-out strategies for pushing her recovery forward and for establishing healthier daily routines within the context of her overall life, where she worked, played, and socialized. For example, having been too embarrassed to be seen in public with a rubber-handled stainless steel cane, she replaced it with a carved wooden one with a marble handle and was thereby liberated to venture out. Having refrained from attending meetings at her condominium because she would become depressed when no one seemed to notice the progress she was making in her recovery, she mastered an approach for evoking positive comments on her successes from others. Having been reluctant to work at improving her mobility, she was able to muster the required effort to develop her capacity in this area once she framed the activities that would promote it as "cane-hiking," recycling a word that echoed an occupation she had loved in the past.

This innovative therapeutic approach, involving a combination of interviews (talking) and action (doing), was described as occupational storytelling and occupational storymaking. Technically, occupational storytelling was defined as a process through which the therapist encourages the stroke survivor to examine the ways in which his or her experience of occupational engagement up to the time of injury or illness had shaped his or her character and was influencing the recovery process. In using it, therapists could come to better understand the motivational systems of their clients. Alternatively, in occupational storymaking, the survivor uses this process of reflection to subsequently become more engaged in occupation to further his or her recovery. The publications that describe this overall approach emphasize collaboration between the therapist and client, through which they develop a shared understanding regarding the future the patient wishes to secure. Additionally, analysis of interview transcripts from the Penny Richardson Study revealed that therapists employing this approach need to master a set of techniques that includes listening carefully, developing empathy, including the ordinary, evoking insights, story analysis and synthesis, occupational coaching, cultural sensitivity, and internalizing a broadened view of activities of daily living (Clark et al., 1996).

Although it built on traditional occupational therapy practice, this intervention approach also broadened it, seeding the conceptualization of occupational therapy as a design process. Implicitly, it required that therapists shift their concentration from discrete occupations about which clients felt passionately to the wider screen that captured ever-changing and diverse life situations, some of which threatened psychosocial, emotional, or physical well-being. The focus was on how patients or clients lived out each day in mutable and culturally contingent circumstances. The design process could entail such components as modifications to the environment, provision or replacement of equipment, formulation of plans for offsetting threats, recycling childhood occupations in more mature formats, and a wide range of other approaches for creating a better person–context fit.

In the end, the Penny Richardson Study demonstrated that both basic and applied research questions could be synergistically addressed within the context of the same study; that occupational science could bring a unique perspective for understanding the everyday emotional, social, and physical challenges of people with disability; that narrative analysis was a powerful method for generating theory on occupation; and, finally, that basic qualitative research (even as circumscribed as one case study) was a potent mechanism for developing theory-driven intervention approaches for the profession of occupational therapy.

The USC Well Elderly Studies— The Emergence and Refinement of the Blueprint for Translational Research and the First Lifestyle Redesign Research Program

The Penny Richardson Study, with its interconnected basic and applied elements, was a precursor to the emergence of the overarching translational research program in occupational science that has since been established at USC. Translational research is defined by the NIH as research that translates the results of basic science into effective treatments. Recently, it has been designated as central to the NIH's mission and, consequently, robust funding streams have been established to support "a stronger research infrastructure" that will "accelerate this critical part of the clinical research enterprise" (NIH, 2009). Arguably, to the extent that basic qualitative research on childhood occupation was applied to develop the occupational storytelling and storymaking intervention approach, the Penny Richardson Study can be labeled translational research, albeit in nascent form according to this definition.

In the next sequence of studies overseen by the first two authors, generically called the USC Well Elderly Research Program, we built on insights garnered through the Penny Richardson Study. Staying on course, we continued to make our way out of the polemics by launching a research program that incorporated basic and applied elements, a mix of qualitative and quantitative methodologies, and the translation of basic research findings (in this case, of the occupational needs of diverse older people living independently) into an effective intervention (now called Lifestyle Redesign). However, we realized that as we implemented the various steps in this research program we were fol-

lowing a sequence that could be depicted in a figure for use by others. With considerable input from Mary Lawlor and other USC faculty, this figure, entitled the "Blueprint for Translational Research," was first published in *Willard and Spackman's Occupational Therapy, 11th ed.* (Clark & Lawlor, 2008). The Blueprint has recently been further refined for publication as Figure 25-2 in this chapter. Today, it continues to guide the USC Division of Occupational Science and Occupational Therapy research enterprise and is most completely illustrated through the USC Well Elderly Research Program.

The First USC Well Elderly Research Study (Blueprint Steps 1 Through 5)

In Step 1, we identify the problem to be worked on. In the early 1990s, the National Institute on Aging (NIA) had identified three priority areas:

1. Prevention

2. Low-income elders

3. Ethnic diversity

Coincidentally, at this time, the first author of this chapter had attended a U.S. Agency for Health Care Policy Research (AHCPR; now renamed the Agency for Healthcare Research and Quality) workshop, the purpose of which was to train allied health professionals in the steps for obtaining NIH and AHCPR funding. Convened in response to an initiative sponsored by Senator Inouye of Hawaii who, having been injured in World War II, was a recipient of rehabilitation services, its aim was to ensure that more research funding was appropriated to physical and occupational therapy scientists. Upon her return from the workshop, the first author was determined to secure funding and organized a team to develop a grant addressing the above NIA priority areas.

This grant was awarded virtually concurrent with the completion of the Penny Richardson Study, with the first author of this chapter as principal investigator. Its overarching aim was to conduct a large-scale randomized controlled trial to compare the efficacy and cost effectiveness of occupational therapy versus a social control intervention in producing positive health outcomes in low income, ethnically diverse older people living in the community. At the time, this focus was of significant public health relevance given the spiraling costs of health care in the nation's older adult population (Orszag & Ellis, 2007). The acquisition of an NIH independent investigator award to fund the study was unprecedented in occupational therapy at the time. Now commonly known as the USC Well Elderly Study (1994–1997), the Research Project Grant (R01) was jointly funded across agencies and institutes including the NIA and the National Center for Medical Rehabilitation Research housed in the National Institute for Child Health and Human Development, both of the NIH; the AHCPR;

Figure 25-2. Blueprint for a translational science research program. (Reprinted with permission from F. A. Clark & M. C. Lawlor; *Willard and Spackman's occupational therapy.* [11th ed.]; E. B. Crepeau, E. S. Cohn, & B. A. Boyt-Schell [Eds.]; Copyright Lippincott Williams & Wilkins; 2009.)

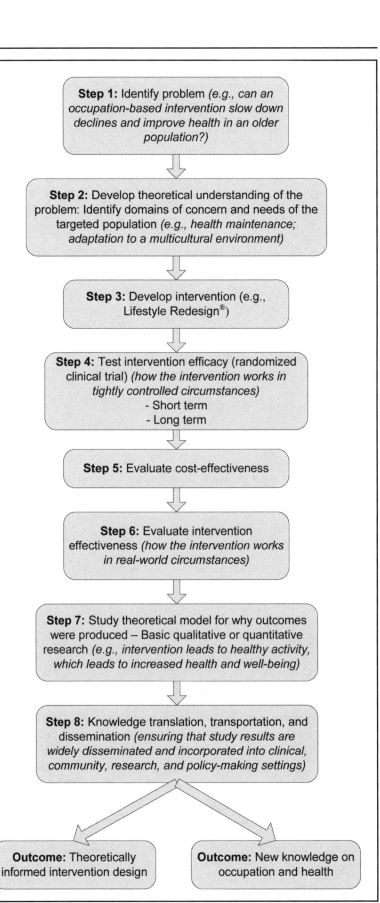

and the American Occupational Therapy Foundation. The investigative team, consisting of three occupational scientists (of whom two are the first two authors of this chapter) who were also occupational therapists, a social psychologist, a biostatistician, a cognitive psychologist, a health economist, and two geriatric physicians, was now positioned to investigate whether occupational therapy relative to a social control intervention could cost effectively slow down declines and improve health in an older population.

Laying the Groundwork: Conducting a Qualitative Needs Assessment

Moving on to Step 2 in the Blueprint, we identified a need to develop a more precise and detailed understanding of the domains of concern and needs of the older people who would be participants in the study to inform subsequent modifications to be made in Step 3 to the occupational therapy intervention protocol. Because a previous meta-analysis that we had completed indicated that occupational therapy was effective in producing a wide range of positive outcomes in various older populations (Carlson, Fanchiang, Zemke, & Clark, 1996), we were reasonably confident that the intervention, as it had been described in the original grant, would produce positive health outcomes. That notwithstanding, we realized that in-depth qualitative research could lead to critical insights and correspondingly to protocol refinements that would be likely to augment the intervention's overall effectiveness.

Qualitative Needs Assessment: Adaptive Strategies of Elders

An ethnographic study of elders with varying degrees of disability, conducted by the second author of this chapter, served as a crucial source of data for refining the intervention protocol (Jackson, 1996). This study was aimed at uncovering the strategies used by elders to remain engaged in meaningful occupations while adapting to the challenges of aging with a disability. The study participants were 20 individuals, aged 60 to 90 years, who had formed an advocacy organization aimed at improving health care for the elderly and educating health care practitioners about the needs and experiences of their older patients. In carrying out this study, the second author attended the group's weekly meetings and outings and conducted interviews with eight of the group's members.

Seven categories of adaptive strategies were revealed through this research. The first and most significant category, Personal Themes of Meaning as Motifs for Occupation, was an approach used by elders to negotiate unwanted physical, emotional, and social changes by engaging in occupations that reflected symbolic themes of meaning that had been important throughout their lives. For example, creative expression through artwork had been a theme of meaning for Edith, but at the time of the interviews, arthritis prevented her from quilting,

one of her most valued creative outlets. In response to this physical challenge, Edith adapted the way she participated in this occupation, by designing the quilts, accompanying her caregiver to buy the fabric, and guiding the caregiver in assembling the materials. For Edith, continuing to engage in a tangible expression of this theme of meaning was crucial to maintaining her quality of life.

The second theme of meaning, Risk and Challenge in Occupation, revealed the innate desire of participants to engage in activities that fostered excitement, challenged their abilities, and offered the possibility of failure. They dismissed the notion that disengagement from such activities was part of the normal aging process. Rather, they interpreted living a "safe" existence without such challenges as a form of deprivation. A third theme, Activity Patterns and Temporal Rhythms, elucidated the ways that the elders created structure and rhythm in their daily routines. Because few of the elders had socially constructed schedules to which they adhered, such as a need to arrive at work or pick up children from school at a certain time, their days tended to be given structure through patterns of occupations that repeated themselves daily or weekly, such as home maintenance tasks, doctor's appointments, or church activities.

A fourth theme, Control, illustrated how elders maintained a sense of independence and autonomy in their lives, even as they sometimes found themselves dependent on others to complete certain tasks for them due to their physical limitations. When relying on others for assistance, elders employed creative strategies to retain control, such as verbally directing others in carrying out activities and maintaining decision-making control over their environment and choice of occupations in which to engage. The fifth theme of meaning was Maintaining Continuity Through Spatial, Social, and Cultural Connectedness, which described how elders preserved stability in their lives despite disruptions such as a change in living situation. This was achieved through reflecting on intergenerational familial bonds, which provided a sense of connectivity with the past and the future; surrounding themselves with objects that evoked memories of the past; reminiscing as a way to reexperience significant events; creating opportunities for spontaneous social interactions to maintain connectedness; and employing technologies such as the telephone and television to maintain ties with the community.

The sixth theme, Acknowledging Identity Through the Celebration of Occupations, was an activity undertaken during the health care advocates' weekly meetings. Each group member shared a significant event from their lives over the past week, which provided an opportunity to celebrate and recognize the importance of events that might on the surface appear commonplace. The seventh and final theme, Advocating Social Change, was the overarching purpose of the health care advocacy group. The group members, angry at their poor treatment within the medical system, channeled their feelings into efforts to transform the health care system that they found disrespectful and oppressive toward the elderly and disabled populations.

Qualitative Needs Assessment: The Domain Study

In addition to the seven themes revealed through the second author's research, we undertook a qualitative study, which we called the Domain Study, to document the life domains and adaptive strategies of significance to older people living in the setting from which we would draw the sample for the randomized controlled trial (Clark et al., 1996). The qualitative research method employed naturalistic inquiry (Lincoln & Guba, 1985) and involved intense interviews of 29 older people until saturation was obtained. What we were interested in uncovering were the domains in which the respondents felt they were most challenged as well as any associated solutions they had devised for dealing with their concerns. In the end, our analyses provided a rich database to guide tailoring of the intervention protocol in accord with the unique and most pressing needs, attributes, values, and life circumstances of the population to be recruited for the study. Of the 10 domains that emerged, several overlapped with typical occupational therapy areas of focus (e.g., activities of daily living, health maintenance). Others were unanticipated but seemed to be of considerable local relevance (e.g., cultural conflict).

The completion of the Domain Study provided the data-based foundation for progressing to Step 3. In this step, we made protocol refinements derived from the findings of the second author's research on adaptive strategies and the Domain Study and produced the version of the intervention to be used in the study. Although the program was comprised of nine modules, it allowed for flexibility and individualization in accord with the unique characteristics of each participant and his or her pressing concerns. Delivery of program content included didactic presentation, group-based peer exchange, direct experience with health-promoting activity, and professional-guided application. In the end, the overarching aim of the intervention was described as enabling each participant to design and implement a personally feasible and healthy lifestyle that is sustainable within his or her life circumstances. Whereas the nine targeted domains were largely derived from the findings of the second author's research and the Domain Study, certain elements of the therapeutic approach including tailoring and individualization echo the genre of therapy that had emerged from the Penny Richardson Study.

Conducting a Randomized Clinical Trial

Once the intervention had been sufficiently refined, the optimal content identified, and the modes of delivery specified, the USC Well Elderly investigative team was poised to take Step 4 and Step 5 in the Blueprint (i.e., to test the outcomes of the intervention through a randomized controlled trial and evaluate its cost effectiveness,

respectively). Although the originally planned sample size for this study was 320, our 98% recruitment success rate resulted in an enrollment of 361 older people. Of these, 122 were randomized to the occupational therapy intervention, 120 to the social control group, and 119 to a no-treatment control group. The participants assigned to the occupational therapy group received the comprehensive, individualized intervention refined in Step 3 (now called Lifestyle Redesign) administered by occupational therapists. During the 9-month intervention phase, these participants developed and implemented individualized plans of health-promoting lifestyle modifications in areas contained in the manual such as safety, diet, activity selection, finances, etc. To ensure that the intervention was being delivered as intended, the first and second authors of this chapter, along with Ruth Zemke and Deborah Mandel, convened weekly fidelity meetings during the intervention phase. What was particularly distinctive about the Lifestyle Redesign intervention was that because it had been informed by the results of the second author's research, the Domain Study, and the Penny Richardson Study, it targeted the unique and complex living circumstances that challenged the participants in their particular social and physical worlds. In contrast, over the same 9-month period, those in the social control program attended a random assortment of activities, much like those typically offered at senior centers, which were overseen by nonprofessionals. The no-treatment control group was tested before, after, and 6 months following the study's intervention phase on outcome measures but received no intervention.

Results of the study indicated that, at the end of the intervention period, being involved in regularly scheduled activity (the social control program) was no more effective in promoting health than not receiving treatment at all (the no-treatment control condition). In contrast, the occupational therapy intervention produced reliable, positive effects on a wide range of health outcomes in the social, physical, and emotional domains (Clark, Azen et al., 1997). Moreover, subsequent analyses revealed that 90% of the occupational therapy program's positive effects persisted 6 months after the treatment phase (Clark et al., 2001) and that the intervention was highly cost effective (Hay et al., 2002). We concluded, based on the pattern of positive findings, that the Lifestyle Redesign intervention slowed down the declines associated with aging and in some cases actually improved health in older people and that it did so with minimal cost outlay relative to other interventions. Upon completion of the first USC Well Elderly Study, we had successfully undertaken the first five steps in the Blueprint.

The first Well Elderly Study went well beyond the Penny Richardson Study by more firmly and comprehensively demonstrating that occupational science could positively impact occupational therapy practice. Because the focus of the intervention was explicitly on occupation, it clearly fell within the conceptual boundaries of occupational science. In its entirety, this research program turned out to be another graphic illustration of our resolution of the polemics that were still plaguing the discipline. First, we incorporated both basic (e.g., to study the life domains of concern of low income, diverse older people) and applied (e.g., to use a database for intervention design and then test the intervention's effectiveness) components. Second, we employed a blend of qualitative and quantitative methodologies as deemed appropriate and, third, we provided some of the most convincing evidence to date of the effectiveness of occupational therapy in producing positive health outcomes with a given population, demonstrating an important advantage of linking occupational science to occupational therapy. Additionally, this research program, because of its comprehensiveness, led to several auxiliary studies and papers that would also further occupational science in areas such as the cultural adaptation of treatment protocols (Jackson et al., 2000), cultural translation of instruments (Azen et al., 1999), and reconceptualizations of how occupational science relates to broader health care concerns in well populations (Clark, 1997) as well as older people (Carlson, Clark, & Young, 1998). When considered together, the Penny Richardson Study and the first USC Well Elderly Study provided an initial picture of the significant contribution occupational science could make to legitimizing occupational therapy and improving the lives of people both with and without significant disabilities.

The Second USC Well Elderly Study (Blueprint Steps 6 and 7)

In Step 6 in the Blueprint, we asked whether the Lifestyle Redesign intervention would be as effective in producing positive health outcomes in diverse older people in less controlled, more complicated real-world circumstances. In the first USC Well Elderly Study, we had tested the intervention's efficacy in that the design incorporated numerous elements that were assumed to maximize the experimental effect (e.g., a relatively homogenous population, limited settings). Effectiveness studies, by contrast, are less tightly controlled and introduce greater variability likely to depress detection of the degree of impact of the intervention (Brekke, Ell, & Palinkas, 2007; Glasgow, Lichtenstein, & Marcus, 2003). To continue the process of translational research, implementation of Step 6 required acquisition of a second large NIH grant. In 2004, we received an R01 grant funded solely by the NIA to, among other aims, test the effectiveness and cost effectiveness of the Lifestyle Redesign intervention within less tightly controlled circumstances. The effectiveness focus of this study, in contrast to the first USC Well Elderly Study, was instantiated by (a) expanding the number and type of sites from 2 to 21, (b) reducing the treatment period from 9 to 6 months, and (c) including proportionally

more older people from the minority populations most at risk for health disparities.

A total of 460 older people enrolled in the study, and because it used a semi-crossover research design it was planned that the entire sample would eventually receive the intervention (Jackson et al., 2009). However, for its intent-to-treat analysis we only compared the health-related outcomes of the evaluable participants assigned to the intervention group ($n = 187$) and control group ($n = 173$) in the first 6 months of study implementation. Within the intervention group, the participants received weekly Lifestyle Redesign group sessions along with up to 12 individualized sessions throughout a 6-month treatment phase. In contrast, those in the control group did not receive an intervention but were pre- and post-tested. The intent-to-treat analysis showed that we were able to replicate the findings of the first USC Well Elderly Study indicating a positive treatment effect on a wide range of health outcomes (Clark et al., 2011). Further, we showed that these results were repeated in secondary analyses of data obtained on the control group after it had crossed over into the intervention phase ($n = 137$) and in the entire sample that was evaluated after having received the intervention ($n = 324$). Finally, results of the second USC Well Elderly Study also demonstrated that, even when delivered under less tightly controlled circumstances, the intervention was proven to be cost effective.

Beyond these findings, the design of this study permitted us to examine the underlying mechanisms that accounted for the positive outcomes. Because of this we could move on to Step 7 in the Blueprint, which entails studying a theoretical model to explain how the outcomes were produced (Jackson et al., 2009). Figure 25-3 depicts the model that was tested in taking this step, which hypothesizes that the intervention effects can be explained through a set of mediating and moderating variables including stress-related biomarkers and measures of healthy activity, active coping, social support, perceived control, and positive reinterpretation-based coping. Because testing the model required measurement of activity as a mediating variable and no suitable instrument was available, our investigative team developed several new activity measurements for the study (Eakman, Carlson, & Clark, 2010). Although not conclusive at this time, initial analyses suggest that the intervention effect is largely mediated through change in activity patterns detectable on the aforementioned instruments. In summary, the design of the second USC Well Elderly Study permitted us to undertake Step 7 in the Blueprint. In completing this step, we were able to generate occupational science theory on the mechanisms that account for the positive outcomes of activity-based interventions such as Lifestyle Redesign and produce new knowledge on the relationships between occupation and other variables to health outcomes.

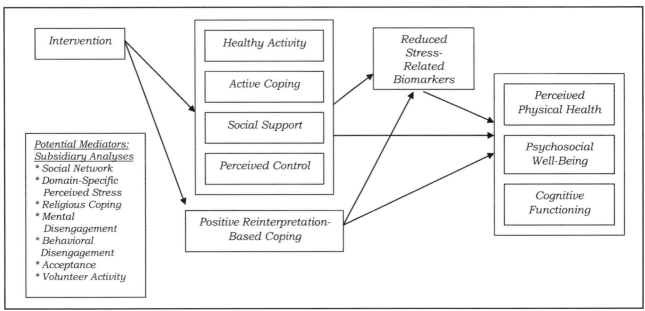

Figure 25-3. Conceptual model of positive effects of activity-based intervention for elders. (© Society for Clinical Trials 2009. Reprinted with permission from Jackson, J., Mandel, D., Blanchard, J., Carlson, M., Cherry, B., Azen, S., ... Clark, F. [2009]. Confronting challenges in intervention research with ethnically diverse older adults: The USC Well Elderly II Trial. *Clinical Trials, 6*[1], 90-101. doi: 10.1177/1740774508101191)

Knowledge Translation, Transportation, and Dissemination of the USC Well Elderly Research Program (Blueprint Step 8)

Step 8 in the Blueprint addresses knowledge translation, transportation, and dissemination (Brekke et al., 2007). This step involves ensuring that the research results are widely disseminated and incorporated on a long-term basis in clinical and community-based settings. The USC Well Elderly Research Program has taken several steps to facilitate this process. First, the first two authors of this chapter have delivered lectures on the findings of the USC Well Elderly Research Program to broad audiences both nationally and internationally. Second, a manual detailing the intervention approach was produced for dissemination (Mandel, Jackson, Zemke, Nelson, & Clark, 1999). Third, the European Network of Occupational Therapy in Higher Education funded the translation of the culturally tailored Lifestyle Redesign Manual in six European nations. Fourth, a pilot study based on the first USC Well Elderly Study was undertaken to explore whether the intervention effects could be replicated in the United Kingdom, and the UK National Institute for Health and Clinical Excellence used the findings of that study, combined with those of the first USC Well Elderly Study, to justify public health guidelines on interventions to promote mental well-being for both primary and residential care of older people. Next, we plan to make the entire USC Well Elderly Research Program database available to other investigators for independent analyses. This database now includes pre, post, and follow-up data

on a wide range of demographic and outcome variables for more than 800 independently living and ethnically diverse older people.

Overall, the USC Well Elderly Research Program has contributed to furthering occupational science in multiple ways. First, it demonstrates that a hybrid research program, with both basic and applied components, can lead to significant breakthroughs in knowledge development and intervention design that help to establish the effectiveness and cost effectiveness of occupational therapy with older populations. Second, it illustrates how diverse research methodologies can be employed to accomplish specific research aims in a tightly integrated research program. Third, it led to instrument development in the domain of activity participation, required for testing theoretical models, and fourth, it established the efficacy, effectiveness, and cost effectiveness of Lifestyle Redesign. This intervention approach is now beginning to be incorporated into public health policy and widely disseminated internationally.

The USC/Rancho Los Amigos National Rehabilitation Center Pressure Ulcer Prevention Studies

Applying the Blueprint to the Issue of Medically Serious Pressure Ulcers in People With Spinal Cord Injury

In the 10-year interim between obtaining funding for the first and second USC Well Elderly Studies, we turned our attention to the problem of the high incidence of medically serious pressure ulcers in people with spinal cord injury. As had been the case in the USC Well Elderly Research Program, we constituted an interdisciplinary team to work on this problem and develop a grant for obtaining needed funding, but in this instance through a partnership between the USC Division of Occupational Science and Occupational Therapy and Rancho Los Amigos National Rehabilitation Center. The investigative team that was assembled consisted of two occupational scientists (who were also occupational therapists), a physiatrist, a plastic surgeon whose practice largely involved flap surgeries for repair of medically serious pressure ulcers, a clinically based occupational therapist, and a social worker who was also spinal cord injured. By this time the Blueprint had been crystallized. For this new study we intended to follow it stringently. We reasoned that just as following the Blueprint had resulted in the design and implementation of a cost-effective occupational therapy intervention for older people, following it could have promise for a similar breakthrough in the area of pressure ulcer prevention.

In undertaking this study we wanted to shift our focus from well populations to people with chronic and severe disability, thereby directly addressing the third polemic, which we previously described. We reasoned that in addressing this serious complication for people with spinal cord injury through the Blueprint, we would be able to transport the research approach we had used with a relatively well population to one with a chronic disability customarily treated by occupational therapists. Those of us on the investigative team who had also worked on the USC Well Elderly Studies were pleased that we would now be producing occupational science that addressed no less than an intractable life-threatening biomedical condition with which all rehabilitation professionals were very familiar. We reasoned that occupational science research aimed at cost-effectively combating this problem could firmly establish that it could lead to substantive innovation in community-based occupational therapy delivery.

In Blueprint Step 1, we conducted an in-depth review of the problem. It revealed that, to date, best practices had not been adequate in reducing the risk of incurring medically serious pressure ulcers in adults with spinal cord injury and that the cost of care was growing exponentially. In a given year, 23% to 33% of the population can be expected to develop such a sore and over the course of a lifetime the percentage rises to 95% (Clark et al., 2006). Such ulcers seriously threaten quality of life, impeding participation in the social and physical world. Typically, treatment for advanced pressure ulcers requires months of bed rest and results in muscle loss due to surgery and concomitant decrease in functional ability as well as hopelessness and depression (Clark & Lawlor, 2008). Ulcers of this severity may also lead to life-threatening infections, which, if they progress, may require surgical repair, with total costs (including hos-

pitalization) of approximately $70,000 per surgery (Clark et al., 2006). Moreover, on a national level, both Healthy People 2010 and the Joint Commission on Accreditation of Healthcare Organizations had identified pressure ulcer prevention as a key priority (Martucci, 2006). After completing Step 1, the team was convinced that this was a research area worthy of investment, one in which there was potential to reduce both the burden of soaring health care costs and the devastating consequences for consumers. A multifaceted, full-fledged, Blueprint-guided occupational science research program seemed optimal for making significant advances in counteracting this problem.

Conducting a Qualitative Needs Assessment

In 2000, for Blueprint Step 2, the Pressure Ulcer Prevention Study (PUPS) team was successful in securing a Field Initiated Research Grant from the National Institute of Disability and Rehabilitation Research to conduct a qualitative study that would provide novel and detailed understandings of the complexity of factors that interact in real-life circumstances to heighten pressure ulcer risk in people with spinal cord injuries. The methodology required that in-depth interviews and participant observation be conducted over an 18-month period with 19 people who had sustained a spinal cord injury and with one person with spinal myelitis. In order to be involved in the study, participants had to have had a history of recurrent development of pressure ulcers.

As was the case in the USC Well Elderly Domain Study, the qualitative findings of this study were analyzed, in part, to identify optimal content and appropriate strategies for a Lifestyle Redesign intervention, in this case focused on the prevention of medically serious pressure ulcers. However, this study went beyond the qualitative approach used in the Domain Study by generating not only descriptive but also relational knowledge. On the descriptive level, the following six content domains were identified for manualization of the intervention:

1. Understanding lifestyle and pressure ulcer risk

2. Taking charge (advocacy)

3. Accessing the physical environment

4. Social networks and meaningful relationships

5. Happiness and personal well-being

6. Planning for the future

However, at more complex levels of analysis, an integrated theoretical framework was formulated to guide the intervention approach.

First, we constructed a number of data-based models of how pressure ulcers developed in daily living contexts of adults with spinal cord injury (Clark et al., 2006). These models underscored the significant amount of complexity and individualization that

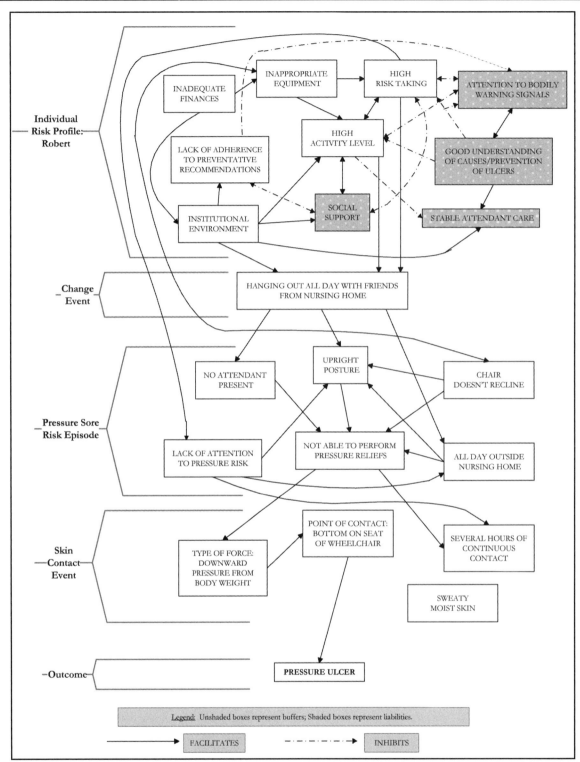

Figure 25-4. Pressure ulcer event sequence. (Reprinted with permission from *Archives of Physical Medicine and Rehabilitation, 87,* Clark, F., Jackson, J., Scott, M., Carlson, M., Atkins, M., Uhles-Tanaka, M., & Rubayi, S., Data-based models of how pressure ulcers develop in daily-living contexts of adults with spinal cord injury, pp. 1516-1525, Copyright [2006], with permission from Elsevier.)

accounted for the emergence of pressure ulcers in particular lives. For example, one model made it possible to depict the various elements that come together in particular pressure ulcer risk episodes. Figure 25-4 is an example. Across such sequences, we found that ulcers were most likely to develop during conditions of change that disrupted the equilibrium of personalized adaptive systems, particularly when the participant was at relatively high risk before the change event. These models were incorporated into the intervention protocol to facilitate therapist analysis of contextual risk-related factors and situations of heightened vulnerability to pressure ulcer development.

Additionally, we employed qualitative data analysis to formulate overarching principles that pertained to lifestyle and pressure ulcer risk in adults with spinal cord injury (Jackson et al., 2010). These principles clarify how risk unfolds in everyday life situations. The first principle is Perpetual Change, which indicates that the threat of developing a pressure ulcer is ever present, even when the person with spinal cord injury is diligently performing a pressure ulcer prevention routine. The second principle, Change/ Disruption of Routine, addresses the danger associated with a change that disrupts risk-relevant conditions that can range from obvious liabilities such as the replacement of a care assistant to seeming minutiae like sleeping on a paper clip left in one's bed sheets. Though on the surface such changes could seem trivial, they were often found to lead to a cascade of detrimental effects. Principle 3 addresses the inevitable Decay of Preventive Behaviors. It suggests that even the most ingrained habitual prevention techniques may attenuate in a nearly imperceptible manner over time, eventually becoming ineffective.

Principle 4, Lifestyle Risk Ratio, posits that those whose risk factor profiles were characterized by more liabilities than buffers were more likely to incur a serious ulcer. This principle suggested that an intervention should include an assessment process through which such risk factor profiles were constructed, attended to, and revised over time as life circumstances change. Principle 5, Individualization, refers to the importance of attending to the unique and complex ways in which factors interact to heighten the risk of developing a pressure ulcer in particular life circumstances. This principle reinforced the idea that a preventive program would need to be individually tailored and context sensitive to be optimally effective. Principle 6 addressed Awareness of Pressure Ulcer Prevention Techniques as well as the Motivational Commitment to Enact Them Consistently, both of which needed to be present to optimally diminish pressure ulcer risk. It implied that an intervention would need to incorporate the development of knowledge and skill along with the building of motivation to put practices learned into action.

Principle 7, Lifestyle Tradeoff, one of our most important discoveries, has led to a renaissance in practice. This principle is also the one that seemed most relevant to issues salient in the prevailing occupational science literature at the time. Fundamentally, each participant in the study was confronted with conflicts between his or her desire to participate in personally meaningful activities and the need to rest in order to care properly for an ulcer. For some participants, engagement in the occupations they loved could become no less than life threatening. This was true for a participant who worked long hours during tax season,

an executive who loved to work hard and then play to relax, and an artist who would go into a flow state and, thereby, forget to do pressure reliefs (Csikszentmihalyi, 1997). Given this principle, it was apparent that an intervention approach needed to identify such potential conflicts between occupation and health and provide assistance in negotiating them. Finally, the last principle, Principle 8, Access to Needed Care, Services, and Support, led us to conclude that advocacy would need to be an essential component of the context-sensitive intervention we would be developing.

These two qualitative studies, though key in building theory on the complex interacting factors that lead to pressure ulcer development, were not the only studies undertaken in Step 2. Dunn, Carlson, Jackson, and Clark (2009) performed a secondary analysis of the data to pinpoint response factors that influenced pressure ulcer progression in the participants. Based on 45 pressure ulcer events contained in the database, they identified eight primary response categories ranging from procrastination to adherence to medical recommendations. Similarly, in their secondary analysis of the data, Fogelberg, Atkins, Blanche, Carlson, and Clark (2009) described the ways in which specific mobility concerns, such as wheelchair adjustments, habituation to new equipment, and lifestyle choices, contributed to the occurrence of pressure ulcer risk episodes.

Developing the Intervention

This extensive body of qualitative findings provided a rich and multifaceted theoretical framework for Step 3, in which the team developed and manualized the Lifestyle Redesign Pressure Ulcer Prevention Program. The manual, as already described, contains six modules with detailed content derived from the previous extensive qualitative analyses. However, beyond this, the intervention is described as being guided by the aforementioned eight principles, and interveners are trained in utilization of the various models that depict pressure ulcer risk episodes. Further, three products were developed based on the data that are specified as resources to be referred to during intervention delivery. These products include the following: (a) hard copy and CD-ROM versions of a rehabilitation professionals' manual and companion manual and (b) online and hard copy versions of a consumer manual, which can be readily accessed at http://www.pressureulcerprevention.com. The rehabilitation professionals' manual includes detailed narratives of the life circumstances that led to pressure ulcer development in the 20 participants in the PUPS study, as well as interactive decision trees and questions regarding certain dilemmas with response options and links to resources on risk-related factors. In contrast, the companion manual and consumer manual summarize recent research on topics relevant to pressure ulcer prevention. Within the framework of the manualized intervention, interveners are trained in the use of the rehabilitation professionals' manual and instructed to encourage consumers to use the consumer manual.

Conducting a Randomized Clinical Trial

Having produced this theoretically driven and resource-rich intervention approach, the Lifestyle Redesign for Pressure Ulcer Prevention Study (LR-PUPS) team is currently undertaking Steps 4, 5, and 6 in the Blueprint. In 2008, we received an R01 grant from the National Center for Medical Rehabilitation Research of the National Institute of Child Health and Human Development to evaluate the efficacy and cost effectiveness of the LR-PUPS intervention in reducing the incidence of medically serious pressure ulcers in people with spinal cord injury and to examine a theoretical model to explain the intervention's outcomes. In this study, 170 people with spinal cord injury who access services at Rancho Los Amigos National Rehabilitation Center are being randomized into the intervention and usual care arms of the study. Participants in the intervention group are receiving a 12-month LR-PUPS intervention and are periodically assessed on a set of outcome measures. Those assigned to usual care are undergoing the same assessments but are not receiving additional services. Divided into two phases, the intervention first involves an intense phase including four preplanned sessions per month followed by a tapered phase in which the preplanned sessions are reduced to two. Throughout the intervention, however, preplanned contacts can be supplemented by incident visits scheduled at times of heightened pressure ulcer risk.

At the time of this writing, 83 participants in the intervention arm and 87 in the usual care control arm have completed the 24-month follow-up period, and we have documented the ways in which risky life circumstances are being targeted through individualization of the manualized intervention (Vaishampayan, Clark, Carlson, & Blanche, 2011) and how these circumstances contribute to additional complexity in conducting a clinical trial (Pyatak et al., 2013). At its conclusion, the results of this study will indicate whether the LR-PUPS intervention is effective in reducing the incidence of pressure ulcers and related surgeries among community-dwelling adults with spinal cord injury and enable theory building on the mechanisms that account for the intervention's outcomes. Secondly, the findings should document whether or not the intervention positively impacts quality of life.

CONTRIBUTION TO OCCUPATIONAL SCIENCE

In this chapter we have outlined the ways in which two integrated sequences of studies guided by our Blueprint for Translational Research, the USC Well Elderly Studies and PUPS, have shaped and furthered occupational science. We have also illustrated that in the process of conducting these research programs we were compelled to address certain tensions regarding the nature of the discipline and its relationship to occupational therapy. In working our way through these polemics, we have shown that occupational science is neither a basic science strictly concerned with the development of theory without regard to its practical applications nor an applied science that only investigates issues with immediate relevance to occupational therapy practice but contains elements of both. The science we do does not stringently adhere to either qualitative or quantitative methodologies as a matter of principle but draws from both research traditions depending on which is most appropriate to answer the question at hand. Our science is not one that addresses only the concerns of well populations or of individuals with chronic disease or disability but encompasses a broad range of stakeholders across multiple populations. And finally, we have made the case that our research programs should not be seen as a drain on the resources of occupational therapy or a distraction from the important work of providing evidence to support the efficacy of our interventions. Rather, we have demonstrated that it has been an asset in attracting resources to develop an evidence base to support our practice profession.

The research programs outlined in this chapter have demonstrated the depth and breadth of occupational science as an academic discipline. They have illustrated the advantages of forging a separate identity from, but maintaining close linkages to, the practice profession of occupational therapy, thus freeing occupational science to develop both basic theoretical knowledge related to human occupation and evidence of its utility as a therapeutic modality. As occupational science has matured over the two decades since its initial founding by scholars at USC and the University of South Australia, its research programs have played an important role in ensuring the relevance of the discipline to multiple stakeholders, thereby helping to secure its future both in the academy and as a partner of the profession of occupational therapy.

IMPLICATIONS FOR PRACTICE

Through a presentation of the Blueprint for Translational Research and the research programs it has guided, this chapter has revealed a mechanism by which basic research on occupation can be used to inform the development of innovative occupational therapy interventions such as the Lifestyle Redesign interventions described herein. This approach to conducting occupational science research developed organically as scholars from USC, including the first and second authors of this chapter, sought to diffuse the tensions surrounding four polemics that threatened to divide the occupational therapy community. The process of conducting research guided by the Blueprint provides a means to resolve these debates about the nature and purpose of occupational science research. Our studies utilize basic research as a foundation to support the development of innovative interventions, which are then evaluated through large-scale efficacy, effectiveness, and cost-effectiveness studies, satisfying clinicians' increasing need for evidence to support our practice. Because the Blueprint approach to conducting research is equally applicable to public health issues facing well populations as well as the concerns of individuals with chronic diseases or disability, we extend the relevance of occupational therapy to new stakeholders while continuing to serve the populations with whom occupational therapists have long been allied. As a science focused on issues related to everyday living, occupational science not only creates a knowledge base pertaining to the life circumstances that impact health outcomes but also translates its new theoretical understandings into innovative interventions.

The occupational science research presented in this chapter has provided occupational therapists with the tools necessary to address the pressing health concerns of the 21st century. As the health care landscape has shifted, reflecting an increase in chronic health conditions brought about in part by lifestyle factors such as poor nutrition, physical inactivity, stress, or social isolation, occupational therapists have an important role to play in addressing these health concerns. To take our rightful place as practitioners who can address these lifestyle factors that contribute to chronic disease, occupational therapists can draw upon evidence-based therapeutic approaches such as those developed in the research programs outlined in this chapter. At the same time, occupational science of the genre we have described makes it possible for occupational therapists to refine existing and implement new therapeutic approaches with the populations they have always served.

LEARNING SUPPORTS

Debates in the Development of Occupational Science

Purpose

This learning support will facilitate students in thinking critically about the polemics that have shaped our academic discipline.

Primary Concepts

Theoretical concepts in occupational science and history of occupational science.

Instructions

1. In a small group, carry out a mock debate between key figures on opposite sides of one of the polemics outlined in this chapter that shaped the development of occupational science.

○ Moderator: Develop a list of questions you will pose to the individuals on each side of the debate. These questions should stimulate discussion by the debate participants on topics relevant to the chosen polemic.

○ Debaters: Prepare by reviewing the primary sources cited in this chapter (e.g., the articles by Mosey, Clark et al., and Carlson and Dunlea with respect to the partition debate). Aim to understand the perspective of the person or people you will be representing and think about how they would counter the arguments of those they disagree with.

Initiating the Research Process— Identifying a Problem

Purpose

This learning support will engage students in the creative process of developing potential topics for research.

Primary Concepts

Experience of conducting research, use of occupational science concepts to inform occupational therapy, and use of the Translational Research Blueprint.

Instructions

1. Think about a health issue that you are interested in knowing more about. It may be something that you have experienced in your own life, heard about in the media, or encountered in your coursework or clinical experiences.

2. Find three to five sources of information that describe aspects of this problem. They may be textbooks, scholarly journal articles, newspaper articles, or other sources.

3. Write a summary of the information you reviewed, including a description of what is already known about the issue and what has yet to be learned. Conclude the summary with one or more potential research questions on your chosen topic that could be answered using the steps outlined in the Translational Research Blueprint.

Conducting Translational Research: Getting to Know the Blueprint

Purpose

This learning support will facilitate a deeper understanding of the process of conducting translational research.

Primary Concepts

Research methodology, becoming an informed consumer of research, and use of the Translational Research Blueprint.

Instructions

1. From an issue of an academic journal or published conference proceedings, select an abstract or journal article describing a research study that interests you.

2. Read the description of the study and determine which step or steps of the Translational Research Blueprint the research study fulfilled.

3. For each of the remaining steps in the Translational Research Blueprint, briefly describe a project that would represent a phase of the research study described in the abstract. In other words, describe how the researchers would have progressed through the Blueprint stages given their particular research question.

ACKNOWLEDGMENTS

We would like to acknowledge Mary Lawlor for her valuable contributions with respect to the theoretical framing of certain portions of the manuscript. We would also like to acknowledge the support of our work by the following agencies: the Division of Maternal and Child Health (#MCH-060745, PI; Cheryl Mattingly); National Institutes of Health (#R01 HD 38878-01A1, PI: Mary Lawlor; #2R01 HD 38878-06, PI: Mary Lawlor; #R01 HD056267-02, PI: Florence Clark; #1 R01 AG11810, PI: Florence Clark); the National Institute of Disability and Rehabilitation Research (#H133G000062, PI: Florence Clark); National Center for Medical Rehabilitation Research of the National Institute for Child Health and Human Development (#1 R01 HD056267-01, PI: Florence Clark); and the National Institute on Aging (#1 R01 AG021108-01A2, PI: Florence Clark).

REFERENCES

Azen, S., Palmer, J. M., Carlson, M., Mandel, D., Cherry, B. J., Fanchiang, S.-P., . . . Clark, F. A. (1999). Psychometric properties of a Chinese translation of the SF-36 Health Survey Questionnaire in the Well Elderly Study. *Journal of Aging and Health, 11*(2), 240-251. doi:10.1177/089826439901100206

Brekke, J. S., Ell, K., & Palinkas, L. A. (2007). Translational science at the National Institute of Mental Health: Can social work take its rightful place? *Research on Social Work Practice, 17*(1), 123-133. doi:10.1177/1049731506293693

Carlson, M. E., & Clark, F. A. (1991). The search for useful methodologies in occupational science. *American Journal of Occupational Therapy, 45*(3), 235-241. doi:10.5014/ajot.45.3.235

Carlson, M. E., Clark, F. A., & Young, B. (1998). Practical contributions of occupational science to the art of successful ageing: How to sculpt a meaningful life in older adulthood. *Journal of Occupational Science, 5*(3), 107-118. doi:10.1080/14427591.1998.9686438

Carlson, M. E. & Dunlea, A. (1995). Further thoughts on the pitfalls of partition: A response to Mosey. *American Journal of Occupational Therapy, 49*(1), 73-81. doi:10.5014/ajot.49.1.73

Carlson, M. E., Fanchiang, S.-P., Zemke, R., & Clark, F. A. (1996). A meta-analysis of the effectiveness of occupational therapy for older persons. *American Journal of Occupational Therapy, 50*(2), 89-98. doi:10.5014/ajot.50.2.89

Clark, F. (1993). Occupation embedded in a real life: Interweaving occupational science and occupational therapy. *American Journal of Occupational Therapy, 47*(12), 1067-1078. doi:10.5014/ajot.47.12.1067

Clark, F. (1997). Reflections on the human as an occupational being: Biological need, tempo, and temporality. *Journal of Occupational Science, 4*(3), 86-92. doi:10.1080/14427591.1997.9686424

Clark, F., Azen, S. P., Carlson, M., Mandel, D., LaBree, L., Hay, J., . . . Lipson, L. (2001). Embedding health-promoting changes into the daily lives of independent-living older adults: Long-term follow-up of occupational therapy intervention. *Journal of Gerontology: Psychological Sciences and Social Sciences, 56B*, 60-63. doi:10.1093/geronb/56.1.P60

Clark, F., Azen, S. P., Zemke, R., Jackson, J., Carlson, M., Hay, J., . . . Lipson, L. (1997). Occupational therapy for independent-living older adults: A randomized controlled trial. *Journal of the American Medical Association, 278*(16), 1321-1326. doi:10.1001/jama.1997.03550160041036

Clark, F., Carlson, M., & Polkinghorne, D. (1997). The legitimacy of life history and narrative approaches in the study of occupation. *American Journal of Occupational Therapy, 51*(4), 313-317. doi:10.5014/ajot.51.4.313

Clark, F., Ennevor, B., & Richardson, P. (1996). A grounded theory of techniques for occupational storytelling and occupational story making. In R. Zemke & F. Clark (Eds.), *Occupational science: The evolving discipline* (pp. 373-392). Philadelphia, PA: F. A. Davis.

Clark, F., Jackson, J., Carlson, M., Chou, C.-P., Cherry, B., Jordan-Marsh, M., . . . Azen, S. (2011). Effectiveness of a lifestyle intervention in promoting the well-being of independently living older people: Results of the Well Elderly 2 Randomized Controlled Trial. *Journal of Epidemiology and Community Health, 66*, 782-790. doi:10.1136/jech.2009.099754

Clark, F., Jackson, J., Scott, M., Carlson, M., Atkins, M., Uhles-Tanaka, M., & Rubayi, S. (2006). Data-based models of how pressure ulcers develop in daily-living contexts of adults with spinal cord injury. *Archives of Physical Medicine and Rehabilitation, 87*, 1516-1525. doi:10.1016/j.apmr.2006.08.329

Clark, F., & Lawlor, M. (2008). The making and mattering of occupational science. In E. Crepeau, E. Cohn, & B. Schell (Eds.), *Willard & Spackman's occupational therapy* (11th ed., pp. 2-14). Philadelphia, PA: Lippincott Williams & Wilkins.

Clark, F. A., Parham, D., Carlson, M. E., Frank, G., Jackson, J., Pierce, D., . . . Zemke, R. (1991). Occupational science: Academic innovation in the service of occupational therapy's future. *American Journal of Occupational Therapy, 45*, 300-310. doi:10.5014/ajot.45.4.300

Clark, F. A., Zemke, R., Frank, G., Parham, D., Neville-Jan, A., Hendricks, C., . . . Abreu, B. (1993). Dangers inherent in the partition of occupational therapy and occupational science. *American Journal of Occupational Therapy, 47*(2), 184-186. doi:10.5014/ajot.47.2.184

Csikszentmihalyi, M. (1997). *Finding flow: The psychology of engagement with everyday life.* New York, NY: Basic Books.

Duchek, J. M., & Thessing, V. (1996). Is the use of life history and narrative in clinical practice fundable as research? *American Journal of Occupational Therapy, 50*(5), 393-396. doi:10.5014/ajot.50.5.393

Dunn, C. A., Carlson, M., Jackson, J. M., & Clark, F. A. (2009). Response factors surrounding progression of pressure ulcers in community-residing adults with spinal cord injury. *American Journal of Occupational Therapy, 63*(3), 301-309. doi:10.5014/ajot.63.3.301

Eakman, A. M., Carlson, M. E., & Clark, F. A. (2010). The meaningful activity participation assessment: A measure of engagement in personally valued activities. *International Journal of Aging and Human Development, 70*(4), 299-317.

Fogelberg, D., Atkins, M., Blanche, E., Carlson, M., & Clark, F. (2009). Decisions and dilemmas in everyday live: Daily use of wheelchairs by individuals with spinal cord injury and the impact on pressure ulcer risk. *Topics in Spinal Cord Injury Rehabilitation, 15*(2), 16-32. doi:10.1310/sci1502-16

Glasgow, R. E., Lichtenstein, E., & Marcus, A. C. (2003). Why don't we see more translation of health promotion research to practice? Rethinking the efficacy-to-effectiveness transition. *American Journal of Public Health, 93*(8), 1261-1267.

Hay, J., LaBree, L., Luo, R., Clark, F., Carlson, M., Mandel, D., . . . Azen, S. P. (2002). Cost-effectiveness of preventive occupational therapy for independent-living older adults. *Journal of the American Geriatrics Society, 50*(8), 1381-1388. doi:10.1046/j.1532-5415.2002.50359.x

Hocking, C. (2000). Occupational science: A stock take of accumulated insights. *Journal of Occupational Science, 7*(2), 58-67. doi:10.1080/14427591.2000.9686466

Jackson, J. (1996). Living a meaningful existence in old age. In R. Zemke & F. Clark (Eds.), *Occupational science: The evolving discipline* (pp. 339-361). Philadelphia, PA: F.A. Davis.

Jackson, J., Carlson, M., Rubayi, S., Scott, M. D., Atkins, M. S., Blanche, E. I., . . . Clark, F. A. (2010). Qualitative study of principles pertaining to lifestyle and pressure ulcer risk in adults with spinal cord injury. *Disability and Rehabilitation, 32*(7), 567-578. doi:10.3109/09638280903183829

Jackson, J., Kennedy, B. L., Mandel, D., Carlson, M., Cherry, B. J., Fanchiang, S.-P., . . . Clark, F. A. (2000). Derivation and pilot assessment of a health promotion program for Mandarin-speaking Chinese older adults. *Aging & Human Development, 50*(2), 127-149.

Jackson, J., Mandel, D., Blanchard, J., Carlson, M., Cherry, B., Azen, S., ..., Clark, F. A. (2009). Confronting challenges in intervention research with ethnically diverse older adults: the USC Well Elderly II Trial. *Clinical Trials, 6*, 90-101. doi:10.1177/1740774508101191

Kielhofner, G. (2002a). *Challenges and directions for the future of occupational therapy.* Keynote address presented at the World Federation of Occupational Therapists Conference, Stockholm, Sweden.

Kielhofner, G. (2002b). UIC's scholarship of practice. *OT Practice, 7*, 11-12.

Kielhofner, G. (2005). Scholarship and practice: Bridging the divide. *American Journal of Occupational Therapy, 59*(2), 231-239. doi:10.5014/ajot.59.2.231

Lincoln, Y. S., & Guba, E. G. (1985). *Naturalistic inquiry.* Newbury Park, CA: Sage Publications.

Mandel, D. R., Jackson, J. M., Zemke, R., Nelson, L., & Clark, F. A. (1999). *Lifestyle redesign: Implementing the Well Elderly Program.* Bethesda, MD: American Occupational Therapy Association.

Martucci, N. (2006). An ounce of prevention: Arresting the occurrence of pressure ulcerations in individuals with disabilities. *Rehab Magazine, 19*(10), 36-39.

Mattingly, C. (1991). The narrative nature of clinical reasoning. *American Journal of Occupational Therapy, 45*(11), 998-1005. doi:10.5014/ajot.45.11.998

Mosey, A. C. (1992). Partition of occupational science and occupational therapy. *American Journal of Occupational Therapy, 46*(9), 851-853. doi:10.5014/ajot.46.9.851

Mosey, A. C. (1993). Partition of occupational science and occupational therapy: Sorting out some issues. *American Journal of Occupational Therapy, 47*(8), 751-754. doi:10.5014/ajot.47.8.751

National Institutes of Health. (2009). *Re-engineering the clinical research enterprise.* Retrieved from http://nihroadmap.nih.gov/clinicalresearch/overview-translational.asp

Orszag, P. R., & Ellis, P. (2007). The challenge of rising health care costs—A view from the Congressional Budget Office. *New England Journal of Medicine, 357*(18), 1793-1795.

Ottenbacher, K. J. (1992). Confusion in occupational therapy research: Does the end justify the method? *American Journal of Occupational Therapy, 46*(10), 871-874. doi:10.5014/ajot.46.10.871

Parham, L. D. (1998). What is the proper domain of occupational therapy research? *American Journal of Occupational Therapy, 52*(6), 485-489. doi:10.5014/ajot.52.6.485

Pyatak, E. A., Blanche, E. I., Garber, S. L., Diaz, J., Blanchard, J., Florindez, L., & Clark, F. A. (2013). Conducting intervention research among underserved populations: Lessons learned and recommendations for researchers. *Archives of Physical and Medical Rehabilitation, 94*(6), 1190-1198. doi: 10.1016/j.apmr.2012.12.009

Vaishampayan, A., Clark, F., Carlson, M., & Blanche, E. (2011). Preventing pressure ulcers in people with spinal cord injury: Targeting risky life circumstances through a community-based intervention. *Advances in Skin & Wound Care, 24*(6), 275-284.

Wilcock, A. A. (1991). Occupational science. *British Journal of Occupational Therapy, 54*(8), 297-300.

Yerxa, E. J. (1991). Seeking a relevant, ethical, and realistic way of knowing for occupational therapy. *American Journal of Occupational Therapy, 45*(3), 199-204. doi:10.5014/ajot.45.3.199

Yerxa, E. J., Clark, F., Frank, G., Jackson, J., Parham, D., Pierce, D., . . . Zemke, R. (1989). An introduction to occupational science: A foundation for occupational therapy in the 21st century. *Occupational Therapy in Health Care, 6*(4), 1-17. doi:10.1300/J003v06n04_04

Zemke, R., & Clark, F. (1996). *Occupational science: The evolving discipline.* Philadelphia, PA: F. A. Davis.

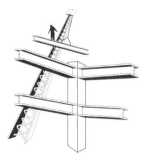

26

Enhancing Occupation-Based Practice at Rancho Los Amigos National Rehabilitation Center

Michele Berro, MA, OTR/L and Lisa Deshaies, OTR/L, CHT

In her Eleanor Clark Slagle Lecture, Suzanne Peloquin proclaimed,

> Time, place, and circumstance open paths to occupation. Occupation fosters dignity, competence, and health. Occupational therapy is a personal engagement. Caring and helping are vital to the work. Effective practice is artistry and science. Our profession takes this stand for the sake of persons and their occupational natures. We engage—we involve and occupy ourselves and commit to mutual promise—so that others may also engage. This is our character; this is our genius; this is our spirit. (2005, p. 623)

The intent of this chapter is to share with the reader our experiences with operationalizing and implementing client-centered and occupation-based practice at our large physical disabilities rehabilitation center. We hope to impart tips, strategies, and lessons learned to assist occupational therapists across practice settings to be truly authentic in their delivery of occupational therapy services.

LITERATURE AND BACKGROUND

A Working Definition of Occupation-Based and Client-Centered Practice

The Occupational Therapy Practice Framework: Domain and Process

The *Framework* (2008) is the American Occupational Therapy Association document that can help with defining and guiding occupational therapy practice. It articulates occupational therapy's unique contribution to the support of health and participation in life through successful engagement in occupation. At the core of the *Framework* is the use of meaningful occupations and the collaboration between client and practitioner as central.

Pierce, D. (Ed.).
Occupational Science for Occupational Therapy (pp. 311-323).
© 2014 SLACK Incorporated.

Occupation-Based Practice

The *Framework* describes three types of therapeutic interventions, including the therapeutic use of occupations and activities. Preparatory methods prepare the client for occupational performance. Examples are splinting and exercise. Purposeful activities allow the client to engage in goal-directed behaviors within a therapeutically designed context that lead to occupation. Practicing vegetable slicing and drawing a straight line are examples. Occupation-based interventions allow clients to engage in actual occupations that are part of their own contexts and that match their stated goals. Preparing a meal and putting on clothes without assistance are some examples of meaningful occupations. Truly occupation-based activities include self-choice, motivation, meaning, purpose, and context.

Client-Centered Practice

A client-centered approach includes active client participation, inclusion of significant others, and identification of the client's goals, priorities, values, and beliefs. It requires a renewed commitment on the part of the therapist to collaborate in order to establish mutually agreed-upon goals from the onset of therapy. This model encourages the client to take responsibility for making choices regarding the types of therapy interventions received. An increased focus on client-perceived outcomes is considered a benchmark of excellence in the provision of health care while at the same time allowing occupational therapists to rediscover their roots in client-centered care.

Maitra and Erway (2006) discussed a perceptual gap that exists between occupational therapists and their clients in relation to stated use of and participation in client-centered practice. Though the majority of therapists claimed to have explained occupational therapy to their clients, involved their clients in the goal-setting process, and addressed clients' goals in treatment, only a small minority of clients reported the same. The article suggests the need for development of a systematic strategy to ensure that occupational therapists and their clients are able to fulfill their roles in client-centered practice. The strategy employed at our rehabilitation facility involves utilizing an occupation-based evaluation that is client centered and then integrating the goals established by the patient into a treatment plan where occupations of choice are practiced as a routine part of the therapy process.

Occupation as Means and Ends

We are convinced that occupational therapists have the best intentions. Yet in many practices there tends to be a focus on impairment reduction and remediation activities that do not directly relate to the patient's stated roles and occupations. What does it mean to be occupational in your approach to practice? According to Gray (1998), it means using purposeful, meaningful, goal-directed interventions that are whole, multidimensional, and performed in context.

Occupation-based practice calls on therapists to engage patients in occupations as both means and ends. Occupational performance activities can be used to remediate physical problems by engaging the patient meaningfully, or they can be the focus of treatment as an end goal. Gray (1998) stated, "Occupation as means refers to the use of therapeutic occupation as the treatment modality to advance someone toward an occupational outcome" (p. 358). When utilizing occupation as means, the challenge is to select activities that are relevant to the end goal and therefore engaging and motivating to the patient.

Gray (1998) described that occupation as ends provides an overarching goal for occupational therapy interventions rather than limiting it to a specific goal or outcome. This philosophy helps the therapist ensure that every aspect of evaluation and treatment is directed toward restoring the client's occupational well-being. "Occupation can be a valuable tool in a person's recovery that does not have to take the place of the healing of the body, but can actually supplement it and enhance it, or even be the catalyst for healing" (Gray, 1998, p. 359).

Acknowledging Barriers to Occupation-Based Practice

We acknowledge that occupation-based practice is not always easy given the numerous challenges that exist in real-life practice settings. Barriers may be related to the environment, the patient, the therapist, or combinations thereof. Some barriers may truly exist (real barriers). Some barriers may not hold true under closer scrutiny (perceived barriers).

Some perceived environmental barriers cited by therapists include lack of supplies and resources, lack of a conducive treatment environment, lack of support from administration or peers, and lack of time to do occupation-based practice. Real barriers are shorter durations of treatment, productivity expectations, increased caseloads, being immersed in a medical model with a focus on reductionist and diagnostic specific treatment, a focus on doing to clients, and incongruent goals and values between therapist and patient.

As for patient-related barriers, cognitive status may limit the patient's ability to participate in the interview process. Communication difficulties, which may include language barriers and aphasia due to stroke or other neurological disorder, may also limit participation. Patients with adjustment to disability issues and coping difficulties at various stages of loss may refuse to engage in the process.

Therapist-related barriers include lack of training in occupation-based evaluation methods and tools, lack of clinical experience, lack of interviewing skills to facilitate goal identification, and lack of commitment to the occupation-based process. Other barriers may include lack of occupational philosophy, professional identity, self-confidence, empowerment, and ongoing self-reflection as well as negative assumptions about a patient's ability to engage in the process.

Some common perceptions, misconceptions, and excuses among therapists are that there is no time to do occupation. Some therapists express concern that clinics are not set up to do occupation, they cannot document on occupation, will not get reimbursed for doing occupation, that occupational therapy colleagues are not doing occupation, or that this intervention will not be sanctioned by department administrators. Therapists assert that patients enjoy engaging in exercise more than in occupation and that their clients will not value the use of occupation. Others claim that families will not understand the use of occupation and that colleagues will not support it. Let's be honest—occupational therapists are the ones who often undervalue occupation—think of it as commonsense and ordinary and not worth paying for.

It is important to think about and focus on what barriers you have control over, what you are able to change in your practice. No one needs to permit you to practice as an occupational therapist or utilize occupation-based evaluation tools or treatment methods. It is a matter of consciously choosing which philosophy will guide your practice. The Rancho story will illustrate this process.

Overview of Rancho Los Amigos National Rehabilitation Center

Rancho is a Los Angeles County Department of Health Services rehabilitation facility with a 210-inpatient bed capacity, primarily serving indigent patients. Inpatient services include stroke, gerontology, brain injury, neurology, spinal cord injury, pediatrics, orthopedics, and acute medicine. Outpatient services include traditional therapy as well as specialty vocational, driver training, and rehabilitation technology programs. Patients range from pediatric to geriatric, speak a variety of languages, and represent many unique cultures. They are socioeconomically diverse, with most having limited resources and social support. Medicaid is the primary insurance. The occupational therapy staff is almost 40 strong, ranging from new graduates to clinicians with more than 30 years of experience.

Rancho began in the late 1800s as a farm for the sick and the poor of Los Angeles County. Many of the early residents suffered from mental illness and it was believed that engagement in activity would help occupy them. They worked the land and were also assigned to a network of "shops" that would teach them a trade such as furniture making and ceramics. Items produced were used or sold for profits, which were contributed back to the farm. The first occupational therapist was hired to work at Rancho in 1926. The inception of the occupational therapy profession and the rehabilitation movement followed parallel tracks that merged and became inseparable at Rancho. With the polio and tuberculosis epidemics in the 1940s,

Rancho became focused on physical rehabilitation and emerged as a leader in the rehabilitation movement. Our rich history is rooted in the philosophy that engagement of mind and body promotes meaningful and productive lives. This held true for the residents of the Rancho farm and endures for our patients today.

THE PROCESS OF STRENGTHENING OCCUPATION-BASED PRACTICE AT RANCHO LOS AMIGOS

Reflecting on Our Practice

In today's fast-paced health care settings, providing creative, individualized, and occupation-based treatment is a growing challenge. Demands such as shrinking budgets, staff shortages, productivity and documentation requirements, packed schedules, limited resources, increased medical acuity of patients, shorter lengths of program, and restrictions on reimbursable services loom large as therapists struggle to best meet their patients' needs. Many facilities are also driven to document progress according to the national standards for rehabilitation as defined by the Inpatient Rehabilitation Facility–Patient Assessment Instrument (IRF-PAI; Uniform Data System for Medical Rehabilitation, 2009). Although the IRF-PAI covers 18 specific areas of function, it leaves little room to address patients' unique individualized goals. These health care trends may limit our practice by leading to reductionist thinking. Such influences and expectations can be in sharp contrast to the philosophy and goals of occupational therapists. Our challenge is to remain true to our roots while pursuing creative occupation-based treatment opportunities within the realities of today's practice.

At Rancho, we asked ourselves how we could better respond to the changing health care trends and the daily demands of our practice environment. We faced many of the same dilemmas that other practitioners struggle with. The paternalistic philosophy of the medical model collided with our own philosophy of patient-directed care. We were also conflicted over the use of the IRF-PAI and its focus on self-care activities as our facility's outcome measure with our wish to show outcomes across a broader range of occupations.

Our desire to overcome the barriers of the health care system led us to reflect on the effectiveness and efficiency of our practice and to search for an outcome measure that reflected our core values. An adjunct purpose was to examine our treatment philosophy and model of practice and to find a client-centered and occupation-based approach on which to base our services. Though the medical model has been predominant at our facility, occupational therapists at Rancho have traditionally focused on occupational performance in the client's context. However, we decided that we needed to make this implicit philosophy explicit by firmly declaring occupational therapy's unique occupation-based approach to patient care and positioning ourselves as leaders in client-centered care on the rehabilitation team.

Methods

Although we did not think of it as a research method at the time, the efforts we made to strengthen the occupation base of our practice are congruent with an action research approach (Stringer, 1999). We collaboratively developed and implemented this change through a series of reflections, discussions, and actions. We began with weekly meetings in our various occupational therapy clinical areas where time was spent reflecting on what staff would want to know about the effects of occupational therapy at our facility. A focus group of occupational therapy department managers, educators, and clinicians who shared a dedicated interest in improving our practice was formed. The group felt that we most needed to focus on functional outcome studies. This would provide clarity for occupational therapy's role, define best practices for effective outcomes, improve the quality of services within our setting, and demonstrate the valuable role of occupational therapists to consumers, other health care providers, and reimbursers.

Review of the Literature in Our Process

Our research process included a review of the literature including occupation-based articles and outcome measures. Articles were identified, reviewed, and discussed. Our literature review included classic and seminal works from Clark (1993), Law et al. (1990), Mattingly and Fleming (1994), Reilly (1962), Trombly (1995), Wood (1996, 1998), Yerxa (1967, 1998), and Zemke and Clark (1996), among others. The literature inspired us to ask several questions of ourselves: What was our current treatment philosophy and model for practice? Were we truly client centered and occupation based? What distinguished us from other disciplines and what is our unique contribution to the rehabilitation team? How could we include our patients in goal setting and the rehabilitation process in a more meaningful way? What could we utilize as an outcome measure that truly reflected occupational therapy's core values? A department philosophy that included occupation-based and client-centered practice began to take shape as a result of answering these questions. A strategic plan for implementing this philosophy subsequently emerged.

Review and Selection of Outcome Measures

Yerxa (1994) challenged us to consider occupational therapy's core values in relation to the type of outcome measure to use. Among these core values were the following:

Occupational therapists help their clients find satisfaction in their daily routine activities, enable their clients to be self-directed, expect patients to be actively involved in determining their own interests and goals, assist patients in gaining more control over their environments, and believe in the importance of people's own subjective experiences in their lives.

The Canadian Occupational Performance Measure (COPM; Law et al., 1990) met these core values because it enlisted clients in the process, was self-directed in allowing patients to state their interests and goals, and was concerned with measuring functional outcomes. It appeared to be the ideal tool and a good fit with our strategic plan to operationalize client-centered and occupation-based practice. We piloted the COPM first with experienced staff. We developed a staff training series on the COPM and required staff to demonstrate competency in its administration. It then became an expectation for all staff to utilize the COPM across diagnostic groups and the inpatient and outpatient continuum. We provided ongoing staff mentoring to ensure staff success with the process, and we explored means to foster and facilitate consistent integration of COPM-identified occupational goals into treatment.

Reflection on Occupation-Based Practice as an Ongoing Process

Staying grounded in occupation involves a process of honest self-reflection. For some staff this comes easier than others. According to Fortune (2000), we lose and confuse our profession's history and identity. We fail to ground practice in occupational philosophies and we resort to "trading occupation for spare parts." We must reclaim our identity as "therapists of occupation" and promote occupational therapy's unique professional identity in our practice. An approach that misses the mark is one where the therapist drives the treatment plan, the therapist makes choices about activities, the therapist does not consult with the client or significant other, and the therapist follows her or his own agenda. Interventions such as dressing boards, graded clothes pins, cone stacking, and peg boards fall short in this regard.

A truly occupation-based activity includes self-choice, motivation, meaning, purpose, and context. Examples include practicing dressing in the client's own clothes, hanging his or her clothes on a line, reaching for items in a cupboard, and preparing a meal using a recipe the client selected. A truly client-centered approach is one that includes active client participation, involvement of significant others, identification of client's goals and priorities, and knowledge of the client's values and beliefs. Upon reflection, for some staff there was a disconnect between what they intended to do and what they actually did.

Redefining Our Practice

In order to redefine our practice, we embraced a treatment philosophy throughout the department that was occupation based and client centered. We broadened our discussions and shared relevant literature and theoretical concepts essential to occupation-based practice. We gained consensus for declaring occupation as the cornerstone that defines and distinguishes who we are to our patients and to the rehabilitation team. We provided staff with an opportunity to practice and hone their interviewing skills. We discussed adjustment to disability issues as they related to specific diagnoses. We talked about the need to create a future typical day with our clients to help them imagine a future beyond their current challenges, to create a demarcation point from the rehabilitation process, and to promote a sense of hope and optimism about engaging in meaningful occupations in the future. We embraced the idea of patients as the experts on themselves and their care.

Therapist and Patient Roles

One of the key theoretical concepts we found most helpful was the use of narrative (Mattingly, 1991). The narrative approach is one that focuses on the patient's illness experience and how disability affects the person's life. It is action centered, not disease centered. It involves "doing with" the patient and the patient as an active partner rather than "doing to" the patient. This approach requires constructing an individualized story of treatment activities rather than a generic one. It provides a meaningful sequence of events that leads to a significant therapeutic experience for the patient. Ultimately, as therapy evolves the patient and the therapist come to share a common story.

Occupational storytelling involves the patient recounting life events through telling a self-story. The therapist elicits information about childhood and adult occupations and inquires about the patient's typical day both past and present. The discussion focuses on the occupation and the meaning it has for the patient as the therapist becomes immersed in a sense of the patient as an occupational being: "Rather than standing apart from and evaluating their patients, in this approach, therapists must engage themselves fully and inextricably in a dialogue with their patients" (Clark, Ennevor, & Richardson, 1996, p. 375).

Occupational storymaking involves the therapist and the patient creating stories as part of therapy. The patient and therapist construct an imaginative future through narrative. The patient begins to engage in meaningful occupations as means and ends. The therapist provides occupational coaching, occupational strategies, ongoing encouragement, and image reconstruction. The patient then begins to visualize her- or himself as an occupational being immersed in activity despite the presence of disability. The therapist instills hope in the patient for a meaningful future and the patient becomes empowered to act as an agent of change. Together the patient and therapist build a bridge from rehabilitation to the community.

Some strategies for implementing occupation-based treatment and reclaiming our identity as therapists of occupation include "being with" clients and understanding what the illness experience means to them. In order to accomplish this, occupational therapists must be astute listeners to truly understand each client's life story, hopes, and dreams. We need to clearly define to our clients what occupational therapy is, our unique perspective and expertise, and how this fits with their needs. We need to help clients know the role we can play in their life story, that we value their opinions, and then empower them to collaborate and drive the process toward recovery and wellness.

Revitalizing Our Practice

Wood (1998) called us to action in her article "It Is Jump Time for Occupational Therapy" when she asked, "Occupation is *in,* but is occupational therapy?" She challenged us to embrace the richness of our work and incorporate all that is unique to our profession in our daily practice.

Occupation-Based Evaluation Tools

At Rancho we adopted several occupation-based evaluations to assist therapists in consistently remaining occupation focused. These include the Occupational Profile, the Typical Day Description, and the COPM. These three evaluations used in combination help to keep therapists grounded in occupation while at the same time helping to explain to the client occupational therapy's unique perspective. Engaging in this process helps to set the stage for treatment that is client centered and occupation based.

The Occupational Profile is part of the *Framework.* It is an unstructured interview in which the goal is for the therapist to identify the client's primary roles, meaningful occupations, contexts in which daily activities occur, important people and support systems in the client's life, and the client's self-identity. The therapist may begin the Occupational Profile, which looks like a dialogue between patient and therapist, while at the same time conducting aspects of the clinical evaluation. The therapist may use phrases such as "Tell me a little bit about yourself" or "Tell me about your life prior to your injury or illness." These probes can yield many interesting facts about the patient that do not necessarily appear in the medical chart. They allow the therapist to connect with the patient on a human level and cultivate the trust and rapport necessary to build a positive therapeutic relationship.

The Typical Day Description is a tool used to gain further insight as to how clients spend their time throughout a 24-hour period, including a more detailed description of the daily activities and occupations they routinely engage in, the specific contexts in which these occur, and the people in their lives who are involved. At Rancho, the Typical Day Description is slightly more structured than the Occupational Profile in that there is a form to complete. On this form, the times of day beginning from early morning to late at night are listed. The task of the therapist is to elicit from the client in a storytelling fashion how his or her day is typically filled with activity. The therapist may say "Describe a typical day prior to your illness or injury" or "Start with when you wake up in the morning and walk me through a normal day until you go to sleep at night." These probes often yield a fuller description of occupations, reveal prominent habits and routines, and highlight their primary interests and their values. During the process we take special note of occupations, context, roles, themes of meaning, and personal projects the client may be engaged in. Themes of meaning may emerge as clients begin to describe their day and list activities. Perhaps the client states that she or he reads the Bible, prays several times and day, and attends church routinely. A theme of spirituality may emerge that can be incorporated into therapy. Another client may describe daily activities of cooking, cleaning, gardening, and child care, and a theme of home and family can be incorporated into an occupation-based treatment plan. Personal projects are those tasks that are often on a person's "To Do" list. Knowledge of these current or previously unfinished projects can provide ideas for therapy and for creating a future typical day.

The COPM is based on the Canadian Model of Occupational Performance. It was first published in 1991 and has been revised several times since. It is a tool used for goal setting and outcome measurement (Law et al., 2005). It is conducted in a semistructured interview format. It has established test–retest reliability between users. The COPM identifies problems in occupational performance in the areas of self-care, productivity, and leisure. It is appropriate for use with various diagnostic groups and across developmental stages. The COPM can be administered to clients or their family members/significant others.

During the COPM interview, a list of occupations is generated that the client is currently having difficulty performing. To help elicit this list, the therapist may ask, "What do you want to be able to do, need to be able to do, or are expected to do at home?" or "What activities are difficult for you to do right now either at home, at work, or in your community?" Up to five occupations are listed and then each is rated by the patient for importance, performance, and satisfaction with performance using a 10-point numeric scale. The rating question for importance is "On a scale of 1 to 10, 1 being not important at all and 10 being extremely important, how important is it for you to be able to do this activity?" For performance the question is "On a scale of 1 to 10, 1 being unable to do the activity and 10 being able to do it extremely well, how well do you feel you are able to perform this activity right now?" Finally, for the satisfaction question, "On a scale of 1 to 10, 1 being not satisfied at all and 10 being extremely satisfied, how satisfied are you with your performance right now?" The COPM is administered at or close to the initial evaluation. Performance and

satisfaction are then scored again at or close to discharge to measure changes in the client's self-perception of occupational performance over the course of therapy. A change score of 2 or more numeric points between initial and discharge COPMs is considered to be clinically significant. This makes the COPM a valuable outcome tool for occupational therapists in assessing, documenting, and reporting the effectiveness of their interventions.

There are many benefits to utilizing the COPM as part of a routine occupational therapy assessment. It is client centered and engages the client in a collaborative manner from the onset of therapy, supporting the notion that the client has equal responsibility for therapy decisions and outcomes. The COPM also incorporates the roles and role expectations of the client. Other benefits are that the process facilitates the negotiation of goals between the client, family, and therapist. It allows the client to participate in prioritizing goals and to reflect on the progress made toward reaching them. It allows the therapist to use the COPM information to influence treatment intervention choices. The COPM demonstrates the impact of occupational therapy through outcome data and provides an opportunity to promote the efficacy of occupational therapy services to administration, other professions, and third-party payers. Perhaps most important, the COPM helps define the role of occupational therapy to the patient while keeping the therapist focused on the patient's occupations and goals.

Some challenges related to the COPM are the abstract nature of the numerical scoring, which may not be easily understood by patients with varying education levels and cultural backgrounds. The tool is difficult to use when patients have low cognition or limited communication abilities such as occurs with aphasia. Challenges can also occur when patients exhibit lack of coping or adjustment to disability. Incongruent goals between patient and therapist or maladaptive goals may also hamper the COPM process. Time constraints may also pose a challenge given shorter lengths of stay and high documentation demands. Another barrier to completing the COPM may be that the client is unwilling to participate in the process. "Why are you asking me about my goals? You are the professional and should be telling me what to do to get better."

Family involvement is an alternative method when traditional methods are not effective. The family is contacted when the patient is unable to participate, when verification of activities and ratings are desired, when negotiation of priorities is needed, or when clarification regarding discharge plans is required. Some advantages of family involvement are that it yields information that we may otherwise be unable to obtain directly from the patient, provides an opportunity for family participation in the therapy process, and enhances collaboration and rapport. Some disadvantages of involving the family may be that the family has a different agenda or inaccurate perceptions of the patient's goals or priorities. The family may also be unwilling or unavailable to participate.

Studying the Outcomes of the Canadian Occupational Performance Measure

Methods

The Occupational Therapy Department at Rancho has been utilizing the COPM as an outcome tool since 1998. Completed COPMs are collected and entered into a computerized database. The data are analyzed on a routine basis with trends and outcomes shared with staff in order to inform our practice. The COPM outcome data between the years 2007 and 2010 will be presented and discussed.

Descriptive Results

Over the 4-year period, 1,097 COPMs were submitted. These COPMs represented inpatients and outpatients with a variety of diagnoses, ages, genders, languages, and ethnicities. More than half of the COPMs were completed by patients who had a stroke, reflecting the largest population of patients seen at our facility. Other diagnoses included brain injury, tetraplegia, paraplegia, and other neurologic and orthopedic conditions. Approximately half of the patients were in the 40- to 59-year-old age range. Sixty percent of the patients were male and 40% were female; 65% of the patients were English speaking, 30% were Spanish speaking, and 5% spoke other languages. More than half of the patients were Hispanic, 20% were Black, 11% were White, 7% were Asian, and 6% were categorized as other. Average length of stay on an inpatient rehabilitation unit was 21.5 days.

The *Framework* was used to categorize the goals listed on the COPM into activities of daily living (ADL), instrumental activities of daily living (IADL), rest and sleep, education, work, play, leisure, and social participation. The study revealed the vast majority of goals mentioned were ADL or IADL related, regardless of diagnosis, age, gender, language, or ethnic differences. In contrast, leisure, work, play, education, social participation, and rest and sleep goals were mentioned far less frequently. Over the 4-year period, 47% of goals were categorized as ADL and 37% were IADL for inpatients, and 26% of goals were categorized as ADL and 47% were IADL for outpatients. When these data were presented to the therapists, they stated that a likely reason for ADL to be mentioned so frequently by inpatients was the immediate need to address activities such as showering and brushing teeth during inpatients' acute hospitalization because patients may have been unable to perform these essential activities for days. Outpatients mentioned a greater number of IADL goals with a greater focus on home skills and community reintegration. The relatively short length of stay for inpatient rehabilitation was also postulated to contribute to ADL goals being predominant. Some suggestions were to have more discussions with the patient and family about the broader role of occupational therapy, making sure to highlight the significance of work, leisure, education, play, social participation, and rest and sleep. It was also mentioned that perhaps patients may need "permission" to explore activities beyond ADL and IADL and be given opportunities to try some of these in the context of therapy.

There were a total of 523 patients with stroke and 96 patients with brain injury. In looking at a potential correlation between the ability to complete the COPM and the patients' IRF-PAI scores related to cognition, we found that the mean score for comprehension was 4.85, for expression it was 4.89, and for problem solving it was 4.57. Data analysis revealed that the comprehension score was the best predictor of the patient's ability to complete the COPM, with a patient scoring 5 or less having a 50% chance of completing the COPM successfully. After reviewing these data, the therapists agreed that a correlation does appear to exist; however, they cautioned that the IRF-PAI is only one predictor of COPM success and despite the patient's IRF-PAI level the COPM should be attempted. Staff suggested using family more frequently to obtain COPM goals and scores when the patient is not able to participate.

According to the COPM manual, change scores are calculated by comparing average ratings for performance and satisfaction from initial to discharge (Law et al., 2005). A difference of 2 or greater is considered a clinically significant change. A negative change would be if a patient's average score at initial was greater than the average score at discharge. Of the 1,097 COPMs the mean change score was 3.43 for performance and 3.71 for satisfaction. We looked at change scores by diagnosis to determine if there were any trends, and found none over the 4-year period. Patients had statistically and clinically significant changes in performance and satisfaction across all diagnostic groups. Age, gender, language, and ethnicity also did not have a significant effect on the patients' change scores. There were very few negative change scores, and these were distributed across all diagnoses.

The Canadian Occupational Performance Measure Study in Summary

As we had hoped, the COPM has been a good fit with our practice. It has been effective across diagnoses, ages, genders, and ethnic backgrounds. It has allowed us to show positive outcomes as a result of occupational therapy intervention. Ongoing data analysis has allowed us to reflect on our practice and implement changes to enhance patient care.

CONTRIBUTION TO OCCUPATIONAL SCIENCE

Occupational science was initiated in order to provide occupational therapy with a knowledge base to strengthen practice (Clark et al., 1991). Clearly, our work in redefining and revitalizing our practice at Rancho contributes to the aspect of occupational science that is focused on occupation in practice. Drawing on works from the occupational science literature provided a theoretical framework in which to approach our practice. Integrating a few key concepts such as narrative, occupational storytelling, and occupational storymaking empowered therapists to become part of a patient's developing life story given the onset of illness or disability. Our ability to utilize these in conjunction with the Occupational Profile, Typical Day Description, and COPM helped us to identify occupations of meaning that might otherwise remain anonymously embedded in daily routines. Instead, we have successfully incorporated them as part of the dialogue and intervention process with our patients. In this way we were able to validate some of the precepts of occupational science as it provided a knowledge base that fundamentally supports our practice.

Suggestions for Your Occupational Therapy Practice

Evaluation

Prioritize and integrate key occupation-based evaluation questions into your routine client interviews. Though impairment-based evaluation must be completed, choose to clinically measure only what you must so that time saved can be used for occupation-based assessments. Start the occupation-based evaluation process while performing clinical measurements. This looks and sounds like an informal dialogue between therapist and patient, but it is an opportunity to gain important insights about the patient's story while establishing therapeutic rapport. Organize occupation-based evaluation tools into a convenient kit containing Typical Day Description forms and COPM forms and rating scale. This kit can be easily transported to various treatment settings such as bedside, clinics, or the patient's home for efficiency and ease of completing the occupation-based evaluation. Include the Typical Day Description and COPM forms in new client charts for ease of use and as a reminder to complete them as part of the initial evaluation. Revise evaluation templates to include adequate space for Occupational Profile information, a Typical Day Description, and COPM goals. It is recommended that this information be placed first on evaluation forms to send a subtle yet powerful message to staff and the treatment team that the patient comes first rather than the diagnosis and medical history.

Enlist patients in the process from the start. This means engaging the patient in goal selection/prioritization and then participating in a specific goal having immediate results. Modify your approach to more easily connect with the patient. Attempt the process several times at different intervals as needed depending on patient readiness. Work to establish rapport and trust between therapist and patient.

Treatment Planning

Use the COPM as a road map for treatment planning. Once a COPM is completed, the goals are established and prioritized and treatment can flow naturally from that point forward. Revisit the COPM routinely to assess whether or not goals are still relevant, determine whether or not goals should be added or deleted, and help the patient see progress toward goals. The COPM can continue to inform the therapist and help to track goals and revise treatment.

Share COPM goals with occupational therapy assistants who may be working with the patient. Encourage them to address patients' stated COPM goals in their treatment sessions. You can also share COPM results with the interdisciplinary team. Distribute a copy of the COPM or a listing of the identified goals in team meetings to establish occupational therapists as the leaders in client-centered care. Sharing this information will help team members to be more aware of the patient's stated goals and is an opportunity for occupational therapy to solicit the team's help in supporting and encouraging the patient to achieve them. It may also be a nice opportunity to plan for co-treatments with other disciplines when this is indicated.

Utilize the COPM to plan customized group activities. Review goals for common themes and design accordingly. Perhaps there is a group of patients who listed cooking, cleaning, or gardening goals. Maybe there is a group who want to return to participating in soccer, basketball, or fishing. Tailor existing groups to individual patient needs or develop new groups based on goals mentioned on the COPM. Devise meaningful home programs using information on the COPM to improve follow-through and adherence outside of the therapy setting.

Treatment Strategies

From the activities mentioned on the COPM, ask the clients and families to bring in personal items from home to be used in treatment such as their own clothing, instruments, pets, grooming supplies, golf clubs, ethnic foods, etc. This allows patients to practice activities with familiar items within the proper context relieving pressure on the therapist or facility to have everything on hand that is needed for treatment. Rearrange clinic areas to look less medical and more home and community like. Exerting these changes allows the therapist to create a mood and send a message to patients and others when they enter the occupational therapy clinic about what happens while they are there.

Use your facility's campus and surrounding community to incorporate occupation. Some examples are the gift shop or snack shop, work sites on campus related to maintenance or tool use, and garden areas to simulate occupations. Community outings to a restaurant, bank, grocery store, beach, or library may all be utilized. Transportation can be addressed through local bus or city services to help patients to understand their options in accessing the community.

Create home living environments to have another venue for practicing occupations in a more conducive setting. A kitchen space, living room, bedroom, baby's room, office, and garden spaces were all created at Rancho with the intention of providing additional opportunities for clients to practice occupations of choice in appropriate settings. Carve out these environments in a spare room or corner of a treatment clinic. Decorate them with home-like items and accessories such as a sofa, bed, lamp, piano, or desk similar to what you might find in a home. Provide a carpeted surface to allow for vacuuming and for practicing mobility. Better yet, arrange to go to the patient's own home, worksite, or community because these offer special opportunities to practice real-life occupations in the actual context.

Create occupation kits (Chisholm, Dolhi, & Schreiber, 2000) to provide ease and efficiency in utilizing occupation in treatment. By looking at our most common COPM activity goals and by talking with staff, a list of needed kits and essential items was generated. Kits assembled included gardening (various hand tools, seed packets, soil, small pots, watering can); letter writing (pens, adaptive writing devices, stationary, cards, envelopes); pet care (food/water bowls, leash, brush); car care (hose, bucket, sponges, detergent); sewing (needle, thread, scissors, buttons, clothing); housecleaning (duster, mop, sponges, vacuum, cleaning products, gloves, bucket); golfing (clubs, balls, tees, artificial putting green); baby care (baby mannequin, diapers, baby clothes, bottle, baby blanket); and home maintenance (hand tools, lightbulbs, plumbing parts). Item donations were solicited by routing lists through the department to see whether anyone had the items at home to donate. Some staff members were willing to purchase items on the list. This method made the cost of the kits minimal and helped them to come together quickly as the result of a group effort. Sturdy clear plastic bins were purchased to house assembled items for each occupation kit. The creation of the kits allowed the therapist to easily retrieve a bin from the storage closet and have everything to perform a particular occupation.

Staff Training

Provide staff training and mentoring in occupation-based evaluation methods. At Rancho, a training series was created. The series began with a range of articles including a review of key occupation-based concepts, adjustment to disability issues, and communication skills. Staff members were asked questions about each article and a discussion was promoted to consider the implications of these ideas in our practice. Principles of effective interviewing were reviewed and practiced through role-playing with peers. The purpose, yields, and procedures for administering the Occupational Profile, Typical Day Description, and COPM were reviewed and there was an opportunity to practice administering each tool. Case studies were provided throughout the training to illustrate key concepts.

Between staff training sessions, homework was given requesting staff to complete a COPM with a patient. A mentor was asked to observe and videotape the interview. The videotaped interviews were used to provide staff with feedback about the effectiveness of their interview and their communication skills, both verbal and nonverbal. A skills checklist was developed to include all of the key elements on the Occupational Profile, Typical Day Description, and COPM. These checklists were completed on each staff person who participated in the training series.

Case Reviews

Hold peer case reviews to brainstorm occupation-based treatment strategies. At Rancho, these are done in area meetings with senior and novice staff. Cases are presented and feedback is provided. A patient review form was developed using *Framework* terminology to ask specific occupation-based questions. The staff members present a case using the patient review form as a guide, which encourages dialogue using client-centered and occupation-based language. Everyone is welcome to provide treatment strategies and intervention ideas. Discussions help to ground all staff in occupation-based practice.

Create a Journal Club

Consider starting a journal club. At Rancho, we also promote occupation-based practice by selecting relevant articles for review at a monthly department-wide meeting. Journal articles are selected and sent to staff along with focused discussion questions to consider as the article is read. A facilitator or discussant will lead the discussion about the quality and merits of the article, solicit thoughts from the group, answer discussion questions, and attempt to apply key concepts to practice at Rancho.

Involve Occupational Therapy Students

Involve fieldwork students in COPM-related projects to promote occupation-based practice. Interns can assist by conducting literature reviews or researching and presenting on key occupational science concepts. Some of the concepts we asked students to research included the use of narrative, occupational storytelling, and occupational storymaking. Additional topics included themes of meaning, personal projects, lifestyle redesign, coping, adjustment, and hope. Reading and discussing these concepts helped to illuminate important aspects of our practice that we wanted to make more explicit and pay more attention to. For example, the concepts of occupational storytelling as a method to elicit

Figure 26-1. Case study initial COPM goals and ratings. I = importance, P = performance, S = satisfaction.

Initial COPM			
Goal	I	P	S
Grasp items with my left hand	10	1	1
Carry things while walking	10	1	1
Hold my grandson in my arms	10	1	1
Push my mom's wheelchair	10	1	1

the patient's story and the idea that the therapist becomes part of the story and then with the patient creates a future story through storymaking as part of the therapeutic process. These concepts highlight the intimacy of the therapeutic relationship and the power of occupational therapy to assist patients in coping and moving on with their lives in a positive way despite a devastating illness or disability.

Students were asked to review COPM goals and put together new occupation kits from commonly mentioned occupations to complement and enhance those already in place within the department. The additional kits provided therapists in the various areas with more occupation choices for use in therapy.

Other Incentives

Introduce low- or no-cost incentives. At Rancho, we created occupational therapy department awards that are presented at our annual Occupational Therapy Month event. They honor the occupational therapist and occupational therapy assistant who most exemplify occupation-based practice in their daily work. We also initiated "Celebrating Occupation" as another feature of our Occupational Therapy Month festivities. Staff members submit occupation-related stories that they have witnessed or conducted during therapy. These stories are read by our department director during our luncheon. This allows staff who are practicing in a client-centered and occupation-based way to be recognized by the entire department for the good work they are doing.

In summary, we empowered staff to embrace occupation as the core of their practice. We created a department where therapists have the freedom to practice as they wish. We developed occupation-based evaluation kits to promote client-centered and occupation-based evaluation, which then becomes a road map to treatment. We created occupation kits to provide ease and efficiency of integrating occupation in practice. We renovated our environment to make it look less medical and more conducive to practicing real-life occupations. We made occupation part of the daily dialogue where everyone is supporting, encouraging, validating, and engaging in occupation-based practice. We invited occupational therapy faculty members and prominent occupational therapy leaders to educate, challenge, and inspire us. We networked with colleagues and presented at various professional conferences to share our ideas and incorporate those from other

facilities. We encourage you to consider some of these strategies as you develop your own practice.

Case Study

We would like to illustrate our use of occupation-based evaluation and treatment methods through this case presentation of Donald. Donald is a 55-year-old Black American male who sustained a right cerebrovascular accident with left hemiplegia as a result of hypertension and poor medication compliance. He was referred to Rancho Los Amigos for outpatient occupational therapy 4 months after his stroke. He had poor balance, requiring a walker for mobility, no functional use of his left upper extremity, and limited abilities to participate in home and community activities.

Occupational Profile

During the initial evaluation, the occupational therapist learned that Donald was living in a single-story home with his elderly mother. He was the father of a 19-year-old daughter and grandfather of her 2-month-old son. Prior to his stroke, Donald was employed in personal security as a bodyguard for celebrities. He often traveled around the world for his job. He worked out frequently at local gyms and spent time at a shooting range.

Typical Day Description

Donald was not able to work or go to the gym but he made an effort to stay as active as possible, stating that staying at home made him feel depressed. He would wake up, eat breakfast that his mother prepared for him, get himself showered and dressed, attend medical and therapy appointments, visit with his daughter and grandson, and spend occasional evenings out with friends going to movies, local restaurants, or clubs that he used to frequent.

Canadian Occupational Performance Measure

Donald was able to identify several activities that he hoped to be able to engage in by the end of his therapy program and an initial COPM was completed (Figure 26-1). The goals he identified were being able to grasp and hold items with his left hand, carry things while walking, hold his grandson in his arms, and push his mother in her wheelchair, which she required for community mobility. During the COPM interview, Donald also mentioned

Discharge COPM		
Goal	P	S
Grasp items with my left hand	6	5
Carry things while walking	5	4
Hold my grandson in my arms	6	10
Push my mom's wheelchair	7	9
Change Score	6	7

Figure 26-2. Case study discharge ratings and change scores. P=performance, S=satisfaction.

being able to walk better and eventually to walk without a cane as other important goals. During subsequent client–therapist interactions, additional therapy themes of home management, community reintegration, and leisure interests emerged and were used to introduce preparatory, purposeful, and occupation-based treatment interventions throughout the course of therapy.

Treatment

Donald's occupational therapy treatment plan included left upper extremity management, home and community skills training, exploration of community resources, referral to vocational rehabilitation, and patient and family education, all aimed toward helping him resume participation in his meaningful occupations and facilitating motor recovery. He engaged in preparatory treatment such as neuromuscular reeducation, trunk and scapular mobilization, range of motion, neuromuscular stimulation, and splinting/positioning for his left arm. Purposeful activities such as sweeping, sports, tabletop games, a group community outing to a museum, swimming at the local YMCA, putting away groceries, gardening, and woodworking also provided opportunities for practice related to goals. Occupation-based treatment utilizing occupations as both ends and means included pushing a wheelchair, carrying items while walking, and holding and carrying a mannequin baby. The therapist utilized a variety of contexts to properly address Donald's needs. The therapy clinic, therapy living environments such as the therapy kitchen and garden, the hospital campus and surrounding community, and Donald's own community served as venues for occupations to be practiced. All of Donald's COPM goals were at one time or another incorporated into his treatment.

Outcomes

Donald demonstrated improved motor control and function of his left arm and was able to use it as a stabilizer in bimanual tasks. He was able to improve his overall balance during transitional movements, progressed to walking with a cane, and was able to push his mother's wheelchair. In addition, he exhibited increased community participation. Most important, he was able to hold his grandson. Donald proudly shared a photo of himself holding the baby with his right arm while using his left arm to help support it. He

was so pleased to have met this goal that he cried tears of joy when telling his therapist. Scores on Donald's discharge COPM (Figure 26-2) were positive, with a change score of 6 for performance and 7 for satisfaction. This clinically significant change not only demonstrated a valuable outcome from occupational therapy but enabled Donald and his therapist to affirm and celebrate his progress together.

Future Plans

> Reflection is the process of critically evaluating our thinking and acting ... to change behaviors so that professional practice is improved. (Stern, Riestall, & Ripat, 2000, p. 147)

Duggan (2005) suggested that reflective practice is key for empowering therapists with a deeper understanding and implementation of client-centered practice. We use this approach to continually revisit our goals, re-evaluate our methods, revise our tools, and engage our staff in the process. We are proud of what our staff has accomplished, but our work is ongoing. We plan to continually reflect on the effectiveness of our evaluation tools, including the Occupational Profile, Typical Day Description, and COPM, to make sure that they remain relevant to our patients and to our practice. We will revise processes and improve efficiencies as needed to meet environmental demands such as increased therapist caseloads and decreased lengths of stay for patients. We plan to continually reflect on how to best solicit patient goals beyond self-care to all areas of occupational performance and how to creatively plan and implement occupation-based treatment. We will encourage each therapist to revisit the COPM routinely as part of the treatment process and revise or add goals as needed.

Other plans include sharing COPM outcomes with staff in a timely manner in order to inform our practice. We hope to create a process for follow-up with patients post-discharge to determine whether outcomes are sustained over time. Data will also be useful to present to administration regarding the value of occupational therapy and to regulatory agencies who are concerned with client-centered practice and patient experience. We plan to continue to share our outcomes and experiences with the occupational therapy community through presentations and publications.

CONCLUSION

In her 1966 Eleanor Clark Slagle Lecture, Elizabeth Yerxa (1967) stated, "Professional authenticity in OT means that the occupational therapist in every professional act defines the profession" (p. 8). Are you practicing authentic occupational therapy in your setting? Authentic occupational therapy involves both the client and the therapist and allows the client to make choices from a range of possibilities presented to him or her by the therapist. It recognizes the mutual and intimate relationship between the client and the therapist and it values the client's ideas and feelings and is "real" in responding to them. We believe authentic occupational therapy involves being occupation based, client centered, and true to our clients, our profession, and ourselves.

Our work is ongoing. Continual personal self-reflection is a necessary part of the process. Practice must continually evolve in response to changes in health care trends and workplace demands. However, in the midst of changes in the health care environment, our ultimate goal and steadfast desire is to remain authentic occupational therapy practitioners. Florence Clark (2005) once said, "Occupational therapy is the unheralded custodian of a sparkling treasure." We think of occupation as a gem. While in our care, we need to safeguard it, polish it, and cherish it always, because occupation gives us a unique perspective and makes ours a special contribution unlike anyone else's. If occupation is at our core and keeps us centered, then we can be assured that our practice is distinctive and authentic.

LEARNING SUPPORTS

Philosophy and Approach to Practice

Purpose

The purpose of this learning support is to assist the student in reflecting on her or his personal philosophy and approach to practice.

Primary Concepts

Concepts addressed are occupation-based practice, client-centered practice, the *Occupational Therapy Practice Framework,* and occupation as means and ends.

Instructions

Think about these concepts as well as your clinical experiences as you answer the following questions:

1. What does it mean to be occupation based? What does it look like? What does it not look like?

2. What does it mean to be client centered? What does it sound like? What does it not sound like?

3. What do you want your practice to look like and sound like?

Integrating the Canadian Occupational Performance Measure Into Real-Life Practice

Purpose

The purpose of this learning support is to help the student integrate the COPM into practice.

Primary Concepts

Concepts addressed are occupation-based and client-centered evaluation and treatment planning.

Instructions

Reflect on the case study with particular attention to establishing therapeutic rapport, integrating the *Occupational Therapy Practice Framework,* and balancing biomechanical and occupation-based treatment as you answer the following questions:

1. How did using the COPM influence care?

2. What did the therapist do to integrate the patient's stated goals? What else could have been done?

3. What role did preparatory, purposeful, and occupation-based activities play in treatment?

4. Had the COPM not been utilized in this case, how might the outcome have been different?

Operationalizing Occupation-Based Practice

Purpose

The purpose of this learning support is to help the student with creative strategies for addressing patient-identified goals in any practice setting.

Primary Concepts

Concepts addressed are occupation-based evaluation and treatment; environmental, patient- and therapist-related barriers; activity contexts; and authentic practice.

Instructions

Reflect on suggestions made for occupational therapy practice and answer the following questions:

1. Imagine a typical inpatient rehabilitation environment. How is this conducive, or not conducive, to addressing occupation-based goals?

2. List five occupation-based and client-centered strategies you can implement in your personal practice in any setting.

3. What can you do to promote occupation-based practice among occupational therapy colleagues and establish occupational therapy as a leader in client-centered practice?

REFERENCES

American Occupational Therapy Association. (2008). Occupational therapy practice framework: Domain and process (2nd ed.). *American Journal of Occupational Therapy, 62*, 625-683. doi:10.5014/ajot.62.6.625

Chisholm, D., Dolhi, C., & Schreiber, J. (2000). Creating occupation-based opportunities in a medical model clinical practice setting. *OT Practice, 5*, CE1-CE7.

Clark, F. (1993). Occupation embedded in a real life: Interweaving occupational science and occupational therapy. *American Journal of Occupational Therapy, 47*, 1067-1078. doi:10.5014/ajot.47.12.1067

Clark, F. (2005, February). *Introduction.* Presented at the Occupational Science Symposium XVII, Los Angeles, CA.

Clark, F., Ennevor, B. L., & Richardson, P. (1996). A grounded theory of techniques for occupational storytelling and story making. In R. Zemke & F. Clark (Eds.), *Occupational science: The evolving discipline* (pp. 373-392). Philadelphia, PA: F.A. Davis.

Clark, F., Parham, D., Carlson, M. E., Frank, G., Jackson, J., Pierce, D., . . . Zemke, R. (1991). Occupational science: Academic innovation in the service of occupational therapy's future. *American Journal of Occupational Therapy, 45*, 300-310. doi:10.5014/ajot.45.4.300

Duggan, R. (2005). Reflection as a means to foster client-centered practice. *Canadian Journal of Occupational Therapy, 72*, 103-112.

Fortune, T. (2000). Occupational therapists: Is our therapy truly occupational or are we merely filling gaps? *British Journal of Occupational Therapy, 63*, 225-230.

Gray, J. M. (1998). Putting occupation into practice: Occupation as ends, occupation as means. *American Journal of Occupational Therapy, 52*, 354-364. doi:10.5014/ajot.52.5.354

Law, M., Baptiste, S., Carswell, A., McColl, M., Polatajko, H., & Pollock, N. (2005). *Canadian Occupational Performance Measure Manual* (4th ed.). Ottawa, Ontario, Canada: CAOT Publications ACE.

Law, M., Baptiste, S., McColl, M., Opzoomer, A., Polatajko, H., & Pollock, N. (1990). The Canadian Occupational Performance Measure: An outcome measure for occupational therapy. *Canadian Journal of Occupational Therapy, 57*, 82-87.

Maitra, K. K., & Erway, F. (2006). Perception of client-centered practice in occupational therapists and their clients. *American Journal of Occupational Therapy, 60*, 298-310. doi:10.5014/ajot.60.3.298

Mattingly, C. (1991). The narrative nature of clinical reasoning. *American Journal of Occupational Therapy, 45*, 998-1005. doi:10.5014/ajot.45.11.998

Mattingly, C., & Fleming, M. (1994). *Clinical reasoning: Forms of inquiry in a therapeutic practice.* Philadelphia, PA: F.A. Davis.

Peloquin, S. M. (2005). Embracing our ethos, reclaiming our heart. *American Journal of Occupational Therapy, 59*, 611-625. doi:10.5014/ajot.59.6.611

Reilly, M. (1962). Occupational therapy can be one of the great ideas of 20th century medicine. *American Journal of Occupational Therapy, 16*, 1-9.

Stern, M., Riestall, G., & Ripat, J. (2000). The use of self-reflection to improve client-centered processes. In G. Fearing & J. Clark (Eds.), *Individuals in context: A practical guide to client-centered practice* (pp. 145-158). Thorofare, NJ: SLACK Incorporated.

Stringer, E. (1999). *Action research.* Thousand Oaks, CA: Sage Publications.

Trombly, C. A. (1995). Occupation: Purposefulness and meaningfulness as therapeutic mechanisms. *American Journal of Occupational Therapy, 49*, 960-972. doi:10.5014/ajot.49.10.960

Uniform Data System for Medical Rehabilitation. (2009). *The FIM System Clinical Guide* (ver. 5.2). Buffalo, NY: Author.

Wood, W. (1996). Legitimizing occupational therapy's knowledge. *American Journal of Occupational Therapy, 50*, 626-634. doi:10.5014/ajot.50.8.626

Wood, W. (1998). It is jump time for occupational therapy. *American Journal of Occupational Therapy, 52*, 403-411. doi:10.5014/ajot.52.6.403

Yerxa, E. J. (1967). Authentic occupational therapy. *American Journal of Occupational Therapy, 21*, 1-9.

Yerxa, E. J. (1994, October). *The "so-what" question: Assessing outcomes of occupational therapy.* Presented at the Occupational Therapy Association of California Annual Conference, Los Angeles, CA.

Yerxa, E. J. (1998). Health and the human spirit for occupation. *American Journal of Occupational Therapy, 52*, 412-418. doi:10.5014/ajot.52.6.412

Zemke, R., & Clark, F. (1996). *Occupational science: The evolving discipline.* Philadelphia, PA: F. A. Davis.

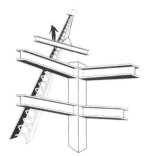

27

The Use of Occupation in Hand Therapy

Donna Colaianni, PhD, OTR/L, CHT and Ingrid Provident, EdD, OTR/L

My personal experience with incorporating more occupation into my therapeutic approach with clients following hand injury improved my clients' outcomes and made interventions more satisfying to me as an occupational therapist. As I pursued postprofessional education, I was motivated to study the effectiveness of occupation-based interventions in hand therapy but was surprised to find that a literature search revealed very little. With such a dearth of research on what seemed to be an important topic, there were many questions to be explored, and this study was my first step on that path. I completed this study as a PhD student at Duquesne University with Dr. Provident as my advisor and co-investigator.

Occupational therapy was founded on the concept that engagement in occupation promotes and restores physical and emotional health (Trombly, 1995). Despite the fact that the profession of occupational therapy is calling for increased use of occupation as a treatment modality, there is little evidence in the literature that occupational therapists working in hand therapy base their practice in occupation (Schier & Chan, 2007). Though some occupational therapists working in hand therapy regard the use of a holistic approach that addresses both physical and psychosocial aspects of hand injuries best practice, they

struggle with the reality of delivering this care (Fitzpatrick & Presnell, 2004).

LITERATURE

Evidence of the Increased Effectiveness of Occupation-Based Treatment in Physical Disabilities

There are few studies that examine the effectiveness of purposeful or occupation-based interventions in hand therapy. Guzelkucuk, Duman, Taskaynatan, and Dincer (2007) compared the effectiveness of therapeutic activities based on activities of daily living (ADL) with therapeutic exercise among a group of 36 participants in a military setting following hand injuries. Both the control and experimental groups participated in therapeutic exercises, including range of motion (ROM) and strengthening exercises. The control group participated in two sessions of exercise daily. The experimental group had one session of exercise and then a second session that consisted of

Pierce, D. (Ed.).
Occupational Science for Occupational Therapy (pp. 325-334).
© 2014 SLACK Incorporated.

25 different therapeutic ADL, including locking and unlocking a door, using a screwdriver, and writing. Participants' active range of motion (AROM), strength, and functional abilities improved to a significantly greater degree and at a faster rate among the group that participated in the ADL program.

In a randomized control trial of 146 hand therapy patients, a gripper or pincher connected to a computer, which either operated a game or instructed the participant to use the gripper or pincher at a comfortable pace, was used. Repetitions performed were significantly greater in the computer game condition than in the computer-directed exercise condition (King, 1992). Jarus, Shavit, and Ratzon (2000) compared the effect of using a computer game with using a machine to make bottle brushes in patients with Colles' fractures. Participants in the group who played computer games demonstrated a significantly higher level of interest in treatment than those in the brush machine group.

Though the evidence for the effectiveness of purposeful or occupation-based interventions in hand therapy is just beginning to emerge, there is a significant body of research regarding the effectiveness of purposeful or occupation-based interventions in physical rehabilitation practice by occupational therapists in settings other than hand therapy. Though these studies did not include typical hand therapy diagnoses, they examined outcomes and capacities of interest to occupational therapists working in hand therapy, such as ROM, pain, activity tolerance, function, repetitions performed, motor learning, and quality of movement.

Occupation-based interventions such as hitting a drum or playing a game increased AROM in individuals with neurologic diagnoses when compared to nonpurposeful activity (Nelson et al., 1996; Van der Weel, Van der Meer, & Lee, 1991). Participating in cooking and craft activities increased activity tolerance among nursing home residents (Dolecheck & Schkade, 1999; Yoder, Nelson, & Smith, 1989). Children with burn injuries reported decreased pain when participating in play-based interventions (Melchert-McKearnan, Deitz, Engel, & White, 2000). Participants with hip fractures experienced improved function after participating in treatment that focused on individually chosen occupation-based activities when compared to participants who participated in biomechanically focused treatment (Jackson & Schkade, 2001). Improved overall outcomes were also seen when using purposeful activities through increased repetitions performed by participants with hemiplegia and burn injuries (Hsieh, Nelson, Smith, & Peterson, 1996; Melchert-McKearnan et al., 2000), improved motor learning among healthy participants (Ferguson & Trombly, 1997), and improved quality of movement among participants following a stroke (Trombly & Wu, 1999).

Component-Focused Practice in Hand Therapy

The medical model and biomechanical frame of reference dominate the field of hand therapy (Fitzpatrick & Presnell, 2004). This results in challenges to the use of occupation-based approaches in hand therapy that are due to a focus on the physiological parts of the human, an accustomed reliance on protocols and prescribed treatment methods (Fitzpatrick & Presnell, 2004; Helm & Dickerson, 1995), and the narrowing of practice due to specialization (Dale et al., 2002; Hoyt Slaymaker, 1986). Pierce (2003) has termed this approach *component-focused practice*. "Component-focused practice addresses the problems of clients through intervention in a very specific area of functioning judged to be the primary barrier to a more desirable occupational pattern" (p. 245). Reliance on predetermined treatment protocols, which are a hallmark of component-focused practice, may be perceived by patients as impersonal and uncaring because they do not take the individual or his or her environment into account. Fixed treatment protocols also focus treatment on the diagnosis instead of the person, leading to dehumanization and client dissatisfaction (Fitzpatrick & Presnell, 2004; Peloquin, 1993). The perception that biomechanical treatment modalities such as exercise are easier affects the treatment choices of occupational therapists working in hand therapy, discouraging the use of individualized occupation-based treatment (Dale et al., 2002; see also Chapter 24).

Specialization in hand therapy appears to increase component-focused practice through a focus on the biomechanical aspects of treatment, such as exercise and modalities (Hoyt Slaymaker, 1986). Novice therapists are especially susceptible to adopting the more structured medical model at the expense of a holistic occupation-based practice (Dale et al., 2002; Hoyt Slaymaker, 1986). The medical model assumes that function is restored when physical signs and symptoms such as pain or decreased ROM are alleviated (Mathiowetz, 1993), causing some occupational therapists who work in hand therapy to delay addressing functional goals until physical symptoms are addressed. However, the assumption that changing underlying physical symptoms changes functional performance is questionable. Only 31% of ADL performance variance can be credited to motor impairment (Trombly, 1995). At best, only modest correlations have been found between components such as pain or ROM and functional performance (Pratt & Burr, 2001; Serlin, Mendoza, Nakamura, Edwards, & Cleeland, 1995). The use of occupation as a treatment modality is proposed to provide more context-specific and generalizable functional outcomes (McLaughlin-Gray, 1998).

The Influence of Logistic Issues in Hand Therapy

Logistic issues in hand therapy settings related to reimbursement (Dale et al., 2002; McColl, 1994) and limited time (Dale et al., 2002; Peloquin, 1993) present occupational therapists in hand therapy settings with challenges to maintaining an occupation-centered approach. Changes in reimbursement, including managed care and the Medicare Prospective Payment System, have placed limits on occupational therapy visits (MacDermid et al., 2002). Health care systems focused on profit, business principles, and efficiency increase caseload demands. Because developing the type of relationship with a client that allows for client-centered and occupation-based care takes time, these restrictions on the number of therapy visits encourage a dehumanized, component-focused, reductionist practice that makes the development of an occupation-based treatment plan difficult (Dale et al., 2002; McColl, 1994; Peloquin, 1993).

METHODS

In order to investigate the effectiveness of occupation as a therapeutic modality for clients with hand injuries, it is vital to understand how occupational therapists currently working in hand therapy make use of the benefits of occupation and negotiate challenges to occupation-based practice. Therefore, the research question that guided this mixed methods survey was "What do occupational therapists working in hand therapy in the United States perceive to be the benefits of and challenges to the use of occupation-based treatments with clients following hand injuries?"

Participants

Participants' e-mail addresses were obtained from the American Society of Hand Therapists (ASHT) Web site for this mixed methods survey. In order to represent a wider variety of experience, 250 certified hand therapists (CHTs) and 250 non-CHTs were randomly selected to be invited to participate in the study, for a total of 500 invitations. Inclusion criteria were registration as an occupational therapist, membership in the ASHT, and an e-mail address included in the "Find a Hand Therapist" section of the ASHT's Web site. Fifty of the 500 e-mail invitations were returned as undeliverable, leaving 450 successfully delivered e-mail invitations. One hundred five participants completed the questionnaire for a total response rate of 23%. Twenty-six non-CHTs participated, for a response rate of 11.5%, and 79 CHTs participated, for a response rate of 35.1%.

Detailed demographics were collected in the survey in order to fully understand the responding sample. The participants' mean age was 43.2 years (standard deviation [SD] = 8.65) with a range of 27 to 59 years. Mean years of experience as an occupational therapist was 18.2 (SD = 8.65) with a range of 4 to 37 years. Ninety-one percent of participants were female ($n = 96$), 8% were male ($n = 8$), and 1% did not reveal their gender ($n = 1$). Seventy-five percent of participants ($n = 79$) were CHTs and 25% ($n = 26$) of participants were non-CHTs. Participants had 13.4 (SD = 6.96) mean years of experience in hand therapy, with a range of 3 to 23 years. The mean number of hours in hand therapy practice per week was 30.8 (SD = 3.99), with a range of 0 to 80 hours. For the CHT participants, the mean years of experience in hand therapy was 14.4 (SD = 6.96), with a range of 5 to 32 years, and for the non-CHT participants it was 10.3 years (SD = 6.96), with a range of 3 to 24 years. The mean number of hours per week in hand therapy practice was 29.5 (SD = 13.11) for the CHTs, with a range of 1 to 60 hours, and 32.4 (SD = 12.72) for the non-CHTs, with a range of 2 to 80 hours.

Data Collection

A review of the literature and pilot testing with four occupational therapists with experience in hand therapy or research contributed to the development of the survey. The use of an online survey permitted a larger sample than would have been possible if individual interviews were completed, although it was not the optimal method for obtaining the in-depth responses that benefit qualitative analysis. The survey consisted of 12 closed-ended and 5 open-ended items. The closed-ended items inquired about participants' demographic information including age, gender, years of experience, hand therapy certification status, how many hours they worked per week, and the frequencies and types of treatments they used. The open-ended items inquired about the participants' thoughts regarding the construct of occupation and occupation-based interventions and included questions such as "How do you define occupation?" "What do you think are barriers to the use of occupation as a treatment modality in hand therapy practice?" and "What do you think are the benefits of using occupation as a treatment modality in hand therapy practice?" All of the 105 participants answered all four of the open-ended questions with responses ranging in length from a few words to several paragraphs. The fifth open-ended question requested additional thoughts and was answered by 54 participants. The study proposal and survey were approved by the institutional review board of Duquesne University.

An e-mail invitation was sent to each participant, explaining the purpose of the study, consent, and risks and benefits and providing a link to the survey. The survey was accessed through an online survey administrator, Zoomerang, which maintained participant anonymity. Participation in the survey was voluntary. At the end of 1 week, a reminder was sent via e-mail, after which the questionnaire was kept open for 1 additional week.

Data Analysis

At the conclusion of the 2-week data collection period, closed-ended responses were entered into SPSS (ver. 13.0, IBM) and analyzed using descriptive statistics to provide background information about the participants. Open-ended responses were analyzed qualitatively for common themes following the strategy described by Creswell (1998). The qualitative analysis began with hand coding of the participants' responses by the primary investigator within the framework of the questions "What are the benefits of the use of occupation-based interventions in hand therapy?" and "What are the challenges to the use of occupation-based interventions in hand therapy?" These 377 coded responses were organized into 20 categories by placing similarly coded statements into categories. The categories were then organized into seven themes. Peer debriefing was accomplished by two additional occupational therapists with experience in qualitative analysis who reviewed and verified the coded responses, categories, and themes. In order to indicate frequency of responses, the number of codes in each category and theme, as well as the percentage of participants contributing to each category, are included in the following results.

Trustworthiness

Pilot testing of the survey instrument promoted face validity. Random selection of participants, as well as the number of respondents ($n = 105$), enhanced the reliability of the study's results. The number of participants allowed a broad expression of perceptions, although some depth of analysis may have been sacrificed by using an online survey. Trustworthiness of the qualitative analysis was enhanced through peer debriefing, which was accomplished through regular and structured discussion of the project between the authors and selected colleagues. Transferability of the qualitative results to the practice settings of readers was enhanced in the study through provision to the reader of adequate description (Creswell, 1998).

Limitations of the Study

The major limitation of this study was that the method of gathering data was not conducive to an in-depth qualitative analysis. Thus, generalization could be limited. The 23% response rate for all participants, including a 35.1% response rate for CHTs and an 11.5% response rate for non-CHTs, also may not reflect the majority of occupational therapists who are functioning as hand therapists. Although all study participants were members of the ASHT, it is possible that they may not be a good representation of occupational therapists working in hand therapy settings. A 75% majority of the participants were CHTs, which may have influenced the results of the study. Additionally, even though the concepts of occupation and occupation-based treatment were defined in the questionnaire, it was apparent that some of the participants did not understand the concept of "occupation as means."

RESULTS

Practice Patterns

Practice patterns for the use of treatment modalities are outlined in Tables 27-1 and 27-2.

The preference for exercise and manual techniques in terms of the percentage of clients with whom the participants used those interventions as well as the average percentage of time the intervention was used within an individual client's typical treatment session are detailed in the tables. Exercises such as AROM, passive resistive exercises (PREs), and Theraputty (Patterson Medical Holdings, Inc.) were used with 61% to 90% of clients. Occupation-based interventions, such as ADL and the use of occupations as an intervention, were used with 41% to 51% of clients. When used, exercise accounted for as much as 41% to 50% of treatment time, and ADL and occupation accounted for 21% to 30%. In general, participants reported using component-focused interventions with more clients and for longer periods of time than occupation-based interventions.

Benefits of Occupation-Based Practice

When asked whether they thought there were benefits of using occupation as a treatment modality in hand therapy practice, 97% of respondents answered yes and 3% answered no. Analysis of the open-ended questions related to the benefits of the use of occupation-based interventions in hand therapy produced the following themes in regard to how therapists explained the value of this approach: facilitating meaningful therapeutic experiences (90 occurrences in the data), facilitating functional activity (57), and facilitating holism (19).

Facilitating Meaningful Therapeutic Experiences

Sixty-six percent of participants indicated that occupation-based treatments facilitate meaningful therapeutic experiences, including the categories motivation and compliance (39 occurrences), meaning for the client (28), relevance (15), and client satisfaction (8). Thirty-six percent of the participants commented on the role that occupation-based treatments played in the compliance of their clients. They reported that occupation-based treatments are intrinsically motivating and give a client, as one therapist stated, "a sense of ownership, if not expertise, in the activity with which he is familiar." One participant noted that the meaningful activity "effectively motivates the patient to focus more on the end result." Another participant reported that clients are better able to build their strength and endurance because "patients are more engaged in a rewarding activity and will participate for a lengthy amount of time [but] exercise may last only 1/2 hour."

Table 27-1

Percentage of Participants' Clients Receiving Specific Intervention (*n*=105)

INTERVENTION	0% TO 10%	11% TO 20%	21% TO 30%	31% TO 40%	41% TO 50%	51% TO 60%	61% TO 70%	71% TO 80%	81% TO 90%	91% TO 100%	NOT USED	WEIGHTED AVERAGE
AROM ex	0	1	0	1	1	1	2	13	16	69	1	81% to 90%
PRE	0	1	4	2	6	10	9	27	23	22	1	61% to 70%
Theraputty	0	2	5	5	12	12	18	20	18	12	1	61% to 70%
JM	4	2	9	9	10	13	16	16	11	11	2	61% to 70%
P stretch	1	4	4	1	9	8	9	21	24	23	1	51% to 60%
Splinting	0	2	11	9	16	13	16	24	7	6	1	51% to 60%
Massage	1	1	1	4	9	12	11	23	21	22	1	61% to 70%
ADL	12	14	10	5	10	6	11	10	7	17	3	41% to 50%
PAMs	4	5	3	6	11	9	11	17	22	16	1	51% to 60%
Activities	11	4	10	10	10	14	8	17	11	8	2	41% to 50%
Crafts	53	16	4	1	6	1	3	1	0	0	20	0% to 10%
Occupations	12	8	16	13	10	6	9	13	10	6	2	41% to 50%

Note. AROM ex=active range of motion exercise, PRE=progressive resistive exercise, JM=joint mobilizations, P stretch=passive stretch, ADL=activities of daily living, PAMs=physical agent modalities, Activities=activities such as clothes pins or pegs.

Table 27-2

Percentage of Client Treatment Time Devoted by Participants to Intervention per Typical Treatment Session (*n*=105)

INTERVENTION	0% TO 10%	11% TO 20%	21% TO 30%	31% TO 40%	41% TO 50%	51% TO 60%	61% TO 70%	71% TO 80%	81% TO 90%	91% TO 100%	NOT USED	WEIGHTED AVERAGE
AROM ex	4	13	12	15	22	7	8	9	4	10	1	41% to 50%
PRE	6	15	26	17	15	8	4	8	3	2	1	31% to 40%
Theraputty	25	30	15	7	11	7	2	3	1	2	2	21% to 30%
JM	30	15	22	13	8	1	8	1	3	1	3	21% to 30%
P stretch	13	24	22	13	13	2	2	8	2	5	1	21% to 30%
Splinting	21	24	17	14	11	3	4	5	1	2	3	21% to 30%
Massage	20	27	23	10	7	2	6	5	4	0	1	21% to 30%
ADL	33	14	22	6	12	3	2	5	3	1	4	21% to 30%
PAMs	20	28	23	12	5	1	6	6	1	1	2	21% to 30%
Activities	30	27	22	6	7	2	3	3	0	3	2	11% to 20%
Crafts	55	9	3	2	3	2	0	1	0	0	30	11% to 20%
Occupation	23	18	20	12	8	8	3	4	4	1	4	21% to 30%

Note. AROM ex=active range of motion exercise, PRE=progressive resistive exercise, JM=joint mobilizations, P stretch=passive stretch, ADL=activities of daily living, PAMs=physical agent modalities, Activities=activities such as clothes pins or pegs.

Participants reported that occupation-based treatment activities that are meaningful to the client are beneficial for different reasons. Twenty-seven percent of the participants stated that meaningful activity promoted client engagement in the therapy process. One participant indicated that the "individual buys into getting improvement or better, because they are performing activities that have meaning to them." One participant reported that clients preferred activities that hold meaning for them, stating, "Patients actually prefer occupation-based interventions if they get to choose the intervention—i.e., adapted golf versus the BTE [Baltimore Therapeutic Equipment] for wrist strengthening."

Fourteen percent of the participants commented that "patients can better relate [occupation-based treatment] to their day to day lives [because] it makes all the medical jargon and exercises translate to real life reasoning." One participant commented on the importance of educating clients on the relevance of occupation-based treatments by saying, "If explained correctly, the patient 'buys in' and fully participates in the treatment, understanding that the ultimate goal is independence." A participant commented that working with activities relevant to the client promotes faster functional recovery because "tasks that relate to patients' interests will help them gain function quicker and will allow them a reward of completion/success." Greater levels of client satisfaction were noted by 8% of participants when using occupation-based interventions because the client experiences, as noted by one participant, an "improved quality of life without waiting for full healing." Another participant noted that "the patients find it more enjoyable." A participant also noted that client satisfaction is improved when the client receives the "psychological benefits of participating in meaningful and satisfying activity."

Facilitating Functional Activity

Forty-six percent of participants reported that occupation-based treatments facilitate functional activity with the following categories: focusing on functional goals (20 occurrences); increasing carryover (15); facilitating subcortical or automatic movement (13); and allowing better assessment of functional performance and necessary adaptations (9). Nineteen percent of participants commented on the importance of occupation-based interventions in ensuring a functionally relevant recovery that is not based on improvement in ROM or strength alone. One participant reported that "occupation is what the hand/upper quadrant is used for. Hand therapy involves, not only return of function within the extremity, but also adaptations to ensure quality of life." The effectiveness of occupation-based interventions in reaching functional goals was illustrated by one participant, who said, "Rote exercise alone cannot increase the functional use of the hand because functional use of the hand involves a varied combination of movements that can only be accomplished using functional tasks." Fourteen percent of therapists participating in the survey also noted improved carryover with the use of occupation-based treat-

ments, with one participant commenting, "I have found that if explained well, the patients generally understand and can apply what they have done in therapy to their personal lives. There is better carryover of the tasks and involvement with their home programs."

Twelve percent of participants commented on the automatic nature of movements that occur as a result of engagement in a purposeful activity, with one participant saying that "the patient then will use desired weak muscles to perform activities they want to perform without realizing they are exercising. By changing activity from cortical to subcortical this then is the beginning of muscle re-education and retraining." Additionally, 9% of the participants indicated that the use of occupation-based interventions allows a better assessment of actual function through better "observation/quantification of patient functional issues than that provided by patient report" and provides "instant feedback on functional status and would allow therapist to modify areas as needed."

Facilitating Holism

Sixteen percent of participants reported that occupation-based treatments facilitate holism within these categories: addressing the client's psychological issues (12 occurrences), being attuned to the theoretical basis of occupational therapy (3), and providing individualized treatment (4). Ten percent of participants indicated that occupation-based interventions addressed psychological issues such as fear, pain, and client confidence in abilities. Occupation-based interventions provided clients with distraction from fear and pain and allowed them to overcome avoidance of using their hand through automatic hand function. One participant commented that "therapy gives the patient a chance to practice occupation and build confidence in their abilities to accomplish functional tasks."

Three percent of participants remarked that the use of occupation-based treatments is consistent with the holistic theoretical base of occupational therapy. One participant stated that occupation-based interventions are "in keeping with our theory base and what will help us define our role and justify what we do in the realm of hand therapy." Participants noted that incorporating occupation-based interventions promotes holism. One participant stated that an occupation-based approach shows the client "that you are treating them as an individual and are interested in improving their specific functional abilities."

Challenges to Occupation-Based Practice

Analysis of the open-ended questions related to challenges to the use of occupation-based interventions in hand therapy resulted in description of the following issues: logistics (98 occurrences), reimbursement (32), credibility (29), and limitations of the client's medical condition or treatment protocol (22).

Logistical Issues

Fifty-one percent of participants reported that logistical issues challenged the use of occupation-based treatments, including limited time (32), limited space (29), limited availability of supplies (20), and the variety of occupations in which people engage (17). Twenty-seven percent of participants reported that lack of space and appropriate facilities was a major challenge to the use of occupation as a treatment modality in hand therapy. One participant said, "We don't have a kitchen set up in our clinic to have patients practice lifting pots and pans or opening jars." Another stated, "My client may need to throw a football 30 yards, or be able to accurately serve a tennis ball. My clinic does not allow me to set up or observe those kinds of goals." Twenty-eight percent of participants commented on how time pressures challenged the use of occupation-based treatment due to the number of clients seen at the same time, heavy case loads, and the limited numbers of visits covered by some insurance companies. "Most [visits are] used up in wound care and obtaining basic ROM and the need to focus on pressing body structure and function issues." The variety of different occupations in which clients might engage also made it difficult to have the necessary equipment or supplies available. Asking the client to bring in supplies from home did not always solve this problem. One participant remarked that:

> Tying flies requires a lot of equipment I don't have, but assumedly the client does. [But] he may not be able to pack it up and bring it all to the clinic so a therapist can observe what difficulty the client may be experiencing. (Colaianni & Provident, 2010)

Reimbursement Issues

Twenty-nine percent of participants reported that reimbursement issues challenged occupation-based practice in hand therapy due to insurance coverage (26 occurrences) and documentation (6). Twenty-four percent of the participants expressed concern that occupation-based treatments would not be covered by insurance companies. One participant stated that "Medicare does not want to pay for things that people enjoy to get back to such as knitting, etc. or any type of hobby or craft, they do not look at it as purposeful." Six percent of the participants also noted the difficulty of documenting occupation-based interventions because the description of context inherent to occupation takes extra time.

Credibility of Occupation-Based Treatments

Twenty-two percent of participants reported challenges to occupation-based practice related to its perceived credibility by different stakeholders: occupational therapists working in hand therapy (16 occurrences), other professionals (10), and clients (3). Fifteen percent of participants reported that part of what limited their use of occupation-based interventions was their own beliefs, including the belief that occupation cannot meet the goals of hand therapy clients, is unnecessary, can be too frustrating for clients, can be too difficult to use, and does not have research support for its use in hand therapy. One participant stated that "purposeful activities do not address end ranges of motion and certainly do not challenge someone to exert maximum strength. Basically, purposeful activities do not emphasize issues of concern to our referring source directly." Another participant said, "Some tasks only take a few seconds to complete (like tying shoes) and therefore would need too many repetitions to increase skill level. [It's] easier and faster to increase strength, endurance, ROM with [PREs]." The current paucity of evidence for the use of occupation-based treatments with hand therapy clients was noted by participants. One participant stated that occupation-based treatment is "thought of as too arts and crafts or not scientific. This is a stigma I do not like about being an OT [occupational therapist]."

Eight percent of therapists providing qualitative data reported that their clients do not understand occupation-based treatments. One participant reported that "the use of occupation-based treatments is sometimes shunned by the patient, as being too low-tech, not 'objective' enough." Two percent of participants also reported a "lack of respect from other professionals and the community" for occupation-based interventions. The attitudes of physicians and administrators were cited as challenges to occupation-based practice. One participant reported that using occupation-based interventions required "convincing the administration that what you are doing isn't 'silly baking activities.'"

Limitations Imposed by the Client's Medical Condition or the Treatment Protocol

The client's stage of healing and restrictions imposed by treatment protocols were cited by 21% of participants as challenges to occupation-based practice (22 occurrences). These participants were particularly concerned with activity restrictions in the acute stage of healing. One participant commented:

> Often patients are in a very acute stage needing to first regain or reestablish lost movement or sensation and the focus is in the resolution of impairments from the injury. … Therefore, the therapist has to be mindful in terms of providing a corresponding activity level which at first obviates the unwanted too excessive motion and then reintroduces it when safe in a graded way. (Colaianni & Provident, 2010)

Summary of Results

In this study of occupation-based practice by hand therapists, 97% of participants believed that occupation-based interventions were beneficial to hand therapy clients due to their facilitation of meaningful therapeutic experiences, functional activity, and holistic care. Interestingly,

91% of the respondents also saw challenges to an occupation-based approach in hand therapy, largely due to the logistics of time pressures, space and supply limitations, and the variety of equipment that would be needed to custom design more personalized interventions. Participants reported using occupation-based interventions with only 41% to 50% of their clients, AROM with 81% to 90% of their clients, and PREs with 61% to 70% of their clients. The participants also spend a lower percentage of time engaging their clients in occupation-based interventions (21% to 30%) than in treatment modalities such as AROM (41% to 50%) or PREs (31% to 40%).

Some participants reported wishing that they could use occupation-based treatments more with their hand therapy clients. One participant said, "I wish I had a more enriched environment in which to engage my clients in occupations." Another participant indicated a lack of good examples of occupation-based hand therapy, stating,

> In my schooling, and I believe in most OT schooling, there is just training to the base skills of hand therapy, but not a good place to practice occupation-based treatment and few good examples to point to. I do not know of one great clinic to point to that really nails the occupation-based treatment ideal. (Colaianni & Provident, 2010)

It is important to address the challenges to occupation-based care in hand therapy settings in order to assist occupational therapists working in hand therapy to use a treatment modality they judge to be beneficial.

CONTRIBUTION TO OCCUPATIONAL SCIENCE

Occupational science is committed to producing knowledge to support occupational therapy practice (Clark et al., 1991). This study offers a detailed examination of occupation-based practice in hand therapy, which is, arguably, one of occupational therapy's most component-focused areas of practice. This knowledge suggests needed occupational science research and demonstration projects that could support more holistic and effective hand therapy practice.

Occupational therapists practicing in hand therapy settings are reluctant to use occupation in their treatments due to many factors. The component-focused approaches common in hand therapy are grounded in the natural sciences of anatomy, physiology, physics, and chemistry. As occupational therapists practicing in hand therapy increasingly understand the science of occupation, they may accept the use of occupation as a treatment approach to a greater degree. Occupational science examines how occupations affect biological and neurobiological processes, which is compatible with the natural science base that appeals to occupational therapists specializing in hand therapy (Amini, 2007). The findings of this study can also assist occupational

scientists in examining the intersection between occupation and the functioning of the upper extremity. "Occupational science can and should become a grounding science for hand therapy practice" (Amini, 2007, p. 12).

IMPLICATIONS FOR OCCUPATIONAL THERAPY

Research and education about the benefits of, and challenges to, the use of occupation-based approaches are vital to helping occupational therapists working in hand therapy to use a treatment modality they judge to be beneficial. Barriers related to space, setting, time, and the cost and availability of supplies may require occupational therapists to think more creatively in order to use occupation-based interventions. However, some of these barriers are not within the control of occupational therapists working in hand therapy. Barriers such as high caseloads and ill-equipped and undersized clinics are often a result of policies set by clinic management for financial reasons. To address the barriers of space, setting, time, and the cost and availability of supplies, continuing education courses that encourage creative thinking and examples of real clinical uses of occupation-based interventions are vital. Demonstration of the effectiveness, particularly the cost effectiveness, of occupation-based interventions through research may also help convince administrators that investing in space, supplies, and staffing would be beneficial.

When addressing barriers related to reimbursement, continuing education courses that assist occupational therapists in appropriately using, documenting, and citing evidence for the effectiveness of occupation as a treatment approach would be helpful. Third-party reimbursement sources would also be more likely to pay for treatments that are submitted with the support of a solid research foundation.

In her 1995 Eleanor Clarke Slagle Lecture, Catherine Trombly discussed the concepts of "occupation as means" and "occupation as ends." Trombly (1995) defined occupation as ends as the concept of occupation as the functional end goal and occupation as means as "the therapy used to bring about changes in impaired performance components" (p. 963). Some participants in this study appeared to view occupation-based hand therapy in terms of occupation as ends instead of both occupation as ends and occupation as means. Perhaps this focus on occupation as ends contributed to the participants' beliefs that insurance companies will not pay for some occupation-based treatment. However, Current Procedural Terminology codes used by Medicare and Medicaid and most insurance companies do allow for the use of activity or occupation-based treatments through the codes for therapeutic activity and ADL as long as a skilled service is being provided. The same factors, such as grading of the exercise, that make AROM exercises skilled services also make properly executed occupation-based treatments skilled services.

Participants perceived barriers related to the credibility of occupation-based interventions among clients, other professionals, and occupational therapists. It appears that many of the participants were not aware of the growing body of research that supports occupation-based approaches to treatment that might assist them with educating clients and other professionals. Clearly, more research on the efficacy of occupation-based treatments for occupational therapy clients with hand injuries is needed. Qualitative studies that explore the client's satisfaction with occupation-based treatments and how hand therapy clients experience meaning during differing treatment modalities would assist in understanding the relative value of occupation-based treatments.

When considering challenges related to the client's medical condition, it should be noted that there are times when uncontrolled movement, whether in the form of exercise or occupation-based activities, would be prohibited by the client's medical condition. Attention to treatment precautions, client acuity, and other sound biomechanical principles should, of course, be included in occupation-based hand therapy approaches. Use of occupation-based interventions in the hand therapy setting should not replace the biomechanical frame of reference and biomechanical forms of treatment, such as physical agent modalities or splinting. Similarly, however, a focus on biomechanical factor should not displace concern with the occupational needs of the client or opportunities to meet those goals through an occupation-based approach. Continuing education courses that incorporate the appropriate grading of activity for use when the client is in the acute stages of healing and research examining the appropriate use of occupation-based treatments in acute stages of healing are also needed.

CONCLUSION

This small study reports the benefits of, and challenges to, the use of an occupation-based approach to hand therapy. For us, it has been one satisfying step on a long road of unanswered questions and needed investigations. Some questions for future research include "What do clinicians mean when they talk about using occupation in hand therapy treatment and how does this compare to definitions in the *Occupational Therapy Practice Framework*?" and "What is the experience of providing occupation-based hand therapy like for the clinician?"

Occupation is the central construct of occupational therapy and has been demonstrated to be a powerful treatment modality in a variety of settings. Occupation has the potential to be a powerful treatment modality in hand therapy as well. McLaughlin-Gray (1998) stated,

"Occupation, when it is applied as activity with wholeness, purpose, and meaning to the person, can also affect him or her psychologically, emotionally, and socially in ways that purposeful activity unrelated to the person cannot" (p. 356). Addressing barriers to the use of occupation-based treatment in hand therapy through research and education is a necessary beginning step to revealing the power of occupation in hand therapy.

LEARNING SUPPORTS

Observe a Clinician

Purpose

The purpose of this activity is to expose you to how occupation is addressed in the clinic and the associated real world successes and pressures.

Primary Concepts

Occupation as means and ends and barriers to the use of occupation.

Instructions

Spend a morning or afternoon observing an occupational therapist working in an area of practice that interests you. While observing, consider the following:

- Does the clinician use everyday occupations (cooking, dressing, work tasks, play, hobbies etc.) as treatment activities (occupation as means)?
- Does the clinician tie the treatments he or she selects to the client's desired occupations (occupation as ends)?
- What is the client's reaction to the chosen treatments?
- Do you observe any barriers to using occupations in treatment in this practice setting?
- Can you think of ways to overcome these barriers?

After the observation, ask the clinician what influences his or her treatment choices, how he or she addresses occupation in treatment, and whether he or she perceives any barriers to using occupation as means during treatment.

Educate Others

Purpose

The purpose of this activity is to familiarize you with the research on the use of occupation in an area of practice that interests you and to disseminate that information to clinicians.

Primary Concepts

Literature review, evidence-based practice, and occupation.

Instructions

Complete a literature search for research on the use of occupation in the setting of interest to you. Create an in-service about the evidence. Invite clinicians to attend or submit the presentation for a local or state occupational therapy conference.

Adding to the Evidence

Purpose

The purpose of this activity is to help you develop research questions about occupation in a practice area of interest to you.

Primary Concepts

Quantitative research, qualitative research, occupation, and occupational science.

Instructions

Reflect on what you discovered when completing the second Learning Support, Educate Others. Consider what questions about the use of occupation in that treatment setting are unanswered. Develop two follow-up research questions about the use of occupation in the setting, with one of a quantitative nature and one of a qualitative nature.

REFERENCES

Amini, D. (2007). Hand therapy and occupational science. *ADVANCE for Occupational Therapy Practitioners, 23*(21), 12.

Clark, F. A., Parham, D., Carlson, M. E., Frank, G., Jackson, J., Pierce, D., . . . Zemke, R. (1991). Occupational science: Academic innovation in the service of occupational therapy's future. *American Journal of Occupational Therapy, 45,* 300-310. doi:10.5014/ajot.45.4.300

Colaianni, D., & Provident, I. (2010). The benefits of and challenges to the use of occupation in hand therapy. *Occupational Therapy in Health Care, 24*(2), 130-146.

Creswell, J. W. (1998). *Qualitative inquiry and research design: Choosing among five traditions.* Thousand Oaks, CA: Sage Publications.

Dale, L., Fabrizio, A., Adhlakha, P., Mahon, M., McGraw, E., Neyenhaus, R., . . . Zaber, J. M. (2002). Occupational therapists working in hand therapy: The practice of holism in a cost containment environment. *Work, 19,* 35-45.

Dolecheck, J. R., & Schkade, J. K. (1999). The extent dynamic standing endurance is affected when CVA subjects perform personally meaningful activities rather than non-meaningful tasks. *Occupational Therapy Journal of Research, 19,* 40-54.

Ferguson, J. M., & Trombly, C. A. (1997). The effect of added-purpose and meaningful occupation on motor learning. *American Journal of Occupational Therapy, 51,* 508-515. doi:10.5014/ajot.51.7.508

Fitzpatrick, N., & Presnell, S. (2004). Can occupational therapists be hand therapists? *British Journal of Occupational Therapy, 67,* 508-510.

Guzelkucuk, U., Duman, I., Taskaynatan, M. A., & Dincer, K. (2007). Comparison of therapeutic activities with therapeutic exercises in the rehabilitation of young adult patients with hand injuries. *Journal of Hand Surgery, 32A*(9), 1429-1435.

Helm, T., & Dickerson, A. (1995). The effect of hand therapy on a patient with a Colles' fracture: A phenomenological study. *Occupational Therapy in Health Care, 9,* 69-77.

Hoyt Slaymaker, J. (1986). A holistic approach to specialization. *American Journal of Occupational Therapy, 40,* 117-121.

Hseih, C. L., Nelson, D. L., Smith, D. A., & Peterson, C. Q. (1996). A comparison of performance in added-purpose occupations and rote exercise for dynamic standing balance in persons with hemiplegia. *American Journal of Occupational Therapy, 50,* 10-15. doi:10.5014/ajot.50.1.10

Jackson, J. P., & Schkade, J. K. (2001). Occupational adaptation model versus biomechanical-rehabilitation model in the treatment of patients with hip fractures. *American Journal of Occupational Therapy, 55,* 531-537. doi:10.5014/ajot.55.5.531

Jarus, T., Shavit, S., & Ratzon, N. (2000). From hand twister to mind twister: Computer aided treatment in traumatic wrist fracture. *American Journal of Occupational Therapy, 54,* 176-182. doi:10.5014/ajot.54.2.176

King, T. I. (1992). Hand strengthening with a computer for purposeful activity. *American Journal of Occupational Therapy, 56,* 635-637. doi:10.5014/ajot.47.7.635

MacDermid, J., Fess, E., Bell-Krotski, J., Cannon, N. M., Evans, R. B., Walsh, R. W., . . . Santore, G. (2002). A research agenda for hand therapy. *Journal of Hand Therapy, 15,* 3-15.

Mathiowetz, V. (1993). Role of physical performance component evaluations in occupational therapy functional assessment. *American Journal of Occupational Therapy, 47,* 225-230. doi:10.5014/ajot.47.3.225

McColl, M. A. (1994). Holistic occupational therapy: Historical meaning and contemporary implications. *Canadian Journal of Occupational Therapy, 61,* 72-77.

McLaughlin-Gray, J. (1998). Putting occupation into practice: Occupation as ends, occupation as means. *American Journal of Occupational Therapy, 52,* 354-364. doi:10.5014/ajot.52.5.354

Melchert-McKearnan, K., Deitz, J., Engel, J. M., & White, O. (2000). Children with burn injuries: Purposeful activities versus rote exercise. *American Journal of Occupational Therapy, 54,* 381-390. doi:10.5014/ajot.54.4.381

Nelson, D. L., Konosky, K., Fleharty, K., Webb, R., Newer, K., Hazboun, V. P., . . . Licht, B. C. (1996). The effects of on occupationally embedded exercise on bilaterally assisted supination in persons with hemiplegia. *American Journal of Occupational Therapy, 50,* 639-646. doi:10.5014/ajot.50.8.639

Peloquin, S. (1993). The patient-therapist relationship: Beliefs that shape care. *American Journal of Occupational Therapy, 47,* 935-942. doi:10.5014/ajot.47.10.935

Pierce, D. (2003). *Occupation by design: Building therapeutic power.* Philadelphia, PA: F.A. Davis.

Pratt, A., & Burr, N. (2001). A review of goniometry use within current hand therapy practice. *British Journal of Hand Therapy, 6,* 45-49.

Schier, J. S., & Chan, J. (2007). Changes in life roles after hand injury. *Journal of Hand Injury, 20,* 57-69.

Serlin, R. C., Mendoza, T. R., Nakamura, Y., Edwards, K. R., & Cleeland, C. S. (1995). When is cancer pain mild, moderate, or severe? Grading pain severity by its interference with function. *Pain, 61,* 277-284.

Trombly, C. (1995). Occupation: Purposefulness and meaningfulness as therapeutic mechanisms. *American Journal of Occupational Therapy, 49,* 960-972. doi:10.5014/ajot.49.10.960

Trombly, C. A., & Wu, C. (1999). Effect of rehabilitation tasks on organization of movement after stroke. *American Journal of Occupational Therapy, 53,* 333-344. doi:10.5014/ajot.53.4.333

Van der Weel, F. R., Van der Meer, A. L. H., & Lee, D. N. (1991). Effect of task on movement control in cerebral palsy: Implications for assessment and therapy. *Developmental Medicine and Child Neurology, 33,* 419-426. doi:10.1111/j.1469-8749.1991.tb14902.x

Yoder, R. M., Nelson, D. L., & Smith, D. A. (1989). Added purpose versus rote exercise in female nursing home residents. *American Journal of Occupational Therapy, 43,* 581-586. doi:10.5014/ajot.43.9.581

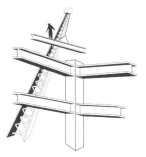

28

Putting Knowledge of Occupation to Work for Youth at Risk

Elaine Fehringer, MA, OTR/L; Amy Marshall, PhD, OTR/L;
Karen Summers, MS, OTR/L; and Doris Pierce, PhD, OTR/L, FAOTA

For 10 years at Eastern Kentucky University (EKU), a group of occupational therapists have worked to develop their understandings of occupation to better meet the needs of youth at risk for poor transitions to productive and satisfying adult lifestyles. In the United States, adolescents are most commonly at risk for poor transitions to adulthood due to disabilities, poor educational attainment, illegal or undesirable juvenile behaviors, or threatening environmental conditions such as abuse and neglect. To us, there was an obvious and beneficial match between these needs and the expertise of occupational therapists. The U.S. Department of Education is concerned about the need for transition supports that improve postsecondary occupational and functional outcomes of students with disabilities. The knowledge base of occupational scientists and therapists in regard to work and independent living for people with disabilities is historical and developed. Occupational therapists are providing services to students with disabilities in schools across the United States, yet only infrequently do they serve these students beyond the elementary grades. We often speculate on why this is. But, more important, we dream of a day when this will not be true. This chapter describes some of the strategies we have used to bring that dream to life.

LITERATURE

Transition Services Defined

According to the Individuals with Disabilities Education Improvement Act ([IDEA] 2004), transition services are designed to result in the improvement of both the academic and functional capacities of the student in the areas of education, employment, and living in the community (Kohler & Field, 2003). Education programs must provide evaluation of, and instruction in, all of these activities, based on the individual student's strengths, needs, interests, and preferences. The purpose of transition programming is to prepare youth with disabilities to become adults leading full and productive lives (IDEA, 2004).

Transition Services for Youth at Risk

All adolescents face many challenges as they transition into adulthood. Vulnerable populations face more challenges than ever before, especially in lean economic times (Osgood, Foster, & Courtney, 2010). School systems are only

Pierce, D. (Ed.).
Occupational Science for Occupational Therapy (pp. 335-346).

legally required to provide transition services to students who receive special education services up to 22 years of age. Unfortunately, other programs, such as juvenile justice systems, who serve vulnerable adolescent populations are not required to prepare students for adulthood. As a result, many of these youth at risk do not acquire the skills they need to become employed or live independently. In order to help these adolescents reach their potential, they need quality transition services (National Center on Education, Disability, and Juvenile Justice, 2007; Osgood et al., 2010).

Best transition practices for youth at risk should be comprehensive and address job, life, and leisure skills based on the adolescent's strengths, preferences, and interests (IDEA, 2004). Successful engagement in these tasks is critical to being a functional adult. In the area of work, students should learn pre-employment skills such as completing job applications, interviewing, career exploration, and life skills as part of work experiences or internships. Instrumental life skills such as budgeting, meal preparation, and self-advocacy are best completed in context and as part of daily activities (Armstrong, Dedrick, & Greenbaum, 2003; Carter, Lane, Pierson, & Glaeser, 2006; Carter & Wehby, 2003; Geenen, Powers, Hogansen, & Pittman, 2007; Stephens & Arnette, 2000). Engaging in these activities in natural settings is the best way for students to prepare for adulthood.

Because all adolescents have their own challenges and interests, a customized transition plan is needed to meet their individualized needs (Bullis, Yovanoff, & Havel, 2004). For example, a student from Appalachia might be a talented artist without realizing that his hobby could become gainful employment. The focus of his individualized transition plan would include identifying potential jobs and skills he would need in order to be prepared for an art career. Unfortunately, limited financial and familial resources are a common challenge for youth at risk (Osgood et al., 2010). If youth are not receiving the support they need at home or in their educational program, how will they develop skills to manage a household or have a career?

Transition Programs for Youth With Disabilities

Students with identified disabilities also face many challenges to building the capacity to lead a quality life. In fact, individuals with disabilities are more likely to be unemployed or underemployed (National Organization on Disability, 2004). As a result of these poor adult outcomes for students with disabilities, legislation now requires special educators to use a student-centered approach to develop a transition plan as part of their individualized education program ([IEP]; IDEA, 2004). Each student's plan should be unique to that student's needs and address goals to improve his or her ability to be employed and live as independently as possible. Although students eligible for special education

services attend both traditional and alternative educational settings, a student in alternative education is four times more likely to have a recognized disability than students at traditional schools (Quinn, Rutherford, Leone, Osher, & Poirier, 2005). In these settings, emotional disturbance is a frequent disability classification.

Stability in placement is necessary for all students to get the maximum education benefit from programming. Sadly, students in juvenile facilities also face the problem of moving frequently between facilities (Hosp, Rutherford, & Griller-Clark, 2001; Pierce, Powell, Marshall, Nolan, & Fehringer, 2009). Frequent transitioning not only impedes a student's ability to prepare for the future but also impairs his or her ability to function academically and socially in a classroom. Students in alternative education settings also deserve quality transition services.

Putting Occupational Science and Therapy Knowledge to Work for Transitioning Youth

Occupational science is a discipline that examines how humans engage in daily activities and the need for this engagement in order to lead happy and healthy lives. Occupations occur throughout everyone's day and across the lifespan in the areas of work, life skills, and play or leisure at home, at school, or in the community (Pierce, 2001). As the transition literature recognizes, adolescents require engagement in all of these areas in order to be prepared for their adult lives (Test et al., 2009). In special education, these skills are referred to as *transition activities.* Transition plans are required to provide "a coordinated set of activities" (IDEA, 34 C.F.R. 300.43[a], 20 U.S.C. 1401[34], 2004). The quality of transition practices would improve, however, if those activities were transformed from a general set of actions into occupations of meaning based on the student's interests, strengths, and preferences. A transition practice guided by occupational science would increase the likelihood of an adolescent engaging in employment, hobbies, and life skills that would result in a productive and satisfying life.

Though the term *occupation* encompasses more than just work activities, most people define themselves by their worker role (Westmorland, Williams, Strong, & Arnold, 2002). Although youth do not yet define themselves through work, adolescence is a crucial time to explore vocational interests. Developing a role in work provides self-esteem and empowerment. Because work is so essential to one's quality of life, adolescents should be taught skills to meet the demands of today's job markets in order to become successful adults. If these vital prevocational services are not provided, the risk of being unemployed or underemployed increases significantly, especially for students with disabilities (National Organization on Disability, 2004).

Like work, the occupations of self-care are critically important to a person's independence and quality of life.

These critical skills of daily living include bathing and dressing, as well as instrumental living skills, such as budgeting, safety, meal preparation, home care, and negotiating the community (American Occupational Therapy Association [AOTA], 2008; Test et al., 2009). Unfortunately, not all youth have adequate opportunities to learn and participate in these vital daily skills. Can you imagine going to a job interview without having clean clothes to wear or trying to focus on learning in a classroom without healthy food?

Leisure Occupations

Though many recognize the need for youth to learn and participate in work and life skills, many do not recognize the need for adolescents to have opportunities to engage in leisure activities. Healthy leisure occupations provide time for youth to socialize, relax, have fun, or develop a career-building hobby. Participating in leisure occupations can teach essential life skills, such as time management and learning to balance other life demands with a favorite leisure occupation. According to Farnworth (1999), adolescents who engage in occupations, especially leisure, improve their health and functioning. When many of the youth in her study left school, their participation in sports and other extracurricular activities decreased and their participation in risky behaviors increased. On the other hand, if youth had opportunities to engage in healthy leisure activities, their at-risk behavior was reduced. Youth who are able to organize their time in order to engage in desired occupations are more likely to have balance in their lives and become productive members of society.

Occupational Therapists Providing Related Services in the Schools

According to the most recent employment survey by the AOTA (2006), approximately 30,000 occupational therapists, or 29% of all therapists, work in school systems. Under No Child Left Behind (2001), occupational therapists are considered pupil services personnel, providing services on an individual basis and through consultation. Although a large number of occupational therapists work in school systems, services are primarily provided to elementary students (AOTA, 2000). In school settings, occupational therapists frequently help young students to engage in academic challenges within their student roles. Though academics are important, many students' education also needs to focus on preparing them to be as functionally independent as possible in work, education, and home settings. Occupational therapists' skills are underutilized in helping students with disabilities to prepare to transition to adulthood. As a result, vulnerable populations are not receiving secondary transition services from some of the most skilled professionals in their schools in the areas of work and daily living skills.

Some occupational therapists have responded to the secondary transition needs of adolescents with disabilities

in their schools. They offer students greater opportunities to participate in practical, real-world activities, resulting in increased functional skills and new roles for students (Michaels & Orentlicher, 2004; Orentlicher & Michaels, 2003a, 2003b; Spencer, Emery, & Schneck, 2003). Because occupational therapists are trained to be focused on the individual's strengths and interests, they use this as the base of the intervention plan. School-based occupational therapy for adolescents should be student centered and occupation based (Phelps & Hanley-Maxwell, 1997; Pierce, Marshall, Cunningham, & Fehringer, 2004).

Occupational therapists are well positioned to help students transition. Occupational therapists can use their expertise in regard to adult work and self-care to prepare youth for their upcoming environments and life contexts (Myers, 2008). All youth face challenges in preparing to engage in adult lifestyles and occupations. Youth at risk have additional obstacles to overcome, including limited resources and opportunities. Occupational therapists can use their knowledge of occupations to help the youth of today face the adult world of tomorrow.

A RESEARCH PROGRAM ON BEHALF OF TRANSITIONING YOUTH

Described below is a chronological account of the efforts of the Youth Research Group of EKU's Occupational Therapy Department over the past decade. There is limited research on the services of occupational therapists to adolescents, especially those in alternative education settings. To support best practice services to adolescents at risk and with disabilities, this team, through a series of studies, is developing occupation-based transition practices for youth.

Starting Out: The Occupational Therapy Program Development Studies

Phase 1: An Effectiveness Pilot

The pilot phase of the program development studies used a mixed methods draft design to examine occupational therapy interventions for youth at risk. Data collection occurred during Spring 2002 at a rural Kentucky alternative school. Team members included four occupational therapists—Ashlyn Cunningham, Leah Dunn, Elaine Fehringer, and Amy Marshall—and the research team leader, Doris Pierce. Twenty-two alternative middle and high school students participated. The purpose of the study was to examine the efficacy of a prototype occupational therapy intervention program for youth at risk. Although some useful instruments were identified, the primary finding was that a program development study was needed initially, rather than an outcomes study. Qualitative data from the pilot were the most useful, including insights on youth occupational patterns and identity, therapist reasoning, and occupation-based practice with youth.

Phases 2 and 3: Participatory Action Research to Develop Programming

The second and third phases of program development research focused on occupation-based, student-centered, cost-effective, and peer group-based interventions for adolescents in alternative educational settings. An action research approach, which uses a cycle of data collection, analysis, and action, was used (Brown & Tandon, 1983; Letts, 2003; Roth & Esdaile, 1999; Stringer, 2007).

Phase 2 took place over one academic year in two alternative schools in Kentucky and was carried out by the same team as in Phase 1. Thirty-two alternative middle school students and 35 alternative high school students participated. Phase 3 tested the program by including a residential juvenile justice setting and an alternative school in a neighboring state. In this phase, participants included the research team leader, Doris Pierce, and four occupational therapists: Elaine Fehringer, Amy Marshall, Jane Shepherd, and Dianne Simons.

Phases 2 and 3: Data Collection

During Phases 2 and 3, the occupational therapists provided audiotaped reflections every other week in response to a set of questions developed by the research team. Initially, questions were straightforward, asking what was working well or not so well. As the project developed, questions were reformulated to center more specifically on central challenges to program development, such as partnering and collaborative goal setting with youth, management of the context of intervention, and planning interventions.

In Phase 2, video and audio interview data were collected from the youth participants who received occupational therapy services. The focus of this effort was to explore the occupational nature of these rural adolescents and to obtain their feedback on services. The interviews elicited descriptions of a typical weekday and weekend, plans for the future, and favorite and least favorite occupations. At the end of the academic year during which services were provided, videotaped student panels of three to five students each provided feedback on the program. In Phase 2 there were also several audiorecorded interviews with school staff, administrators, state agency staff, and occupational therapists nationally known for their expertise in working with youth at risk, gaining further feedback on the program.

Phases 2 and 3: Analysis

Video- and audiotaped interviews, as well as therapist reflections, were transcribed as necessary, reviewed by the team to produce coding categories, and coded and retrieved using computer-assisted qualitative data analysis software. Following coding, memos were produced for use in semi-weekly team meetings to generate programming improvements. These innovations were then evaluated in therapist reflections. Some coding categories proved useful throughout the study, requiring repeat analysis as further data were generated, and others were collapsed together as broader relations were discovered.

Phases 2 and 3: Results

The focus of the final phase was refinement of occupational therapy programming. The teens' identities were used to shape peer group interventions that focused on exploring their occupational selves, used student interests to select activities, and used gender identity in group management. Optimal qualities of occupations used as interventions were that they be fun, promote success, be hands-on, result in a product, and be interactive, collaborative, and self-directed.

The team's emerging understanding of the occupational identities of the rural youth they served was grounded in the fact that, at this age, they had limited personal insight. Leisure interests were few and focused on home and family. Boys were often involved in paid work, and girls were more involved in unpaid work and chores, yet both groups had significant responsibilities. The future plans of the adolescents were sometimes unrealistic and vague. They generally had difficulty succeeding in traditional school settings. Disability was evident but largely unidentified.

In the program, occupational therapists attempted to place students in a position of power over their own lives or to "liberate" them from their current school situations, which were often punitive and used strict behavioral codes. This occurred through "choices within structure," or the use of temporal, spatial, and sociocultural strategies to maintain therapist control while increasing student ownership of, and collaboration in, the development of intervention activities (Marshall, Pierce, & Fehringer, 2005).

The Practical Living Program

The Practical Living Program was a significant outcome. Its name comes from a primary content area of Kentucky's core curriculum. Program themes identified by the alternative school students as important areas of intervention included daily living skills, healthy leisure choices, and pre-vocational/vocational exploration. Therapists drew heavily on their research into the daily lives of these rural adolescents in their offering of a "palette" of activity choices with the three main areas of the program. In addition to these primary intervention themes, underlying issues surrounding social participation played a key role in intervention planning. Adolescents' negative personal identities, limited future identities, and limited social communication skills impacted their abilities to participate in the occupational therapy interventions. Thus, these areas required attention in the design and provision of services.

It was through active, group-based assessments and shared goal setting that students identified areas for intervention that would be beneficial to all members of the group. The collaboration and input of the adolescents in activity planning were encouraged through student-centered assessments. Planning for activities occurred at the end of each session during a reflection period, when students were asked what activities they would like to do the following week. Evaluation instruments included an interest collage, time-use pie chart, Holland's Self-Directed Search, and a goals checklist, among others.

Providing Rural Interdisciplinary Services to Youth With Mental Health Needs

In 2004, the EKU Department of Occupational Therapy was awarded the Providing Rural Interdisciplinary Services to Youth With Mental Health Needs (PRISYM) grant: a $1 million, 3-year federal interdisciplinary training grant funded by the Health Resources and Services Administration. It was developed to serve rural Appalachian adolescents with mental health needs and their families, address disparities in health services in eastern Kentucky, and respond to the training needs of health professional students at EKU. PRISYM trained occupational therapy, psychology, and social work students to provide interdisciplinary, culturally sensitive services to rural Appalachian youth with mental health needs. PRISYM created experiences in partnership with two multicounty Kentucky mental health service regions in order to prepare graduates more likely to enter rural practice.

Methods

PRISYM used an approach that rested on the following: an interdisciplinary leadership team, which included the project director, Doris Pierce; coordinators for each discipline, Stephanie Adams, Amy Marshall, and Sandra Medley; a research coordinator, Amy Marshall; directors from the two partnering state mental health regions, Kari Collins and Jill West; a representative from state mental health services, Michelle Blevins; representatives from both youth and parent advocacy groups, Carol Cecil and Carmilla Ratliff; and expert consultants, Alan Banks and Anne Blakeney. Throughout the project, the leadership team and student trainees collaborated in using an action research approach to training and service program development by completing interview studies: in Year 1, focusing on the advantages and disadvantages of rural practice; in Year 2, on the barriers to services to rural Appalachian adolescents with mental health needs; and in Year 3, on suggested changes or additions in regard to preparing students for rural practice.

Results

A cycle of action research was used throughout PRISYM for improvements in didactics, development of training sites, improving the focus on culturally sensitive care to rural Appalachian youth and families, and planning for sustainability. PRISYM developed a best practice model of interdisciplinary service provision to youth with mental health needs in eastern Kentucky, new training sites were developed, and there was increased recruitment and retention of health care practitioners (Pierce et al., 2008).

In order to promote the sustainability of the services and partnerships that were initiated during PRISYM, the EKU Department of Occupational Therapy also sought out and developed a partnership with the Kentucky Educational Collaborative for State Agency Children (KECSAC). KECSAC is a statewide collaborative that provides funding and technical support to state agencies, school districts, and local programs to ensure that state agency children receive an education comparable to other Kentucky students. They contract with 54 Kentucky school districts and oversee 105 individual programs serving more than 21,000 state agency children annually (KECSAC, 2008). Approximately half of KECSAC programs are within the juvenile justice system.

Direct and indirect occupational therapy services were provided to three KECSAC programs. Level I fieldwork opportunities were developed for occupational therapy students within KECSAC schools. Services were shaped by the specific needs of each school, including assessment and evaluation of selected youth, occupational therapy interventions with groups or individual students, supervision and supported placement for occupational therapy and social work students, policy development, advocacy activities, and collaborative research.

Statewide Description of Transition of Kentucky Educational Collaborative for State Agency Children Youth

The frequent transitions of state agency youth between schools, homes, and communities can result in youth disengagement and poor adult outcomes (Malmgren & Gagnon, 2005). As the relationship between the occupational therapy researchers of the Youth Research Group and KECSAC continued to develop, KECSAC requested that the team conduct research to identify and describe the key components of successful transitions of state agency students. Members of the research team included Norman Powell and Ronnie Nolan, Director and Associate Director of KECSAC, and Elaine Fehringer, Amy Marshall, and Doris Pierce of the EKU Occupational Therapy Department.

Methods

Over a year of shared design, data collection, analysis, and write-up, the team produced statistical and theme-based descriptions of youth transition as perceived by youth and administrators in KECSAC programs. Survey data from all 105 program administrators were analyzed to produce a statistical summary of a variety of key aspects of transitions and student demographics. Qualitative data from the study included 1-hour focus group interviews that included most administrators of the 105 programs within nine simultaneous focus groups, a 1-hour focus group interview with KECSAC's three program improvement specialists, five focus groups of five youth each, 10 in-depth interviews with individual youth, on-site individual interviews of program directors, and the annual site reports and site transition plans for all programs. Qualitative data analysis used a grounded theory, constant comparative approach. Trustworthiness was ensured through collaborative team analysis and multiple member checks.

Results

The statistical description of youth transition patterns illustrated the following: movement of youth between KECSAC programs and traditional educational settings; movement out of educational settings into nonschool outcomes; the length of stay in nontraditional educational programs; and student characteristics such as types of disability, ethnicity, gender, and age.

Overall, the qualitative analysis highlighted the degree to which, in these nontraditional state agency schools, transition is viewed much more narrowly than intended under IDEA (2004). For these administrators and youth, *transition* referred almost entirely to entry and discharge from that state agency setting, rather than as a focus on planning for the adolescent's transition to positive adult outcomes. Qualitative themes focused entirely on more internal programmatic issues, such as difficulties with obtaining student records at entry and poor collaboration between intervention and education staff. A distinct need for schools that are transferring students to improve coordination and communications, as well as developing a culture more receptive to arriving students, was described. The results also indicated the critical importance of student–adult relationships in these alternative schools, especially in light of the degree to which home schools actively stigmatized students returning from alternative school placements. A one-on-one relationship with a caring adult who valued them was of great importance to youth. If their educational experiences are to result in successful adult lives, state agency youth are in critical need of individualized planning and supports to navigate through their highly frequent interschool transitions (Pierce et al., 2009).

Kentucky Educational Collaborative for State Agency Children: Building Enhanced Strategies for Transition

The KECSAC Building Enhanced Strategies for Transition (BEST) study (Marshall, Powell, Pierce, Nolan, & Fehringer, 2012) was developed in response to the findings of the previous study, which identified and described key components of transition in KECSAC students. The BEST Study worked in collaboration with the staff and students of five KECSAC education programs to develop exemplary transition practices as models for other state agency programs. Research team members included Elaine Fehringer, Amy Marshall, Rebecca Painter, Norman Powell, Karen Summers, and Doris Pierce. The study, funded by the Kentucky Departments of Education and Juvenile Justice, developed model transition practices for KECSAC youth in two state residential detention centers, a private residential mental health facility, an adolescent day treatment center, and (for contrast) a semiprivate laboratory school located on EKU's campus.

Methods

Action research was used to encourage participants at all sites to develop and improve transition practices that were perceived to be the most important to them at their site. In addition to the action research approach at each of the five sites, the study used grounded theory to seek a cross-site understanding of emerging changes in transition services (Charmaz, 2006).

Emerging Results

As this chapter was being prepared, data from this study were still being analyzed. Each research site was also in the process of disseminating their findings to other KECSAC programs. One of the regional detention centers developed a transition manual, which clearly defined stages that youth move through while at the detention center, to be used as a model for other juvenile detention centers in the state. The other juvenile detention center wanted to help students improve ACT scores in order to be admitted to and receive funding from the community college system. A software program to improve reading speed and comprehension was adopted for use during the fall semester to better prepare students taking the ACT in the spring months. One facility built a statewide network of advocates for state agency youth throughout schools that provides a safety net for students returning from state agency schools to their home schools, including a recognizable logo denoting "safe spaces" in schools where someone is available for help or support, a resource guide for students in crisis, and professional development for school district educators. In the day treatment program, training was provided for educators and administrators to strengthen the process for students transitioning from the local day treatment to their traditional schools, including policies for constructive behavior management. The semiprivate, non-KECSAC laboratory school, which was included in the study primarily to enhance the contrast in the constant comparative method, worked to incorporate transition services into their school's curricula, developed work and community connections for students soon to graduate, and fostered opportunities for peer mentoring among students. The KECSAC BEST Study is committed to statewide dissemination of the transition program innovations produced in this research.

Summary of a Research Program on Behalf of Transitioning Youth: What Next?

A Growth in Perspective and Research Capacity

In the years that the Youth Research Group has worked together, we have greatly refined our understanding of youth at risk and transition. We are now envisioning a model of occupational therapy practice with transitioning youth. We have greater insight into the relative effectiveness of different strategies for advancing our dream of occupational therapy transition services for adolescents. We have grown our own skills, our state and national partnerships, and our education of occupational therapy students in regard to the challenges and strategies to youth transitions to satisfying and productive postsecondary lives.

Research Underway

As we prepare this chapter, the KECSAC BEST Study is in write-up, led by Amy Marshall. Karen Summers has just concluded a 2-year action research study supporting a group of therapists in an Arizona school district in developing occupational therapy secondary transition services at the request of the Arizona Department of Education and with the support of the AOTA and the IDEA Partnership. Doris Pierce has launched a 2-year, mixed methods occupational therapy transition services outcomes study, supported by the Ohio Department of Education's Office of Exceptional Children. Elaine Fehringer is designing a study focused on the transition service needs of rural adolescent mothers.

As a Team

We continue to share our work where we think it will best advance our dream. We try to write more than we talk. Our opportunities to present and network with new collaborators are so great that we have to make hard choices. We divide and conquer on that one. Working together as a team, with fresh data and a new research design, has always been more energizing for us than the writing up of results. But we remind ourselves of what we are trying to accomplish, and then the value of the writing time is clear. Perhaps our most important message is that, over 10 years of shared work, with modest funding but gargantuan determination, with discovered allies and each other, we are gradually and incrementally making a difference for youth at risk through research.

CONTRIBUTIONS TO OCCUPATIONAL SCIENCE

The sequence of research reported here contributes to occupational science in several ways. Primarily, it highlights the strong match of an understanding of the occupational patterns and occupational needs of youth at risk to the existing potential for occupational therapists in school settings to build the readiness of adolescents with disabilities for their transitions to employment and independent living in adulthood. There are gaps in the occupational science literature that would support such services. To make occupation-based services to adolescents with disabilities more available and effective, research describing typical adolescent development of adult life skills is needed. A continued growth of knowledge regarding the therapeutic use of occupation will also, of course, be useful in practice with adolescents. Studies that specifically target engagement in independent living and employment would be invaluable.

Results of this research begin to address these gaps. The program development studies provide a description of weekday and weekend routines in Appalachian youth placed in alternative educational settings. The Practical Living Program provides a peer-based and inexpensive format for addressing age-appropriate independent living skills, prevocational exploration and job skills, and the discovery of healthy leisure opportunities to replace risky behaviors. The PRISYM project produced many lessons in regard to interdisciplinary collaboration as an approach to the injustices of inadequate services to rural youth with mental health needs. The statewide study of transition needs of youth in nontraditional educational settings in Kentucky developed our understanding of the needs of youth at risk for additional, legally mandated supports in order to meet the occupational demands of living a productive adulthood, as well as identifying the dynamic educational settings that would be key to any efforts to rectify the lack of transition service to youth in nontraditional educational settings. The KECSAC BEST Study provided examples and guidance in how this can be done.

Overall, the interest of our team in the occupational needs of youth at risk sensitizes us to the need for more descriptive and predictive occupational science knowledge for this age group. It also fires us to continue in our work to design occupation-based interventions that will be effective in addressing these needs and injustices. It is our hope that this research offers demonstration programs that will inspire other occupational scientists and therapists to put occupation to work for youth in the schools, communities, and nations in which they work and live.

IMPLICATIONS FOR PRACTICE

Viewing Occupation-Based Practice Through a Youth at Risk Lens

Occupational therapists have long known the importance of engagement in occupation in order to foster the development of habits, roles, and routines (AOTA, 2008).

The adolescents in the studies reported here were in need of experiences that would allow them to develop ways of acting and thinking that lead to the "habits, routines, roles and rituals" (ATOA, 2008, p. 641) so necessary to make a successful transition to adulthood. Unlike their adult counterparts, these clients do not have skills that they are relearning; intervention with this group is aimed at habilitation rather than rehabilitation. Occupational therapists believe that people change, adapt, and become when they participate in occupations that are relevant and meaningful (AOTA, 2008; Wilcock, 1999). The truth and wisdom of this became apparent as the researchers in the program development studies engaged youth at the greatest risk for poor transitions to adulthood in activities of daily living, prevocational skills, work, and leisure experiences. In order to plan effective services, the occupational therapists found that they needed to use student-centered assessments and valued, culturally appropriate, age-matched, and occupation-based interventions. An important factor for coming to understand the youths' needs and strengths was opportunities for individual and social participation in a variety of contexts.

Occupational Therapists Bring Skills for Bridging Systems

This group of clients presents with complex needs that must be addressed in multiple contexts. One of the lessons learned from PRISYM was that services to youth with mental health needs are spread across several systems, yet no single system is accountable for youth outcomes. Because occupational therapists have training that spans medical, educational, and social systems, they are uniquely positioned to be an integral contact and coordinator for the interprofessional team that seeks to ensure good transitions between settings and into productive adult lifestyles.

Matching an Occupational Science Perspective to Occupational Therapy Practice

Occupational science informs occupational therapy practice about typical occupational patterns and rhythms of "time use, habits, skills, and self-organization" (Pierce, 2003, p. 6). When knowledge from occupational science research becomes embedded into the practice of occupational therapy, occupation-based and client-centered services flow naturally. As occupational science research is conducted and reported, that knowledge undergirds occupational therapy practice by illuminating the central function of the use of meaningful occupation—the beauty and power of ordinary and routine acts of everyday life. As Mattingly (1998) so eloquently stated, "even the most mundane moments can have their poetry and that poetry might be the most important thing a [therapy] session offers" (p. 18). In the youth at risk population, mastery of daily living skills and developing concepts of future employment and legal leisure is poetry that is paramount in making a successful transition to adulthood. Mastering these "everyday occupations" (Hasselkus, 2011) of grooming, budgeting, menu planning and meal preparation, laundry and clothing management, constructing a résumé, filling out a job application, and providing volunteer services can incrementally move challenged youth toward an independent adult life.

An Occupation-Based Approach to Interventions for Youth

The Practical Living Program was an outgrowth of the three-phase program development study described earlier in this chapter. It was intended to produce occupation-based, cost-effective, student-centered, and peer-based interventions for this population. And it did. But along the way, we discovered much more than we had anticipated.

During the program development studies, we began to understand the meaning of the term *client-centered* in a way that focused not on the individual tailoring of one-to-one interventions but on assessments and interventions that were collaborative with groups of youth and tailored to their age and culture. We learned to focus on assessment and goal setting that was shared. We began to skillfully manage adolescent group interactions, attending closely to gender dynamics and delicately balancing between adolescent leadership and maintaining effective orderliness within our allotted time.

From assessments such as the time-use pie chart and the interest collage, as well as interviews with the adolescents, we realized that students in these alternative education classrooms were similar to their peers in regular education classrooms in terms of interests (video games, Internet, social networking, texting) and in constructing fantasy futures (basketball star, country music star). Yet, many were also starkly different in their time-use patterns. At a research site in rural Appalachia, youth reported a significant amount of adult-level household responsibilities and care for younger siblings. They were often engaged in fishing and hunting that provided food to their families. They played board games or "shot hoops" at home. They often spent leisure time with siblings and cousins, rather than unrelated neighborhood peers. Understanding the cultural character of the occupations of these adolescents supported the effectiveness of interventions designed to appeal strongly to their interests and habits.

Adolescents in this alternative school also had an exaggerated shift toward nocturnal habits, even for adolescents. A majority indicated that they usually did not go to sleep until between 3:00 a.m. and 5:00 a.m. and needed to rise by 6:00 a.m. for a long bus ride to school. During the school day, they were sleepy and apathetic toward the academic packets they were to quietly complete in their individual study carrels. Therapists found that adolescents in this low arousal state responded quite well to peer-based, novel, active, and personally valued activities.

State Agency Youth: A Population Unnoticed by Occupational Therapy?

The statewide study of transition in state agency schools showed that students in alternative education move frequently between settings. Frequent moves mean that the paperwork, including an IEP that may or may not include occupational therapy services, often does not arrive at a setting until after a student has moved on. In the study, 34% of students in Kentucky's state agency schools had identified disabilities. From our observations of these youth, we suspect that the percentage of students with disabilities in these settings would be much higher if full screenings were provided to all students. Given this finding, school-based occupational therapists should assume that there are students in those settings who require services, rather than assuming that if a student is not receiving referrals there are no student needs. Further, students who do have IEPs and move to state agency schools are often considered ineligible for services by the occupational therapists at the home school and so are denied services even if they are still enrolled within their home county. In actuality, home districts are responsible for providing or funding services to students in state agency schools, regardless of the location of that state agency school. If there are several therapists working for a district, one therapist should be identified and take responsibility for frequent program contacts, advocate for the legal mandate to plan for transition needs, and find out when new students have transitioned in and check their IEP or assess as necessary.

Adolescents in the Schools: Where Are Occupational Therapy Services?

Our work in these programs has taught us that most adolescents who could benefit from occupational therapy do not have an IEP or, if there is an IEP, occupational therapy is not identified on it. Occupational therapists in school systems tend to focus on younger children and the acquisition of motor skills necessary for success in elementary school. As students age, children or young adolescents with motor, sensory, learning, and emotional and behavioral disorders are discharged from occupational therapy despite their functional and transition readiness needs. It is imperative that school-based therapists begin to understand early in their interactions with all students with disabilities the capacities they hold to meet the needs of students who will eventually be transitioning to adulthood. In elementary school, while working on handwriting, the occupational therapist should be assessing whether hand-

writing is going to be a viable option for communication in work and community settings. If it is judged to be a more functional strategy, the therapist should immediately begin working with the student to develop technology skills that will help him or her become competitive in school and social environments. For students nearing middle school, goals should begin to shift away from motor and sensory issues and toward skills of readiness for adulthood. The automatic discharge of students from occupational therapy services by age or by movement to a middle or high school building is not only illogical, it is unethical.

Linking to Core Content in the Schools

Another lesson learned from the studies was the importance of linking all provided services to the core content standards set by the state department of education where the therapist is working. A visit to the state department of education's Web page is an easy way to be informed about the state's core content standards. In the state where the research was done, we discovered that the state required local education agencies to assess the usual academic areas but had also identified practical living, healthy leisure, and prevocational skills as core content. These three areas were a perfect fit to an occupational therapist's skill set.

A Big Future for Occupational Therapists Working With Adolescents

It is time that occupational therapist respond to the transition service needs that exist in adolescent populations in traditional and nontraditional schools. A significant percentage of students in alternative education programs have both identified disabilities and great challenges in preparing them to transition successfully from student to competent adult. Many students in these programs also have unidentified disabilities and are at even higher risk for making a poor transition to adulthood. Students with identified disabilities in traditional schools have a need for occupational therapists to begin thinking more broadly about their potential services, drawing on their depth of knowledge of work, daily life skills, and social inclusion.

LEARNING SUPPORTS

Peer Group, Student-Centered, Occupation-Based Assessments

Purpose

The goal of this learning support is for students to analyze how group-based activities can be used as assessment data for planning effective interventions for youth at risk.

Primary Concepts

- Social needs of teens support group-based assessment

- Interests of typical teens guide student-centered assessment and intervention

- Nocturnal shift in sleeping patterns of adolescents require novel activities

Instructions

1. In this chapter, the research team found that few published assessments to identify needs and guide intervention existed. This research team chose to use the pie of life and a vocational interest collage to assess time-use patterns and current interests. Based on your understanding of group theory and activities, select five group activities and analyze those activities for the assessment data that might be discovered. How might the activity reveal values and interests? What contexts (social, virtual, spiritual, spatial, temporal, cultural, etc.) might be discovered by having youth engage in this activity?

2. In a group of two or three, share your chosen activities, further analyze the activities, and then select two activities to use as assessments to guide intervention for a group of 14- to 17-year-old males placed in a residential detention facility or a group of 13- to 17-year-old females who are pregnant and living in a residential educational facility.

3. Give your rationale for selecting each activity. Use theory to guide your thinking. What occupations or life skills do you expect to get information about by using this activity? Knowing that teenagers have a shift in sleep patterns, describe how you will address the need for novel activities. Often group dynamics in these classrooms present challenges to running group activities. What group dynamics among the youth might you need to anticipate and prepare for during the activity?

4. From your expected assessment data, plan two intervention sessions for each of the identified groups above.

Understanding the Linkage Between Occupational Science Foundational Knowledge, Occupational Therapy's Role as a Related Service to Youth in Alternative Education Programs, and State Core Content

Purpose

The goal of this learning support is to for students to develop understanding of the linkages between occupational science foundational knowledge, occupational therapy

as a related service in education systems, and how services provided to youth in alternative education programs must align with the State Department of Education core content.

Primary Concepts

- Interests, sleep patterns, physical and emotional development, educational and social demands of typical youth

- Related services and educational relevance

- State-defined core content for grades K through 12

Instructions

1. Go to your state department of education's Web site and search for the K through 12 academic standards (sometimes called *core content* or *core content for assessment*). You will usually find standards that address art, science, language, math, history, health or physical education, and prevocational and life skills. Read through the standards and identify those standards that are a strong fit between occupational therapy and the state standards.

2. Identify concepts from occupational science foundational knowledge that support occupational therapy's involvement as a related service for youth with special needs. Citing the standards that fit with your preparation as an occupational therapist, write a memo to the special education director of your district proposing weekly group-based services for youth in a high school special education classroom.

3. Identify one standard of interest to you and develop group-based, weekly intervention sessions for youth at risk who, due to truancy or random drug screens or behaviors, have been moved from special education services in the traditional school to an alternative education program in your district (e.g., for a math class you might design a cooking activity a teen would enjoy and reinforce the concept of fractions by using the recipe). Design 1 month of weekly 50-minute interventions, specifying goals, materials, ways of organizing the group, and real products the teens can consume or take home.

Interviewing as Assessment: Individual or Focus Group?

Purpose

The purpose of this learning support is to give the student an opportunity to compare and contrast two different types of interviewing: individual or group-based.

Primary Concepts

- Semistructured interviews

- Data collection techniques for individual or group-based interviews

- Transcription of data

Instructions

1. With a partner, develop an interview guide for an individual interview to discover a typical teen's weekday and weekend time use and current interests. Interview guides should include introduction of your purpose for the interview and opening questions to help put the person at ease. Next, prepare 8 to 10 questions with additional probes for each question to guide you through collecting information about the person that will give you a full picture of the adolescent as an occupational being and allow you to construct an occupational profile.

2. Individually, you and your partner will each interview a teen using your questions. Decide how you are going to collect the data. Will you record the interview? Will you write notes as you interview? Set up and conduct the interview.

3. Analyze what you learned about each teen in terms of large chunks of information such as sleep patterns, education strengths and dislikes, leisure interests, etc.

4. Join one other dyad of interviewers and report what you learned about your two interviewees. Listen to their report. Then construct a set of 10 questions to elicit additional information you would like to know now that you have analyzed your individual interviews.

5. As a foursome, conduct a focus group with at least four youth. Record the focus group. Have the focus group last for no more than 1 hour. Divide the tape into four sections; each team member will transcribe a portion of the audiorecording to text. When fully transcribed, combine the sections into one document. All four should then read the whole document.

6. Write a reflection paper on the strengths of individual and focus group interviews. Discuss the inherent weakness of each type. Discuss your reaction to transcribing your section of the focus group.

ACKNOWLEDGMENTS

The team would like to acknowledge the youth who have participated in our studies for their inspiration and willingness to consider and collaborate in regard to their occupations; the Kentucky Educational Collaborative for State Agency Children, which endorsed the capacities of occupational therapists to serve and study the transition readiness of the state agency children of Kentucky; PRISYM's Interdisciplinary Leadership Team, which pursued innovative services to underserved rural youth; Rebecca Painter and Norman Powell for their collaboration on the KECSAC BEST Study; and Dianne Simons and Jane Shepherd of Virginia Commonwealth University, who provided an additional site to Phase 3 of the program development studies.

REFERENCES

American Occupational Therapy Association. (2000). Standards of practice for occupational therapy. *American Journal of Occupational Therapy, 52,* 866-869. doi:10.5014/ajot.2010.64S106

American Occupational Therapy Association. (2006). *Your career in occupational therapy: Workforce trends in occupational therapy.* Bethesda, MD: AOTA Press.

American Occupational Therapy Association. (2008). Occupational therapy practice framework: Domain and process (2nd ed.). *American Journal of Occupational Therapy, 62,* 625-683. doi:10.5014/ajot.62.6.625

Armstrong, K., Dedrick, R., & Greenbaum, P. (2003). Factors associated with community adjustment of young adults with serious emotional disturbance: A longitudinal analysis. *Journal of Emotional and Behavioral Disorders, 11*(3), 66-76. doi:10.1177/106342660301100201

Brown, L. D., & Tandon, R. (1983). Ideology and political economy in inquiry: Action research and participatory research. *The Journal of Applied Behavioral Science, 32,* 277-294. doi:10.1177/002188638301900306

Bullis, M., Yovanoff, P., & Havel, E. (2004). The importance of getting started right: Further examination of the facility-to-community transition of formerly incarcerated youth. *Journal of Special Education, 38*(2), 80-94. doi:10.1177/00224669040380020201

Carter, E., Lane, K., Pierson, M., & Glaeser, B. (2006). Self-determination skills and opportunities of transition-age youth with emotional disturbance and learning disabilities. *Exceptional Children, 72,* 333-346.

Carter, E., & Wehby, J. (2003). Job performance of transition-age youth with emotional and behavioral disorders. *Exceptional Children, 69,* 449-465.

Charmaz, K. (2006). *Constructing grounding theory: A practical guide through qualitative analysis.* Thousand Oaks, CA: Sage Publications.

Farnworth, L. (1999). Time use and leisure occupations of young offenders. *American Journal of Occupational Therapy, 54,* 315-325. doi:10.5014/ajot.54.3.315

Geenen, S., Powers, L., Hogansen, J., & Pittman, J. (2007). Youth with disabilities in foster care: Developing self-determination within a context of struggle and disempowerment. *Exceptionality, 15*(1), 17-30. doi:10.1080/09362830709336923

Hasselkus, B. R. (2011). *The meaning of everyday occupation* (2nd ed.). Thorofare, NJ: SLACK Incorporated.

Hosp, M. K., Rutherford, J. R. B., & Griller-Clark, H. (2001). Incarcerated youth with disabilities: Their knowledge of transition plans. *Journal of Correctional Education, 52,* 126-130.

Individuals with Disabilities Education Improvement Act of 2004, Pub. L. No. 108-446 (2004).

Kentucky Educational Collaborative for State Agency Children. (2008). *KECSAC Annual Census: 2008.* Richmond, KY: Author.

Kohler, P., & Field, S. (2003). Transition-focused education: Foundation for the future. *The Journal of Special Education, 37*(3), 147-183. doi:10.1177/00224669030370030701

Letts, L. (2003). Occupational therapy and participatory research: A partnership worth pursuing. *American Journal of Occupational Therapy, 57,* 77-87. doi:10.5014/ajot.57.1.77

Malmgren, K. W., & Gagnon, J. C. (2005). School mobility and students with emotional disturbance. *Journal of Child and Family Studies, 14,* 299-312. doi:10.1007/s10826-005-5058-0

Marshall, A., Pierce, D., & Fehringer, E. (2005, October). *Liberating structures: Occupational therapy and at-risk youth.* Paper presented at the Society for the Study of Occupation, Potomac, MD.

Marshall, A., Powell, N., Pierce, D., Nolan, R., & Fehringer, E. (2012). Youth and administrator perspectives on transition in Kentucky's state agency schools. *Child Welfare, 91*(2), 95-116.

Mattingly, C. (1998). *Healing dramas and narrative plots: The narrative structure of experience.* New York, NY: Cambridge University Press.

Michaels, C., & Orentlicher, M. (2004). The role of occupational therapy in providing person-centered transition services: Implications for school-based practice. *Occupational Therapy International, 11,* 209-228.

Myers, C. (2008). Descriptive study of occupational therapists' participation in early childhood transitions. *American Journal of Occupational Therapy, 62,* 212-220. doi:10.5014/ajot.62.2.212

National Center on Education, Disability, and Juvenile Justice. (2007). Transition aftercare. Retrieved from http://www.edjj.org/

National Organization on Disability. (2004). Landmark disability survey finds pervasive disadvantages. Retrieved from http://www.nod.org/index.cfm?fuseaction=Feature.showFeature&FeatureID=1422

No Child Left Behind Act, Pub. L. No.107-110, 115 Stat. 14425, 20 U.S.C. 6301 *et seq.* (2001).

Orentlicher, M. L., & Michaels, C. A. (2003a). Enlisting occupational therapy practitioners in supporting students in transition from school to adult life: Part I. *Developmental Disabilities Special Interest Section Quarterly, 26*(2), 1-4.

Orentlicher, M. L., & Michaels, C. A. (2003b). Enlisting occupational therapy practitioners in supporting students in transition from school to adult life: Part II. *Developmental Disabilities Special Interest Section Quarterly, 26*(3), 1-4.

Osgood, D., Foster, E., & Courtney, M. (2010). Vulnerable populations and the transition to adulthood. *Transition to Adulthood, 20,* 209-229. Retrieved from http://www.futureofchildren.org

Phelps, L., & Hanley-Maxwell, C. (1997). School-to-work transitions for youth with disabilities: A review of outcomes and practices. *Review of Educational Research, 67,* 197-226. doi:10.3102/00346543067002197

Pierce, D. (2001). Untangling occupation and activity. *American Journal of Occupational Therapy, 55,* 138-146. doi:10.5014/ajot.55.2.138

Pierce, D. (2003). *Occupation by design.* Philadelphia, PA: F. A. Davis.

Pierce, D., Marshall, A., Adams, S., Cecil, C., Garrett, B., Huff, M., & Ratliff, C. (2008). Training for interprofessional services to Appalachian adolescents with mental health needs: Lessons learned from PRISYM. In C. B. Royeen, G. M. Jenson, & R. A. Harvan (Eds.), *Leadership in interprofessional health education and practice* (pp. 367-390). Boston, MA: Jones and Bartlett Publishers.

Pierce, D., Marshall, A., Cunningham, A., & Fehringer, E. K. (2004, May). *Initiating programming for at-risk youth in your district.* Paper presented at the American Occupational Therapy Association Annual Conference, Minneapolis, MN.

Pierce, D., Powell, N., Marshall, A., Nolan, R., & Fehringer, E. (2009). *Kentucky youth at risk transitions: A report to the Commonwealth.* Richmond, KY: Eastern Kentucky University.

Quinn, M., Rutherford, R., Leone, P., Osher, D., & Poirier, J. (2005). Youth with disabilities in juvenile corrections: A national survey. *Exceptional Children, 71,* 339-345.

Roth, L. M., & Esdaile, S. A. (1999). Action research: A dynamic discipline for advancing professional goals. *British Journal of Occupational Therapy, 62*(11), 498-506.

Spencer, J. E., Emery, L. J., & Schneck, C.M. (2003). Occupational therapy in transitioning adolescents to post-secondary activities. *American Journal of Occupational Therapy, 57,* 435-441. doi:10.5014/ajot.57.4.435

Stephens, R. D., & Arnette, J. L. (2000). *From the courthouse to the schoolhouse: Making successful transitions.* Retrieved from http://www.ncjrs.gov/pdffiles1/ojjdp/178900.pdf

Stringer, E. T. (2007). *Action research: A handbook for practitioners* (3rd ed.). Thousand Oaks, CA: Sage Publications.

Test, D., Mazzotti, V., Mustain, A., Fowler, C., Kortering, L., & Kohler, P. (2009). Evidence-based secondary transition predictors for improving postschool outcomes for students with disabilities. *Career Development for Exceptional Individuals, 32,* 160-181. doi:10.1177/0885728809346960

Westmorland, M. G., Williams, R., Strong, S., & Arnold, E. (2002). Perspectives on work (re)entry for persons with disabilities: Implications for clinicians. *Work, 18*(1), 29-40.

Wilcock, A. (1999). Reflections on doing, being and becoming. *Australian Occupational Therapy Journal, 46,* 1-11. doi:10.1046/j.1440-1630.1999.00174.x

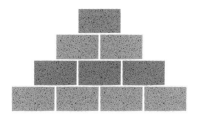

Occupational Science for Occupational Therapy
A Look Into the Future

Doris Pierce, PhD, OTR/L, FAOTA

THE STRENGTHS OF OCCUPATIONAL SCIENCE FOR OCCUPATIONAL THERAPY

Since its launch in 1989, occupational science has grown remarkably. Its capacity to honor its founding promise to produce a knowledge base to strengthen occupational therapy is greater now than ever before. As described here, the maturing discipline has built over time, developing four interdependent levels of knowledge of occupation, each with unique research intents: descriptive, relational, predictive, and prescriptive. Although still young, the science is increasingly productive of research, publications, and original concepts. Occupational science degrees are being awarded at the baccalaureate and doctoral levels. An international array of organizations supports the disciplinary culture of the science. Its disciplinary journal has been in place for 20 years. The strengths of occupational science are remarkable.

The outstanding research gathered here illustrates the potential of occupational science to carry occupational therapy into greater theoretical depth, into an unparalleled uniqueness of professional insights into the lives of its clients, and into enhanced effectiveness in supporting their participation in desired occupations. To continue to grow along this path, occupational science can be expected to open an increasing number of academic programs and to continue to produce original disciplinary concepts through research at all four levels. Occupational science and occupational therapy will continue into the future in what Clark (2006) has termed a "symbiotic" relationship (p. 172).

THE PERSISTENCE OF THE PARTITION OF OCCUPATIONAL SCIENCE FROM OCCUPATIONAL THERAPY

When occupational science was launched, it prompted a highly unusual response—a published debate in occupational therapy's premiere journal over the proposal that

Pierce, D. (Ed.).
Occupational Science for Occupational Therapy (pp. 347-350).
© 2014 SLACK Incorporated.

occupational science be partitioned off from occupational therapy. Although that particular exchange seemed to give a logical victory to occupational science, forces promoting the partition of the science from the profession remain strong. This persistent barrier prevents occupational therapy from more directly profiting from occupational science.

Partition Persists in the Polarized View of Occupational Science Research as Basic and Occupational Therapy Research as Applied

Unfortunately, occupational science and occupational therapy are still considered by many to be distinct and unrelated endeavors. It is much simpler to think of occupational science as basic descriptive research on occupation and occupational therapy as a completely different focus on the applications of occupation in practice. This polarized view is actually fairly congruent with that proposed at the debut of occupational science (Clark et al., 1991). It may even have been helpful to the infant discipline to have some separation from occupational therapy in its early years, insulating the new science from the trends, politics, and pressures of the profession while it explored and developed initial concepts. Since that time, however, occupational science has become more complex, addressing all levels of research, from descriptive to prescriptive. Still, that initial dichotomy persists, supporting partition of the discipline from the profession.

Partition Is Strengthened by Reverse Snobbery

Occupational science arose from a predominantly female health care profession (Pierce, 2012). Because occupational therapy is so accustomed to consuming the theories and research of more mature and masculine disciplines, giving respect to a more grassroots and female discipline is, to some degree, inconceivable. I think of this as reverse snobbery. It was best expressed by Groucho Mark when he said, "I wouldn't want to be a member of a club that would have me" (Pierce, p. 305). Instead of encouraging and recognizing the fresh and focused work that emanates from our original discipline, occupational therapy continues to emulate, envy, and overvalue the work of outside disciplines that only marginally address occupation. The dependence of occupational therapy on extradisciplinary-trained scholars to fill its academic departments increases this tendency of occupational therapy to look outside itself for science it can respect. Such ingrained attitudes strengthen the partition of occupational science from occupational therapy.

Partition Recently Increased Due to the Narrowed Editorial Stances of Key Journals

Partition of occupational science from occupational therapy within publishing venues has grown over the years. This is largely due to the increasingly disparate editorial policies of the *Journal of Occupational Science* and the *American Journal of Occupational Therapy*, which has created a critical gap, a deformation, in the published occupational science discourse.

As occupational science has evolved, it has moved from its original conceptualization as a more descriptive science (Clark et al., 1991) to a science that also examines the relations of occupation to other phenomena, predicts its larger patterns, and studies its prescriptive uses. The *Journal of Occupational Science*, first published in 1993, began with an editorial policy congruent with that debut vision in combination with the vision of occupational science held by Ann Wilcock. Although occupational science has changed dramatically over 20 years, the editorial stance of the *Journal* has not. That is, occupational science as published in the *Journal of Occupational Science* is primarily Level 2, relational research, or Level 1, descriptive research. Extradisciplinary research that may help to explain occupation is especially welcomed by the *Journal*. Level 4, prescriptive applications of occupation are absolutely not accepted and there is no particular interest in publishing works in regard to occupational therapy. This editorial stance is certainly within the prerogatives of the *Journal*'s editorial board. Because the *Journal of Occupational Science* is the only disciplinary journal, however, this strongly supports the partition of occupational science from occupational therapy.

The partition has been further exacerbated by the movement of the *American Journal of Occupational Therapy* away from occupational science in recent years. In the past, the *American Journal of Occupational Therapy* has been open to different types of research and has offered special issues in which occupational scientists were highly involved in published disciplinary work useful to occupational therapy. That has dramatically changed. The *American Journal of Occupational Therapy* now strictly prioritizes Level 4, outcomes research. The reason for this editorial policy shift is that occupational therapy is experiencing what has been called "an outcomes panic" (Lieberman & Scheer, 2002, p. 345). For the premiere journal of the profession, the need for evidence of effectiveness has supplanted any need for research on occupation at the descriptive, relational, or predictive levels. This is understandable, but unfortunate. Occupational therapy has always adeptly employed complex theory as a primary tool for moving between the biomedical business of health care and the intimate worlds of clients. Such a narrow editorial focus is not responsive to that need.

In combination, the editorial stances of these two key journals dramatically increase the partition of occupational science from occupational therapy. One journal has failed to change in step with the expansion of the discipline it represents, excluding a highly significant portion of occupational science research from our only disciplinary journal. The other has rapidly narrowed to a strategic focus that excludes most of occupational science. The result is that occupational scientists whose work could be beneficial to occupational therapy must scramble among less widely disseminated occupational therapy journals in order to publish. Some occupational scientists abandon their commitment to disseminate knowledge to occupational therapy, contributing instead outside to disciplines whose journals value their work. Others abandon their commitment to any type of occupational science research beyond occupational therapy outcomes, in order to continue their commitment to publish research useful to, and widely disseminated within, occupational therapy.

For occupational science to overcome partition and flourish in its efforts to contribute to occupational therapy, a broader publishing venue is required. An integrative and repeated conversation, in regard to how different types of occupational science research may be related to each other and how they support practice, is badly needed.

Preventing Epistemic Closure

Occupational therapy, and thus the science it has birthed, operates simultaneously on two epistemic planes. That is, we use two ways of knowing the world. This requires a philosophical poise, sophistication, and tolerance not usually required of scientists or practitioners. In fact, it often confuses us. Instead of one correct set of base assumptions, as is more typical of a science, a continual negotiation between two contrasting worldviews is required in occupational science (Hocking et al., 2008; Pierce & Frank, 1992; Rudman & Huot, 2012; Yerxa, 2009; see also Chapter 11). This echoes the skill with which master therapists move between the expectations of systems of medical or educational practice and the unique ways in which each client may see his or her everyday life.

Occupational science and occupational therapy deliberately use and value the subjective, emic, or personal perspectives held by individuals in regard to their own occupations (Wood, 1995; Yerxa, 1983, 1991, 1992). At the same time, the discipline and the profession also encompass etic, objective, or systemic perspectives on occupation that are not accessible to everyday individuals, are often drawn from extradisciplinary theories, and address broader perspectives such as the influence of culture (Dickie, Cutchin, & Humphry, 2006). This nimble philosophy is a gift. It provides us with capacities to bridge between worlds that are not readily available to other disciplines and professions (see Chapter 24).

Occupational science is, and will probably always be, at risk of abandoning this demanding gift. Over occupational therapy's history, different forces have pushed and pulled, lobbying for changes in the profession's underlying values (Kielhofner & Burke, 1977; Yerxa, 1983). Now, as occupational science encounters and explores various extradisciplinary theories, it is confronted with similar arguments that it should abandon its valuing of the emic, individual, and subjective perspective on occupation that it has inherited from its humble occupational therapy roots in order to assume a broader, more etic philosophical stance that is in alignment with current social science theories (Dickie et al., 2006; Hocking, 2012; Magalhaes, 2012). Rather than allowing the science to be enriched, challenged, and developed by negotiating between two epistemologic levels, some insist on a forced choice. The rejection of occupation as an experience that is also owned, interpreted, and authored by our clients and research participants is being celebrated as an "emerging paradigm shift" (Kinsella, 2012, p. 70).

It is critical that occupational science resist this pressure toward epistemic closure, just as occupational therapy has done over its history. Abandoning one set of philosophical assumptions as less correct can only narrow our vision of what occupational science may become in the future. It would be premature. Further, it is not necessary. Ceasing to study and value the perspectives of individuals will hamper the fit of occupational science to the knowledge base needs of occupational therapists as they work with individuals. It may even be that the true value of occupational science's historical contribution to the universe of knowledge will spring from this unique and demanding philosophy.

Honoring Our Promise

As I have argued elsewhere, it is critical that occupational science honor its promise to respond to occupational therapy's needs for a unique science that informs practitioners in regard to the profession's central construct—occupation (Pierce, 2012). Although many discoveries along the way may require investigation that, at times, seems only distantly related to practice, that is the way of science and scientists. Passions and trends, insights and transformations, continual critical reflection and conversation in regard to what has come before, in order to push ahead—that is the nature of a vital discipline. Occupational therapy is only beginning to understand what occupational science will offer to the field. Education, practice, and research will all be energized and revolutionized by the new science. Occupational science should, in turn, recognize how fortunate it is in its alliance with occupational therapy, which endows its research work with a social relevance and positive impact that might be envied by any social science.

CONCLUSION

A new era is arriving in occupational therapy. It will be led by the students of today, whose occupational science-based understanding of their practice will equip them to go beyond what therapists before them could envision. Occupational science is under rapid construction across four interdependent levels, driven by the passions of its researchers for a rich diversity of topics. We cannot know what that future holds. What we do know is that the discipline will strengthen the profession and that the profession will, as always, turn that strength to the benefit of its clients.

REFERENCES

Clark, F. (2006). One person's thoughts on the future of occupational science. *Journal of Occupational Science, 13*, 167-179.

Clark, F. A., Parham, D., Carlson, M. E., Frank, G., Jackson, J., Pierce, D., …, Zemke, R. (1991). Occupational science: Academic innovation in the service of occupational therapy's future. *American Journal of Occupational Therapy, 45*, 300-310. doi:10.5014/ajot.45.4.300

Dickie, V., Cutchin, M., & Humphry, R. (2006). Occupation as a transactional experience: A critique of individualism in occupational science. *Journal of Occupational Science, 13*, 83-93. doi:10.1080/14427591.2006.9686573

Hocking, C. (2012). Occupations through the looking glass: Reflecting on occupational scientists' ontological assumptions. In G. Whiteford & C. Hocking (Eds.), *Occupational science: Society, inclusion, participation* (pp. 54-66). Oxford, United Kingdom: Wiley-Blackwell.

Hocking, C., Pierce, D., Shordike, A., Wright-St Clair, V., Bunrayong, W., Vittayakorn, S., & Rattakorn, P. (2008). The promise of internationally collaborative research for studying occupation: The example of the older women's food preparation study. *OTJR: Occupation, Participation and Health, 28*(4), 180-190. doi:10.3928/15394492-20080901-02

Kielhofner, G., & Burke, J. (1977). Occupational therapy after 60 years: An account of changing identity and knowledge. *American Journal of Occupational Therapy, 31*, 675-688.

Kinsella, E. (2012). Knowledge paradigms in occupational science: Pluralistic perspectives. In G. Whiteford & C. Hocking (Eds.), *Occupational science: Society, inclusion, participation* (pp. 69-85). Oxford, United Kingdom: Wiley-Blackwell.

Lieberman, D., & Scheer, J. (2002). AOTA's evidence-based literature review project: An overview. *American Journal of Occupational Therapy, 56*, 344-349. doi:10.5014/ajot.56.3.344

Magalhaes, L. (2012). What would Paulo Freire think of occupational therapy? In G. Whiteford & C. Hocking (Eds.), *Occupational science: Society, inclusion, participation* (pp. 8-22). Oxford, United Kingdom: Wiley-Blackwell.

Pierce, D. (2012). Promise. *Journal of Occupational Science, 19*, 298-311. doi:10.1080/14427591.2012.667778

Pierce, D., & Frank, G. (1992). A mother's work: Two levels of feminist analysis. *American Journal of Occupational Therapy, 46*, 972-980.

Rudman, D. L., & Huot, S. (2012). Conceptual insights for expanding thinking regarding the situated nature of occupation. In M. Cutchin & V. Dickie (Eds.), *Transactional perspectives on occupation* (pp. 51-64). New York, NY: Springer.

Wood, W. (1995). Weaving the warp and weft of occupational therapy: An art and science for all times. *American Journal of Occupational Therapy, 49*(1), 44-50. doi:10.5014/ajot.49.1.44

Yerxa, E. (1983). Audacious values: The energy source for occupational therapy practice. In G. Kielhofner (Ed.), *Health through occupation* (pp. 149-152). Philadelphia, PA: F. A. Davis.

Yerxa, E. (1991). Seeking a relevant, ethical, and realistic way of knowing for occupational therapy. *American Journal of Occupational Therapy, 45*, 199-204. doi:10.5014/ajot.45.3.199

Yerxa, E. (1992). Some implications of occupational therapy's history for its epistemology, values, and relation to medicine. *American Journal of Occupational Therapy, 46*, 79-83. doi:10.5014/ajot.46.1.79

Yerxa, E. (2009). Infinite distance between the I and the it. *American Journal of Occupational Therapy, 63*(4), 490-497. doi:10.5014/ajot.63.4.490

Financial Disclosures

Dr. Karen Atler has no financial or proprietary interest in the materials presented herein.

Dr. Carolyn M. Baum receives royalties on the Activity Card Sort from AOTA Press.

Michele Berro has no financial or proprietary interest in the materials presented herein.

Dr. Catana Brown receives royalties for the Test of Grocery Shopping Skills, which is published by AOTA Press.

Dr. Wannipa Bunrayong has no financial or proprietary interest in the materials presented herein.

Dr. Florence A. Clark has no financial or proprietary interest in the materials presented herein.

Dr. Donna Colaianni has no financial or proprietary interest in the materials presented herein.

Dr. Lisa Tabor Connor has no financial or proprietary interest in the materials presented herein.

Dr. Susan Corr has no financial or proprietary interest in the materials presented herein.

Lisa Deshaies has no financial or proprietary interest in the materials presented herein.

Joanne Phillips Estes has no financial or proprietary interest in the materials presented herein.

Elaine Fehringer has no financial or proprietary interest in the materials presented herein.

Dr. Erin R. Foster has no financial or proprietary interest in the materials presented herein.

Dr. Betty Risteen Hasselkus has no financial or proprietary interest in the materials presented herein.

Dr. Mary W. Hildebrand has no financial or proprietary interest in the materials presented herein.

Dr. Claudia List Hilton has no financial or proprietary interest in the materials presented herein.

Dr. Clare Hocking has no financial or proprietary interest in the materials presented herein.

Dr. Jeanne Jackson has no financial or proprietary interest in the materials presented herein.

Dr. Hans Jonsson has no financial or proprietary interest in the materials presented herein.

Dr. Gillian King has no financial or proprietary interest in the materials presented herein.

Dr. Sheama Krishnagiri has no financial or proprietary interest in the materials presented herein.

Dr. Mary Law has no financial or proprietary interest in the materials presented herein.

Dr. Amy Marshall has no financial or proprietary interest in the materials presented herein.

Dr. Phyllis J. Meltzer has no financial or proprietary interest in the materials presented herein.

Dr. Matthew Molineux has no financial or proprietary interest in the materials presented herein.

Alexandra Palombi has no financial or proprietary interest in the materials presented herein.

Dr. Doris Pierce has no financial or proprietary interest in the materials presented herein.

Dr. Pollie Price has no financial or proprietary interest in the materials presented herein.

Dr. Ingrid Provident has no financial or proprietary interest in the materials presented herein.

Dr. Elizabeth A. Pyatak has no financial or proprietary interest in the materials presented herein.

Dr. Phuanjai Rattakorn has no financial or proprietary interest in the materials presented herein.

Dr. Melisa Rempfer receives royalties for the Test of Grocery Shopping Skills, which is published by AOTA Press.

Dr. Wendy Rickard has no financial or proprietary interest in the materials presented herein.

Dr. Charlotte Brasic Royeen has no financial or proprietary interest in the materials presented herein.

Dr. Debbie Laliberte Rudman has no financial or proprietary interest in the materials presented herein.

Dr. Anne Shordike has no financial or proprietary interest in the materials presented herein.

Dr. Diane L. Smith has no financial or proprietary interest in the materials presented herein.

Dr. Jenny Strong has no financial or proprietary interest in the materials presented herein.

Karen Summers has no financial or proprietary interest in the materials presented herein.

Soisuda Vittayakorn has no financial or proprietary interest in the materials presented herein.

Dr. Gail Whiteford has no financial or proprietary interest in the materials presented herein.

Dr. Alison Wicks has no financial or proprietary interest in the materials presented herein.

Dr. Timothy J. Wolf has no financial or proprietary interest in the materials presented herein.

Dr. Wendy H. Wood has no financial or proprietary interest in the materials presented herein.

Dr. Valerie A. Wright-St Clair has no financial or proprietary interest in the materials presented herein.

Dr. Elizabeth J. Yerxa has no financial or proprietary interest in the materials presented herein.

Index